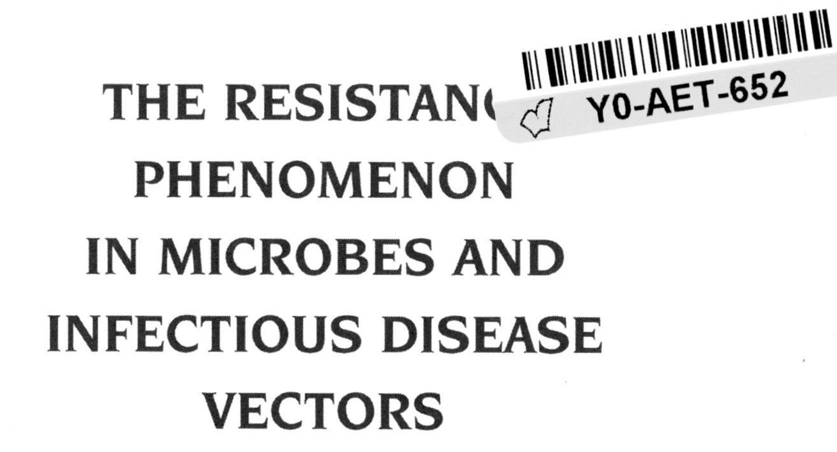

THE RESISTANC PHENOMENON IN MICROBES AND INFECTIOUS DISEASE VECTORS

Implications for Human Health and Strategies for Containment

Workshop Summary

Stacey L. Knobler, Stanley M. Lemon, Marjan Najafi, and Tom Burroughs, *Editors*

Forum on Emerging Infections

Board on Global Health

INSTITUTE OF MEDICINE
OF THE NATIONAL ACADEMIES

THE NATIONAL ACADEMIES PRESS
Washington, D.C.
www.nap.edu

THE NATIONAL ACADEMIES PRESS 500 Fifth Street N.W. Washington, DC 20001

NOTICE: The project that is the subject of this workshop summary was approved by the Governing Board of the National Research Council, whose members are drawn from the councils of the National Academy of Sciences, the National Academy of Engineering, and the Institute of Medicine.

Support for this project was provided by the U.S. Department of Health and Human Services' National Institutes of Health, Centers for Disease Control and Prevention, and Food and Drug Administration; U.S. Agency for International Development; U.S. Department of Defense; U.S. Department of State; U.S. Department of Veterans Affairs; U.S. Department of Agriculture; American Society for Microbiology; Burroughs Wellcome Fund; Eli Lilly & Company; Pfizer; GlaxoSmithKline; and Wyeth-Ayerst Laboratories.

This report is based on the proceedings of a workshop that was sponsored by the Forum on Emerging Infections. It is prepared in the form of a workshop summary by and in the name of the editors, with the assistance of staff and consultants, as an individually authored document. Sections of the workshop summary not specifically attributed to an individual reflect the views of the editors and not those of the Forum on Emerging Infections. The content of those sections is based on the presentations and the discussions that took place during the workshop.

International Standard Book Number: 0-309-08854-2
Library of Congress Number 2003005451

Additional copies of this report are available for sale from the National Academies Press, 500 Fifth Street, N.W., Box 285, Washington, DC 20055; (800) 624-6242 or (202) 334-3313 (in the Washington metropolitan area); Internet, http://www.nap.edu.

For more information about the Institute of Medicine, visit the IOM home page at: www.iom.edu.

Printed in the United States of America.

The serpent has been a symbol of long life, healing, and knowledge among almost all cultures and religions since the beginning of recorded history. The serpent adopted as a logotype by the Institute of Medicine is a relief carving from ancient Greece, now held by the Staatliche Museen in Berlin.

Cover: The background for the cover of this workshop summary is a photograph of a batik designed and printed specifically for the Malaysian Society of Parasitology and Tropical Medicine. The print contains drawings of various parasites and insects; it is used with the kind permission of the Society.

"Knowing is not enough; we must apply.
Willing is not enough; we must do."

—Goethe

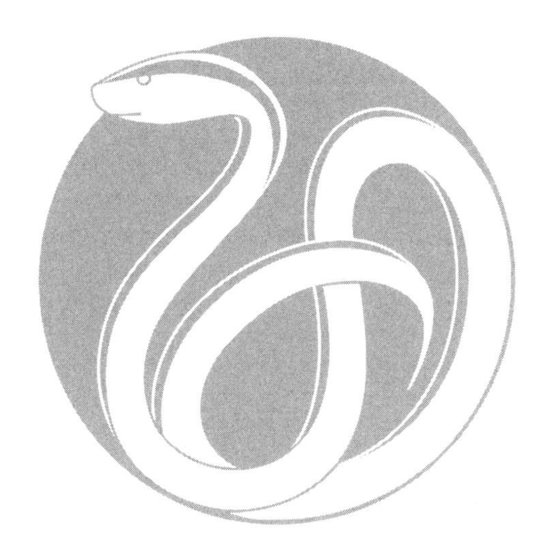

INSTITUTE OF MEDICINE

OF THE NATIONAL ACADEMIES

Shaping the Future for Health

THE NATIONAL ACADEMIES

Advisers to the Nation on Science, Engineering, and Medicine

The **National Academy of Sciences** is a private, nonprofit, self-perpetuating society of distinguished scholars engaged in scientific and engineering research, dedicated to the furtherance of science and technology and to their use for the general welfare. Upon the authority of the charter granted to it by the Congress in 1863, the Academy has a mandate that requires it to advise the federal government on scientific and technical matters. Dr. Bruce M. Alberts is president of the National Academy of Sciences.

The **National Academy of Engineering** was established in 1964, under the charter of the National Academy of Sciences, as a parallel organization of outstanding engineers. It is autonomous in its administration and in the selection of its members, sharing with the National Academy of Sciences the responsibility for advising the federal government. The National Academy of Engineering also sponsors engineering programs aimed at meeting national needs, encourages education and research, and recognizes the superior achievements of engineers. Dr. Wm. A. Wulf is president of the National Academy of Engineering.

The **Institute of Medicine** was established in 1970 by the National Academy of Sciences to secure the services of eminent members of appropriate professions in the examination of policy matters pertaining to the health of the public. The Institute acts under the responsibility given to the National Academy of Sciences by its congressional charter to be an adviser to the federal government and, upon its own initiative, to identify issues of medical care, research, and education. Dr. Harvey V. Fineberg is president of the Institute of Medicine.

The **National Research Council** was organized by the National Academy of Sciences in 1916 to associate the broad community of science and technology with the Academy's purposes of furthering knowledge and advising the federal government. Functioning in accordance with general policies determined by the Academy, the Council has become the principal operating agency of both the National Academy of Sciences and the National Academy of Engineering in providing services to the government, the public, and the scientific and engineering communities. The Council is administered jointly by both Academies and the Institute of Medicine. Dr. Bruce M. Alberts and Dr. Wm. A. Wulf are chair and vice chair, respectively, of the National Research Council.

www.national-academies.org

FORUM ON EMERGING INFECTIONS

ADEL MAHMOUD (*Chair*), President, Merck Vaccines, Whitehouse Station, New Jersey

STANLEY LEMON (*Vice-Chair*), Dean, School of Medicine, The University of Texas Medical Branch, Galveston, Texas

DAVID ACHESON, Chief Medical Officer, Center for Food Safety and Applied Nutrition, Food and Drug Administration, Rockville, Maryland

STEVEN BRICKNER, Research Advisor, Pfizer Global Research and Development, Pfizer Inc., Groton, Connecticut

GAIL CASSELL, Vice President, Scientific Affairs, Eli Lilly & Company, Indianapolis, Indiana

GORDON DEFRIESE, Professor of Social Medicine, University of North Carolina, Chapel Hill, North Carolina

CEDRIC DUMONT, Medical Director, Department of State and the Foreign Service, Washington, DC

JESSE GOODMAN, Deputy Director, Center for Biologics Evaluation and Research, Food and Drug Administration, Rockville, Maryland

RENU GUPTA, Vice President and Head, U.S. Clinical Research and Development, and Head, Global Cardiovascular, Metabolic, Endocrine, and G.I. Disorders, Novartis Corporation, East Hanover, New Jersey

MARGARET HAMBURG, Vice President for Biological Programs, Nuclear Threat Initiative, Washington, DC

CAROLE HEILMAN, Director, Division of Microbiology and Infectious Diseases, National Institute of Allergy and Infectious Diseases, National Institutes of Health, Bethesda, Maryland

DAVID HEYMANN, Executive Director, Communicable Diseases, World Health Organization, Geneva, Switzerland

JAMES HUGHES, Assistant Surgeon General and Director, National Center for Infectious Diseases, Centers for Disease Control and Prevention, Atlanta, Georgia

SAMUEL KATZ, Wilburt C. Davison Professor and Chairman Emeritus, Duke University Medical Center, Durham, North Carolina

PATRICK KELLEY, Colonel, Director, Department of Defense Global Emerging Infections System, Walter Reed Army Institute of Research, Silver Spring, Maryland

MARCELLE LAYTON, Assistant Commissioner, Bureau of Communicable Diseases, New York City Department of Health, New York, New York

JOSHUA LEDERBERG, Raymond and Beverly Sackler Foundation Scholar, The Rockefeller University, New York, New York

CARLOS LOPEZ, Research Fellow, Research Acquisitions, Eli Lilly Research Laboratories, Indianapolis, Indiana

LYNN MARKS, Global Head of Infectious Diseases, GlaxoSmithKline, Collegeville, Pennsylvania

STEPHEN MORSE, Director, Center for Public Health Preparedness, Columbia University, New York, New York

MICHAEL OSTERHOLM, Director, Center for Infectious Disease Research and Policy and Professor, School of Public Health, University of Minnesota, Minneapolis, Minnesota

GARY ROSELLE, Program Director for Infectious Diseases, VA Central Office, Veterans Health Administration, Department of Veterans Affairs, Washington, DC

DAVID SHLAES, Executive Vice President for Research and Development, Idenix, Cambridge, Massachusetts

JANET SHOEMAKER, Director, Office of Public Affairs, American Society for Microbiology, Washington, DC

P. FREDRICK SPARLING, J. Herbert Bate Professor Emeritus of Medicine, Microbiology, and Immunology, University of North Carolina, Chapel Hill, North Carolina

MICHAEL ZEILINGER, Infectious Disease Team Leader, Office of Health and Nutrition, U.S. Agency for International Development, Washington, DC

Liaisons

ENRIQUETA BOND, President, Burroughs Wellcome Fund, Research Triangle Park, North Carolina

NANCY CARTER-FOSTER, Director, Program for Emerging Infections and HIV/AIDS, U.S. Department of State, Washington, DC

EDWARD McSWEEGAN, National Institute of Allergy and Infectious Diseases, National Institutes of Health, Bethesda, Maryland

Staff

STACEY KNOBLER, Director, Forum on Emerging Infections

MARJAN NAJAFI, Research Associate

LAURIE SPINELLI, Project Assistant *(until June 2002)*

BOARD ON GLOBAL HEALTH

DEAN JAMISON *(Chair)*, Senior Fellow, Fogarty International Center, National Institutes of Health, Bethesda, Maryland
YVES BERGEVIN, Chief, Health Section, UNICEF, New York, New York
PATRICIA DANZON, Professor, Health Care Systems Department, University of Pennsylvania, Philadelphia, Pennsylvania
RICHARD FEACHEM, Executive Director, Global Fund to Fight AIDS, Tuberculosis and Malaria, Geneva, Switzerland
NOREEN GOLDMAN, Professor, Woodrow Wilson School of Public and International Affairs, Princeton University, Princeton, New Jersey
MARGARET HAMBURG, Vice President for Biological Programs, Nuclear Threat Initiative, Washington, DC
GERALD KEUSCH, Director, Fogarty International Center, National Institutes of Health, Bethesda, Maryland
ARTHUR KLEINMAN, Maude and Lillian Presley Professor of Medical Anthropology/Professor of Psychiatry and Social Medicine, Harvard Medical School, Boston, Massachusetts
ADEL MAHMOUD, President, Merck Vaccines, Whitehouse Station, New Jersey
JOHN WYN OWEN, Secretary, Nuffield Trust, London, United Kingdom
ALLAN ROSENFIELD, Dean, Mailman School of Public Health, Columbia University, New York, New York
SUSAN SCRIMSHAW, Dean, School of Public Health, University of Illinois at Chicago, Chicago, Illinois
DONALD BERWICK *(IOM Council Liaison)*, Clinical Professor of Pediatrics and Health Care Policy, Harvard Medical School, Boston, Massachusetts
DAVID CHALLONER (*IOM Foreign Secretary*), Vice President for Health Affairs, University of Florida, Gainesville, Florida

Staff

JUDITH BALE, Director
PATRICIA CUFF, Research Associate
STACEY KNOBLER, Study Director
MARJAN NAJAFI, Research Associate
KATHERINE OBERHOLTZER, Project Assistant
JASON PELLMAR, Project Assistant
MARK SMOLINSKI, Study Director
LAURIE SPINELLI, Project Assistant *(until June 2002)*

Reviewers

All presenters at the workshop have reviewed and approved their respective sections of this report for accuracy. In addition, this workshop summary has been reviewed in draft form by independent reviewers chosen for their diverse perspectives and technical expertise, in accordance with procedures approved by the National Research Council's Report Review Committee. The purpose of this independent review is to provide candid and critical comments that will assist the Institute of Medicine (IOM) in making the published workshop summary as sound as possible and to ensure that the workshop summary meets institutional standards. The review comments and draft manuscript remain confidential to protect the integrity of the deliberative process.

The Forum and IOM thank the following individuals for their participation in the review process:

Steven Brickner, Pfizer, Inc., Groton, Connecticut
Keith Klugman, Emory University School of Public Health, Atlanta, Georgia
David Ofori-Adjei, University of Ghana, Accra, Ghana
Clyde Thornsberry, Focus Technologies, Inc., Franklin, Tennessee
Mary Wilson, Harvard School of Public Health, Boston, Massachusetts
Kathleen Young, Alliance for Prudent Use of Antibiotics, Boston, Massachusetts

The review of this report was overseen by Melvin Worth, M.D., Scholar-in-Residence, the National Academies, who was responsible for making certain that an independent examination of this report was carried out in accordance with institutional procedures and that all review comments were carefully considered. Responsibility for the final content of this report rests entirely with the editors and individual authors.

Preface

The Forum on Emerging Infections was created in 1996 in response to a request from the Centers for Disease Control and Prevention and the National Institutes of Health. The goal of the Forum is to provide structured opportunities for representatives from academia, industry, professional and interest groups, and government[1] to examine and discuss scientific and policy issues that are of shared interest and that are specifically related to research and prevention, detection, and management of emerging infectious diseases. In accomplishing this task, the Forum provides the opportunity to foster the exchange of information and ideas, identify areas in need of greater attention, clarify policy issues by enhancing knowledge and identifying points of agreement, and inform decision makers about science and policy issues. The Forum seeks to illuminate issues rather than resolve them directly; hence, it does not provide advice or recommendations on any specific policy initiative pending before any agency or organization. Its strengths are the diversity of its membership and the contributions of individual members expressed throughout the activities of the Forum.

[1]Representatives of federal agencies serve in an ex officio capacity. An ex officio member of a group is one who is a member automatically by virtue of holding a particular office or membership in another body.

ABOUT THE WORKSHOP

Resistance in microbes—bacterial, viral, or protozoan—to therapeutics is neither surprising nor new. It is, however, an increasing challenge as drug resistance accumulates and accelerates, even as the drugs for combating infections are reduced in power and number. Today some strains of bacterial and viral infections are treatable with only a single drug; some no longer have effective treatments. The disease burden from multi-drug-resistant strains of tuberculosis, malaria, hepatitis, and HIV is growing in both developed and developing countries.

Infections caused by resistant microbes may fail to respond to treatment, resulting in prolonged illness and greater risk of death. Treatment failures also lead to longer periods of infection, which increase the numbers of infected people moving into the community and thus expose the general population to the risk of contracting a resistant strain of infection. When infections become resistant to first-line antimicrobials,[2] treatment has to be switched to second- or third-line drugs, which are nearly always much more expensive and sometimes more toxic as well. In many countries, the high cost of such replacement drugs is prohibitive, with the result that some diseases can no longer be treated in areas where resistance to first-line drugs is widespread. Most alarming of all are diseases where resistance is developing for virtually all currently available drugs. Even if the pharmaceutical industry were to step up efforts to develop new replacement drugs immediately, current trends suggest some diseases will have no effective therapies within the next ten years.

More recently, the challenges of resistance are compounded by growing concerns about the possible use of biological weapons leading to large-scale disease outbreak or exposure. The ability to respond effectively to such exposures could be significantly compromised by the introduction of drug-resistant pathogens. The use of prophylactic drugs or therapies on large populations may also contribute to the development of drug resistance and thus increase both the immediate and longer-term challenges of treating infectious diseases.

A number of trends in human behavior increasingly contribute to the emergence of resistance to antimicrobial agents. Host behaviors such as noncompliance with recommended treatment and self-medication are among the most complicit problems associated with the development of resistance. However, the duration of therapy for most acute infections has

---

[2]In this report, antibiotics are defined as substances (not limited to those produced from microorganisms) that can kill or inhibit the growth of bacteria, while antimicrobials are substances that destroy or inhibit the growth of pathogenic groups of microorganisms, including bacteria, viruses, protozoa, and fungi.

been determined empirically by treatment outcome, and more research is required on the effect of a reduction of treatment duration on the risk of the emergence of resistance. Other factors contributing to the rise in antimicrobial resistance include over-prescribing by physicians, failure to control the spread of infection in hospitals and long-term care facilities, and the overuse of antimicrobials in animals used for food products.

These trends are currently outpacing scientific discovery to counter resistant pathogens. However, one promising aspect of such factors in the emergence of resistance is their amenability to change, which may be accomplished through public education, appropriate training, political action, and domestic and international regulation.

Beyond the development of resistance in microbes, the ever-increasing resistance of disease vectors to biological and chemical pesticides looms as another complicating factor in efforts to control and eliminate the emergence of infectious diseases. Resistance to insecticides has appeared in the major insect vectors from every genus (e.g., mosquitoes, sand flies, ticks, fleas, and lice). Resistance has developed to every chemical class of insecticide, including microbial drugs and insect growth regulators. Insecticide resistance is predicted to have an increasing and profound effect on the reemergence of most vector-borne diseases. And where resistance has not contributed to disease emergence, it is expected to threaten disease control. Malaria control programs that already face complex challenges presented by multi-drug-resistant strains of the parasite are additionally undermined by vector mosquito populations that show increasing resistance to the pyrethroid-treated bed nets used to reduce malaria transmission.

Resistance is a natural response of microbes and other organisms to selective pressure from antimicrobial and other biological and chemical countermeasures. Adaptive mechanisms in the organisms permit survival and the development of genetic resistance. While the emergence of resistance cannot be eliminated, the rate and extent of its occurrence can be contained. In order to contain the threats posed to human health by resistance, it is important to determine the magnitude and trends of resistance and to define the relative importance of different contributing factors, such as therapeutic, behavioral, economic and social, and health systems factors, as well as veterinary and agricultural misuse. Based on this understanding it may be possible to develop effective methods to contain resistance in different settings.

Through invited presentations and participant discussion, the February 6–7, 2002, Forum workshop explored the causes and consequences of the resistance phenomenon. The Forum discussion also examined the scientific evidence supporting current and potential strategies for containment of resistance in microbes, vectors, and animal and human hosts. Additionally, the methods and measures of a response for industry, federal regulation, domestic and international public health, federal and academic research, and the private health care sector were debated.

ORGANIZATION OF WORKSHOP SUMMARY

This workshop summary report is prepared for the Forum membership in the name of the editors, with the assistance of staff and consultants, as a collection of individually authored papers. Sections of the workshop summary not specifically attributed to an individual reflect the views of the editors and not those of the Forum on Emerging Infections' sponsors or the Institute of Medicine (IOM). The contents of the unattributed sections are based on the presentations and discussions that took place during the workshop.

The workshop summary is organized within chapters as a topic-by-topic description of the presentations and discussions. Its purpose is to present lessons from relevant experience, delineate a range of pivotal issues and their respective problems, and put forth some potential responses as described by the workshop participants. The Summary and Assessment chapter discusses the core messages that emerged from the speakers' presentations and the ensuing discussions. Chapter 1 is an introduction and overview of the resistance phenomenon. Chapters 2 to 7 begin with overviews provided by the editors, followed by the edited presentations made by the invited speakers. Appendix A is an authored paper describing the consequences of antimicrobial use in agriculture. Appendix B presents the workshop agenda. Appendix C is a list of information resources on resistance. Appendixes D, E, and F contain the executive summaries of three government reports on the topic of antimicrobial resistance. Appendix G presents Forum member and speaker biographies.

Although this workshop summary provides an account of the individual presentations, it also reflects an important aspect of the Forum philosophy. The workshop functions as a dialogue among representatives from different sectors and presents their beliefs on which areas may merit further attention. However, the reader should be aware that the material presented here expresses the views and opinions of those participating in the workshop and not the deliberations of a formally constituted IOM study committee. These proceedings summarize only what participants stated in the workshop and are not intended to be an exhaustive exploration of the subject matter.

ACKNOWLEDGMENTS

The Forum on Emerging Infections and the IOM wish to express their warmest appreciation to the individuals and organizations who gave valuable time to provide information and advice to the Forum through participation in the workshop.

The Forum is indebted to the IOM staff who contributed during the course of the workshop and the production of this workshop summary. On behalf of the Forum, we gratefully acknowledge the efforts led by Stacey Knobler, director of the Forum, and Marjan Najafi, research associate, coeditors of this report, who dedicated much effort and time to developing this workshop's agenda, and for their thoughtful and insightful approach and skill in translating the workshop proceedings and discussion into this workshop summary. We would also like to thank the following IOM staff and consultants for their valuable contributions to this activity: Tom Burroughs, Laurie Spinelli, Judith Bale, Mark Smolinski, Katherine Oberholtzer, Patricia Cuff, Jennifer Otten, Clyde Behney, Bronwyn Schrecker, Sally Stanfield, Sally Groom, Michele de la Menardiere, and Beth Gyorgy.

Finally, the Forum also thanks sponsors that supported this activity. Financial support for this project was provided by the U.S. Department of Health and Human Services' National Institutes of Health, Centers for Disease Control and Prevention, and Food and Drug Administration; U.S. Department of Defense; U.S. Department of State; U.S. Department of Veterans Affairs; U.S. Department of Agriculture; American Society for Microbiology; Burroughs Wellcome Fund; Eli Lilly & Company; Pfizer; GlaxoSmithKline; and Wyeth-Ayerst Laboratories. The views presented in this workshop summary are those of the editors and workshop participants and are not necessarily those of the funding organizations.

Adel Mahmoud, Chair
Stanley Lemon, Vice-Chair
Forum on Emerging Infections

Contents

Summary and Assessment

The emergence of resistance to therapeutics is not a new phenomenon among microbes—whether viral, bacterial, or protozoan. Following the introduction and subsequent widespread use of penicillin, the first major "miracle" antibiotic, in the early 1940s, microbiologists soon discovered that a number of bacterial strains had become resistant to this antibiotic. Over the years, successive introductions of new classes of antimicrobial[1] drugs have been followed, often quickly, by the emergence of resistant microbes. Nor is the emergence of microbial resistance to therapeutics surprising, as these pathogens follow the same general rules—including survival of the fittest—that guide evolution among all organisms. However, they are capable of evolving much more rapidly than higher, multicellular organisms, due to their simpler genomes, capacity for inter-species exchange of genetic elements encoding for resistance, and much shorter generation times.

What is perhaps most notable today is the increasing degree to which microbial resistance has become an important health threat—and the continuing failure of the nation, indeed the world, to mount an adequate response. Drug resistance is accumulating and accelerating, thereby reduc-

[1]In this report, antibiotics are defined as substances (not limited to those produced from microorganisms) that can kill or inhibit the growth of bacteria, while antimicrobials are substances that destroy or inhibit the growth of pathogenic groups of microorganisms, including bacteria, viruses, protozoa, and fungi.

ing in number and power the drugs available for combating infectious diseases. Resistance to available therapies is a major confounding factor in effective treatment of human pathogens that account for the majority of the global infectious disease burden—malaria, tuberculosis, and AIDS. Today, some pathogenic strains of bacteria that were previously readily amenable to antibiotic therapy have become resistant to all available antibiotics, while strains of many other serious pathogens are now resistant to all but one easily administered drug, placing them on the brink of being untreatable. Coupled with the unrelenting emergence of antimicrobial resistance among common pathogens, there is a growing sense that drug discovery efforts are yielding fewer and fewer truly new leads toward novel classes of antimicrobial agents. This raises the specter of a real shift in the balance of the battle being fought by health professionals against a wide array of infectious agents.

Concerns about microbial resistance are further compounded by the possibility, made vivid during autumn 2001, that terrorists or a rogue nation might use biological weapons to trigger large-scale disease outbreaks. The ability to respond effectively to such events could be significantly compromised by the purposeful introduction of genetically engineered drug-resistant pathogens. Furthermore, the use of prophylactic antimicrobials or biologics in large populations of humans and/or animals in response to such a threat also may hasten the development of drug resistance and thus compound the risks of both immediate and longer-term problems in treating infectious diseases.

The Forum on Emerging Infections convened a two-day workshop discussion—the subject of this summary—to take a fresh look at a variety of issues related to microbial resistance. The goal was not to lament continuing shortcomings, but to reconsider our understanding of the relationship between microbes, disease vectors, and the human host, and to identify possible new strategies for meeting the challenge of resistance. Central to the discussion was an exploration of the many similarities inherent in the emergence of resistance to antimicrobial drugs, and the development of resistance to pesticides among insect vectors of serious pathogens such as the malaria parasite.

FRAMING THE ISSUE

Drug-resistant bacterial, viral, and protozoan pathogens pose a serious and growing menace to all people, regardless of age, gender, or socioeconomic background—a picture that holds true for developed and developing nations alike. Indeed, microbial resistance threatens to reverse many of the therapeutic miracles of the past half century. A rapidly expanding list of antimicrobial-resistant organisms is affecting us in a variety of ways.

The vast majority of infections that people acquire in hospitals, for example, are caused by bacterial agents, such as *Staphylococcus aureus*, that are resistant to penicillin. In many hospitals in the United States, nearly half of these penicillin-resistant staphylococci are also resistant to second-generation, penicillinase-resistant drugs, such as methicillin. Compounding matters, the antibiotic vancomycin, currently one of the few available treatments for methicillin-resistant staphyloccocal infections, is now showing increasing signs of losing ground as vancomycin resistance becomes ever more common among the most frequent infectious agents in hospitals (i.e., staphylococci, streptococci, pneumococci, enterococcus, and *Clostridium difficile*). Indeed, since this workshop, two different strains of *S. aureus* with full-fledged vancomycin resistance mediated by the vanA gene were isolated in the United States. Moreover, bacteria are now beginning to appear that are resistant to linezolid, introduced in 2000 for the treatment of vancomycin-resistant infections.

Drug-resistant microbes also are becoming more common in the community. At least five major bacterial pathogens,[2] including *Streptococcus pneumoniae*, which remains a major worldwide cause of pneumonia, meningitis, sepsis, and otitis media, and *Mycobacterium tuberculosis*, which causes tuberculosis, have developed resistance to a number of drugs. This problem is further compounded by the ability of microbes to share important resistance genes within and across bacterial species via a variety of genetic transfer mechanisms.

Infections caused by resistant microbes that fail to respond to treatment result in prolonged illness and greater risk of death. When infections become resistant to first-line antimicrobials, treatment must be switched to second-line or even third-line drugs, which are sometimes more toxic than the drugs they replace. Treatment failures also lead to longer periods of infection, and this factor increases the numbers of infected people moving from hospitals into the community. Moreover, even healthy patients colonized with drug-resistant, hospital-acquired bacterial flora may be discharged from hospitals. Both phenomena enhance the likelihood that resistant pathogens will spread into the community.

In addition to its direct threat to human health, microbial resistance exacts an economic cost that can trigger adverse health consequences. Treating individuals with alternative drugs is nearly always much more expensive than conventional treatment. In some settings, the drugs needed to treat multi-drug-resistant forms of tuberculosis, for example, are more than 100-fold more expensive than the standard drug regimen used to treat nonresistant forms of the bacteria. In many resource-poor countries, the

[2]Staphylococci, enterococci, pneumococci, tuberculosis, and salmonella.

high cost of such replacement drugs is prohibitive, with the result that some diseases are no longer treated in areas where resistance to first-line drugs has become widespread.

The added costs of treating drug-resistant infections also place a burden on society. For example, the American Society for Microbiology estimated in 1995 that health care costs associated with treatment of resistant infections in the United States amounted to more than $4 billion annually—a figure then equivalent to approximately 0.5 percent of total U.S. health care costs. It is clear, however, that this figure significantly underestimates the actual cost of resistance, since it includes only direct health care costs and excludes an array of other costs, such as lost lives and lost workdays. Moreover, these costs are expected to increase considerably given increasing rates of microbial resistance. The bottom line: coping with microbial resistance diverts a significant amount of dollars from other areas of the health care enterprise.

Although the emergence of microbial resistance cannot be stopped—since nature provides pathogenic organisms with too many mechanisms for survival—the challenge is to transform this growing threat into a manageable problem. Over the past 10 years, a number of organizations, domestic and international, public and private, have provided recommendations and options for addressing microbial resistance. Some common recommendations have included improving surveillance for emerging resistance problems, prolonging the useful life of current antimicrobial drugs (through parsimonious use, attention to completion of prescribed courses of therapy, or use as part of combination therapies that may be less likely to permit development of resistance), developing new drugs, and using other important measures (such as improved vaccines, diagnostics, and infection-control methods) to prevent or limit the spread of microbial resistance.

Despite the urgency of the problem, however, converting these ideas into widespread practice has not been simple or straightforward, and accomplishments to date have been insufficient, according to a January 2001 report by a U.S. government multiagency task force. Yet, recent years have brought encouraging signs of progress made and progress possible. At perhaps the most fundamental level, there is greater recognition—within government, the health care and research communities, the pharmaceutical industry, and society at large—that antimicrobial resistance is a major problem, and that this problem can be solved only with wide-ranging and coordinated actions. Such recognition is increasingly international. For example, the World Health Organization (WHO) recently declared antimicrobial resistance to be one of the top issues in global health.

MICROBE RESISTANCE

To manage microbial resistance over the long term, a sea change is needed in how we view the ecology and evolution of infection. The emergence of resistance must be recognized as an integral part—not an aberrant part—of the ecology of microbial life. Developing a fuller understanding of how microbes evolve when faced with drugs that threaten their survival may lead to innovative ways to bring them under control. While we once concentrated primarily on developing chemicals to use in an all-out war aimed at eradicating pathogens—a strategy almost guaranteed to promote microbial resistance—it may be possible now to devise treatment approaches that make an organism's genetic bent work in our favor.

"Smarter" approaches to drug discovery might seek compounds to which changes in the structures of the microbial targets (proteins or nucleic acids) that are required for resistance to the drug also lead to a loss of function, or the development of combinations of drugs with mutually incompatible resistance mechanisms. Although arrived at serendipitously, the combination of AZT and lamivudine shows such activity when used for treatment of AIDS, while another nucleoside analog, adefovir, appears to be incapable of stimulating the emergence of resistance in its target virus, hepatitis B virus, most likely because mutations in the viral polymerase that would confer resistance render the enzyme inactive. Such examples suggest what might be possible with continuing advances in understanding the structure-activity relationships of new compounds. However, this is predicated on acquiring a more detailed understanding of the structure and function of the microbial targets of various therapeutic agents, and increasingly more sophisticated structure-aided (i.e., "rational") approaches to drug design.

Case Studies of Antimicrobial Resistance

Workshop speakers presented updates on the genetics and ecology of several important pathogens. Among the microbes and infectious diseases discussed:

The bacterial strains staphylococci, enterococci, and pneumococci are ancient evolutionary companions of humans. In modern times, they have taken on major roles in microbial resistance. The various types of staphylococci, taken together, are among the most frequent causes of nosocomial, or hospital-acquired, infection, while enterococci are ranked second. *S. pneumoniae* is one of the most frequent causes of community-acquired infection.

Recently, scientists have acquired detailed information concerning how these various bacteria develop drug resistance. In staphylococci, one key change is that the mechanism of resistance is no longer considered to be the product of a single resistance gene. Rather, there is an entire stress-response pathway involving a central resistance gene and a number of auxiliary genes, all of which are essential for the bacteria to optimize resistance. Halting the function of any of these genes will reduce the microbe's propensity to develop drug resistance. Thus, there may be more targets than previously suspected for developing drugs to fight this microbe.

Malaria remains one of the leading killers in the developing world. The traditional first-line drug for treating the disease was chloroquine. Its widespread use, however, has led to increasing microbial resistance. For years, scientists struggled to understand how malaria parasites develop resistance. They have now identified a single gene as the culprit and pinpointed a particular type of mutation at a specific location in the gene as being critical in the development of resistance. Researchers are now using this knowledge to explore new drugs that precisely target the resistance mechanism.

Schistosomiasis, a debilitating disease caused by a parasitic worm that is transmitted to humans from snails, remains a public health problem in many regions, including Africa, the Middle East, Asia, and South America. For many of the species that infect humans, there is only one effective drug available: praziquantel. However, this drug has been in use for more than 20 years, and concern is increasing that resistance has emerged, or will soon emerge, in the parasite. This means planning must now focus on extending the drug's useful life and on developing new drugs before resistance emerges fully.

Workshop participants outlined a number of specific issues and priorities that will aid in better understanding microbial resistance and mitigating its impact on human health:

- Recognize that microbial infection, evolution, and resistance is an integral part of the ecology of life, and develop a fuller understanding of how microbes evolve when faced with drugs that threaten their survival.
- Develop therapeutic agents that are "engineered" to make evolution work in favor of humans, rather than in favor of microbes.
- Pursue drug-development strategies that will lead to therapeutics that are less likely to provoke additional waves of resistance. One strategy would be to develop narrow-spectrum drugs that will not challenge the entire microbial world each time they are used in therapy.
- Develop therapeutic interventions that target the "ecological reservoirs" of bacterial pathogens, particularly drug-resistant strains.
- Use drugs prudently in all patient care settings and in national and international disease-control programs, especially when a drug has not yet triggered widespread microbial resistance. Model programs for surveillance of antimicrobial resistance on a global scale also will be important to monitor and anticipate the emergence of resistance and begin developing alternative drugs and treatment programs.

VECTOR RESISTANCE

Beyond the development of resistance in pathogenic microbes, the ever-increasing resistance of disease vectors (the insects and arachnida that pass pathogens to humans) to chemical and biological pesticides looms as another complicating factor in efforts to control the emergence of infectious diseases. Resistance to insecticides has appeared in every major species of vector—including mosquitoes, ticks, fleas, lice, and sand flies—and various vectors have developed resistance to every class of pesticide. Where resistance has not contributed to disease emergence, it is expected to threaten disease control. A prime example was the emergence of DDT resistance in the mosquito species that serves as a vector for the transmission of malaria among humans. Widespread emergence of DDT resistance contributed heavily to derailing WHO's global efforts to eradicate the disease, setting back malaria control by decades. Malaria control programs that already face complex challenges presented by multi-drug-resistant strains of the parasite are additionally undermined by mosquito populations that show increasing resistance to the pyrethroid-treated bed nets commonly used to reduce malaria transmission.

Workshop participants agreed that scientists studying microbial resistance can learn much from the work of those studying these aspects of vector control, including how to prevent vectors from developing resistance to pesticides. Likewise, policy makers developing programs to control the spread of microbial resistance can benefit by examining the successes and failures of current pest-control programs. The underlying principles, pitfalls in control strategies, and possible approaches to solutions to resistance are not necessarily all that different.

One promising strategy discussed is to develop an integrated approach to control efforts. In the field of vector control, such coordinated efforts are called integrated pest management, or IPM. Although a number of factors, including cost, have prevented IPM from being adopted on a widespread basis, its potential remains clear. Tackling a pest problem in numerous ways at once—including the use of pesticides in a timely manner at select locations—will likely yield more thorough and longer-lasting control than would result from any single method applied individually.

Speakers also cited the value of developing and applying mathematical models to help understand complex aspects of resistance, including efforts to control the emergence of resistance, in both pests and pathogens. One advantage of modeling is that it enables researchers to conduct experiments that would be impossible, too expensive, or unethical to conduct otherwise. Models can serve a variety of purposes, including examining trends in data, exploring questions of population dynamics, developing and testing different management options, and generating new hypotheses for study.

Although scientists studying microbial resistance are increasingly using mathematical models, there currently is little interdisciplinary work involving scientists studying insecticide resistance. One primary reason for this gap is that bacterial population genetics differ substantially from the population genetics of most pest organisms. Still, there is much to be gained by cross-fertilization between the disciplines. It is important that modelers in both arenas become familiar with the results and efforts of the other. Such cooperation will help form a more complete understanding of the resistance phenomenon.

Workshop participants described a range of actions that can help improve vector-control efforts and minimize the spread of microbial resistance:

- Expand surveillance programs to monitor the susceptibility of vector populations to pesticide resistance. Once data have been gathered, it is crucial that the results be interpreted practically, in terms of control efficiency, so that effective strategies for remediation can be undertaken.
- Promote the use of integrated pest management programs, which in most cases are more effective than "single shot" programs in controlling pest populations and minimizing their resistance to chemical control agents.
- Foster multidisciplinary research efforts involving scientists studying microbial resistance and those studying various aspects of vector control, including how to prevent vectors from developing resistance to pesticides.
- Expand and apply knowledge of the basic molecular mechanisms underlying resistance to insecticides in order to develop novel control strategies that can truly manage resistance.
- Develop and apply mathematical models to help understand complex aspects of resistance, including efforts to control the emergence of resistance, in both pests and pathogens. Researchers studying microbial resistance and those studying insecticide resistance can benefit by working together.
- Examine the successes and failures of current pest-control programs when developing public policies aimed at controlling the spread of microbial resistance.

FACTORS CONTRIBUTING TO THE EMERGENCE OF RESISTANCE

To best meet the problem of microbial resistance, it is necessary to understand not only the scientific basis of how organisms become resistant but also the social and administrative practices that contribute to the emergence of resistance. A variety of factors have been identified, and important advances continue to be made in understanding their roles and how they might be mitigated.

Among the leading forces at work in the United States and other developed countries is the over-prescription of antimicrobials, particularly antibiotics, by physicians. Such overuse is fueled, in part, by patient expectations and demands. Growing patient awareness of antimicrobial agents (sometimes generated by direct-to-consumer marketing and not necessarily accompanied by understanding) sets up an expectation among patients that they should receive such drugs, even in the absence of appropriate indications. A variety of factors—including diagnostic uncertainty, lack of opportunity for patient follow-up, pressure to minimize length of office visits that precludes proper patient education, and lack of knowledge regarding optimal therapies—may influence a physician's response to patient demands. Meanwhile, in many developing countries, antimicrobial agents are readily available and can be purchased as a commodity without the advice or prescription of a physician or other trained health care provider. In such settings, drugs are often of questionable quality, with less than full potency, thereby possibly promoting the emergence of resistant pathogenic organisms—whether simply colonizers or in fact those involved in producing disease—in people taking them.

Hospitals also are fertile breeding grounds for microbial resistance. The combination of highly susceptible immunosuppressed patients (e.g., AIDS patients, cancer patients, or transplant recipients) who lack the basic immune mechanisms so essential to elimination of pathogens, intensive and prolonged antimicrobial use, close proximity among patients, and multiple invasive procedures have resulted in hospital-acquired infections that are highly resistant to available therapeutics. Large hospitals and teaching hospitals generally experience more problems with drug-resistant microbes, probably because they treat greater numbers of the sickest patients and those at highest risk of becoming infected. The failure of health care workers to practice simple control measures that have been known for decades (e.g., hand washing) frequently contributes to the spread of infection in hospitals.

Some common types of human behavior increasingly play a role in promoting resistance. Such behaviors as failure to complete recommended treatment or self-medication are among the most frequent factors associated with the development of resistance. Noncompliance occurs when individuals forget to take medication, prematurely discontinue the medication as they begin to feel better, or realize that they are unable to afford a full course of therapy. Self-medication with antimicrobials almost always involves unnecessary, inadequate, and ill-timed dosing—creating an ideal environment for microbes to adapt rather than be eliminated. As mentioned above, in many countries, antimicrobials are also readily available to consumers without a medical prescription. Moreover, in some countries, problems of noncompliance and self-medication are magnified because significant amounts of the available antimicrobials (particularly antibiotics) are poorly manufactured, counterfeit, or have exceeded their effective lifetimes and are thus less than fully effective.

Another important contributing factor is the overuse of antimicrobial agents in animals raised commercially for food, such as poultry, pigs, and cows. According to one estimate, approximately 40 percent of the 50 million pounds of antibiotics produced in the United States in 1998 was given to animals, either for therapeutic use or to promote growth. Overuse of these agents can lead to the development of drug-resistant microbes (largely bacteria, such as salmonella and campylobacter) that subsequently are transmitted to humans, usually through food products. Concern also is growing about the role played by the accumulation of low levels of antimicrobials derived from consuming animal products in the emergence of resistant pathogens among humans.

Workshop participants cited a number of specific initiatives that could help to control the emergence of resistance:

- Expand efforts to prevent hospital-acquired infections. Important activities include surveillance, outbreak investigation and control, sterilization and disinfection of equipment, and proper confinement of patients infected with resistant microbes.
- Enforce infection control measures among health care workers in acute and long-term care facilities, and other environments such as child care facilities.
- Improve physicians' prescribing practices through such means as education, formulary restrictions, multidisciplinary drug utilization evaluation, and computerized decision support systems. In all cases, the commitment and participation of the prescribing clinician and the health care institution are essential. Hospitals and clinics may derive direct financial benefits from such improved prescription practices.
- Ensure that patients comply with recommended drug therapies. This is one of the most important lessons that evolutionary biology can contribute to health management—that when it comes to the evolution of resistant diseases, half measures can increase problems of resistance.
- Expand research efforts to determine the effectiveness of short-course antimicrobial therapy for acute and self-limiting infections.
- Tailor education and intervention programs to specific communities and countries, especially in the developing world, since cultural factors will greatly determine their success.

• Conduct research to better understand the social and behavioral determinants that influence the emergence of resistant pathogens.

• Prevent misuse and overuse of antimicrobial agents in agriculture. This should include identifying critical control points along the continuum of food production. For example, management changes carried out at the farm level will not prevent the transfer of pathogenic organisms if there is significant contamination post-harvest or in the processing of food.

• Expand public education efforts to explain why treatment with antibiotics is not always the best medicine. In addition, numerous household products now contain antimicrobial agents that can encourage the selection of resistant organisms; education efforts are needed to explain that the same level of protection can be obtained with standard soap and household disinfectants.

EMERGING TOOLS AND TECHNOLOGY FOR COUNTERING RESISTANCE

The issue of how to counter microbial resistance continues to grow more complex. The traditional means to overcoming resistance problems has been to extend the useful life of current classes of antimicrobial drugs, often by developing slightly different chemical derivatives, or to develop wholly new classes of drugs that are not yet subject to resistance. However, the first route often provides marginal gains at best. And while completely novel classes of antimicrobials were discovered and subsequently introduced rapidly into clinical practice during the 1940s and 1950s, only a single new chemical class of antibiotics has emerged during the past several decades. Looking forward, many at the workshop viewed the antimicrobial pipeline as dismally empty.

Workshop participants described a variety of efforts to gain better understanding of the genetics and biochemistry of pathogens and the molecular mechanisms by which they develop resistance to antimicrobials. The genomics revolution, in particular, may be opening promising new avenues for exploration, but the pharmaceutical pipeline has yet to be populated with new classes of compounds under development. The promise seems present, but it has yet to be realized.

One class of antibiotics that has received considerable attention is the β-lactams. These drugs, which include penicillin, methicillin, oxacillin, and the newer cephalosporins comprise particularly important classes of antibacterials. Scientists have now demonstrated that nature has devised at least four strategies by which bacteria can develop resistance to β-lactam antibiotics. Of these, the most prevalent is the occurrence of certain enzymes, called β-lactamases, that break apart critical components of the drugs. Moreover, four distinct and independent mechanisms have evolved for the catalytic functions of these enzymes. Individually, the enzymes have undergone additional diversification. These observations provide strong evidence that random mutation and selection lead along different evolutionary tangents depending on the environment a pathogen finds itself in, the genetic composition of the organism, and the resources available to it.

Other research groups are taking a radically different approach to drug design. Nearly all bacteria enter humans at a mucous membrane site, such as the upper and lower respiratory tract or the intestines. These membranes thus act as reservoirs for many pathogenic bacteria. To date, however, there are essentially no drugs that can control pathogens on mucous membranes. Because of the fear of developing resistance, antibiotics are not indicated for control of the "carrier state" of pathogenic bacteria in most instances. This means physicians must wait for infection to occur before treating the patient. Yet, it is clear that by reducing or eliminating such human reservoirs of infection, the incidence of disease in the community will in turn be markedly reduced. Some scientists are now exploring the potential use of enzymes derived from viruses that infect bacteria (Yes, even bacteria are subject to infections themselves!) that may have the capacity to treat or prevent certain bacterial infections by safely and specifically destroying the pathogenic microbes on mucous membranes, in spinal fluid, or possibly in other closed compartments. For example, lytic enzymes derived from bacteriophage that are specific for *S. pneumoniae* and *S. aureus* could be administered nasally to control these organisms in people who spend time within institutions where such infections are rampant, such as day care centers, hospitals, and nursing homes.

However, getting promising candidate drugs to market is a long and expensive venture. As part of the current regulatory approval process, drug developers must evaluate whether their candidate achieves a clinical cure; that is, whether a person receiving the agent becomes free of symptoms. But this marker of success may not correlate with the extent to which the drug killed and eliminated the pathogen. If the pathogen persists, despite improvements in the signs and symptoms of infection, then conditions are ripe for the emergence of resistance.

This conundrum may be addressed by critically examining the pharmacokinetics and pharmacodynamics of new drugs using a technical approach known as PK/PD. PK/PD is built on taking regular cultures from a person receiving a therapeutic agent, and determining at which point pathogenic microbes are no longer present. In this way, the technology offers a direct measure of the agent's ability not only to cure the patient but also to eliminate the pathogen. PK/PD will not replace current evaluations of drug efficacy. But conducting a complementary PK/PD analysis, which can be done with a relatively small number of patients studied intensively but at a modest cost, can provide data that may indicate how likely a drug candidate is to stimulate the emergence of microbial resistance.

Workshop participants highlighted a range of actions that will help in developing new tools and technologies for countering resistance. These included:

- Expand research to prolong the useful life of current antimicrobial drugs and to develop new drugs, especially those with minimal potential for triggering antimicrobial resistance.
- Identify and eliminate any economic or regulatory "disincentives" that act to discourage pharmaceutical companies from undertaking research in this area. In some cases, creating positive economic incentives to encourage such research may be warranted.
- Ensure that the regulatory process provides a clear and feasible path for gaining approval of new therapeutic agents. This effort should include identifying and adopting ways to keep the cost of clinical trials required by regulation as low as safety allows.
- Develop ways to assess the potential emergence of microbial resistance as a part of traditional clinical trials. One promising approach may be to examine the pharmacokinetics and pharmacodynamics of new drugs as a complementary aspect of drug trials.
- Expand the development of a variety of non-drug-related measures (such as improved vaccines, diagnostics, and infection-control methods) to prevent or limit the spread of microbial resistance.
- Conduct research to better understand the interactions among pathogens, medical devices, and human hosts, and to develop rapid, reliable diagnostic techniques to identify the presence of infection, the specific infecting organism, and its antimicrobial susceptibilities.
- Explore alternative approaches to the application of therapeutics, such as alternating drug regimens. Both in medicine and agriculture, cyclic use of chemical control agents can often retard the evolution of resistance.

STRATEGIES TO CONTAIN THE DEVELOPMENT AND CONSEQUENCES OF RESISTANCE

Given the complexity of microbes—and their evolutionary drive to survive—it follows that managing the varied problems associated with microbial resistance will require a richly interwoven response. Workshop participants stressed that this response will require participation by individuals, organizations, and governments at the local, state, national, and international levels.

The primary blueprint for federal actions in the United States is the *Public Health Action Plan to Combat Antimicrobial Resistance*, issued in

2001 by a multiagency task force led by the Centers for Disease Control and Prevention (CDC), the Food and Drug Administration (FDA), and the National Institutes of Health. The task force developed a plan with input from state and local health agencies, universities, professional societies, pharmaceutical companies, health care delivery organizations, agricultural producers, consumer groups, and other members of the public. This plan will be implemented incrementally, in collaboration with these and other partners, as resources become available. The task force is now developing a second part of the plan, which will identify actions that more specifically address international issues.

The domestic action plan has four focus areas: surveillance, prevention and control, research, and product development. Among proposed efforts to improve surveillance, the plan calls for developing and implementing a coordinated national plan for monitoring antimicrobial resistance; ensuring the availability of reliable drug susceptibility data; tracking patterns of antimicrobial drug use; and monitoring antimicrobial resistance in agricultural settings. Efforts to improve prevention and control include extending the useful life of antimicrobial drugs through policies that discourage overuse and misuse; improving diagnostic testing practices; and preventing infection transmission through improved infection-control methods and use of vaccines. Expanded research also will be critical, as basic and clinical research provide the fundamental knowledge necessary to develop appropriate responses to antimicrobial resistance emerging in hospitals, communities, farms, and the food supply.

The plan calls for increasing understanding of microbial physiology, ecology, genetics, and mechanisms of resistance; augmenting the existing research infrastructure to support a critical mass of researchers in antimicrobial resistance and related fields; and translating research into clinically useful products, such as novel approaches to detecting, preventing, and treating antimicrobial-resistant infections. Strategies include fostering product development to ensure that researchers and drug manufacturers are focused on current and projected gaps in the arsenal of antimicrobial drugs, vaccines, and diagnostics and of potential markets for these products; stimulating the development and appropriate use of products for which customary market incentives are inadequate; and optimizing the development and use of veterinary and related agricultural products that reduce the transfer of resistance to pathogens that can infect humans.

Various federal agencies already are implementing parts of the action plan. The FDA, as part of its mandated regulatory responsibility, has played and continues to play an important role in ensuring that drugs and other chemical agents used in humans and in animals being raised for human consumption do not pose unacceptable health risks, including risks that may arise as a result of antimicrobial resistance. For example, the agency has developed a Framework Document that proposes a modified approval process for antimicrobials used in animals. The process is intended to ensure the human safety of such antimicrobials by prioritizing them according to their importance in medicine and establishing required mitigation actions with increasing resistance.

The FDA also uses a variety of other approaches to address the issue of antimicrobial resistance. For example, its Center for Drug Evaluation and Research searches for ways to enhance the available approaches to the development of new antibiotics. Among other efforts, the FDA is fostering early communication with pharmaceutical companies, using the product-labeling system to help educate physicians and other health care workers about antimicrobial resistance, and exploring methods for using data collected in clinical trials to make reliable inferences about a drug's potential to trigger antimicrobial resistance.

The CDC is active in promoting and implementing surveillance efforts, prevention and control activities, and applied research, including prevention research. One prevention and control effort, for example, focuses on health care settings, where infection with resistant organisms—many of them resistant to multiple drugs—has become a major patient safety concern. The agency has initiated the Campaign to Prevent Antimicrobial Resistance in Health Care Settings, a nationwide effort that targets front-line clinicians, patient care partners, health care organizations, purchasers, and patients. Its general goals include informing clinicians, patients, and other stakeholders about the escalating problem of antimicrobial resistance in health care settings; motivating interest in and acceptance of interventional programs to prevent resistance; and providing clinicians with tools to support needed practice changes.

The campaign centers around four basic strategies that clinicians can use to prevent antimicrobial resistance. These strategies include preventing infections so as to directly reduce the need for antimicrobial exposure and the emergence and selection of resistant strains; diagnosing and treating infections properly, which will benefit patients and decrease the opportunity for development and selection of resistant microbes; using antimicrobials wisely, since optimal use will ensure proper patient care while avoiding overuse of broad-spectrum antimicrobials and unnecessary treatment; and preventing transmission of resistant organisms from one person to another by emphasizing the importance of infection control. The CDC is now developing similar programs that target other groups of high-risk patients, including hospitalized children, geriatric, obstetrical, critical-care, and surgical patients as well as nursing home residents and those on dialysis.

International organizations also are stepping up efforts to contain antimicrobial resistance. Of particular note, the WHO in 2001 issued the *WHO Global Strategy for Containment of Antimicrobial Resistance*. Its portfolio of actions are intended for use by national governments and health systems, patients and communities, prescribers and dispensers, hospitals, pharmaceutical companies and marketers, growers of food-producing animals, and international organizations and partnerships concerned with containing antimicrobial resistance. The plan details a comprehensive framework of interventions designed to reduce the disease burden and the spread of infection, improve access to and improve use of appropriate antimicrobial agents, strengthen health systems and their surveillance capabilities, introduce and enforce regulations and legislation, and encourage the development of new drugs and vaccines.

Much of the responsibility for implementing WHO's strategy will fall on individual countries, and some of them—especially in the developing world—will need assistance. One such effort is being conducted by the Rational Pharmaceutical Management Plus Program, directed by a nongovernmental organization supported by the U.S. Agency for International Development. In conjunction with several partners, the program is developing a systematic approach to designing national-level efforts to contain antimicrobial resistance. This approach will provide a framework by which various stakeholders, working with technical consultants when necessary, can assess policies, drug use, and levels of resistance in their countries, and then tailor a range of strategies for advocacy, policy development, and systems change. Although this approach is generic, its implementation likely will be country-specific and unfold in distinct ways, according to circumstances in each country. Whatever its specific character, it is anticipated that the systematic approach will result in an increased level of awareness about this issue, heightened activity among local health organizations, and the introduction of stronger policies to monitor and contain the spread of antimicrobial resistance.

In light of the increasing magnitude of the problem, many workshop participants noted the need for implementing a vigorous, comprehensive attack on antimicrobial resistance. Too many studies have highlighted the problem—with their conclusions and recommendations remaining largely unfulfilled. Participants also suggested a number of specific issues and priorities that will help in containing the development and consequences of antimicrobial resistance:

- Complete implementation of the *Public Health Action Plan to Combat Antimicrobial Resistance*. This will require providing adequate funding across a range of public agencies and private organizations.
- Continue implementation of the *WHO Global Strategy for Containment of Antimicrobial Resistance*. Special priority should be given to the development of national legislation that eliminates the distribution of antibiotics without prescription from a trained health care provider; educa-

tion directed at distributors and consumers as well as prescribers of antibiotics; infection control to prevent the dissemination of resistant strains; quality assurance of antibiotics and other medicines; and the establishment of functional and sustainable laboratories for antibiotic resistance surveillance.

- Implement and expand surveillance efforts, at all levels, to ensure early detection of antimicrobial resistance problems. In the United States, disease reporting is mandated by state laws, but most states do not require reporting of drug susceptibility information, and the completeness of reporting varies. Some current surveillance systems need enhancement using updated laboratory and informatics technologies.
- Expand professional education and training, such as through expanded use of the CDC's "12 Steps to Prevent Antimicrobial Resistance" programs aimed primarily at front-line clinicians dealing with high-risk patients. Professional societies also can take a more active role in promoting education for their members.
- Conduct economic studies of antimicrobial resistance to complement scientific and epidemiological studies. Such studies can both inform the policy making process and suggest ways to provide incentives to individuals and institutions, such as hospitals, to adopt practices that will help limit the spread of antimicrobial resistance.

Stanley M. Lemon, M.D.
Dean of Medicine
The University of Texas
Medical Branch at Galveston

1

Introduction

MICROBIAL RESISTANCE: ADOPTING AN EVOLUTIONARY APPROACH

Resistance of infectious microorganisms to therapeutics is a serious—and growing—health threat in the developed and developing world alike. Introductions of new classes of antimicrobial drugs have been followed, often quickly, by the emergence of resistant microorganisms. Drug-resistant pathogens are now commonplace in hospitals and other health care settings, and they are increasingly found in communities as well. Compounding the problem, drug discovery efforts are yielding fewer truly new leads toward novel classes of antimicrobial agents.

In addition to the direct effect of antimicrobial resistance on human health, there also is an economic cost. In one estimate, for example, the hundreds of thousands of penicillin-resistant and methicillin-resistant infections that occur in the United States each year add roughly $30 billion to the national health care bill. Higher costs that result from antimicrobial resistance are particularly burdensome for developing nations, and in some cases effective therapies are now priced out of practical reach.

One major factor contributing to the emergence of drug-resistant microbes is the increase in the sheer volume of antimicrobial agents, particularly antibiotics, being used today. By one analysis, between 35 million and 50 million pounds of antibiotics are produced annually in the United States alone, for medical use in humans as well as agricultural use in a variety of animals and plants. Recent years also have seen an explosion of household products that contain antibacterial agents. This "antibacterial craze" defies the critical message that washing with soap and water is sufficient to provide hygiene to healthy individuals. Moreover, some studies indicate that bacteria emerging with resistance to these chemicals show decreased susceptibility to a number of antibiotics.

The unrelenting spread of antimicrobial resistance has been recognized for some time, with a number of public and private organizations issuing reports calling for action by the health care community, governments, and the public. The World Health Organization (WHO), for example, has declared antimicrobial resistance to be one of the top three issues in global health. Yet, efforts to manage antimicrobial resistance have, in general, remained insufficient in the face of the magnitude of the problem.

Not only are more—and better coordinated—efforts required. There also is a need to view antimicrobial resistance in a fundamentally different way. Where we once concentrated primarily on developing chemicals to eradicate pathogens, we now need to pay closer attention to the ecology and evolution of infection. Developing a fuller understanding of how microbes evolve when faced with drugs that threaten their survival may lead to innovative ways to bring them under control.

Indeed, genetics and evolutionary science hold some important lessons. Over the past 10 years, for example, scientists have expanded their knowledge of the breadth and complexity of the genetics of antimicrobial resistance. Hundreds of genes have been identified that render a variety of microbes resistant to a variety of drugs. These findings are encouraging laboratories, both public and private, to step up efforts to define new resistance genes and investigate their biochemical activity.

Evolutionary science has grown in sophistication and predictive power, and a body of theory and practical observation now exists that suggests possible strategies for helping to solve some of the problems that arise from the continued "arms races" between humans and microbes. For example, a number of ways have been demonstrated to slow down the evolution of drug resistance. These approaches include, among others, drug overkill strategies that reduce a microbe's potential for genetic mutation, direct observation therapy to ensure that patients complete their full courses of treatment, and alternating use of various antibiotic drugs to lessen the genetic pressure that promotes resistance. Another promising avenue beginning to be explored involves developing drugs that "engineer" a microbe's genetic mutations in a way that imposes a fitness cost and renders the pathogen less able to survive or evolve in its human host.

Use of such tactics follows from the realization that fighting infectious disease is only part of the health care battle. Suppressing the emergence of these diseases also should be an integral part of the agenda to foster the long-term promotion of human health.

ARMS RACES AND ANTIMICROBIAL RESISTANCE: USING EVOLUTIONARY SCIENCE TO SLOW EVOLUTION

Stephen R. Palumbi, Ph.D.

Department of Organismic and Evolutionary Biology
Harvard University, Cambridge, MA

A Thomson's gazelle can run like lightning late for a train: a fact that meshes beautifully with the prime place that this fleet animal holds on the menu of the world's fastest cat—the cheetah. The predator-prey drama unfolds with dinner on one side and death on the other, and the evolutionary dynamics that drive this system are very clear. Both cheetah and gazelle are in an arms race: where evolutionary change of the predator drives either compensatory change in the prey—or extinction. Any increase in gazelle speed or maneuverability exerts evolutionary pressure on the cheetah to notch up its own speed. The result of this arms race is a steady escalation of running ability, until both players challenge the maximum performance their basic construction will allow. Escalation caused by predator-prey arms races is a normal expectation of evolutionary models. Similar dynamics play out in many aspects of human-disease interactions, and similar evolutionary predictions have been validated many times.

Antibiotics exert a powerful evolutionary force, driving infectious bacteria to evolve powerful defenses against all but the most recently invented drugs. For example, when penicillin first became available in the middle 1940s, most infections caused by *Staphylococcus aureus* could be easily cured by a dose of 10,000 units (Neu, 1994). But by the late 1940s resistant strains were reported, and were so common by the early 1960s that hospitals in North America switched treatment strategies to the more powerful, and more expensive drug, methicillin (see Table 1-1). Methicillin resistance, discovered for the first time in Cairo in 1961, has spread so that by 2000, it rendered about 50 percent of the hospital-acquired infections of *S. aureus* resistant to the drug. Vancomycin, called the drug of last resort, cured these more powerful infections, but cases of resistance are increasing. In 1999, the FDA approved linezolid to treat vancomycin-resistant infections. The first linezolid-resistant bacteria are currently making the rounds.

This classic arms race between the evolutionary potential of bacteria and the industrial power of the modern pharmaceutical industry results in two important features of modern health care. First, antibiotic treatments are not static—they change over time as new strains of bacteria evolve and spread. Second, the substitution of treatments generally results in steady escalation of treatment costs. Generic amoxicillin is a standard treatment for childhood infections, with a cost of $4–$24. But so many strains of

TABLE 1-1 The History of Our Ongoing Race with *Staphylococcus aureus*

1943	penicillin available
1947	first resistant strains reported
1960s	switch to methicillin
1961	methicillin-resistant strain found in Cairo
1980s	methicillin resistance rising, vancomycin used as last resort
1992	15% methicillin-resistant
1996	35% methicillin-resistant
2000	50% methicillin-resistant
2002	vancomycin resistance reported

SOURCE: Garrett, 1994; Palumbi, 2001a; CDC, 2002a.

bacteria have evolved beta-lactamase enzymes that destroy the antibiotic that new formulations also include a beta-lactamase inhibitor, clavulanic acid. The resulting mixture, co-amoxyclav, has an augmented price of $64–$172 according to the Consumers Union of the United States (2001).

Overall these increases can have a substantial impact on health care costs. For example, if a hospital patient becomes infected with *S. aureus*, and the strain is resistant to penicillin, then the average hospital bill increases by about $9,000 in the United States (Abramson and Sexton, 1999). Should the strain prove to be resistant to methicillin as well, then the cost increase triples to $27,000. These costs add up to substantially increased expenditures in local hospitals: in the New York city area, costs of treating resistant *S. aureus* exceeded $400 million in 1999 (Rubin et al., 1999). The hundreds of thousands of penicillin-resistant and methicillin-resistant infections in the United States add to the national health care bill by an estimated $30 billion (Palumbi, 2001b).

Rapid Escalation of HIV

Probably one of the world's fastest evolving human diseases is also one of the clearest examples of arms races in health care and the escalation that results. Human immunodeficiency virus (HIV-1) has one of the fastest mutation rates on record due to a high error rate in its main genome-copying enzyme reverse transcriptase. The practical result of this high rate of mutation is that every infection of a new individual results in a unique evolutionary trajectory as the virus mutates into many slightly different forms. HIV is not a single infection, but a welter of different infections termed a quasi-species (Crandall, 1999).

This variation fuels rapid HIV evolution in response to two different sources of selection. This first source is the immune system of the person

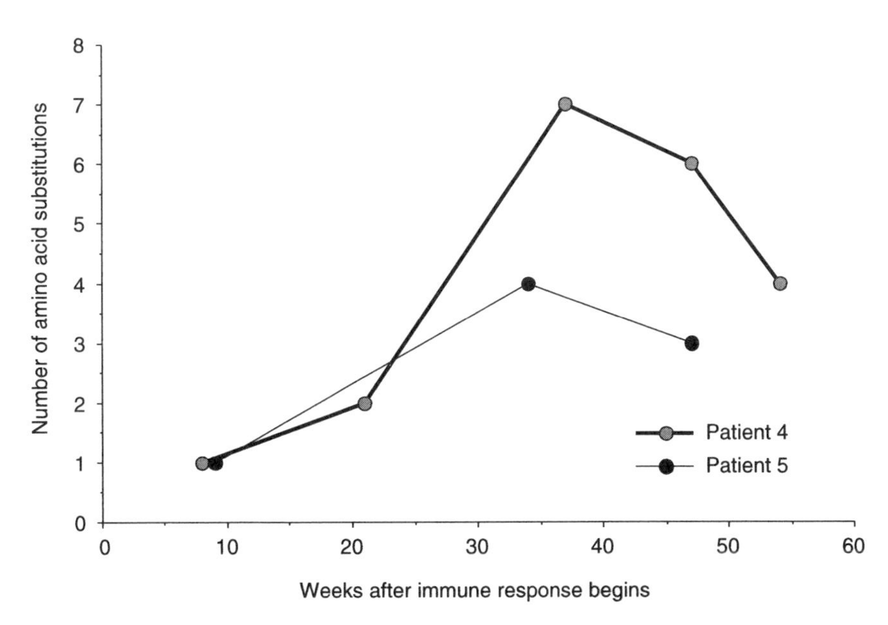

FIGURE 1-1 Rapid evolution of amino acid sequence of HIV coat proteins after the start of the immune response to infection. Within months, coat proteins evolve to evade immune detection. SOURCE: Wolinsky et al., 1996.

harboring the disease, which responds to HIV infection the way it should: by mounting a vigorous defense. But even though the immune system targets and destroys the first infective virus, by the time this defense is activated, the virus has mutated into so many forms that some of them evade immune detection. Mere weeks after the start of the immune response, amino acid evolution in the coat proteins that cover the viral shell has begun (see Figure 1-1). The cycle of immune targeting and viral escape repeats many times, each cycle representing a turning of the arms race wheel. Because the cellular hosts of HIV are T cells, which play an important role in the immune system, each arms race cycle reduces the strength of the immune system, eventually resulting in an immune collapse, and the onset of acquired immune deficiency syndrome (AIDS).

This is only the first of two major arms races with HIV. The second ignites when antiretroviral drugs are used to combat the virus. In every case, HIV evolves so quickly in response to this strong selection that antiretroviral drugs, used singly, have only a short window of effectiveness. For example, AZT was one of the first effective anti-HIV drugs. At first it worked well to reduce viral loads and to remove circulating viral RNAs from the bloodstream. This was because the reverse transcriptase enzyme

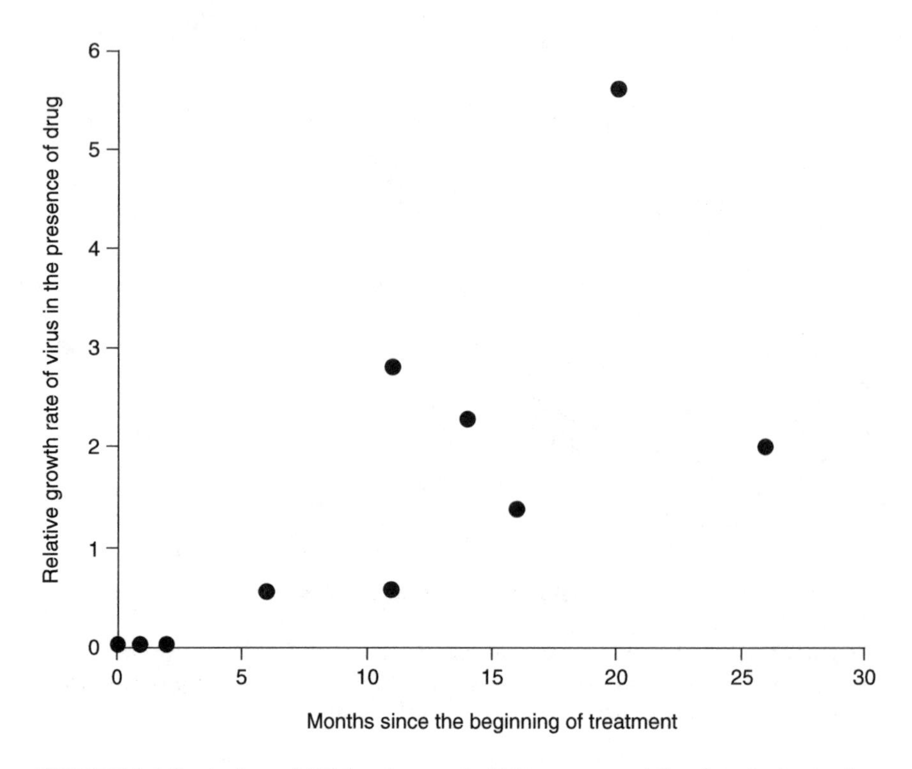

FIGURE 1-2 Evolution of AZT resistance in HIV occurs rapidly after the beginning of treatment. SOURCE: Larder and Kemp, 1989.

used AZT instead of the normal DNA precursors when it copied viral RNA into DNA, and these altered DNA copies were non-functional (Palumbi, 2001a). But within 6–18 months, HIV levels rose in AZT-treated patients, and the virus no longer responded to the drug (see Figure 1-2). Studies conducted in vitro showed that HIV quickly evolved the ability to grow in the presence of AZT. Further studies showed that four amino acid substitutions were required to confer virtual immunity of HIV to AZT, and that these same four amino acid substitutions occurred independently in patient after patient (see Figure 1-3). Not only is this an excellent, experimental demonstration of convergent evolution, but it also shows the ability of selection and mutation to combine to produce rapid HIV evolution within each infected individual.

HIV also evolves quickly in the presence of other drugs to become resistant. In fact there is no single drug to which HIV has not been able to evolve resistance. Ignoring this widespread and pervasive evolution would be a fatal mistake.

The global cost of this rapid evolution must also not be ignored, be-

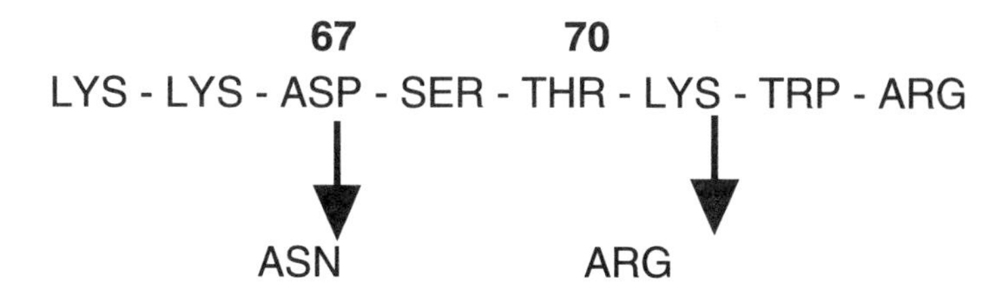

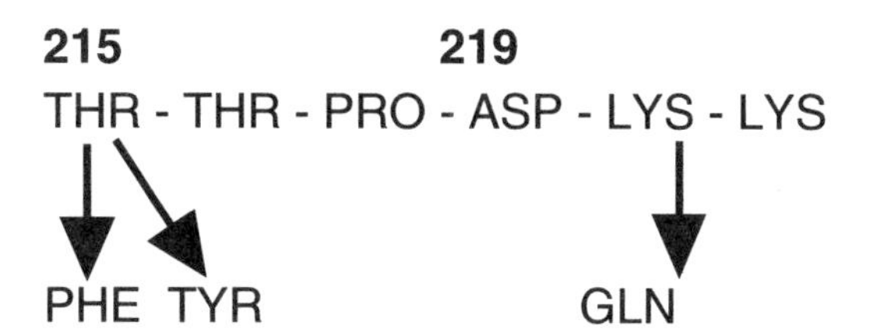

FIGURE 1-3 Four amino acid substitutions in the reverse transcriptase enzyme are sufficient to confer strong AZT resistance. These four substitutions occur in different order but accumulate in independent cases of the evolution of resistance. SOURCE: Larder and Kemp, 1989.

cause HIV evolution demands huge payments in human lives and health care expenditures. AZT is relatively cheap to produce, and if not for evolution of resistance, we would have substantially overcome HIV years ago by deploying this and other anti-retrovirals. Instead, HIV evolution prevents us from using simple drug treatment strategies, and HIV sufferers in North America and Europe rely on triple-drug therapy to stall the progress of the disease. This treatment is expensive (about $15,000–$20,000 a year per patient in the United States in 2000 [Bozzette et al., 2001]), and contributes $6 billion–$8 billion to U.S. annual health care costs (Palumbi, 2001b). Such high costs are impossible to meet in many developing nations, especially those in Africa that are the epicenter of the global HIV epidemic. In this case, the escalation of costs during the arms race with HIV results in a disease which is only temporarily manageable medically and entirely unmanageable economically.

Escalation and Global Medical Care

Other human diseases are evolving so quickly that they too are more and more expensive to treat, causing grave concerns about the ability to treat them in poor populations. Tuberculosis (TB) is relatively easy to cure as long as a patient takes a long enough dose of the appropriate antibiotics. But because treatment demands a six-month drug course, it is common for people to cease taking the proper antibiotics before a cure is effected. Relapses after a partial drug course are common, and the strain of TB that re-emerges has a much higher chance of being resistant (Lewis, 1995). These resistant strains can take up to 200 days in a hospital to cure, at a cost that far exceeds the cost of curing the original, non-resistant strain. Likewise, malaria (Hastings and Mackinnon, 1998), leprosy (Honore and Cole, 1993), as well as a host of other bacteria like *Enterococcus faecium* (Schentag et al., 1998) have evolved strains that are expensive to treat. All these outcomes result from the same basic evolutionary mechanism of arms races and escalation.

Antibiotic resistance and other evolutionary responses to medical treatment parallel the evolution of resistance in insect pests, agricultural weeds, and fisheries populations under strong selective mortality (Palumbi, 2001b). Such evolutionary changes have long been heralded, but there has been little in the way of coordinated response to this threat. In some sense this lack of coordinated response stems from the failure of medical, agricultural, and public health industries to realize that insect and bacterial resistance are based on the same evolutionary principles, and therefore can be addressed in the same fundamental ways. Over the past few decades, evolutionary science has grown in sophistication and predictive power, and has produced a body of theory and practical observation that can be used to help solve some of the problems of arms race escalation outlined above. Certainly, this approach cannot invent new drugs or roll back resistance, but it can help in important ways.

Evolutionary Science and Arms Races

From the standpoint of evolutionary science, arms races can be understood as the outcome of antagonistic coevolution, where evolutionary change in one species induces change in a second that induces more change in the first. This positive feedback loop is common whenever one species causes mortality in a second, but it is not inevitable. Furthermore, the rate and the direction of coevolution can be changed. As a result, understanding the evolutionary machinery that drives arms races can provide clues about how to throw a wrench in the works. Over the last decade, a number of different ways to slow down, halt, or reverse arms races have been invented and tried. In some cases, these efforts have paid off well to reduce the problems of antibiotic resistance, and can provide some clues about efforts that may be valuable in the future.

Drug Overkill

If we are in an arms race with HIV and it is one of the most quickly evolving organisms known, why has there been recent victory over HIV? What stopped the HIV race? Current medical care in the United States emphasizes administration of triple drug therapy, the combined administration of reverse transcriptase inhibitors and protease inhibitors (Ho, 1995). This approach has reduced deaths due to HIV by several-fold since 1996, and it has greatly slowed the evolution of this disease within patients (Wong et al., 1997). But how?

Triple drug therapy works to slow evolution because it is a drug overkill strategy. The combination of drugs is so potent that even among the enormous numbers of viruses circulating in the bloodstream, none possesses the genetic mutations necessary to allow the virus to grow. Essentially, there is no variation among viruses for the ability to grow in the presence of triple drug therapy. Evolution is fueled by variation, and where there is none, evolution halts. As a result, in overkill strategies, not only are the viruses quelled by potent drugs, but their ability to evolve resistance defenses is seriously curtailed.

Unfortunately, this strategy for HIV has not effected any cures. It is sufficient to keep the virus in check and to prevent its rapid evolution, but it has not yet led to the cure of anyone with HIV. This means that our current drug strategy is best viewed as a temporary measure to slow down the HIV rampage while a more permanent solution is found.

Direct Observation Therapy

Hidden within the success of drug overkill strategies lies the reason for the failure of many less powerful antimicrobial approaches. If complete inhibition of viral growth explains slow HIV evolution during triple-drug treatment, then partial treatment can easily be seen as a major impetus to the evolution of resistance. This is one of the most important lessons that evolutionary biology can contribute to health management—that when it comes to the evolution of resistance diseases, half measures can kill.

To see why this is true, imagine that a population of bacteria in an infection varies in the susceptibility of individual cells to a drug, and that some cells die in the presence of a drug dose more quickly than others (see Figure 1-4). The median life span of infectious cells in the presence of the drug is about 6.5 days in this example. If treatment stops after this time, half the cells have died, but the other half survive, going on to reproduce. Assuming their offspring inherit their drug survival abilities, then the median life expectancy of the half that are left increases to about 9 days. A 10-day drug course eliminates 80 percent of the cells, but the survivors have a median drug resistance time of about 12 days.

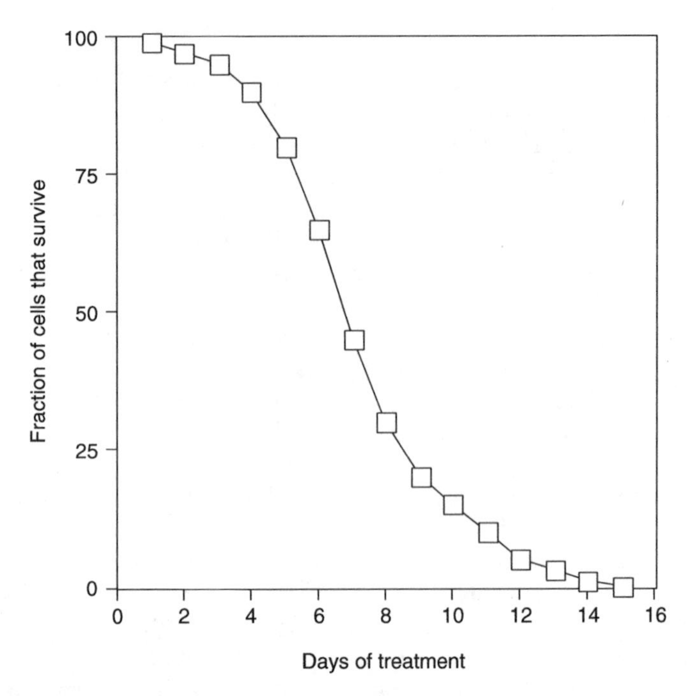

FIGURE 1-4 Hypothetical relationship between survival of a population of infectious cells and the length of a drug treatment regimen. The graph and subsequent discussion assume wide, genetically based variation in susceptibility in the original population, and no heterogeneity in drug exposure.

The increase in survival time among infectious cells after a drug treatment is called the "response to selection," and it increases with the severity of the selection and the heritability of the trait in question. Only when the complete drug course is taken, and all the infectious cells in the body have been eliminated does the response to selection drop. At this point, selection is 100 percent, no cells are left to start a new generation (unless there is reinfection from outside), and evolution cannot proceed. Although this is a hypothetical example, and the response to a drug course may not be as smooth as depicted in Figure 1-4, the overall point is that the result of selection is always a more robust population, unless mortality is complete, or heritability is low.

These considerations show why there is an increasing call for rigorous adherence to antibiotic treatment protocols, and why partial doses of antibiotics are contributing so heavily to the evolution of drug resistance. Prolonged treatment with antimicrobials is also important because of their impact on commensal flora. Even judicious use of antimicrobials will not completely halt evolution of resistance because such evolution could also occur in normal bacterial flora that is exposed to antimicrobials during treatment of a pathogenic disease, or in pathogenic organisms inhabiting the outside environment. High titres of antimicrobials in soils or water, for example, may select for resistance (Ash et al., 2002). In management of tuberculosis, strict treatment protocols include six or more months of antibiotic use, largely because the slow-growing TB bacteria have a long drug survival time. To reduce the evolution of resistance caused by failure to complete such long courses, Direct Observation Therapy uses a protocol in which TB drugs are delivered daily to outpatients, who then take the drugs under observation. Such assurance of a complete TB treatment greatly reduces the rate of relapse, slows the evolution of resistance, and decreases the cost of treating resistant TB. It has been used in developing countries as well as in urban centers in the United States to help stem TB epidemics. The basic principle applies to any infectious disease for which a partial antibiotic dose would generate a strong evolutionary response to selection. The strategy slows arms races because it breaks the evolutionary cycle.

Integrated Pest Management

Attempts to slow the evolution of resistance are not restricted to medicine. Insect resistance to pesticides is a growing problem (Georghiou, 1986) in which arms races generate escalation in the strength and concentrations of insecticides used by farmers. Control failures result in increased pesticide use, potential environmental damage, and expensive crop losses. Reducing the speed of evolution in these cases can result from reducing the selection imposed by insecticides, a reduction that can be accomplished by using alternative tactics—besides chemical treatment—to control populations. Alternatives like using traps, baits, or an insect predator such as a praying mantis, or using crop rotations to prevent buildup of particular pest species can all postpone the need for chemical spraying, and therefore reduce the selection imposed by pesticides, and thus reduce the evolution of resistance. In these cases, overall insect mortality might remain high. But because the mortality sources are variable, the response to selection caused by any single mortality agent is smaller, and the evolution that results is slower.

In hospitals, integrated pest management can be called hand washing—the use of physical antimicrobial measures to reduce populations of potential infectious agents. These approaches do not supplant the use of antibiotics, but they reduce their use, saving them for times and places in which antibiotic drugs are absolutely required. Because antibiotic use is lower, selection for resistance is lower. Consider the result of using spray antibiotics to sterilize hospital instruments or other equipment. Each application acts as an opportunity for selection of bacterial populations for increased resistance. But when those same instruments are comprehensively sterilized with heat, there is no selection for antibiotic resistance.

Alternating Antibiotic Use

The general principle of diversifying the force of selection can apply to antimicrobial use if a suite of different agents are employed so that the selection against any single one of them is lessened. Like the above example in which antimicrobial use is lessened through application of other disinfectant techniques, selection for resistance to any one antimicrobial can sometimes be lessened through alternating use of different drugs. Both in medicine and agriculture, cyclic use of chemical control agents lessens the evolution of resistance. For herbicides, for example, many farmers are discouraged from using the same herbicide more than two growing seasons in a row, because otherwise resistant weeds crop up too often.

Likewise, some hospitals have tried cycling among different antibiotics in an attempt to reduce the evolution of resistance, and reduce the costs of treating resistant infections. In these cases, drug use is switched on a prescribed schedule, often resulting in reduced infections, reduced incidence of resistance, or reduced costs (see Table 1-2). Emerging theory helps design treatment protocols that limit resistance (Bonhoeffer et al., 1997), although substantial questions about how to implement these strategies remain.

Fitness Costs of Resistance

Trade-offs in adaptation are a consistent theme in evolutionary science—adaptation to favor one attribute (like flight in birds) may have a high cost (e.g., large mass allocation to flight muscles) or lead to parallel changes that may be deleterious in some cases (like hollow and brittle bones). In cases in which flight was no longer adaptive—like predator-free oceanic islands—these fitness costs of flight are reversed, and birds have

TABLE 1-2 Responses to Antibiotic Cycling in Hospitals Trying to Reduce Costs of Treating Resistant Infections

Target	Response	Study
Gentamicin resistance	Improvement	Gerding et al., 1991
Ceftazidime resistance	Reduced infection	Kollef et al., 1997
Ceftazidime resistance	Reduced drug use	Kollef et al., 2000
Multi-drug resistance	No improvement	Dominguez et al., 2000
Ciprofloxacin resistance	Reduced infection	Gruson et al., 2000

evolved flightlessness (a feature that is not necessarily a good strategy after humans discover these islands, as the dodo and many flightless New Zealand moas found out).

In the case of antimicrobial resistance, the evolution of mechanisms to evade drug actions might be highly costly or generate parallel, deleterious change. Enzymes that degrade or pump antibiotics are expensive to produce. Ribosomes that are resistant to tetracycline may be slower to synthesize proteins. If this were generally true, then cessation of use of an antibiotic would result in the de-evolution of resistance because cells that did not have resistant abilities would be favored. In such cases, we could reverse the course of evolution by shelving the drug for a while.

Although antibiotic resistance mechanisms that impose a fitness cost are known, in general fitness costs of antibiotic resistance are fairly small. In some experiments, resistant and non-resistant bacterial strains have been grown together in the absence of antibiotics for thousands of generations without the resistantless strains taking over. Such cases generate problems because once established, these "cheap" resistance mechanisms are difficult to eradicate. Antibiotic cycling protocols detailed above will not necessarily work to reduce the evolution of these strategies, and other approaches like Integrated Pest Management will have similarly reduced effectiveness.

We cannot change the nature of resistant mutations, and therefore cannot engineer the evolution of mutations that happen to have fitness costs. However, one avenue to explore is the development of new antibiotics for which a resistance mechanism would pose a fitness cost. The choice to develop and deploy an antibiotic rests on many different features of its performance, but one feature that might be taken more heavily into account is the nature and cost of mutations that provide resistance. Given that resistance is inevitable, those antibiotics that impose a fitness cost on resistant strains might be most valuable in the long term—both from a public health and from an economic point of view.

Conclusions

Evolutionary arms races provide a valuable conceptual framework in which to understand the nature of the current crisis in antimicrobial resistance, and understand the evolutionary principles involved. Even if co-evolutionary changes are inevitable as a result of antimicrobial arms races, there are strategies that can be used to slow down their advance, and perhaps curtail the evolution of resistance. Current examples of successful deceleration of evolution include drug overkill strategies, direct observation therapy, integrated pest management, and antibiotic cycling. Use of these tactics follows from the realization that fighting infectious disease is only part of the health care battle. In addition, fighting the evolution of these diseases must be part of the agenda for long-term human health care.

ANTIBIOTIC RESISTANCE 1992–2002: A DECADE'S JOURNEY

Stuart B. Levy, M.D.

Center for Adaptation Genetics and Drug Resistance
Tufts University School of Medicine, Boston, MA

This overview briefly examines the status of antibiotic resistance over a 10-year perspective which is described more fully in the second edition of *The Antibiotic Paradox* (Levy, 2002a).

In 1992, I warned about ominous events, like the emergence of vancomycin-resistant *Staphylococcus aureus* or the widespread appearance of *Streptococcus pneumoniae* resistant to multiple drugs, or fluoroquinolone-resistant *E. coli* (Levy, 1992). It is no surprise now that these are actual events—but what else has happened over the past decade?

While there are many factors involved in the emergence of antibiotic resistance, the two major ones still operate today: the *antibiotic*, which encourages selection and evolution of resistant strains, and the *resistance genes* which are acquired by bacteria or appear by mutation.

Over the past ten years, investigators have identified many additional transferable resistance genes. In 1992 there were 25 TEM-like β-lactamases described. Currently, the β-lactamase website (http://www.lahey.org/studies/webt.stm) lists over 100. In 1992, tetracycline resistance determinants numbered 12; in 2002, there are 35. Ten years ago, there were perhaps two or three types of multi-drug efflux pumps. Now, there are five (Alekshun and Levy, 2000). These new genetic findings represent growing knowledge of the breadth and complexity of antibiotic resistance.

These findings indicate that new drug resistance determinants are reaching clinically detectable levels under the selection of continued antibiotic misuse. Scientists are stimulated to evaluate, clone, and genetically define them. These efforts represent an increased interest in resistance—not nearly enough, but more than before. It is heartening to see laboratories defining new resistance genes and investigating their biochemical activity.

Over the past decade, the use of antibiotics has continued to increase, even though the actual quantity is still controversial. By my estimate there are between 35 and 50 million pounds of antibiotics being produced in the United States (Levy, 2002a). Some groups have said that animals use half this amount. Others say that almost 25 million pounds go to animals and that people use less than 5 million pounds (Mellon et al., 2001). Studies are underway to try to quantitate antibiotic use. In that context, an estimated

260 million prescriptions for antibiotics were filled in outpatient pharmacies in the United States in 1996 (Hutchinson, 1998). This figure does not include hospital use. Therefore, a considerable amount of pressure is being exerted on the natural microbial environment by the antibiotics provided to humans, animals, and plants, including the spraying of antibiotics on fruit trees.

One area in which antibiotic usage has decreased is in aquaculture. In 1992 there were no FDA regulations on how antibiotics were to be provided to the fish industry (Levy, 1992). There was no government mark on a piece of fish that identified whether it did or did not come from a fishery using antibiotics. Today the aquaculture industry has decreased the use of antibiotic-impregnated feeds by as much as four-fold (Levy, 2002a). Part of the reason for this change is in response to outside pressure; part is linked to improved hygiene and increased use of vaccines. The industry uses public areas to raise the fish. The seas, ponds, and other waters are overseen by ecology groups which have little tolerance for environmental pollution and put forth great efforts in protecting the environment.

An area that has also broadened over the decade is the genetics of resistance. We have heard about transposons, plasmids, and bacteriophages before, but a newer genetic entity has reached greater recognition in the last decade—the "integron." Showing structural resemblance to transposons, integrons carry different genes, including those for antibiotic resistance, in a series behind a single promoter from which expression of all the genes downstream occurs. Integrons capture and integrate cassettes of antibiotic resistance genes and other genes via an integrase. The genes are joined in tandem, producing a single element mediating resistance to multiple antibiotics. The integron has been shown to be responsible for multi-drug resistance in a large number of gram-negative bacteria and helps explain the multi-drug resistance phenomenon of the current and previous decade.

At the end of the 1980s and continuing into the 1990s, vancomycin-resistant enterococci (VRE) bearing a large plasmid-borne transposon began to appear in hospital patients. The situation has worsened over the past decade. Virtually every hospital in the United States encounters VRE. It was expected that this genetic element would enter *S. aureus,* largely because transfer had been shown on mouse skins in the laboratory of W. Noble in London (Noble et al., 1992). But it did not happen quickly over the ensuing years, and, actually, not until just this year (2002).

Two different strains of *S. aureus* with full-fledged vancomycin resistance mediated by the vanA gene were isolated in the United States. The first was identified in a patient in Michigan in July (Centers for Disease Control and Prevention [CDC], 2002a) and the second in a patient in Pennsylvania in October (CDC, 2002b). Thus the drastic event feared a decade ago is now a reality. We can wonder what the future will bring in terms of other vanA-resistant *S. aureus* clinical isolates and how wide the determinant has already spread among staphylococci.

Before this current emergence, hospitals saw *S. aureus* strains that were heterogeneously resistant or homogeneously resistant to vancomycin by chromosomal mutation. These so-called vancomycin intermediate resistant strains, or "VISA," have appeared in Japan, the United States, and elsewhere. Although the clinical laboratory tests (e.g., MIC values) might not designate these strains as fully resistant, patients bearing them have failed vancomycin therapy. Thus, they are clinically vancomycin-resistant.

In the beginning of the last decade, the fluoroquinolone family of antibiotics was a small group. Today there are more than a dozen different members of this family used worldwide. Initially, these agents were provided for serious multi-drug-resistant infections. Eventually, as resistance emerged to other first-line antibiotics, (for instance, in *E. coli* urinary tract infections), the fluoroquinolones became much more widely used in the community. Following closely on the heels of this increased use was the emergence of fluoroquinolone resistance. There are strains of *E. coli* in Southeast Asia, China, and even in the United States, that are resistant to greater than 250 μg/ml of the drug—the result of multiple mutations in the target genes, the topoisomerases, in combination with increased expression of multi-drug efflux pumps. What happened is something few could have predicted—the emergence of many different mutations producing a clinically relevant fluoroquinolone resistance in gram-negative bacteria.

Among the staphylococci, fluoroquinolone resistance was detected relatively soon after the introduction of the first fluoroquinolones. Gram-positive bacteria, including *S. aureus,* emerged with target gene mutations and/or efflux pumps. These mutations when present in a strain make the newer generation fluoroquinolones (designed to treat gram-positive bacteria) less effective and render the strains one or two mutational steps from full-fledged resistance.

In London, ciprofloxacin resistance in *Salmonella typhi* rose from just a few percent in 1996–1997 to about 25 percent in 1998 and 1999 (Threlfall and Ward, 2001). Many of the strains initially came from outside the United Kingdom, but were propagated and spread by fluoroquinolone use within the United Kingdom. This finding raises grave concerns that ciprofloxacin may not remain effective as a drug of last resort in those parts of the world where resistance to other antibiotics, namely ampicillin, chloramphenicol, and co-trimoxazole, has eliminated these drugs as effective treatment for typhoid fever.

In the United States, the CDC described four patients in Minnesota and North Dakota who died from a methicillin-resistant *S. aureus* (MRSA) infection whose resistance was not recognized early (CDC, 1999). MRSA, while well known among hospital patients, is not commonly found in the community. The unique feature of the so-called "community-acquired MRSA" was that they were resistant chiefly to β-lactam antibiotics, which included methicillin, but not other antibiotic classes like vancomycin, or the aminoglycosides.

For the physicians in the community, the first thought was to use a penicillin. No one expected that MRSA was the infectious cause in these children. The number of community-acquired MRSA strains is increasing: in one Chicago hospital, the rate per 100,000 admissions was 10 in 1988–1990, rising to 259 in 1993–1995 (Herold et al., 1998).

Also in the community, there has been a steady rise in antibiotic-resistant pneumococci. Just recently, the CDC reported an 11-month-old girl from a community in Georgia with refractory otitis media caused by a pneumococcus resistant to six different antibiotics (CDC, 2002c). She required hospitalization. The infection was traced to a day-care center where many other children were colonized with the same organism. This was not an urban environment with heavy antibiotic usage, but rather a small community. However, antibiotic usage there was largely without guidelines. Importantly, the pneumococcal vaccine, which covered the organism involved, had not been introduced.

Today, many different multi-drug-resistant bacteria, including both gram-negative and gram-positive bacteria, cause problems in communities as well as hospitals (see Table 1-3). These resistant organisms affect the health of our larger populations.

What else has happened to encourage resistance?

TABLE 1-3 Clinical Problems of Multi-Drug Resistance

Hospital-acquired disease organisms	Community-acquired disease organisms
Gram-negative	**Gram-negative**
Acinetobacter sp.	*Escherichia coli*
Citrobacter sp.	*Neisseria gonorrhoeae*
Enterobacter sp.	*Salmonella typhi*
Escherichia coli	*Salmonella typhimurium*
Klebsiella sp.	
Pseudomonas aeruginosa	**Gram-positive**
Serratia marcescens	Enterococcus sp.: VRE
	Mycobacterium tuberculosis
Gram-positive	
Enterococcus sp.: VRE	*Staphylococcus aureus: MRSA*
Coagulase-negative staphylococci	*Streptococcus pneumoniae*
Staphylococcus aureus: MRSA;VISA;VRSA	*Streptococcus pyogenes*

SOURCE: Levy, 2002b.

Antibacterials is a common name given to surface agents (otherwise known as biocides) contained within household products which inhibit a variety of microbes. Some act quickly like alcohols, peroxides, and chlorinated products. Others, such as triclosan or benzalkonium chloride, leave residues. The latter encourage the selection of resistant organisms. In 1992 there were 23 such products on the market; in 1999, *The New York Times* estimated 700 of these items marketed for households. The public is amassing these antibacterials in their homes in a variety of products. Why? To some extent it is in response to fear of the "super bug," the multi-drug-resistant bacterium. The other pressure is to protect the family against infectious organisms caused by food. "I want to do what is best for my child," is commonly expressed. While these reasons cannot be criticized, the public needs to be informed that the same protection is provided by using standard soap and disinfectants.

The antibacterial craze demonstrates a couple of problems. For one, it defies the message that washing with soap and water is sufficient to provide hygiene to healthy individuals. Today's public believes one has to add an antibacterial chemical to gain a health benefit from washing. This opinion does not help our cause against antibiotic misuse and the emergence of resistance.

Secondly, bacteria emerging with resistance to these chemicals can show decreased susceptibility to antibiotics. A Japanese group reported a few years ago that MRSA selected in the laboratory for half the susceptibility to a biocide, benzalkonium chloride, showed a dramatic increase in resistance to a wide spectrum of β-lactam antibiotics (Akimitsu et al., 1999). Susceptibility to other antibiotics was either unchanged or changed minimally. This phenotype, that is, predominantly β-lactam resistance, is strikingly similar to the community-acquired MRSA strains. Is it possible that disinfectants, not β-lactam antibiotics, selected these resistant bacteria?

S. aureus is one of the principal organisms targeted by triclosan in the hospital. But decreased susceptibility to triclosan is emerging in MRSA isolated from hospitals (Suller and Russell, 2000). This evolution will curtail this important use, fail to protect from transmission of disease, and create more resistance problems. A mutation in the target gene of triclosan activity, *fabI* (enoyl reductase) affects other drugs besides triclosan (McMurry et al., 1998). Given the multi-drug efflux pumps in *E. coli* and *S. aureus*, overexpression of one of these pumps, like in *E. coli* and Pseudomonas (Chuanchuen et al., 2001), could contribute to resistance mediated by a *fabI* mutation. These pumps export antibiotics as well. So, one selects a resistance mechanism affecting both antibacterials and antibiotics.

What does the future look like? What is happening today that provides optimism for the future?

When we entered the 1990s, the only in-depth analysis of antibiotic use and resistance was a report from an NIH Fogarty International Center-supported Task Force effort in 1983–1986 (Levy et al., 1987). Over 100 physicians, scientists, and public health and industry representatives from all over the world discussed the imminent problems of resistance through six task forces. Although the report urged that something be done about the problem, the effort was disregarded and even downplayed under the guise that the problem was being overstated. Some influential critics from industry believed that such an activity cast wrongful doubts on the efficacy of their antibiotic products. The report was not accepted as hoped—as a call to action by physicians, consumers, and public health officials.

More recently in 1995, the U.S. Office of Technology Assessment (OTA) released an assessment of the resistance problem in the United States just before the Office was closed (OTA, 1995). It stated the obvious—resistance was a mounting public health problem stemming from antibiotic misuse. The report particularly was noteworthy because Congress was showing interest at last. Since then, there have been reports from other professional and government groups including the American Society for Microbiology (ASM, 1995), the Society for Hospital Epidemiology of America (Shlaes et al., 1997), the American College of Physicians-American Society of Internal Medicine (ACP-ASIM, 2001), and the House of Lords Select Committee on Science and Technology (1998). We have learned something from these efforts, but up until now, they have had little impact on the problem.

Somewhat greater success has been achieved by The Alliance for Prudent Use of Antibiotics (APUA), founded in 1981, working in conjunction with its 35 country chapters on research and education concerning antibiotic use and resistance. For 20 years, it has championed the improved use of antibiotics globally. Recently, the organization synthesized the efforts of various expert groups—25 reports over the past 15 years—as a background and foundation for WHO's *Global Strategy for Containment of Antimicrobial Resistance* (WHO, 2001). The APUA document was published along with the WHO report in 2001 (APUA, 2001).

APUA has created materials to educate the consumer about antibiotics and resistance. Its "antibiotic" brochure has been translated into several languages and has been disseminated to almost a million people. The newsletter, translated into Russian and Spanish, reaches thousands quarterly. The CDC has also published a pamphlet for patients, which appeals to the consumer to stop demanding and stockpiling antibiotics.

The most important thing that has happened in this past decade is the wider awareness and response to the resistance problem. The WHO General Assembly selected resistance as one of the three major health problems facing the world today. The ACP-ASIM has chosen antibiotic resistance as its clinical theme for 2000–2002.

Are we going to see a difference? I hope so, but forums like this one have to define practical ways in which change can occur. We do not need more reports; we need action.

The pharmaceutical companies left the antibiotic field in the mid-1980s, came back to it in the mid-1990s, but appear to be leaving it again now. Antibiotics are difficult and costly to develop. Sales may not reach the minimum of $500 million to $1 billion per year to maintain the interest of the large pharmaceutical companies. This is a sad situation, complicated by the fact that many large companies have merged to form even larger ones. Thus, the creativity and competition that occurred among companies before is greatly diminished as, for instance, three companies become one. It is more likely now that new antibiotics will come from the smaller biopharmaceutical groups that make firm commitments to the discovery efforts. Big pharmaceutical companies join when the drug is far enough along that the risk is minimized.

Vaccination has made another big impact over the last decade. The involvement of *Haemophilus influenzae type B* in otitis media and meningitis has been curtailed with the use of the conjugate vaccine. We must expand acceptance of vaccination with the pneumococcal conjugate. A recent report looked at the effects of the vaccine coverage on invasive disease and found the vaccine to be very effective (Black et al., 2001). While less than 20 percent were fully vaccinated, a much larger percent of the individuals had reduction in invasive disease indicating that there was a "herd effect." If we can get the vaccine to more communities, patients like that little 11-month-old girl from Georgia can be protected. We would greatly reduce pneumonia and prevent fatal meningitis. We also would decrease the initial choice of an antibiotic for a suspected bacterial etiology (e.g., pneumococcus) of upper respiratory disease like otitis media. Providing vaccines against both *H. influenzae* and *S. pneumoniae* would make a viral cause of the illness more acceptable and antibiotics less prescribed.

Another initiative at APUA is the Global Advisory on Antibiotic Resistance Data (GAARD), which includes the large surveillance systems of Bristol-Myers Squibb (SENTRY), GlaxoSmithKline (ALEXANDER), Focus Technology, and, most recently, AstraZeneca (MYSTIC) and Bayer. Large amounts of data on drug-bug combinations are collected which can be helpful to public health officials. APUA was able to catalyze an agreement between the companies funding these projects to meet periodically and discuss and share the data. The project provides antibiotic susceptibility surveillance information on large numbers of clinical isolates and allows early changes in susceptibility to be revealed, such as the decreased susceptibility of *Haemophilus influenzae* to fluoroquinolones detected at 0.1 percent (Travers et al., 2001).

Another project that has recently been completed, also by APUA, is an in-depth examination of the impact of animal use of antibiotics on human public health and the environment (APUA, 2002). The FAAIR (Facts About Antibiotics in Animals and the Impact on Resistance) project brings scientific evidence to the policy debate regarding use of antibiotics for animals. A unique feature of this report is its broader perspective. It looks at the ecological impact of animal use, not just the direct animal-to-consumer path of transmission. Antibiotics provided to animals for therapy, prophylaxis, or as growth promotion, select resistant organisms which can spread to farm dwellers, as well as food consumers.

The important, but often lost, message is that antibiotics affect more bacteria than the targeted pathogen. They will decimate entire microbial communities that are exposed. Those that are resistant become reservoirs of antibiotic resistance genes.

In fact, an antibiotic provided to humans, plants, or animals does not stay with the treated individual nor is it always readily degraded. It eventually passes into the environment in some form at some level, which explains the detection of drugs in municipal waters, streams, and agricultural fields (Kolpin et al., 2002). We can now speak not only of antibiotic effects during therapy, but effects "after therapy" (Levy, 2001, 2002a). Since resistance does not often emerge in the person while on the antibiotic, I suggest that much resistance occurs outside the treated person or animal. Perhaps it would be considered unrealistic, but what an advantage there would be to develop an antibiotic that does its treatment, but then self-destructs.

With this point in mind and focusing on the environment, APUA and University of Illinois, funded by the National Institute of Allergy and Infectious Diseases, began the Reservoirs of Antibiotic Resistance (ROAR) project. The aim is to look for the genes of resistance harbored in natural environments as they may evolve as future clinical treatment problems.

Can we reverse the resistance problem? It may take a long time for a bacterium to lose a transposon or a mutation, but one way to reverse resistance is to encourage the susceptible commensal organisms to return. Such was the basis for reversal of macrolide resistance among *Streptococcus pyogenes* in Finland when physicians stopped the use of erythromycin (Seppala et al., 1997). It was not due to loss of resistance from a particular *S. pyogenes*, but, rather, by replacement with other susceptible strains.

In addition to the various scientific challenges that must be met, we also need to devise new public policies and procedures that will help minimize the emergence of antimicrobial resistance. For example, I have been suggesting for a number of years that the Food and Drug Administration (FDA) create an entirely separate category for antibiotics, apart from other drugs. Antibiotics are the only type of therapeutic agents that have societal effects beyond their physiological effects, so it is logical for them to have their own official category, complete with its own set of regulatory requirements. The FDA would then be better positioned to devise unique incentives that encourage the pharmaceutical industry to pursue the development of new antibiotics, to market antibiotics prudently, and to conduct surveillance efforts to see that any incipient antimicrobial resistance is contained. As we use antibiotics in this decade, we should be thinking more ecologically. Let our treatments be directed at the causative agents and less destructive of the broad microbial environment.

REFERENCES

Abramson MA and Sexton DJ. 1999. Nosocomial methicillin-resistant and methicillin-susceptible *Staphylococcus aureus* primary bacteremia: at what cost? *Infection Control and Hospital Epidemiology* 20:408–411.

ACP-ASIM (American College of Physicians-American Society of Internal Medicine). 2001. Principles of Appropriate Antibiotic Use Position Papers. *Annals of Internal Medicine* 134:479–529.

Akimitsu N, Hamamoto H, Inoue R, Shoji M, Akamine A, Takemori K, Hamasaki N, Sekimizu K. 1999. Increase in resistance of methicillin-resistant *Staphylococcus aureus* to beta-lactams caused by mutations conferring resistance to benzalkonium chloride, a disinfectant widely used in hospitals. *Antimicrobial Agents and Chemotherapy* 43:3042–3043.

Alekshun MN and Levy SB. 2000. Bacterial drug resistance: response to survival threats. In: Storz G, Heugge-Aronis R, eds. *Bacterial Stress Responses*. Washington, DC: ASM Press. Pp. 323–366.

APUA (Alliance for the Prudent Use of Antibiotics). 2001. *Antibiotic Resistance: Synthesis of Recommendations by Expert Policy Groups*. WHO/CDS/CSR/DRS/2001.10. Geneva: WHO.

APUA. 2002. The need to improve antimicrobial use in agriculture: ecological and human health consequences. *Clinical Infectious Diseases* 34 (Suppl 3):S71–S144.

Ash RJ, Mauck B, Morgan M. 2002. Antibiotic resistance of gram-negative bacteria in rivers, United States. *Emerging Infectious Diseases* 8:713–716.

ASM (American Society for Microbiology). 1995. Report of the ASM task force on antibiotic resistance. *Antimicrobial Agents and Chemotherapy* Suppl:S1–S23.

Black SB, Shinefield HR, Hansen J, Elvin L, Laufer D, Malinoski F. 2001. Postlicensure evaluation of the effectiveness of seven valent pneumococcal conjugate vaccine. *Pediatric Infectious Diseases Journal* 20:1105–1107.

Bonhoeffer S, Lipsitch M, Levin B. 1997. Evaluating treatment protocols to prevent antibiotic resistance. *Proceedings of the National Academy of Sciences* 94:12106–12111.

Bozzette SA, Joyce G, McCaffrey D, Leibowitz A, Morton S, Berry S, Rastegar A, Timberlake D, Shapiro M, Goldman D. 2001. Expenditures for the care of HIV-infected patients in the era of highly active antiretroviral therapy. *New England Journal of Medicine* 344:817–823.

CDC (Centers for Disease Control and Prevention). 1999. Four pediatric deaths from community-acquired methicillin-resistant *Staphylococcus aureus*—Minnesota and North Dakota, 1997–1999. *Morbidity and Mortality Weekly Report* 48:707–710.

CDC. 2002a. *Staphylococcus aureus* resistant to vancomycin—United States, 2002. *Morbidity and Mortality Weekly Report* 51:565–567.

CDC. 2002b. Vancomycin-resistant *Staphylococcus aureus*—Pennsylvania, 2002. *Morbidity and Mortality Weekly Report* 51:902.

CDC. 2002c. Multidrug-resistant *Streptococcus pneumoniae* in a child care center—Southwest Georgia, December 2000. *Morbidity and Mortality Weekly Report* 50:1156–1158.

Chuanchuen R, Beinlich K, Hoang TT, Karkhoff-Schweizer RR, Schweizer HP. 2001. Cross-resistance between triclosan and antibiotics in *Pseudomonas aeruginosa* is mediated by multidrug efflux pumps: exposure of a susceptible mutant strain to triclosan selects *nfxB* mutants overexpressing MexCD-OprJ. *Antimicrobial Agents and Chemotherapy* 45:428–432.

Consumers Union of the United States. 2001. Super-germ alert: how to avoid antibiotic use and misuse. *Consumer Reports* 66:60–61.

Crandall K, ed. 1999. *The Evolution of HIV*. Baltimore: Johns Hopkins University Press.

Dominguez EA, Smith TL, Reed E, Sanders CC, Sanders WE Jr. 2000. A pilot study of antibiotic cycling in a hematology-oncology unit. *Infection Control and Hospital Epidemiology* 21(1 Suppl):S4–8.

Garrett L. 1994. *The Coming Plague: Newly Emerging Diseases in a World out of Balance*. New York: Farrar, Straus and Giroux.

Georghiou GP. 1986. The magnitude of the resistance problem. In: *Pesticide Resistance: Strategies and Tactics for Management*. Washington, DC: National Academy Press. Pp. 14–43.

Gerding DN, Larson TA, Hughes RA, Weiler M, Shanholtzer C, Peterson LR. 1991. Aminoglycoside resistance and aminoglycoside usage: ten years of experience in one hospital. *Antimicrobial Agents and Chemotherapy* 35:1284–1290.

Gruson D, Hilbert G, Vargas F, Valentino R, Bebear C, Allery A, Bebear C, Gbikpi-Benissan G, Cardinaud JP. 2000. Rotation and restricted use of antibiotics in a medical intensive care unit. Impact on the incidence of ventilator-associated pneumonia caused by antibiotic-resistant gram-negative bacteria. *American Journal of Respiratory and Critical Care Medicine* 162:837–843.

Hastings IM and Mackinnon MJ. 1998. The emergence of drug-resistant malaria. *Parasitology* 117:411–417.

Herold BC, Immergluck LC, Maranan MC, Lauderdale DS, Gaskin RE, Boyle-Vavra S, Leitch CD, Daum RS. 1998. Community-acquired methicillin-resistant *Staphylococcus aureus* in children with no identified predisposing risk. *Journal of the American Medical Association* 279:593–598.

Ho D. 1995. Time to hit HIV, early and hard. *New England Journal of Medicine* 333:150–151.

Honore N and Cole ST. 1993. Molecular basis of rifampin resistance in *Mycobacterium leprae*. *Antimicrobial Agents and Chemotherapy* 337:414–418.

House of Lords Select Committee on Science and Technology. 1998. Seventh Report. [Online]. Available: http://www.parliament.the-stationery-office.co.uk/pa/ld199798/ldselect/ldsctech/081vii/st0701.htm.

Hutchinson JM. 1998. More than 160,000,000 antibiotic prescriptions in the USA. Abstract O-22 In: Abstracts of the 38th Interscience Conference on Antimicrobial Agents and Chemotherapy, San Diego, September 24–27, 1998.

Kollef MH, Vlasnik J, Sharpless L, Pasque C, Murphy D, Fraser V. 1997. Scheduled change of antibiotic classes: a strategy to decrease the incidence of ventilator-associated pneumonia. *American Journal of Respiratory and Critical Care Medicine* 156:1040–1048.

Kollef MH, Ward S, Sherman G, Prentice D, Schaiff R, Huey W, Fraser VJ. 2000. Inadequate treatment of nosocomial infections is associated with certain empiric antibiotic choices. *Critical Care Medicine* 28:3456–3464.

Kolpin DW, Furlong ET, Meyer MT, Thurman EM, Zaugg SD, Barber LB, Buxton HT. 2002. Pharmaceuticals, hormones, and other organic wastewater contaminants in U.S. streams, 1999–2000: a national reconnaissance. *Environmental Science and Technology* 36:1202–1211.

Larder BA and Kemp SD. 1989. Multiple mutations in HIV-1 reverse transcriptase confer high-level resistance to zidovudine (AZT). *Science* 246:1155–1158.

Levy SB. 1992. *The Antibiotic Paradox: How Miracle Drugs Are Destroying the Miracle.* New York: Plenum Publishing.

Levy SB. 2001. Antibiotic resistance: consequences of inaction. *Clinical Infectious Diseases* 33:S124–S129.

Levy SB. 2002a. *The Antibiotic Paradox: How the Misuse of Antibiotics Destroys Their Curative Powers.* Boston: Perseus Books.

Levy SB. 2002b. The 2000 Garrod lecture: factors impacting on the antibiotic resistance process. *The Journal of Antimicrobial Chemotherapy* 49:25–30.

Levy SB, Burke JP, Wallace CK. 1987. Antibiotic use and antibiotic resistance worldwide. Report of a study sponsored by the Fogarty International Center of the National Institutes of Health, 1983–1986. *Reviews of Infectious Diseases* 9 Supplement 3:S231–316.

Lewis R. 1995. The rise of antibiotic-resistant infections. *FDA Consumer* 29:11–15.

McMurry LM, Oethinger M, Levy SB. 1998. Triclosan targets lipid synthesis. *Nature* 394:531–532.

Mellon M, Benbrook C, Benbrook KL. 2001. *Hogging It.* Cambridge, MA: Union of Concerned Scientists.

Neu HC. 1994. Emerging trends in antimicrobial resistance in surgical infection: a review. *European Journal of Surgery Supplement* (573)7–18.

Noble WC, Virani Z, Cree RG. 1992. Co-transfer of vancomycin and other resistance genes from *Enterococcus faecalis* NCTC 12201 to *Staphylococcus aureus. FEMS Microbiology Letters* 72:195–198.

OTA (Office of Technology Assessment). 1995. *Impacts of Antibiotic-Resistant Bacteria.* Washington, DC: OTA.

Palumbi SR. 2001a. *The Evolution Explosion: How Humans Cause Rapid Evolutionary Change.* New York: WW Norton.

Palumbi SR. 2001b. Humans as the world's greatest evolutionary force. *Science* 293:1786–1790.

Rubin RJ, Harrington C, Poon A, Dietrich K, Greene J, Moidussin A. 1999. The economic impact of *Staphylococcus aureus* infection in New York City hospitals. *Emerging Infectious Diseases* 5:9–18.

Schentag JJ, Hyatt JM, Fitzpatrick P, Paladino JA, Birmingham MC. 1998. Infection control and changes in the antibiotic formulary for management of epidemic and endemic vancomycin-resistant *Enterococcus faecium. Hospital Practice 1998 Special Report*:22–36.

Seppala H, Klaukka T, Vuopio-Varkila J, Muotiala A, Helenius H, Lager K, Huovinen P. 1997. The effect of changes in the consumption of macrolide antibiotics on erythromycin resistance in group A streptococci in Finland. Finnish Study Group for Antimicrobial Resistance. *New England Journal of Medicine* 337:441–446.

Shlaes DM, Gerding DN, John JF, Craig WA, Bornstein DL, Duncan RA, Eckman MR, Farrer WE, Greene WH, Lorian V, Levy S, McGowan JE Jr, Paul SM, Ruskin J, Tenover FC, Watanakunakorn C. 1997. Society for Healthcare Epidemiology of America and Infectious Diseases Society of America Joint Committee on the Prevention of Antimicrobial Resistance: Guidelines for the Prevention of Antimicrobial Resistance in Hospitals. *Infection Control and Hospital Epidemiology* 18:275–291.

Suller MT and Russell AD. 2000. Triclosan and antibiotic resistance in *Staphylococcus aureus. Journal of Antimicrobial Chemotherapy* 46:11–18.

Threlfall EJ and Ward LR. 2001. Decreased susceptibility to ciprofloxacin in *Salmonella enterica* serotype Typhi, United Kingdom. *Emerging Infectious Diseases* 7:448–450.

Travers K, Stelling J, Levy SB, Miller L, Souder B, Jones R. 2001. Emerging geographically diverse *Haemophilus influenzae* isolates with reduced susceptibility to fluoroquinolones: a GAARD report. Late breaker session at the 41st Interscience Conference on Antimicrobial Agents and Chemotherapy, Chicago, December 16–19, 2001.

WHO (World Health Organization). 2001. *Global Strategy for the Containment of Antimicrobial Resistance.* WHO/CDS/CSR/DRS/2001.2. Geneva: WHO.

Wolinsky SM, Korber BTM, Neumann AU, Daniels M, Kunstman KJ, Whetsell AJ, Furtado MR, Cao Y, Ho DD, Safrit JT, Koup RA. 1996. Adaptive evolution of human immunodeficiency virus-type 1 during the natural course of infection. *Science* 272:537–541.

Wong JK, Hezareh M, Gunthard HF, Havlir DV, Ignacio CC, Spina CA, Richman DD. 1997. Recovery of replication-competent HIV despite prolonged suppression of plasma viremia. *Science* 278:1291–1295.

2

Microbe Resistance

OVERVIEW

Since the discovery and subsequent widespread use of antimicrobials, a variety of pathogenic viruses, bacteria, protozoa, and helminths have developed numerous mechanisms that render them resistant to some—and, in certain cases, to nearly all—antimicrobial agents. The focus of this session of the workshop was on exploring some of the latest information emerging about how various important pathogens develop resistance to drugs and how such resistance might be overcome.

The bacterial strains staphylococci, enterococci, and pneumococci pose some of the most serious problems in terms of antimicrobial resistance. Scientists have now acquired detailed information about how these bacteria develop drug resistance. In staphylococci, for example, optimization of resistance depends on the operation of a complex pathway involving a central resistance gene and a number of auxiliary genes. Thus, developing drugs that specifically target any of these genes holds potential for reducing the microbe's drug resistance. A second novel intervention would target the ecology of these types of bacteria. For example, penicillin-resistant strains of pneumonia bacteria have been found to breed prolifically in the nasopharynx of preschool-age children, particularly those who attend day care centers. Devising interventions to limit antimicrobial exposure might help reduce the genetic propensity of these bacteria to develop drug resistance.

Malaria and schistosomiasis are major health threats in the developing world. Chloroquine was historically the primary drug for treating malaria, but its widespread use has led to increasing microbial resistance. Scientists have now identified a particular type of mutation at a specific location on a single gene as being critical in the development of resistance, and efforts are now under way to develop new drugs that target this resistance mechanism. Praziquantel is the only drug now available to treat schistosomiasis. Since the drug has been in use for more than two decades, concerns are mounting that the parasitic worms that transmit the disease from snails to humans are beginning to become resistant. Among the immediate needs, praziquantel's effectiveness can be prolonged by more selective use, with treatment targeted only to those people at greatest risk for heavy infection and morbidity, as well as by the use of integrated disease management practices, such as snail control, health education, and improved sanitation. At the same time, new drug development needs to continue in anticipation of the eventual failure of praziquantel efficacy.

Influenza is a global threat to health. Vaccines represent the first line of defense against the flu, with a new vaccine being developed and distributed each year in response to the changing genetic composition of the causative virus. Still, vaccines are not a total answer, and several classes of antiviral drugs have been developed to treat infected individuals. Two antivirals—amantadine and rimantadine—have been around since the 1960s. Although effective in some circumstances, both types of drugs suffer from drug-resistance problems. Another family of newer drugs, called neuraminidase inhibitors, shows even more promise, as these formulations appear to pose a reduced risk of triggering resistance. A major problem, however, is that the pharmaceutical companies that produce these newer drugs are not making enough doses to cover medical needs in the event—certain to happen at some point—that a highly modified and virulent form of the influenza virus emerges from the animal world and spreads among the human population worldwide.

Adding to concerns about antimicrobial resistance is the possibility that terrorists or a rogue nation might use "bioweapons" to expose large numbers of people to genetically engineered drug-resistant pathogens in order to trigger large-scale disease outbreaks. This scenario was brought into sharp perspective in autumn 2001 by the intentional distribution through the U.S. mail of envelopes containing spores of *Bacillus anthracis*. One issue considered during this session involved the effects of exposure to both anthrax and ionizing radiation at the same time, conditions that military personnel, in particular, might someday face. Based on a recent study in mice, scientists have been able to identify some fundamental factors that contribute to increased susceptibility to bacterial infections in general, and to *B. anthracis* in particular, after ionizing radiation, as well as to make some general recommendations about effective methods of therapy and prophylaxis following such combined exposures.

NEW STRATEGIES AGAINST MULTI-DRUG-RESISTANT BACTERIAL PATHOGENS

Alexander Tomasz, Ph.D.

The Rockefeller University, New York, NY

A major impact of the "chemical warfare" that humanity has been waging against the microbial world on an escalating scale since the discovery of antibiotics is the emergence of a vast variety of resistance mechanisms that have moved into virtually all pathogenic species—viruses, bacteria, and protozoa alike. This emergence has occurred with a swiftness that, on an evolutionary scale, is truly remarkable.

The rapid progression from a uniformly antibiotic-sensitive bacterium to a uniformly antibiotic-resistant species is well demonstrated by the case of *Staphylococcus aureus,* which is a primary agent of hospital-acquired infections. In the early 1940s, when penicillin was introduced into therapy, all strains of staphylococci were highly sensitive to this antibiotic. In less than a decade, *S. aureus* acquired the penicillinase-based resistance mechanism from an unknown "extra species" source. Penicillin resistance spread across the entire species with the "plasmid epidemic," and by the late 1950s penicillin was useless against *S. aureus*.

The final stage of this remarkable and sweeping genetic change, propelled by the pressure of antibiotic use, is documented in a recent study conducted in Portugal (Sá-Leão et al., 2001). Screening the *S. aureus* nasal flora recovered from 1,000 young and healthy volunteers who had never received antibiotics showed that 97 percent of the *S. aureus* colonizing these individuals produced penicillinase and were resistant to penicillin (Sá-Leão et al., 2001). Clearly, the extra-species drug-resistance gene penicillinase has become a domesticated genetic component of *S. aureus* without causing any survival deficit to the cells. The penicillin-resistant *S. aureus*, which was originally associated only with patients in hospitals, has managed to move into the community within 50 years of its appearance on the scene.

Equally fast was the response of *S. aureus* and other staphylococci to the introduction in 1959 of semisynthetic β-lactam antibiotics, such as methicillin. The first methicillin-resistant *S. aureus* (MRSA) was detected in the United Kingdom in 1961 (Jevons, 1961). By the 1990s, MRSA had become a globally spread pathogen, making the management of nosocomial *S. aureus* infections complicated and expensive.

Essentially the same phenomena were observed in *Streptococcus pneumoniae*, one of the major community-acquired pathogens of our era. *S. pneumoniae* are responsible for a series of potentially life-threatening diseases that together cause an estimated 1 million to 3 million deaths worldwide annually. The first penicillin-resistant pneumococci (PRSP) were detected in 1965 (Hansman et al., 1974), followed by increasing numbers of reports on the detection of resistant strains. By the mid-1990s, penicillin-resistant strains had spread globally.

In both MRSA and PRSP, antibiotic resistance has unfolded in stages, on a rapid time and geographic scale. Initial detection of MRSA and PRSP was followed by reports on geographic spread. Next came reports on the increase in resistance level and in the frequency of resistant isolates. Eventually, multi-drug-resistant strains carrying resistance traits to different classes of antimicrobial agents also began to appear.

In 1993, a small group of international experts, including microbiologists, physicians, and public health personnel, gathered at Rockefeller University for a workshop to survey data on the accelerating spread of multi-drug-resistant pathogens (Tomasz, 1994). By this time, the specter of untreatable bacterial infections had appeared on the horizon as a clear possibility. Strains of common community-acquired and nosocomial pathogens equipped with multi-drug-resistant traits had been identified, with some clinical isolates retaining susceptibility to only a single antimicrobial agent.

The workshop participants identified a number of specific genetic events which, if they occurred, could precipitate a genuine public health crisis. Examples of such events include the acquisition of high-level vancomycin resistance among MRSA or pneumococci, and the acquisition of β-lactamase plasmid by group A streptococci. The alarm sounded at the workshop was recently echoed by the World Health Organization (WHO): "Increasingly drug-resistant infections in rich and developing nations alike are threatening to make once treatable diseases incurable (WHO, 2000). Tables 2-1 and 2-2 illustrate the multi-drug resistance phenomenon: the strikingly successful adaptation of two major human pathogens—*S. aureus* and *S. pneumoniae*—to a planetary environment that became saturated with highly toxic substances due to the immense quantities of antimicrobial agents deployed in human and veterinary medicine, in agribusiness, and in virtually the entire biosphere.

What can one do in this situation? Clearly the backlash of multi-drug resistance has caught the pharmaceutical chemists and infectious diseases specialists by surprise. In retrospect, it seems that the antibiotic era had two interrelated "cardinal sins." One sin was the neglect and sometimes complete abandonment of preventive measures in favor of a single-minded antibiotic strategy against bacterial infections. The second was the failure to seriously consider consequences of the fact that the overwhelming major-

TABLE 2-1 Development of Multi-Drug Resistance by *S. aureus* and *S. epidermidis* (S: susceptible, R: resistant)

	S. aureus ATCC 6538 (1930)	MRSA Brazilian epidemic clone (1994)	Methicillin-resistant *S. epidermidis* New York Hospital (1996)
Amikacin	S	R	R
Amp/Sulbactam	-	R	R
Ampicillin	S	R	R
Cephalothin	S	R	R
Cefotaxime	S	-	-
Chloramphenicol	S	R	R
Ciprofloxacin	S	R	R
Clindamycin	S	R	R
Erythromycin	S	R	R
Gentamicin	S	R	R
Imipenem	S	R	R
Oxacillin	S	R	R
Rifampin	S	R	R
Vancomycin	S	S	S
Teicoplanin	S	S	-
Tetracycline	S	R	R
Trimeth/Sulfa	S	R	-
Mupirocine (topical)	S	R	R

ity of both the most effective antibiotics and resistance mechanisms are actually products of the microbial world. Antibiotics are produced in tiny quantities and on a microscopic scale by some microbes—presumably for the control of the "quorum" of their habitat—and the producer microbes also invented self-protective resistance mechanisms against their own products. The reintroduction of these highly toxic agents into the biosphere in enormous quantities was a major violation of this quorum sensing. It has amplified local wars among microbes to a global conflict between human and microbe, a chemical warfare in which both offensive and defensive (resistance) armaments came from the microbial world (Tomasz, 2000).

The current genomic revolution may offer clues for the production of new antimicrobial agents that would not have been invented by the microbial world during evolution. Development and introduction of such novel agents would be a welcome development indeed. However, it would be naïve to think that the microbial world already "awakened" by the antimicrobial armaments race would simply submit to such new onslaughts. Antibiotic-resistance mechanisms have emerged rapidly in the past, even against completely synthetic agents, such as trimethoprim and fluoro-

TABLE 2-2 Development of Multi-Drug Resistance by *S. pneumoniae* and *Enterococcus faecium* (S: susceptible, R: resistant)

	S. pneumoniae D39 (1949)	*S. pneumoniae* 6B Dallas, Texas (1992)	*Enterococcus faecium* (VRE) (Tn5482) Memorial Hospital (1996)
Amikacin	S	-	R
Amp/Sulbactam	S	R	R
Ampicillin	S	R	R
Cephalothin	S	-	R
Cefotaxime	S	R	-
Chloramphenicol	S	R	S
Ciprofloxacin	S	R	R
Clindamycin	S	R	R
Erythromycin	S	R	R
Gentamicin	S	-	R
Imipenem	S	S	R
Oxacillin	S	R	R
Rifampin	S	-	R
Vancomycin	S	S	R
Teicoplanin	S	S	R
Tetracycline	S	R	S
Trimeth/Sulfa	S	R	R
Mupirocine (topical)	S	-	-

quinolones. Thus, a possible deployment of new antimicrobial agents would not solve the basic dilemma of the antimicrobial armaments race that originates from its erroneous core philosophy: namely, the indiscriminate killing of bacteria by wide-spectrum antimicrobial agents. The fallacies of this philosophy have been pointed out repeatedly (Tomasz, 2000).

There are a number of antimicrobial strategies, not yet exploited, that would be more discriminatory and therefore less likely to provoke another wave of drug resistance. The pharmaceutical industry's traditional approach to drug development has been either to find new wide-spectrum drugs against bacterial targets or to reconfigure old drugs against targets that became inaccessible due to drug resistance. Examples of these two strategies would be the development of new classes of fluoroquinolones and the semisynthetic modification of β lactams to accommodate the penicillinase-based resistance mechanism.

However, there are at least two completely different strategies that offer promise. The first strategy would target the resistance phenotype; the second would target the ecology of resistant bacteria.

Recent studies have shown that in both MRSA and PRSP, high-level antibiotic resistance requires more than the presence of the central drug-resistance determinant (the *mecA* gene in the case of MRSA, and the mosaic PBP genes that encode low affinity binding proteins in PRSP). Expression of an optimal high-level antibiotic-resistant phenotype also requires the assistance of a number of additional genetic determinants, the functioning of which is critical for the generation of antibiotic resistance, although the protein products of these genes do not react with the antimicrobial agent. Transposon mutagenesis of a highly methicillin-resistant MRSA strain has identified over 20 such "auxiliary genes" (De Lencastre et al., 1999). Inactivation of these genes had no effect on the transcription of the resistance gene *mecA* to its gene product (the low affinity penicillin binding protein PBP2A), yet phenotypic resistance of the bacteria was drastically reduced. Recent observations in PRSP identified a similar phenomenon. Inactivation of the small pneumococcal operon *murMN*, responsible for the production of branched structured components in the bacterial cell wall, caused a complete collapse of the penicillin resistant phenotype in spite of the fact that the primary resistance determinants (the low affinity PBPs) remained unchanged in the mutant bacteria (Filipe and Tomasz, 2000).

These observations indicate that reversal of drug resistance is possible by two completely different ways: either by inactivation of the central genetic determinant and its gene product, or by inactivation of the products of auxiliary genes (see Figure 2-1). It follows that auxiliary genes represent novel types of antibacterial targets. Compounds capable of inactivating the products of these genes should represent synergistic agents that together with β-lactam antibiotics would render resistant bacteria sensitive again to these classical antimicrobial agents.

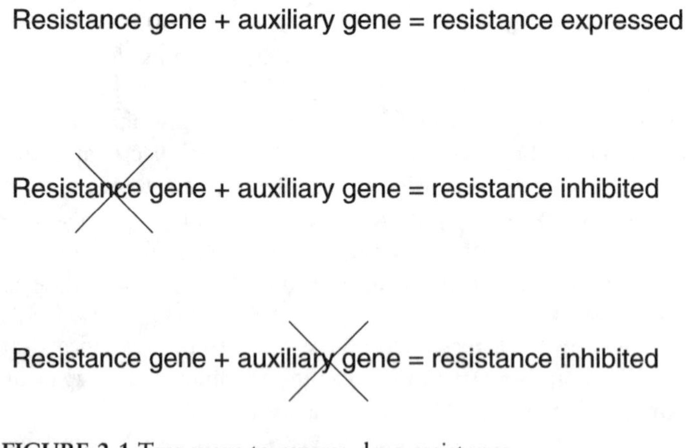

Resistance gene + auxiliary gene = resistance expressed

~~Resistance~~ gene + auxiliary gene = resistance inhibited

Resistance gene + ~~auxiliary~~ gene = resistance inhibited

FIGURE 2-1 Two ways to reverse drug resistance.

A major roadblock to development of such agents, however, is that this approach seems to collide head-on with the central philosophy of the pharmaceutical industry, which is only willing to invest in the development of wide-spectrum antimicrobial agents that can assure a market in the range of $1 billion a year. Clearly, the types of agents described here would be specific for the particular bacterial pathogen and therefore would be outside such marketing interest. While the position of "big pharma" on this issue is based on complex economic realities, I believe that the future points in a different direction: the development of highly specific narrow-spectrum agents, the deployment of which would not challenge the entire microbial world each time they are used in therapy. Such development will be hastened by current progress in devising highly sensitive molecular techniques for rapidly detecting and identifying bacterial pathogens—a capability that may lie in the not too distant future. With rapid and safe diagnostics at hand, the use of wide-spectrum antimicrobial agents should be reserved to special cases only because of their indiscriminate challenge to both harmful and harmless bacteria.

A second novel intervention with bacterial pathogens, particularly drug-resistant strains, would target the ecology of these bacteria. Recent observations indicate that the overwhelming majority of diseases caused by resistant strains of *S. aureus* are linked to a surprisingly few epidemic clones or genetic lineages that have immense geographic spread (Oliveira et al., 2002) and that appear to combine in their genetic backgrounds not only determinants of antibiotic resistance but also genes that assure ecological success (i.e., spread and colonization) of the bacteria (see Figure 2-2). Similar observations also have been made for penicillin-resistant *S. pneumoniae* (Sá-Leão et al., 2000). Clearly, identification of determinants of epidemicity may provide completely new targets—vaccines or chemical agents—against specific multi-drug-resistant clones that are responsible for most of the hardships of resistant disease.

Following up on this ecological reasoning raises questions related to the ecological reservoirs of bacterial pathogens, particularly the drug-resistant clones. It has been clearly shown that in the case of PRSP a major sanctuary and breeding ground of drug-resistant strains is the nasopharynx of preschool-age children, particularly those who attend day care centers. All children have immature immune systems. When this natural condition is combined with the close contact among children that is characteristic of day care centers, the high frequency of viral respiratory diseases in such centers, and the use (and misuse) of immense quantities of antimicrobial agents, the result is the creation of a bona fide "factory" of resistant pneumococci (Sá-Leão et al., 2000). Similar studies could not identify a comparable reservoir of MRSA among healthy carriers (Sá-Leão et al., 2001).

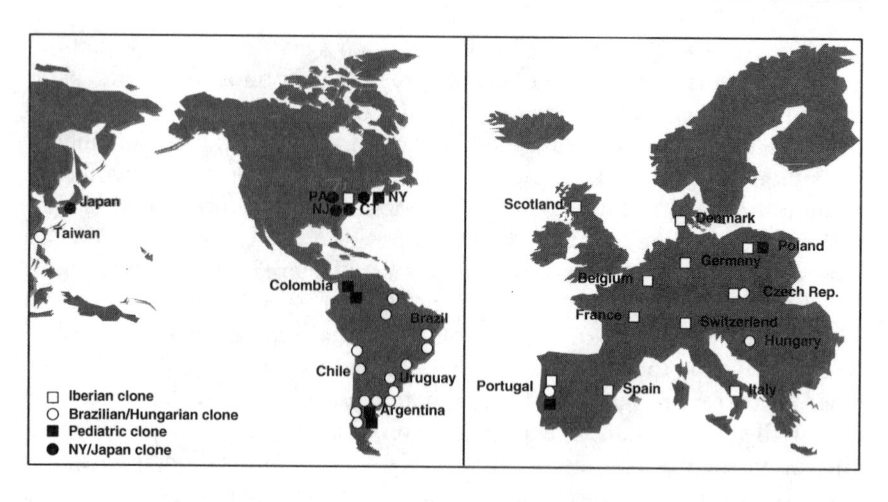

FIGURE 2-2 Geographic spread of pandemic MRSA clones.

Rather, it seems that for resistant staphylococci the ecological reservoir is the hospital itself.

A novel and potentially effective intervention to reduce the spread of resistant forms of these two important pathogens would involve intervention at the level of their ecological reservoirs—namely, lowering the carriage rate of resistant bacteria. The European Community has recently initiated such a major project (EURIS, European Resistance Intervention Study), which is aimed at identifying the most effective intervention strategies by which carriage of resistant pneumococci could be reduced among children attending day care centers in member countries (Sá-Leão et al., 2000). An analogous attempt for MRSA would zero in on the hospital itself by introducing rigorous infection-control measures, such as those that have been successfully tested and advocated by several recent studies (Farr and Jarvis, 2002; Pittet, 2002).

MALARIA AND THE PROBLEM OF CHLOROQUINE RESISTANCE

Thomas E. Wellems, M.D., Ph.D.

Laboratory of Malaria and Vector Research
National Institute of Allergy and Infectious Diseases
National Institutes of Health, Bethesda, MD

The discovery of chloroquine nearly 70 years ago had a considerable impact against the morbidity and mortality of malaria. This impact had such effect that chloroquine became recognized as one of the most successful and important drugs ever deployed against an infectious disease. Massive use of the drug, however, eventually produced resistant malaria strains (Peters, 1989). First reports of chloroquine resistance were with *Plasmodium falciparum*, the species responsible for the most acute and deadly form of human malaria (Payne, 1987). By the 1970s, resistant *P. falciparum* strains were established in South America, India, Southeast Asia, and Papua New Guinea. Africa was spared until the late 1970s, when resistance was detected in Kenya and Tanzania, seeding the spread of resistance across the continent within a decade (Peters, 1987). In the absence of a replacement drug with the low cost and reliability of chloroquine, the morbidity and mortality from malaria resurged in Africa (Greenberg et al., 1989; Trape et al., 1998).

Molecular Basis of Chloroquine Action and Resistance

Chloroquine interrupts hematin detoxification in malaria parasites as they grow within their host red blood cells (Chou et al., 1980) (see Figure 2-3).

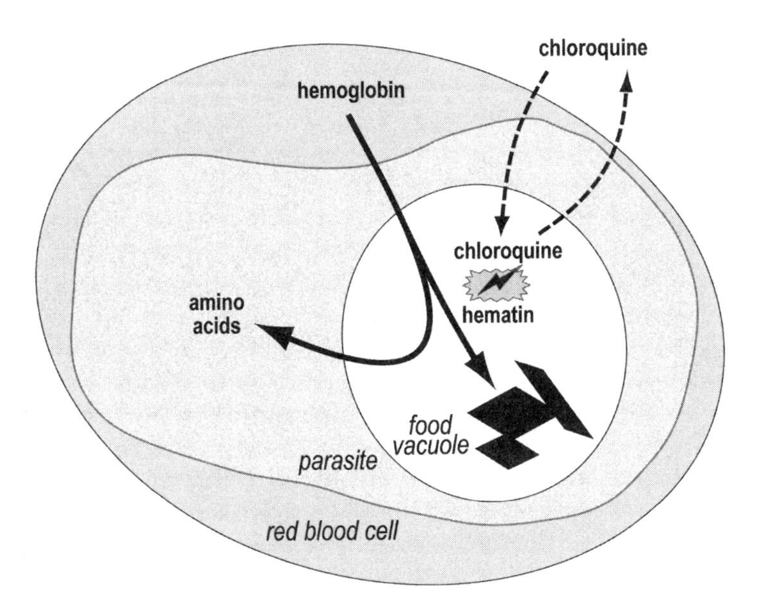

FIGURE 2-3 The pathway of hemoglobin digestion and hematin polymerization in a *P. falciparum*-infected red blood cell. Chloroquine accumulates in the acid digestive food vacuole of sensitive parasites and interferes with polymerization. Chloroquine-resistant parasites reduce this accumulation and thereby reduce drug toxicity.

Hematin, a toxic ferriprotoporphyrin product released from digested host hemoglobin, is normally detoxified in the parasite's acid food vacuole by polymerization into innocuous pigment crystals (Dorn et al., 1998). Chloroquine interferes with polymerization and poisons the parasite by complexing with hematin and adsorbing to the growing faces of the crystals (Sullivan et al., 1996; Pagola et al., 2000).

Chloroquine-resistant *P. falciparum* survives drug exposure by reducing the accumulation of chloroquine in the digestive food vacuole (Verdier et al., 1985). The mechanism of this reduction, not yet established, may involve changes in digestive vacuole pH or a direct effect on drug flux across the digestive vacuole membrane.

Chloroquine resistance results from multiple mutations in PfCRT, a *P. falciparum* protein located at the parasite's digestive vacuole membrane (Fidock et al., 2000). PfCRT contains 10 predicted transmembrane segments and has a structure consistent with a transporter or channel (Nomura et al., 2001) (see Figure 2-4). Although the exact patterns of PfCRT mutations differ according to the geographic origin of chloroquine-resistant parasites, all of these patterns include a key substitution for lysine at position

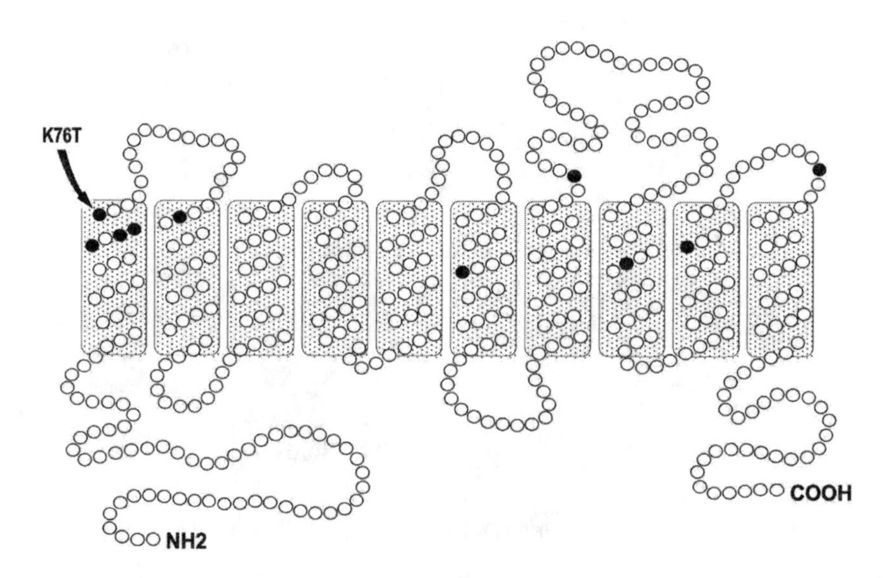

FIGURE 2-4 Schematic representation of PfCRT and positions of mutations associated with chloroquine resistance. The critical K76T mutation occurs in the first of the ten predicted transmembrane domains. Filled circles show the positions of all other PfCRT mutations that have been identified in different chloroquine-resistant isolates. These mutations may compensate for the K76T change or help maintain critical functional properties of the PfCRT molecule in resistant parasites.

76. This substitution is universally K76T in naturally resistant *P. falciparum*. In drug pressure experiments, chloroquine-resistant parasites have been selected that carry alternative K76I and K76N substitutions in PfCRT, but such changes have not been detected outside the laboratory (Cooper et al., 2002). These results suggest that loss of lysine's positive charge at PfCRT position 76 is a central feature of the chloroquine resistance mechanism.

The fact that K76T is always found in the context of additional PfCRT mutations suggests that this key substitution requires accommodative or compensatory adjustments elsewhere in the protein. Different patterns of mutations can evidently serve in these adjustments, as characteristic PfCRT types occur in the Eastern and Western hemispheres (Fidock et al., 2000; Carlton et al., 2001; Wellems and Plowe, 2001). At least four independent foci of chloroquine resistance have been deduced from these PfCRT types: two in South America; one in Southeast Asia that eventually spread to Africa; and one in or near Papua New Guinea with the same substitutions as a South American form. Drug pressure has driven population sweeps of chloroquine-resistant *P. falciparum* from these foci into nearly all malaria regions (Wootton et al., 2002) (see Figure 2-5). An exception in these sweeps is Central America, where *P. falciparum* populations are still sensitive to chloroquine and may be isolated by a genetic or transmission restriction against the entry of resistant strains.

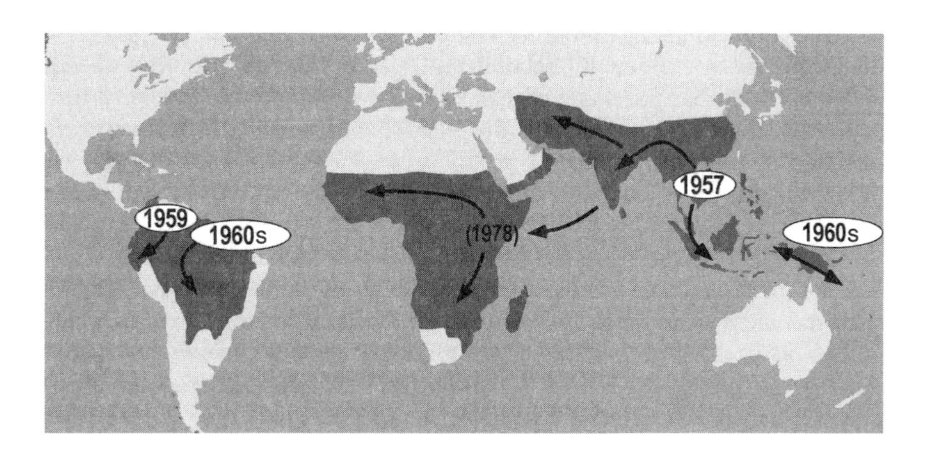

FIGURE 2-5 Map of the spread of chloroquine-resistant *Plasmodium falciparum* from four foci identified by PfCRT alleles and polymorphic markers.

Role of PfCRT Mutations and Malaria Immunity in Chloroquine Treatment Outcomes

Epidemiological investigations have confirmed the association of chloroquine treatment failures with the PfCRT K76T mutation. In a study in Mali, this mutation and other possible markers of resistance were evaluated against chloroquine treatment outcomes in cases of uncomplicated malaria (Djimdé et al., 2001).The PfCRT K76T mutation was found in 100 percent of the chloroquine treatment failures, compared to a baseline prevalence of 41 percent K76T in patients before treatment. However, not all infections with chloroquine-resistant parasites persisted or recurred after chloroquine treatment: 27 percent of patients with these infections showed clinical resolution of symptoms and parasitological clearance. These clearances after drug treatment correlated with age, consistent with an important influence of immunity that develops in children over time from repeated malaria episodes (Djimdé et al., 2001; Wellems and Plowe, 2001).

The association between mutant PfCRT and chloroquine treatment outcomes has also been evaluated in the Cameroon (Basco and Ringwald, 2001), Sudan (Babiker et al., 2001), Mozambique (Mayor et al., 2001), and Papua Indonesia (Maguire et al., 2001), where chloroquine-sensitive and -resistant *P. falciparum* strains both remain common; and in Brazil (Vieira et al., 2001), Uganda (Dorsey et al., 2001a), Laos (Pillai et al., 2001), Thailand, and Papua New Guinea (Chen et al., 2001), where chloroquine-resistant parasites now predominate. Results from these studies support a universal association of the PfCRT K76T mutation with chloroquine treatment failures and show that additional factors including immunity can affect the outcome resistant infections after treatment.

The importance of immunity in treatment outcome has recently been demonstrated in a rodent model of drug-resistant malaria. Results with this model showed that rodents with partial immunity from previous infections benefited from drug treatment and cleared resistant *Plasmodium yoelii* parasites (Cravo et al., 2001).

Other Factors That May Affect Rates of Chloroquine Treatment Failure

The uptake, distribution, and metabolism of chloroquine can have a significant effect on treatment outcomes. Concentrations of chloroquine and its principal monodesethylchloroquine (mono-DEC) metabolite are reported to exhibit inter-individual variations that can influence classifications of resistance in vivo (Hellgren et al., 1989).

Chloroquine resistance lines that have been adapted to in vitro culture conditions frequently show differences in laboratory measures of chloroquine response (as measured by IC_{50} values). The question is often raised whether these in vitro variations might be associated with additional *P. falciparum* determinants that can modulate the effect of PfCRT mutations and increase treatment failure rates. The Pgh-1 P-glycoprotein encoded by the *pfmdr1* gene is a possible example of such a determinant (Cowman et al., 1991). Certain substitutions in Pgh-1 can affect the chloroquine IC_{50}s of parasites resistant (but not sensitive) to chloroquine and are associated with in vitro mefloquine and quinine responses (Reed et al., 2000). Pgh-1 N86Y is a widespread polymorphism in Asia and Africa that has been associated with chloroquine-resistant strains in some studies but not in others (Dorsey et al., 2001b). In Mali, a 50 percent prevalence of Pgh-1 N86Y in patients before treatment rose to 86 percent (17 percent mixed type) in cases of chloroquine failure (Djimdé et al., 2001). However, multivariate analyses of PfCRT K76T and Pgh-1 N86Y showed no independent effect of Pgh-1 N86Y on treatment failure rates and no strengthening of the association of PfCRT K76T with these failure rates. These results indicate that the Pgh-1 N86Y polymorphism does not have an important effect in chloroquine treatment failure but may relate to fitness adaptations in response to physiological changes from PfCRT mutations.

Whether clinical chloroquine resistance might be affected by other Pgh-1 polymorphisms or modulatory determinants elsewhere in the *P. falciparum* genome will require additional epidemiological studies of candidate mutations and case treatment outcomes. Such studies will also help clarify uncertainties about the relative importance of the different factors that modulate in vitro drug responses in the laboratory and factors that affect treatment failure rates in vivo.

Points of Observation and Recommendation

- Tests that rapidly detect the PfCRT K76T molecular marker have several advantages and applications in the surveillance of chloroquine-resistant *P. falciparum*. By making use of PCR-amplified DNA from small blood spots on filter paper, tests that are now available significantly reduce the time, labor, cost, and operative limitations of in vivo or in vitro assays with live parasites. Molecular marker data from large numbers of blood samples can therefore be efficiently collected and used in treatment policy decisions where the prevalence of resistant strains is unknown or changing. Fresh malaria outbreaks or drug-resistant epidemics are important situations that can benefit from such data. PfCRT K76T surveillance may also be useful in regions where chloroquine use has been stopped because of problems with resistance. Such surveillance may detect declining rates of chloroquine resistance, perhaps allowing the reconsideration of chloroquine in combination with other antimalarial drugs.
- The importance of the interface between drug action and immunity

is highlighted by the relief from chloroquine-resistant malaria that immune individuals can often experience after treatment. Chloroquine is therefore still commonly used as a first-choice drug by malaria-experienced individuals in regions of drug resistance, especially where supplies of alternative drugs are expensive and must be targeted to young children and malaria-naive patients who lack protective immunity. An interesting question is whether vaccines will be able to improve therapeutic responses against malaria. Better understanding of the interface between drug action and immunity will help address this possibility.

- New drugs that act on hematin but are not subject to the chloroquine resistance mechanism should be of great benefit. Indeed, certain 4-aminoquinoline compounds with side chain variations, such as short- and long-chain analogs of chloroquine (De et al., 1996; Ridley et al., 1996) and amodiaquine derivatives (Hawley et al., 1996), are known to be effective against chloroquine-resistant parasites. This may be because the chloroquine resistance mechanism is sensitive to the side chain structure of chloroquine while the inhibition of hematin polymerization depends largely on π-π recognition between the 7-chloro-substituted quinoline ring and hematin μ-oxodimers (Vippagunta et al., 1999). Hematin remains attractive as a target because it is a molecule the parasite cannot mutate. The search for new compounds with desirable pharmacokinetic profiles, low toxicity, and low production costs will be helped by improved understanding of the resistance mechanism at the molecular level.

- Chemosensitizing agents that can be co-administered with chloroquine may have promise against chloroquine-resistant *P. falciparum*. Several studies have shown that resistance can be partially reversed by a range of structurally diverse agents that include calcium antagonists such as verapamil, various tricyclic compounds, and some plant alkaloids (Martin et al., 1987; Rasoanaivo et al., 1996). One of these compounds, chlorpheniramine, has been combined with chloroquine and tested in a study of African children (Sowunmi et al., 1997). The combination was suggested to have some benefit against chloroquine-resistant infections but requires further study. Better understanding of the mechanism by which chloroquine-chemosensitizing agents act may provide new leads for drug development.

- *Plasmodium vivax* causes a debilitating form of malaria less fatal than *P. falciparum* but nevertheless still responsible for tremendous impact on the economy and life in afflicted regions. Despite comparable exposure of *P. vivax* and *P. falciparum* to chloroquine pressure, no *P. vivax* strain was reported to be chloroquine-resistant until 1989 (Rieckmann et al., 1989). Resistant *P. vivax* is present today in several regions of Southeast Asia (Baird et al., 1997), and some evidence suggests that it also occurs in South America (Whitby, 1997). Although chloroquine is thought to have the same action on hematin in *P. vivax* and *P. falciparum*, chloroquine resistance in these two major agents of malaria differs in that the homolog of the PfCRT transporter in *P. vivax* does not have reading-frame mutations associated with chloroquine treatment failures (Nomura et al., 2001). Investigations of *P. vivax* determinants responsible for resistance are presently limited by the lack of a practical in vitro culture system and genetic crosses for linkage mapping. These tools of investigation are needed. Advances against chloroquine-resistant malaria, including diagnostics and analogs of chloroquine against the different forms of *P. vivax* and *P. falciparum*, will benefit from basic research in this direction.

DRUG RESISTANCE IN TREATMENT OF SCHISTOSOMIASIS

Charles H. King, M.D., M.S.

Case Western Reserve University School of Medicine and
University Hospitals of Cleveland, Cleveland, OH

The Worm Challenge

The helminthic parasites, commonly referred to as "worms," are among the most common of human infections. Worldwide, over 1 billion people are infected with *Ascaris* roundworms, 1.2 billion carry hookworm, and an estimated 200 million people are infected with blood flukes of *Schistosoma* spp. (WHO, 1993; Chan, 1997). Although worm infections are rarely lethal, they produce a significant spectrum of disease and disability, ranging from moderate exercise intolerance up to severe anemia and organ damage, with the resulting loss of millions of productive life-years globally (de Silva et al., 1997). Poor sanitation favors the simultaneous transmission of many parasites, and it is common for one person to harbor infection with multiple worms of many different helminth species. What is more, even after successful treatment, symptomatic, high-level worm infection may return in as few as three to six months after cure.

The 1970s and 1980s saw the development of a number of safe and effective oral anthelmintics including mebendazole, albendazole, ivermectin, and praziquantel. Together, these broad-spectrum agents proved capable of giving effective treatment for almost any human helminth infection. The economics of treating human worms were not favorable, however. The limited resources of the developing countries, where worms are endemic, coupled with the significant overhead required to provide repeated drug therapy, severely limited the fundamental demand for these drugs. Although wide-scale, population-based programs were recommended by the WHO as the best means of controlling helminth-related diseases, in practice, many health ministries chose to focus on other priorities.

With the initially limited use of anthelmintics, serious drug resistance was not observed and was not thought to be a problem. An unfortunate consequence of the drugs' initial success, combined with their limited use, was the disinclination of pharmaceutical researchers to pursue additional, new classes of anthelmintic drugs for human use. Both antiparasitic drug use and the roster of available anthelmintic drugs remained stable until the 1990s, when national and international programs began to provide widespread treatment for onchocerciasis and lymphatic filariasis. Newer programs, now being implemented, aim to provide widespread "deworming" of children at risk (Partnership for Child Development, 1997). These, too, will greatly expand the human use of anthelmintic drugs, raising the concern that resistance to anthelmintics will soon be with us.

Common Threads of Drug Resistance in Helminths and Bacteria

In a sense, anti-parasite drug treatment poses many of the same challenges found in treating multiply-resistant bacterial infections:

1. A single, often expensive agent is used for almost all therapy;
2. Older, alternative drugs are being dropped from production;
3. With limited market potential, new drug development is not perceived as a priority;
4. Pathogen isolates with intermediate-level drug resistance are beginning to be found in heavily treated areas.

As a result, clinically significant resistance to our best anthelmintics is expected to occur in the near future (Brindley, 1994).

Unique Features of Drug Resistance in Helminths: The Schistosomiasis Experience

How does the problem of drug resistance differ for helminthic infections? In practical terms, anthelmintic resistance is difficult to detect, because we have no easy means of performing in vitro culture and sensitivity testing for worms. Early, low-level resistance will be difficult to detect, after which the typically rapid shift from 10 percent to 90 percent resistance will come as a surprise to many practitioners.

In parasitic infections such as schistosomiasis, treatment does not have to be fully curative to control disease—the antischistosomal drug praziquantel is accepted as "highly effective" even though it is never 100 percent effective in eliminating infection (King and Mahmoud, 1989). Its therapeutic effect is obtained because, in schistosomiasis, unlike bacterial, viral, or even malarial infection, the pathogen does not reproduce within the human body (King, 2001). With substantial *suppression* of infection, the net result is effective prevention of disease (Warren, 1982).

Complicating the search for praziquantel resistance, the clinical efficacy of praziquantel therapy varies spontaneously from person to person. Host immune responses are essential to the anti-schistosomal effect of the drug, and their effectiveness appears to vary from strain to strain and from person to person. Further, not all stages of the schistosome parasite are drug-sensitive (Cioli, 1998)—if a person is infected with both the praziquantel-sensitive adult worm stages and with praziquantel-insensitive immature worms (schistosomula), examination three months after treatment may show a "persistently" positive egg count, suggesting drug failure. In fact, the eggs detected at three months post-treatment are likely to be due to the maturation and mating of these initially insensitive immature forms, which are now grown to adulthood and are fully susceptible to praziquantel retreatment (Gryseels et al., 2001).

In contemplating the phenomenon of bacterial drug resistance, the functional ecosystem for the emerging resistant strain is the individual human body. Although there is potential for spread to other humans, the foremost factor in the survival of a resistant bacterium is its success within the treated human host. By contrast, schistosomes divide their life cycle between free-living forms (miracidia, cercariae), a form parasitic for snails (sporocysts), and the forms parasitic for humans (schistosomula larvae and adult schistosomes) (Sturrock, 2001). The transmission of schistosomiasis is integrally linked both to environmental factors and to human susceptibility factors (King, 2001). For schistosomes, reproductive success depends on many more external environmental factors, and the emergence or persistence of resistant strains requires relative success in all aspects of its life cycle.

There is an uneven distribution of worm burden across infected human populations (King et al., 2000). Even in a highly endemic area, most people harbor light infections, while a small minority (5–10 percent) harbor very heavy worm burdens. For schistosomes, reproduction requires obligate sexual mating. The clustering of parasite distribution means that worm mating tends to be nonrandom. This phenomenon, combined with a long generation time (6–12 months), undoubtedly results in the slowing of the spread of resistance traits in schistosomiasis.

Experience with Drug Resistance in Schistosomiasis

Hycanthone

In the 1970s and early 1980s, the drug hycanthone was used as population-based treatment for *Schistosoma mansoni.* Lab studies in animals indicated 10–20 percent of worms survived therapy, and it was found that the progeny of these survivors were resistant to hycanthone (Cioli and Pica Mattoccia, 1984). Further study indicated that the resistance trait was heritable, autosomal recessive, inducible by drug exposure, and not intrinsic (Brindley, 1994). Hycanthone was ultimately withdrawn for safety reasons before resistance became a clinically significant issue, but concern remained over the relative ease with which resistance occurred.

Concern About Praziquantel

Over the last several years, reports have begun to emerge of evident praziquantel "failures" in treating schistosomiasis mansoni. Given the baseline variability in praziquantel cure rates, as described above, there was considerable debate about the implications of these reported failures. In a new focus in Senegal, reports of very low cure rates (<40 percent) in large-scale treatment of *S. mansoni* raised concerns about declining drug efficacy (Cioli, 1998; Gryseels et al., 2001). Eventually, the apparently poor response to praziquantel at this site was found to be due to ongoing heavy reinfection, but the event elicited international concern and prompted the European Community to found a concerted action network on "Patterns of praziquantel usage and monitoring of possible resistance in Africa" to periodically review the issue (Renganathan and Cioli, 1998).

Laboratory studies have identified tolerant and relatively resistant *S. mansoni* strains from clinical isolates. Some *S. mansoni* strains taken from Egyptian subjects who failed multiple courses of praziquantel therapy demonstrated moderate- to high-level resistance to praziquantel therapy (William et al., 2001). Of note, this resistance phenotype is sometimes lost in later generations after serial passaging in mice. It was noted that tolerant strains are less fecund, releasing fewer eggs per adult worm pair (Fallon et al., 1997). Reports also indicate that at the life cycle stage of asexual multiplication, which occurs in the intermediate snail host, tolerant strains produce fewer of the cercarial forms that are infectious for humans (William et al., 2001). Although these studies suggest that low-level praziquantel resistance is already present in the field environment, they also indicate that tolerant strains are less fit to compete with drug-sensitive schistosomes. To date, such resistance is very uncommon, and does not affect the continuing recommendation that praziquantel be used in mass treatment programs for schistosomiasis (Bennett et al., 1997).

Is this tolerance universal? Review of our own long-term (eight-year) experience in treating urinary schistosomiasis due to *S. haematobium* in Kenya does not show a similar pattern (King et al., 2000). Although there is year-to-year variation in cure rates, there have been no treated participants who have failed to eliminate their infection after repeated praziquantel therapy. Furthermore, children who became reinfected after the start of the treatment program had the same curative response to praziquantel as children who were treated for the first time.

In order to address the reasons why resistance was not observed, we turned to mathematical modeling of resistance transmission, using a dynamic model in which the features of parasite clustering and sexual reproduction could be incorporated. Our modeling analysis indicated that there were several features of the parasite/drug treatment ecology that were likely to explain the absence, so far, of any clinically apparent resistance. First, there was incomplete exposure of the parasite population to the drug—our school-based program left adult age groups untreated so that 25–50 percent of worms went unexposed, creating a "refuge" for sensitive worm genes (Van Wyk, 2001); second, emergence of clinically detectable resistance was estimated to require 7 to 10 generations, and, given the 6- to 12-month generation time for *S. haematobium*, there was probably not sufficient time for this to occur; third, if the resistance trait is recessive or polygenic, sexual reproduction was predicted to slow its emergence by several generations; and fourth, crowding effects on fecundity in heavily infected humans was likely to delay the transmission of resistance genes as well. Most important, reduced reproductive fitness of the resistant strains was seen to substantially delay the arrival of clinically significant levels of drug resistance (King et al., 2000).

Conclusions Based on Field Experience and Modeling Analysis

Praziquantel resistance is not yet a clinical reality, but it is expected to emerge within the next 10 years (King et al., 2000). Resistance becomes more likely as drug usage becomes more widespread (Bennett et al., 1997; Van Wyk, 2001). Praziquantel's pivotal role in schistosomiasis therapy means that we must find means to extend its useful life span. In addition, drugs must be developed to replace praziquantel when praziquantel resistance begins to dominate at the clinical level (Doenhoff et al., 2000).

For now, praziquantel's effectiveness can be prolonged by more selective use, with treatment targeted only to those patients at greatest risk for heavy infection and morbidity. Resistance can also be delayed by the use of integrated disease management techniques, including snail control, water development, health education, sanitation, alternative drug use, and, possibly, by the development of effective vaccination strategies.

Immediate Needs

Loss of praziquantel effectiveness could become an operational catastrophe for schistosomiasis control programs. For now, there are several immediate needs that must be addressed. The new wave of inexpensive generic formulations needs to be monitored for potency and for quality, so that subtherapeutic praziquantel dosing does not become the norm (Doenhoff et al., 2000). Operational research programs should be implemented, employing effective sampling techniques for field monitoring in order to detect and quickly report treatment failures. Desktop decision tools are needed to optimize the impact of treatment programs, and backup plans are needed for production of the WHO-designated "essential drugs," oxamniquine and metrifonate, when praziquantel effectiveness declines significantly. Finally, new drug development needs to continue in anticipation of the eventual failure of praziquantel efficacy.

In summary, it is now essential that, as national and international control programs become a reality, the value of praziquantel is not prematurely lost. Prudent use will extend the usefulness of this very safe and effective drug. However, such measures will only delay and not prevent the eventual emergence of drug resistance. It is imperative that public health planners and health providers anticipate the emergence of praziquantel resistance, and the final need for alternative agents.

BACTERIAL INFECTION IN IRRADIATED MICE: THERAPY AND PROPHYLAXIS (ANTHRAX, A SPECIAL CONSIDERATION)[1]

Thomas B. Elliott, Ph.D.[2]

Armed Forces Radiobiology Research Institute, Bethesda, MD

Military personnel will be exposed to common infectious agents and may be exposed to biological weapons and ionizing radiation. Ionizing radiation depresses hemopoiesis in bone marrow and compromises innate and acquired immune responses. Neutropenia and thrombocytopenia contribute to the reduced innate responses. Consequently, concurrent infection and sublethal irradiation are synergistic (Elliott et al., 1990).

The number of leukocytes and thrombocytes in blood of mice given 6.5 Gy ^{60}Co gamma photons is shown *versus* time in days after irradiation in Figure 2-6 (Elliott et al., 1990). The leukocytes decline rapidly to almost

[1]For additional data and analysis on the findings of this research, see Brook et al., 2001a.

[2]Studies of this nature are complex and require the cooperation of many persons. Contributors to studies of post-irradiation infections during the past several years include: GD Ledney, I Brook, GS Madonna, RA Harding, WE Jackson, III, GB Knudson, MO Shoemaker, SS Bouhaouala, RE Ruiz, J Deen, CE Inal, S Leppla, J Rogers, SJ Peacock, YA Golubeva, BT Gnade, JH Thakar, AFRRI ^{60}Co Radiation Staff, Veterinary Staff, and Graphics Staff.

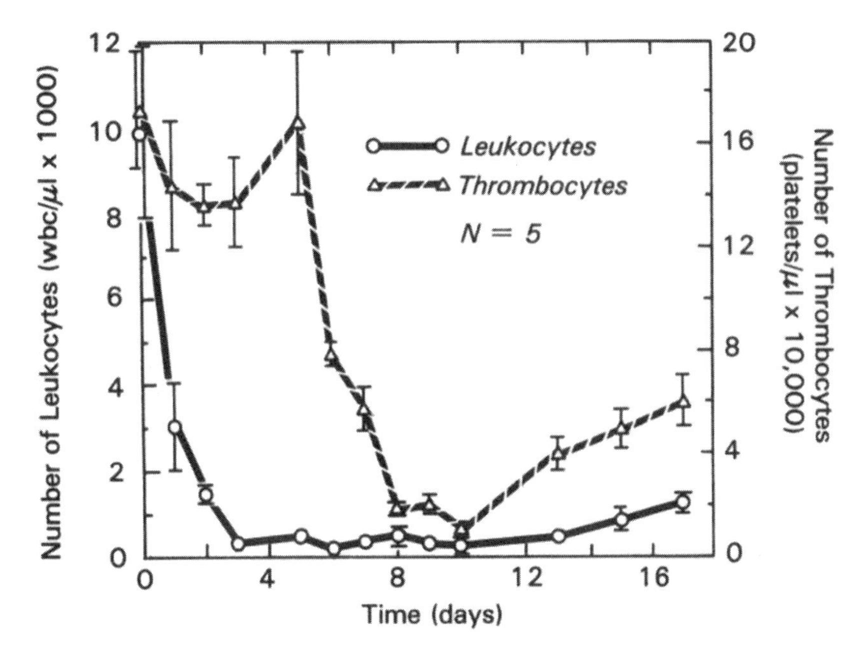

FIGURE 2-6 The number of leukocytes and thrombocytes in blood of B6D2F_1/J female mice given 6.5 Gy ^{60}Co gamma photons is shown *versus* time in days after irradiation. SOURCE: Elliott et al., 1990.

undetectable concentration by Day 3. They remain low for almost two weeks, when they begin a gradual recovery. The thrombocytes remain stable for approximately 5 days, and then decline to a low concentration between 8–10 days and then begin to recover.

The gastrointestinal mucous layer is reduced within 3 days in gamma-photon-irradiated mice. The resident enteric microflora change and, thereby, resistance to colonization with exogenous bacteria is reduced. As shown in Figure 2-7, the indigenous microflora decline from 10^{10-12} CFU/g to 10^{4-6} CFU/g within 4 days (Brook et al., 1988). Whereas the anaerobic bacteria (primarily *Bacteroides* species) remain low for over two weeks following irradiation, facultative bacteria, primarily the *Enterobacteriaceae*, in the ileum recover to 10^9 CFU/g by Day 12. Bacteria translocate from intestines 5–8 days after lethal doses of gamma radiation.

We developed animal models of infection following irradiation to evaluate efficacy of therapeutic agents against endogenous and exogenous infections following sublethal and lethal doses of ionizing radiation (Brook et al., 1999). In particular, we developed a model to assess susceptibility of irradiated mice to a biological warfare (BW) agent, *Bacillus anthracis* spores,

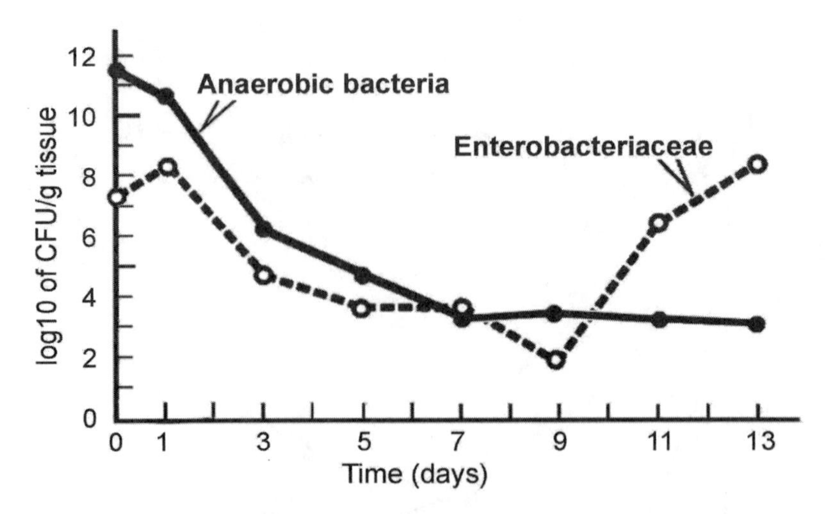

FIGURE 2-7 Indigenous intestinal microflora decline from $10^{10\text{-}12}$ CFU/g to $10^{4\text{-}6}$ CFU/g within 4 days in irradiated mice. SOURCE: Brook et al., 1988.

which were inoculated intratracheally in a measured dose to simulate inhalation of an aerosol (Brook et al., 2001a).

There are several reasons for performing these studies in an animal model. We need to limit and control the variable factors. Animal models offer a compromise between clinical reality and experimental simplicity. They include the complex pathophysiological and immunological interactions and features of infectious disease, which cannot be mimicked together in vitro. We use whole-body, acute doses to simulate real worst-case military scenarios, whereas whole-body, acute doses are not commonly used in human medicine. In oncology, radiation therapy is focused and partial-body. For transplantations, irradiation is whole-body, but fractionated by giving one-tenth of the total dose per session, and almost always (90–95 percent of cases) chemotherapy is provided during the intervals between radiation sessions in order to ablate the bone marrow.

Microbiology of *B. anthracis*-Induced Polymicrobial Sepsis

The experimental design for collecting scheduled microbiological specimens from sublethally irradiated mice that were challenged with intratracheal *B. anthracis* Sterne spores, is shown in Figure 2-8. Following irradiation and spore challenge, we collected tissues aseptically from five mice per treatment group, which were euthanized at scheduled times after spore challenge. We cultured homogenized lung and spleen as well as blood.

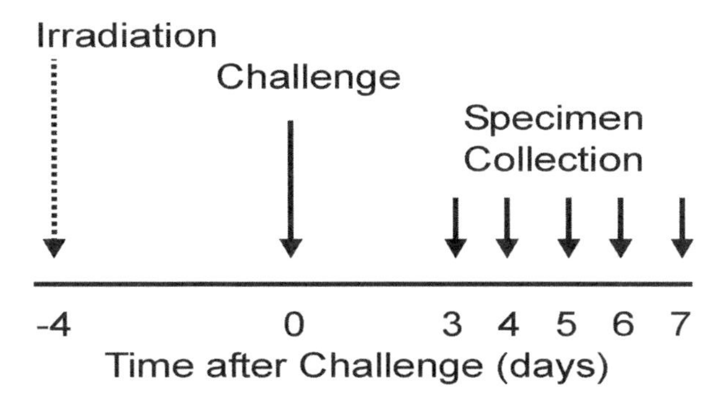

FIGURE 2-8 The experimental design for collecting scheduled microbiological specimens from irradiated and challenged mice.

When we gave mice only a 0-, 3-, 5-, or 7-Gy dose of gamma photons, no bacteria were isolated from tissues. When we gave mice only a dose of *B. anthracis* Sterne spores, we only isolated *B. anthracis* from tissues. But when we gave mice a dose of spores four days after irradiation, we isolated not only *B. anthracis*, but several other bacterial species as well (e.g., *Enterococcus faecalis, Erysipelothrix rhusiopathiae, Staphylococcus* sp., *Acinetobacter lwoffi, Enterobacter cloacae, Klebsiella pneumoniae,* and *Escherichia coli*)—as many as three species in a single animal—which caused a polymicrobial sepsis. This is a unique finding in sublethally irradiated mice, in our experience, which complicates successful antimicrobial therapy for anthrax following irradiation (Brook et al., 2001a).

To summarize the susceptibility of irradiated mice to infectious agents, ionizing radiation impairs innate immune responses, decreases colonization resistance of endogenous bacteria, and reduces the threshold of sepsis caused by exogenous bacteria.

Following lethal doses, ionizing radiation induces translocation of endogenous bacteria from intestines to the bloodstream. Furthermore, combined sublethal radiation and *Bacillus anthracis* spores decrease the threshold for translocation of intestinal bacteria and the consequent bacteremia. Animals develop a polymicrobial infection caused by exogenous *B. anthracis* together with endogenous enteric gram-positive and gram-negative bacteria. This is a unique finding.

Antimicrobial Therapy for Sepsis After Irradiation

The successful management of post-irradiation sepsis is a difficult challenge (Brook et al., 1988; Brook and Elliott, 1991). Antimicrobial agents together with basic clinical support are fundamental. Quinolones have been recommended for preventing sepsis by selective decontamination of the intestinal tract. Although anti-gram-positive antibiotics could be used to supplement other antimicrobial agents, it is imperative that the anaerobic microflora in the intestine not be suppressed because ionizing irradiation reduces them by several logarithms and they are required to provide colonization resistance.

Selected non-specific biological response modifiers (BRMs), which enhance innate immunity by inducing cytokines naturally, or specific BRMs, such as cytokines, could augment specific antimicrobial agents, but this combined approach to therapy following irradiation remains essentially experimental (Peterson et al., 1994). Probiotics, such as specific strains of *Lactobacillus*, might also offer an advantage by enhancing colonization resistance and restoring the intestinal microflora.

Factors that influence therapy for post-irradiation infection include: (i) reduced innate immune responses, particularly the decreased number of phagocytic cells; (ii) the pathogenesis of microorganisms; (iii) coverage by selected bactericidal (not bacteriostatic) antimicrobial agents, which cover facultative gram-positive and gram-negative (but not anaerobic) bacteria; (iv) the half-life of the selected antimicrobial agent (which in turn determines the dose schedule); (v) the route of administration (oral is optimal following irradiation, especially for large numbers of casualties); and (vi) the starting time and duration of antimicrobial therapy.

The general principles of pharmacokinetics and pharmacodynamics must be considered as well. Figure 2-9 shows the concept that the concentrations of the selected antimicrobial agents must remain above the threshold minimum bactericidal concentration to achieve successful therapy after irradiation because of the absence of an effective innate response and to maintain as high an area under the curve divided by the MBC (AUBC) as practical. That is, in principle, the higher the AUBC, the greater the cidal effect against the bacteria.

Selection of an effective antimicrobial chemotherapeutic regimen also depends upon (i) the cidal mechanisms of action of the selected agents, whether by inhibiting formation of cell wall, interrupting cell membrane function, interfering with DNA function or replication, inhibiting protein synthesis, or antagonizing metabolism, and (ii) microbial drug resistance of bacteria, whether by selection of a pre-existing genetic ability in a population or by mutation, which changes the genetic ability of the microorganism. For antimicrobial therapy for sepsis after irradiation, second-generation quinolones, either ciprofloxacin or levofloxacin, are recommended as the first choice, third- or fourth-generation cephalosporins, either ceftriaxone (third-generation) or cefepime (fourth-generation) as a second choice, or aminoglycosides, either gentamicin or amikacin, as a third choice,

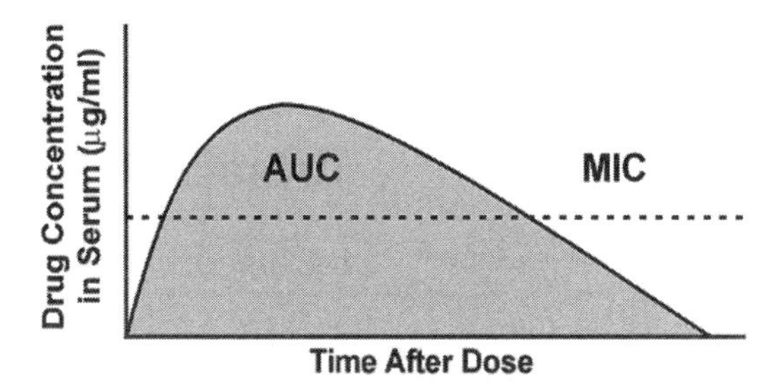

AUC = area under the curve
MIC = minimum inhibitory concentration
MBC = minimum bactericidal concentration

AUC/MIC = AUIC
AUC/MBC = AUBC

FIGURE 2-9 Concept of the relationship between pharmacokinetic factors, minimum inhibitory concentration (or minimum bactericidal concentration) of an antimicrobial agent and the area under the curve *versus* time after administration of the drug.

with or without amoxicillin or vancomycin as an adjunct, for a duration of 21 days (Brook and Ledney, 1992).

Experimental Antimicrobial Therapy for *B. anthracis* Sterne-Induced Polymicrobial Sepsis After Irradiation

The currently recommended treatment for anthrax for up to 60 days is the quinolone, ciprofloxacin i.v., penicillin G i.v., or the tetracycline, doxycycline i.v. (Dixon et al., 1999; Inglesby et al., 1999). Figure 2-10 depicts our experimental design for evaluating antimicrobial therapeutic agents against *B. anthracis* Sterne infection in sublethally irradiated (7 Gy) B6D2F_1/J female mice. Antimicrobial agents were given for 7, 14, or 21 days after intratracheal spore challenge (Elliott et al., 2002).

To determine the effect of starting time of therapy on survival, irradiated mice, 12 per group, were given 7.8×10^8 CFU *B. anthracis* Sterne spores i.t. Penicillin G, 62.5 mg i.m., was started 6, 24, or 48 hours after spore challenge and continued for 7 days through day 11. Survival was prolonged when penicillin was started 6 or 24 hours after challenge, but when penicillin G therapy was delayed for 48 hours, survival was essentially the same as the control (Elliott et al., 2002).

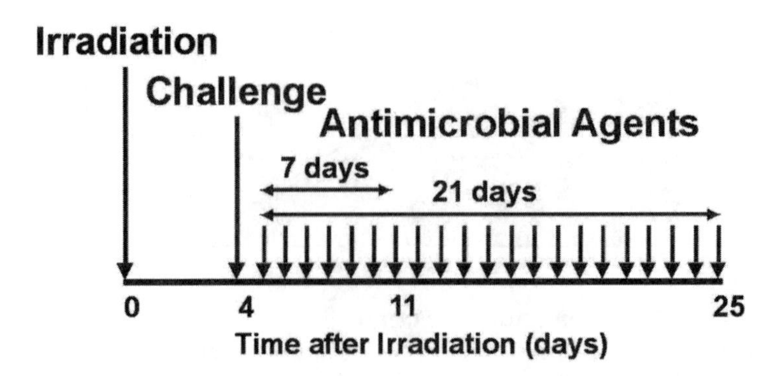

FIGURE 2-10 An experimental design for evaluating antimicrobial therapeutic agents against *B. anthracis* Sterne infection in sublethally irradiated (7 Gy) B6D2F_1/J female mice. SOURCE: Elliott et al., 2002.

To compare survival following therapy with penicillin and the two quinolones, ofloxacin and trovafloxacin, irradiated mice, 19 or 20 per group, were given 4.1×10^8 CFU *B. anthracis* Sterne spores i.t. The quinolone ofloxacin, 40 mg/kg p.o., and penicillin G, 125 mg i.m., were given either separately or in combination, and the quinolone, trovafloxacin, 20 mg/kg, was given either s.c. or p.o. Administration of the agents was started 24 hours after i.t. spore challenge. No control mice survived. Survival was 20 and 25 percent in mice given ofloxacin or penicillin G separately. When these two agents were combined, survival was increased to 55 percent. Survival in mice that were given trovafloxacin p.o. or s.c. was 95 and 100 percent, respectively (Elliott et al., 2002).

To evaluate efficacy of macrolides against *B. anthracis* infection, irradiated mice, 20 per group, were given 1.8×10^8 CFU *B. anthracis* Sterne spores i.t. Mice were given doses of macrolides s.c. or p.o., which were based on allometric scaling to 10 times the equivalent doses in humans, starting 24 hours after i.t. spore challenge for 14 days through day 18. Sterile water was given either s.c. or p.o. to control groups of mice. Azithromycin (AZM, 50 mg/kg) was given either s.c. or p.o. Clarithromycin (CLR, 150 mg/kg) and erythromycin (ERY, 500 mg/kg) were given only p.o., and the quinolone, trovafloxacin (TVA, 20 mg/kg) was given p.o. for comparison with previous results and as a sort of "positive" control. Only one of 40 water-treated control mice survived. Few mice that were given the macrolides survived (between 0 and 15 percent). Survival was 80 percent in mice given trovafloxacin for comparison. The macrolides may be ineffective because they tend to accumulate in tissues and, so, concentrations in serum are low (Elliott et al., 2002).

Antimicrobial Resistance in *B. anthracis* Sterne in Vitro

We have not observed a change in antimicrobial susceptibility in *B. anthracis* Sterne against penicillin G, ciprofloxacin, levofloxacin, and vancomycin during the course of 21 days of antimicrobial therapy. However, we evaluated the potential for *B. anthracis* Sterne to develop antimicrobial resistance in vitro by passing growth of the bacteria sequentially in minimally inhibiting concentrations of quinolones and doxycycline. Each drug was diluted two-fold as depicted in Figure 2-11. A 0.1-ml amount of a suspension of bacteria, which contained approximately 2.0×10^7 CFU *B. anthracis* Sterne, was added to each tube in the series and allowed to incubate at 35°C. The MIC was determined by visual observation of microbial growth at 24 and 48 hours.

The highest subinhibitory concentration of each antimicrobial agent in which microbial growth was observed was then used as the inoculum for the next series of dilutions. This macrodilution method (Davies et al., 1999) was performed in duplicate with each antimicrobial agent for 21 serial passages to simulate 21 days of therapy.

The graph in Figure 2-12 shows the results from the evaluation with alatrofloxacin, a prodrug of trovafloxacin. The MIC began to increase four times or greater than the initial MIC by the ninth passage. So, it appears that a subpopulation of *B. anthracis* Sterne possesses the propensity to develop resistance against alatrofloxacin in vitro. Results with ciprofloxacin,

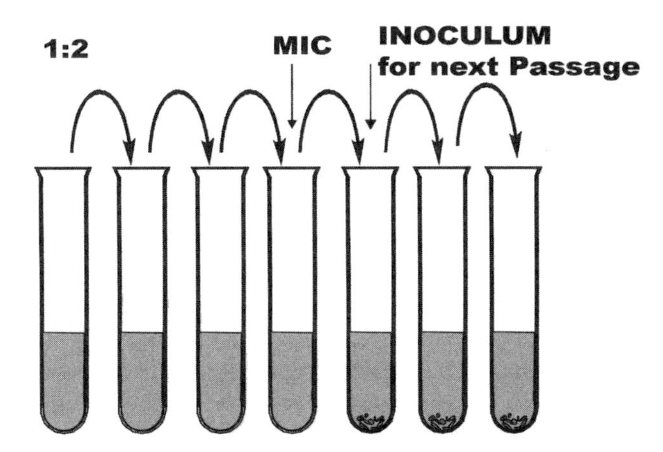

FIGURE 2-11 Two-fold macrodilution of an antimicrobial agent in vitro to determine minimum inhibitory concentration (MIC) of the drug against a strain of bacteria.

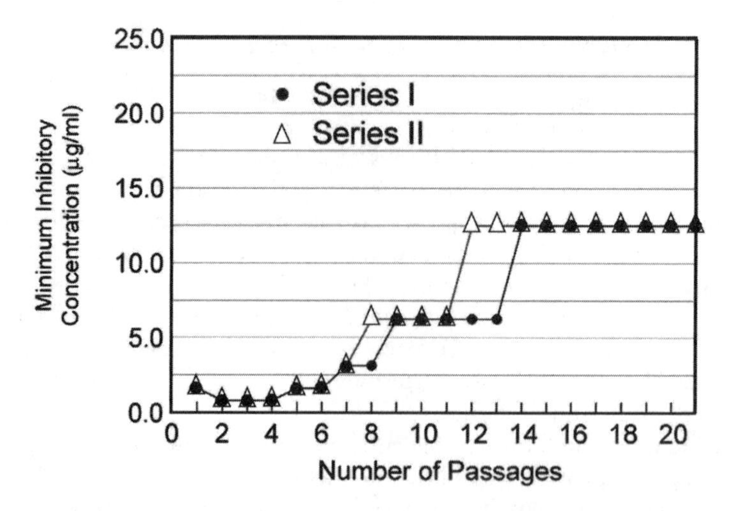

FIGURE 2-12 Change in minimum inhibitory concentration of alatrofloxacin against *Bacillus anthracis* Sterne in brain heart infusion during the course of 21 serial passages of the microorganism performed in duplicate. SOURCE: Elliott, unpublished data; Brook et al., 2001b.

gatifloxacin, and ofloxacin were similar but we observed only a minimal increase of the MIC for doxycycline. Cross-susceptibility was also determined with the cultures from the twenty-first passage among the quinolones. All substrain isolates that were grown in the presence of one quinolone were also resistant to the other quinolones (Brook et al., 2001b).

Antimicrobial agents alone are not likely to resolve infection by *B. anthracis*, particularly following irradiation, because pathogenesis and death from *B. anthracis* is mediated by lethal and edema toxins together with a polymicrobial sepsis. Therefore, once the toxins are formed, antimicrobial agents alone are not adequate to prevent mortality. By extending the general approach to treating sepsis following irradiation, successful management of anthrax following irradiation will include the following elements discussed below.

New quinolones are effective against both *B. anthracis* and endogenous bacteria. Agents with a wide spectrum of activity and high concentration in serum are more effective than agents with limited spectrum (e.g., penicillin and early quinolones) or low serum concentration (e.g., macrolides). *Bacillus anthracis* could develop antimicrobial resistance with prolonged therapy. Vaccination early during therapy or injection of anti-serum could be a valuable adjunct to inactivate lethal and edema toxins. The standard, initial vaccination requires three injections two weeks apart. Horse anti-serum was used during the treatment of victims of the release of virulent *B.*

anthracis spores in Sverdlovsk, USSR, in 1979, but the patients died, so anti-serum seems to have limited value (Abramova et al., 1993).

Summary

We demonstrated (i) that low-level, acute radiation combined with endemic and BW agents, *B. anthracis* in particular, increases mortality synergistically; (ii) improved, effective therapy, that is, recent quinolones, to control *mixed, polymicrobial infection* with intestinal bacteria, which is induced by *B. anthracis* spore challenge after irradiation; and (iii) development of antimicrobial resistance in vitro in *B. anthracis* Sterne.

REFERENCES

Abramova FA, Grinberg LM, Yampolskaya OV, Walker DH. 1993. Pathology of inhalational anthrax in 42 cases from the Sverdlovsk outbreak of 1979. *Proceedings of the National Academy of Sciences* 90:2291–2294.

Babiker HA, Pringle SJ, Abdel-Muhsin A, Mackinnon M, Hunt P, Walliker D. 2001. High-level chloroquine resistance in Sudanese isolates of *Plasmodium falciparum* is associated with mutations in the chloroquine resistance transporter gene *pfcrt* and the multi-drug resistance gene *pfmdr1*. *Journal of Infectious Diseases* 183:1535–1538.

Baird JK, Leksana B, Masbar S, Fryauff DJ, Sutanihardja MA, Suradi, Wignall FS, Hoffman SL. 1997. Diagnosis of resistance to chloroquine by *Plasmodium vivax*: timing of recurrence and whole blood chloroquine levels. *American Journal of Tropical Medicine and Hygiene* 56:621–626.

Basco LK and Ringwald P. 2001. Analysis of the key *pfcrt* point mutation and in vitro and in vivo response to chloroquine in Yaoundé, Cameroon. *Journal of Infectious Diseases* 183:1828–1831.

Bennett JL, Day T, Liang FT, Ismail M, Farghaly A. 1997. The development of resistance to anthelmintics: A perspective with an emphasis on the antischistosomal drug praziquantel. *Experimental Parasitology* 87:260–267.

Brindley PJ. 1994. Drug resistance to schistosomicides and other anthelmintics of medical significance. *Acta Tropica* 56:213–231.

Brook I and Elliott TB. 1991. Quinolone therapy in the prevention of mortality after irradiation. *Radiation Research* 128:100–103.

Brook I and Ledney GD. 1992. Quinolone therapy in the management of infection after irradiation. *Critical Reviews in Microbiology* 18:235–246.

Brook I, Elliott TB, Harding RA, Bouhaouala SS, Peacock SJ, Ledney GD, Knudson GB. 2001a. Susceptibility of irradiated mice to *Bacillus anthracis* Sterne by the intratracheal route of infection. *Journal of Medical Microbiology* 50:702–711.

Brook I, Elliott TB, Ledney GD. 1999. Infection after ionizing irradiation. In Zak O, Sande MA, eds. *Handbook of Animal Models of Infection: Experimental Models in Antimicrobial Chemotherapy*. San Diego: Academic Press. Pp. 151–161.

Brook I, Elliott TB, Pryor HI 2nd, Sautter TE, Gnade BT, Thakar JH, Knudson GB. 2001b. In vitro resistance of *Bacillus anthracis* Sterne to doxycycline, macrolides, and quinolones. *International Journal of Antimicrobial Agents* 18:559–562.

Brook I, Walker RI, MacVittie TJ. 1988. Effect of antimicrobial therapy on bowel flora and bacterial infection in irradiated mice. *International Journal of Radiation Biology* 53:709–716.

Carlton JM, Fidock DA, Djimdé A, Plowe CV, Wellems TE. 2001. Conservation of a novel vacuolar transporter in *Plasmodium* species and its central role in chloroquine resistance of *P. falciparum*. *Current Opinion in Microbiology* 4:415–420.

Chan MS. 1997. The global burden of intestinal nematode infections: 50 years on. *Parasitology Today* 13:438–443.

Chen N, Russell B, Staley J, Kotecka B, Nasveld P, Cheng Q. 2001. Sequence polymorphisms in *pfcrt* are strongly associated with chloroquine resistance in *Plasmodium falciparum*. *Journal of Infectious Diseases* 183:1543–1545.

Chou AC, Chevli R, Fitch CD. 1980. Ferriprotoporphyrin IX fulfills the criteria for identification as the chloroquine receptor of malaria parasites. *Biochemistry* 19:1543–1549.

Cioli D. 1998. Chemotherapy of schistosomiasis: an update. *Parasitology Today* 14:418–422.

Cioli D and Pica Mattoccia L. 1984. Genetic analysis of hycanthone resistance in *Schistosoma mansoni*. *American Journal of Tropical Medicine and Hygiene* 33:80–88.

Cooper RA, Ferdig MT, Su X, Ursos LM, Mu J, Nomura T, Fujioka H, Fidock DA, Roepe PD, Wellems TE. 2002. Alternative mutations at position 76 of the vacuolar transmembrane protein PfCRT are associated with chloroquine resistance and unique stereospecific quinine and quinidine responses in *Plasmodium falciparum*. *Molecular Pharmacology* 61:35–42.

Cowman AF, Karcz S, Galatis D, Culvenor JG. 1991. A P-glycoprotein homologue of *Plasmodium falciparum* is localized on the digestive vacuole. *Journal of Cell Biology* 113:1033–1042.

Cravo P, Culleton R, Hunt P, Walliker D, Mackinnon MJ. 2001. Antimalarial drugs clear resistant parasites from partially immune hosts. *Antimicrobial Agents and Chemotherapy* 45:2897–2901.

Davies TA, Pankuch GA, Dewasse BE, Jacobs MR, Applebaum PC. 1999. In vitro development of resistance to five quinolones and amoxicillin-clavulanate in *Streptococcus pneumoniae*. *Antimicrobial Agents and Chemotherapy* 43:1177–1182.

De D, Krogstad FM, Cogswell FB, Krogstad DJ. 1996. Aminoquinolines that circumvent resistance in *Plasmodium falciparum* in vitro. *American Journal of Tropical Medicine and Hygiene* 55:579–583.

de Lencastre H, Wu SW, Pinho MG, Ludovice AM, Filipe SR, Gardete S, Sobral R, Gill S, Chung M, Tomasz A. 1999. Antibiotic resistance as a stress response: complete sequence of a large number of chromosomal loci in *Staphylococcus aureus* strain COL that impact on the expression of resistance to methicillin. *Microbial Drug Resistance* 5:163–175.

de Silva NR, Chan MS, Bundy DA. 1997. Morbidity and mortality due to ascariasis: re-estimation and sensitivity analysis of global numbers at risk. *Tropical Medicine and International Health* 2:519–528.

Dixon TC, Meselson M, Guillemin J, Hanna PC. 1999. Anthrax. *New England Journal of Medicine* 341:815–826.

Djimdé A, Doumbo OK, Cortese JF, Kayentao K, Doumbo S, Diourté Y, Dicko A, Su X, Nomura T, Fidock DA, Wellems TE, Plowe CV. 2001. A molecular marker for chloroquine-resistant *falciparum* malaria. *New England Journal of Medicine* 344:257–263.

Doenhoff M, Kimani G, Cioli D. 2000. Praziquantel and the control of schistosomiasis. *Parasitology Today* 16:364–366.

Dorn A, Vippagunta SR, Matile H, Jaquet C, Vennerstrom JL, Ridley RG. 1998. An assessment of drug-haematin binding as a mechanism for inhibition of haematin polymerisation by quinoline antimalarials. *Biochemical Pharmacology* 55:727–736.

Dorsey G, Kamya MR, Singh A, Rosenthal PJ. 2001a. Polymorphisms in the *Plasmodium falciparum pfcrt* and *pfmdr-1* genes and clinical response to chloroquine in Kampala, Uganda. *Journal of Infectious Diseases* 183:1417–1420.

Dorsey G, Fidock DA, Wellems TE, Rosenthal PJ. 2001b. Mechanisms of quinoline resistance. In: Rosenthal PJ, ed. *Antimalarial Chemotherapy: Mechanisms of Action, Resistance, and New Directions in Drug Discovery*. Totowa, NJ: Humana Press. Pp. 153–172.

Elliott TB, Brook I, Harding RA, Bouhaouala SS, Shoemaker MO, Knudson GB. 2002. Antimicrobial therapy for *Bacillus anthracis*-induced polymicrobial infection in ^{60}Co-γ-irradiated mice. *Antimicrobial Agents and Chemotherapy* 46:3463–3471.

Elliott TB, Brook I, Stiefel SM. 1990. Quantitative study of wound infection in irradiated mice. *International Journal of Radiation Biology* 58:341–350.

Fallon PG, Mubarak JS, Fookes RE, Niang M, Butterworth AE, Sturrock RF, Doenhoff MJ. 1997. *Schistosoma mansoni*: maturation rate and drug susceptibility of different geographic isolates. *Experimental Parasitology* 86:29–36.

Farr BM and Jarvis WR. 2002. Would active surveillance cultures help control health care-related methicillin-resistant *Staphylococcus aureus* infections? *Infection Control and Hospital Epidemiology* 23:65–68.

Fidock DA, Nomura T, Talley AK, Cooper RA, Dzekunov SM, Ferdig MT, Ursos LM, Sidhu AB, Naudé B, Deitsch KW, Su X, Wootton JC, Roepe PD, Wellems TE. 2000. Mutations in the *P. falciparum* digestive vacuole transmembrane protein PfCRT and evidence for their role in chloroquine resistance. *Molecular Cell* 6:861–871.

Filipe SR and Tomasz A. 2000. Inhibition of the expression of penicillin resistance in *Streptococcus pneumoniae* by inactivation of cell wall muropeptide branching genes. *Proceedings of the National Academy of Sciences* 97:4891–4896.

Greenberg AE, Ntumbanzondo M, Ntula N, Mawa L, Howell J, Davachi F. 1989. Hospital-based surveillance of malaria-related paediatric morbidity and mortality in Kinshasa, Zaire. *Bulletin of the World Health Organization* 67:189–196.

Gryseels B, Mbaye A, De Vlas SJ, Stelma FF, Guisse F, Van Lieshout L, Faye D, Diop M, Ly A, Tchuem-Tchuente LA, Engels D, Polman K. 2001. Are poor responses to praziquantel for the treatment of *Schistosoma mansoni* infections in Senegal due to resistance? An overview of the evidence. *Tropical Medicine and International Health* 6:864–873.

Hansman D, Devitt L, Miles H, Riley I. 1974. Pneumococci relatively insensitive to penicillin in Australia and New Guinea. *Medical Journal of Australia* 2:353–356.

Hawley SR, Bray PG, O'Neill PM, Naisbitt DJ, Park BK, Ward SA. 1996. Manipulation of the N-alkyl substituent in amodiaquine to overcome the verapamil-sensitive chloroquine resistance component. *Antimicrobial Agents and Chemotherapy* 40:2345–2349.

Hellgren U, Kihamia CM, Mahikwano LF, Bjorkman A, Eriksson O, Rombo L. 1989. Response of *Plasmodium falciparum* to chloroquine treatment: relation to whole blood concentrations of chloroquine and desethylchloroquine. *Bulletin of the World Health Organization* 67:197–202.

Inglesby TV, Henderson DA, Bartlett JG, Ascher MS, Eitzen EM, Friedlander AM, Hauer J, McDade J, Osterholm MT, O'Toole T, Parker G, Perl TM, Russell PK, Tonat K. 1999. Anthrax as a biological weapon: medical and public health management. *Journal of the American Medical Association* 281:1735–1745.

Jevons MP. 1961. "Celebenin"-resistant staphylococci. *British Medical Journal* 1:124–125.

King CH. 2001. Epidemiology of schistosomiasis: determinants of transmission of infection. In: Mahmoud AAF, ed. *Schistosomiasis*. London: Imperial College Press. Pp. 115–132.

King CH and Mahmoud AA. 1989. Drugs five years later: praziquantel. *Annals of Internal Medicine* 110:290–296.

King CH, Muchiri EM, Ouma JH. 2000. Evidence against rapid emergence of praziquantel resistance in *Schistosoma haematobium*, Kenya. *Emerging Infectious Diseases* 6:585–594.

Maguire JD, Susanti AI, Krisin, Sismadi P, Fryauff DJ, Baird JK. 2001. The T76 mutation in the *pfcrt* gene of *Plasmodium falciparum* and clinical chloroquine resistance phenotypes in Papua, Indonesia. *Annals of Tropical Medicine and Parasitology* 95:559–572.

Martin SK, Oduola AM, Milhous WK. 1987. Reversal of chloroquine resistance in *Plasmodium falciparum* by verapamil. *Science* 235:899–901.

Mayor AG, Gómez-Olivé X, Aponte JJ, Casimiro S, Mabunda S, Martinho D, Barreto A, Alonso PL. 2001. Prevalence of the K76T mutation in the putative *Plasmodium falciparum* chloroquine resistance transporter *(pfcrt)* gene, and its relation to chloroquine resistance in Mozambique. *Journal of Infectious Diseases* 183:1413–1416.

Nomura T, Carlton JM, Baird JK, del Portillo HA, Fryauff DJ, Rathore D, Fidock DA, Su X, Collins WE, McCutchan TF, Wootton JC, Wellems TE. 2001. Evidence for different mechanisms of chloroquine resistance in two *Plasmodium* species that cause human malaria. *Journal of Infectious Diseases* 183:1653–1661.

Oliveira DC, Tomasz A, de Lencastre H. 2002. The secrets of success of a human pathogen: molecular evolution of pandemic clones of methicillin-resistant *Staphylococcus aureus. Lancet Infectious Diseases* 2:180–189.

Pagola S, Stephens PW, Bohle DS, Kosar AD, Madsen SK. 2000. The structure of malaria pigment β-haematin. *Nature* 404:307–310.

Partnership for Child Development. 1997. Better health, nutrition, and education for the school-aged child. The Partnership for Child Development. *Transactions of the Royal Society for Tropical Medicine and Hygiene* 91:1–2.

Payne D. 1987. Spread of chloroquine resistance in *Plasmodium falciparum. Parasitology Today* 3:241–246.

Peters W. 1987. Resistance in human malaria IV: 4-aminoquinolines and multiple resistance. In: *Chemotherapy and Drug Resistance in Malaria.* London: Academic Press. Pp. 659–786.

Peters W. 1989. Changing pattern of antimalarial drug resistance. *Journal of the Royal Society of Medicine* 82 Suppl 17:14–17.

Peterson VM, Adamovicz JJ, Elliott TB, Moore MM, Madonna GS, Jackson WE 3rd, Ledney GD, Gause WC. 1994. Gene expression of hematoregulatory cytokines is elevated endogenously following sublethal γ-irradiation and is differentially enhanced by therapeutic administration of biological response modifiers. *Journal of Immunology* 153:2321–2330.

Pillai DR, Labbe AC, Vanisaveth V, Hongvangthong B, Pomphida S, Inkathone S, Zhong K, Kain KC. 2001. *Plasmodium falciparum* malaria in Laos: chloroquine treatment outcome and predictive value of molecular markers. *Journal of Infectious Diseases* 183:789–795.

Pittet D. 2002. Promotion of hand hygiene: magic, hype, or scientific challenge? *Infection Control and Hospital Epidemiology* 23:118–119.

Rasoanaivo P, Ratsimamanga-Urverg S, Frappier F. 1996. Reversing agents in the treatment of drug-resistant malaria. *Current Medicinal Chemistry* 3:1–10.

Reed MB, Saliba KJ, Caruana SR, Kirk K, Cowman AF. 2000. Pgh1 modulates sensitivity and resistance to multiple antimalarials in *Plasmodium falciparum. Nature* 403:906–909.

Renganathan E and Cioli D. 1998. An international initiative on praziquantel use. *Parasitology Today* 14:390–391.

Ridley RG, Hofheinz W, Matile H, Jaquet C, Dorn A, Masciadri R, Jolidon S, Richter WF, Guenzi A, Girometta MA, Urwyler H, Huber W, Thaithong S, Peters W. 1996. 4-aminoquinoline analogs of chloroquine with shortened side chains retain activity against chloroquine-resistant *Plasmodium falciparum. Antimicrobial Agents and Chemotherapy* 40:1846–1854.

Rieckmann KH, Davis DR, Hutton DC. 1989. *Plasmodium vivax* resistant to chloroquine? *Lancet* 2:1183–1184.

Sá-Leão R, Santos Sanches I, Couto I, Alves CR, de Lencastre H. 2001. Low prevalence of methicillin-resistant strains among *Staphylococcus aureus* colonizing young and healthy members of the community in Portugal. *Microbial Drug Resistance* 7:237–241.

Sá-Leão R, Tomasz A, Santos Sanches I, Brito-Avô A, Vilhelmsson SE, Kristinsson KG, de Lencastre H. 2000. Carriage of internationally spread epidemic clones of *Streptococcus pneumoniae* with unusual drug resistance patterns in children attending day care centers in Lisbon, Portugal. *The Journal of Infectious Diseases* 182:1153–1160.

Sowunmi A, Oduola AM, Ogundahunsi OA, Falade CO, Gbotosho GO, Salako LA. 1997. Enhanced efficacy of chloroquine-chlorpheniramine combination in acute uncomplicated falciparum malaria in children. *Transactions of the Royal Society of Tropical Medicine and Hygiene* 91:63–67.

Sturrock RF. 2001. The schistosomes and their intermediate hosts. In: Mahmoud AAF, ed. *Schistosomiasis*. London: Imperial College Press. Pp. 7–83.

Sullivan DJ, Gluzman IY, Russell DG, Goldberg DE. 1996. On the molecular mechanism of chloroquine's antimalarial action. *Proceedings of the National Academy of Sciences* 93:11865–11870.

Tomasz A. 1994. Multiple-antibiotic-resistant pathogenic bacteria. A report on the Rockefeller University workshop. *New England Journal of Medicine* 330:1247–1251.

Tomasz A. 2000. Lessons from the first antibiotic era. In: Andrew PW, Oyston P, Smith GL, Stewart-Tull DE, eds. *Fighting Infection in the 21st Century*. Society for General Microbiology Millenium Meeting Symposium Volume. Oxford, UK: Blackwell Science. Pp. 198–216.

Trape JF, Pison G, Preziosi MP, Enel C, Desgrees du Lou A, Delaunay V, Samb B, Lagarde E, Molez JF, Simondon F. 1998. Impact of chloroquine resistance on malaria mortality. *Comptes Rendus de l'Académie des Sciences. Série III, Sciences de la Vie* 321:689–697.

Van Wyk JA. 2001. Refugia—overlooked as perhaps the most potent factor concerning the development of anthelmintic resistance. *Onderstepoort Journal of Veterinary Research* 68:55–67.

Verdier F, Le Bras J, Clavier F, Hatin I, Blayo MC. 1985. Chloroquine uptake by *Plasmodium falciparum*-infected human erythrocytes during in vitro culture and its relationship to chloroquine resistance. *Antimicrobial Agents and Chemotherapy* 27:561–564.

Vieira PP, das Gracas Alecrim M, da Silva LH, González-Jiménez I, Zalis MG. 2001. Analysis of the PfCRT K76T mutation in *Plasmodium falciparum* isolates from the Amazon region of Brazil. *Journal of Infectious Diseases* 183:1832–1833.

Vippagunta SR, Dorn A, Matile H, Bhattacharjee AK, Karle JM, Ellis WY, Ridley RG, Vennerstrom JL. 1999. Structural specificity of chloroquine-hematin binding related to inhibition of hematin polymerization and parasite growth. *Journal of Medicinal Chemistry* 42:4630–4639.

Warren KS. 1982. Selective primary health care: strategies for control of disease in the developing world. I. Schistosomiasis. *Reviews of Infectious Diseases* 4:715–726.

Wellems TE and Plowe CV. 2001. Chloroquine-resistant malaria. *Journal of Infectious Diseases* 184:770–776.

Whitby M. 1997. Drug resistant *Plasmodium vivax* malaria. *Journal of Antimicrobial Chemotherapy* 40:749–752.

WHO (World Health Organization). 1993. *The Control of Schistosomiasis: Second Report of the WHO Expert Committee*. Geneva: WHO.

WHO. 2000. *Overcoming Antimicrobial Resistance: WHO Report on Infectious Diseases 2000*. [Online]. Available: http://www.who.int/infectious-disease-report/2000/.

n S, Sabra A, Ramzy F, Mousa M, Demerdash Z, Bennett JL, Day TA, Botros S. 2001. tability and reproductive fitness of *Schistosoma mansoni* isolates with decreased sensitivity to praziquantel. *International Journal of Parasitology* 31:1093–1100.
tton JC, Feng X, Ferdig MT, Cooper RA, Mu J, Baruch DI, Magill AJ, Su XZ. 2002. Genetic diversity and chloroquine selective sweeps in *Plasmodium falciparum*. *Nature* 418:320–323.

3

Vector Resistance

OVERVIEW

One way to help stem the spread of antimicrobial resistance is to reduce the number of cases of disease that must be treated with therapeutic agents, thereby reducing the selective pressure that often leads to such resistance. Toward this goal, insecticides play a major role in controlling major disease vectors—the arthropods that pass pathogens to humans.

The use of insecticides, however, presents a problem parallel to the use of antimicrobials—the chemical agents themselves frequently promote resistance among the vectors they are intended to control. Indeed, resistance to insecticides has appeared in every major species of arthropod vectors—including mosquitoes, ticks, fleas, lice, and sand flies—and various vectors have developed resistance to every class of pesticide. The focus of this session of the workshop was an examination of the role that vectors play in a variety of diseases and how management efforts are being used to better control vector populations.

Malaria represents a classic example of the difficulties associated with vector-control efforts. In 1955, the World Health Organization (WHO) called for the global eradication of malaria through the use of DDT. However, the mosquitoes that carry the disease soon developed resistance to DDT, and in 1976 WHO shifted its goal from eradication to control. The resistance problems continued with the switch to newer insecticides, such as the organophosphates and pyrethroids. Many experts maintain that new insecticides, coupled with the development and implementation of various other control measures, will be needed to regain long-term control over the mosquitoes that spread malaria. Some experts, however, argue that DDT has unfairly been declared an unacceptable hazard, and that it can play an important—and significantly larger—role in controlling not only malaria but also such other widespread diseases as dengue.

Research on resistance among vectors now takes two basic approaches. One approach is to study the molecular mechanisms involved. Scientists already have a relatively good understanding of the basic mechanisms underlying resistance to commonly used insecticides, and they are now using recently developed molecular techniques to begin to dissect these mechanisms at the DNA level. The next challenge will be to use this molecular understanding to develop novel vector-control methods that avoid or minimize resistance problems.

The second approach to research involves resistance management—that is, developing and implementing control methods that minimize the likelihood that vectors will evolve strong resistance to important insecticides. Two such promising control strategies are alternating the use of different insecticides and applying them in mosaic patterns over a given geographic area. Scientists are now conducting, in Mexico, a large-scale trial of these two strategies, compared to the use of DDT or a pyrethroid insecticide used in the conventional manner. Information from such trials may enable scientists and policy makers to establish rational strategies for long-term insecticide use.

Expanding the use of integrated pest management, or IPM, also holds promise for improving vector-control programs. Tackling a pest problem in numerous ways at once—including the use of pesticides in a timely manner at select locations—will likely yield more thorough and longer-lasting control than would result from any single method applied individually.

Developing and applying mathematical models can provide a solid basis for identifying new ways to effectively control the emergence of resistance among vector populations—and also to identify methods that are not effective. Among their benefits, models enable researchers to examine trends in data, explore questions of population dynamics, compare various management options, and generate new hypotheses for study. A major roadblock to progress in this area is the lack of interdisciplinary work among modelers studying insect resistance and those studying antimicrobial resistance in pathogens. Indeed, increased scientific collaboration across disciplines could foster scientific progress in numerous areas related to antimicrobial resistance. Likewise, policy makers developing programs to control the spread of antimicrobial resistance among pathogens could benefit by examining the successes and failures of current vector-control programs.

INSECTICIDE RESISTANCE IN INSECT VECTORS OF HUMAN DISEASE

Janet Hemingway, Ph.D.
Liverpool School of Tropical Medicine
Liverpool, United Kingdom

Insecticides play a central role in controlling major vectors of diseases. In 1955 the WHO Assembly proposed the global eradication of malaria with DDT. However, the shift from malaria eradication to control in 1976 was prompted by the appearance of DDT resistance in many mosquito vectors. The resistance problems continued with the switch to newer insecticides such as the organophosphates (OPs), carbamates, and pyrethroids. Operationally, many control programs have now switched from blanket spraying of house interiors to focal use of insecticides on bednets. Focal spraying reduces the amount of insecticide used, but also limits the choice of insecticides to pyrethroids due to the need for rapid insect kill and high mammalian safety margin.

Today the major emphasis in research into resistance is on the molecular mechanisms of resistance, and rational resistance management, with a view to controlling the spread and development of resistant vector populations. The level of resistance in insect populations is dependent on the amount and frequency of insecticides used, and the inherent characteristics of the insect species selected. For example, for decades tsetse flies have been controlled by DDT treatment, but resistance has never developed in this species; the same is true of triatomid bugs. In both species the major factor influencing insecticide resistance development is the life cycle of the insect pest, in particular the long life cycles for the bugs, and the production of very small numbers of young by the tsetses. Mosquitoes, in contrast, have all the characteristics suited to rapid resistance development including short life cycles and abundant progeny.

Vector Resistance

The major mosquito vectors span the *Culex, Aedes,* and *Anopheles* genera. *Culex* are the vectors of filariasis and Japanese encephalitis, *Aedes* of dengue, dengue hemorrhagic fever, and yellow fever, and *Anopheles* of malaria. The range of many of these species is still expanding.

DDT was first introduced for mosquito control in 1946. In 1947 the first cases of DDT resistance occurred in *Aedes* (Brown, 1986). Since then over a hundred species of mosquito have become resistant to one or more insecticide (WHO, 1992). Insecticides used for malaria control have included γ-benzine hexachloride (BHC), organophosphorus, carbamate, and pyrethroid insecticides. Other insecticide groups, such as the benzylphenyl ureas and *Bacillus thuringiensis* (Bti), have had limited use against mosquitoes.

γ-BHC/dieldrin resistance is still widespread, despite the lack of use of these insecticides for many years. OP resistance, in the form of either broad-spectrum resistance or malathion-specific resistance, occurs in many vectors (Hemingway, 1982, 1983; Hemingway and Georghiou, 1983; Herath et al., 1987). OP resistance is widespread in all the major *Culex* vectors (Hemingway and Karunaratne, 1998) and pyrethroid resistance occurs in *C. quinquefasciatus* (Chandre et al., 1998). Pyrethroid resistance is widespread in *Ae. aegypti* (Hemingway et al., 1989) and cases of OP and carbamate resistance also occur in this species (Mourya et al., 1993). The development of pyrethroid resistance in *An. gambiae* is particularly important given the recent emphasis on the use of pyrethroid impregnated bednets for malaria control (Vontas et al., 2001).

The peridomestic vectors of *Leishmania* are primarily controlled by insecticides throughout their range. The control of these sandflies is often a by-product of anti-malarial housespraying. The only insecticide resistance reported to date in sandflies is to DDT (El-Sayed et al., 1989).

The body louse *Pediculus humanus* has developed widespread resistance to organochlorines (Brown and Pal, 1971), is malathion-resistant in parts of Africa (WHO, 1992), and has "low-level" resistance to pyrethroids in several regions (Fine, 1963). Resistance to DDT and lindane occurs in the human head lice in Israel, Canada, Denmark, and Malaysia (WHO, 1992). Permethrin has been extensively used for head lice control since the early 1980s. The first reports of control failure with this insecticide were in the early 1990s in Israel (Mumcuoglu et al., 1995), the Czech Republic (Rupes et al., 1994), and France (Chosidow et al., 1994).

The *Simulium damnosum* complex, vectors of onchocerciasis, have been subjected to long-term insecticide-based control in West Africa since 1974. Temephos resistance prompted a switch to chlorphoxim, but resistance to this insecticide occurred within a year (Hemingway et al., 1991). Resistance in Simulium is currently being managed by a rotation of temephos, Bti, and permethrin, the insecticide usage being determined by the rate of water discharge in the major breeding sites of these vectors.

The Biochemistry of Resistance

Insecticide Metabolism

Three major enzyme groups are responsible for metabolically based resistance to organochlorines, OPs, carbamates, and pyrethroids. DDT-dehydrochlorinase is a glutathione S-transferase (Clark and Shamaan, 1984). Esterases are involved in OP, carbamate, and pyrethroid resistance. Monooxygenases are involved in the metabolism of pyrethroids, carbamate, and the activation and/or detoxication of OPs.

Esterase-Based Resistance: The esterase-based resistance mechanisms have been most extensively studied in *Culex* mosquitoes and the aphid *Myzus persicae*. Broad-spectrum OP resistance is conferred by the elevated esterases, which act by rapidly binding and slowly turning over the insecticide (Kadous et al., 1983). Two common esterase loci, *est*α and *est*β, are involved in *Culex* (Vaughan et al., 1997). In *C. quinquefasciatus* the most common elevated esterase phenotype involves est$\alpha 2^1$ and est$\beta 2^1$ (Vaughan and Hemingway, 1995). Smaller numbers of *Culex* have elevated estβ1 alone, elevated estα1 alone, or co-elevated estβ1 and estα3 (DeSilva et al., 1997; Hemingway and Karunaratne, 1998). Differences of up to 1,000-fold in the inhibition kinetic constants of these esterases in resistant and susceptible insects occur for the oxon analogues of various OPs (Karunaratne et al., 1995). The superiority of insecticide binding in enzymes from resistant insects suggests that there has been a positive insecticide selection pressure to maintain elevation of favorable esterase.

In contrast to the situation in *Culex* a number of *Anopheles* species have a non-elevated esterase mechanism that confers resistance specifically to malathion through increased rates of metabolism (Hemingway, 1982, 1983, 1985; Malcolm and Boddington, 1989).

Glutathione S-Transferase-Based Resistance: GSTs are multifunctional enzymes that detoxify a large range of xenobiotics. They catalyze the nucleophilic attack of reduced glutathione (GSH) on the electrophilic centers of lipophilic compounds. Multiple forms of these enzymes have been reported for the mosquito, housefly, *Drosophila*, sheep blowfly, and grass grub (Clark et al., 1984; Clark et al., 1985; Toung et al., 1990).

There are at least three families of insect GST and all have a role in insecticide resistance. In *Ae. aegypti* at least two GSTs are elevated in DDT-resistant insects (Grant and Matsumura, 1989), while in *An. gambiae* a large number of different class III GSTs are elevated (Prapanthadara et al., 1993). The *Ae. aegypti* and *An. gambiae* GSTs in resistant insects are constitutively over-expressed. The GST-2 of *Ae. aegypti* is over-expressed in all tissues except the ovaries of resistant insects (Grant and Hammock, 1992).

Monooxygenase-Based Resistance: The monooxygenases are a complex family of enzymes involved in the metabolism of xenobiotics. The P^{450} monooxygenases are the rate-limiting enzyme step in the chain. P^{450}s are involved in the metabolism of virtually all insecticides, leading to activation of OPs, or, more generally, detoxication. Elevated monooxygenase activity is associated with pyrethroid resistance in *An. stephensi*, *An. gambiae* (Vulule et al., 1994), and *C. quinquefasciatus* (Kasai et al., 1998).

Target Site Resistance

The OPs, carbamates, organochlorines, and pyrethroids all target the nervous system. Newer classes of insecticides are now coming onto the market place for vector control, but the high cost of developing and registering them inevitably means that insecticides are developed initially for the agricultural market and then utilized for public health vector control, where their activities and safety profile are appropriate. Compounds targeting the nicotinic acetylcholine receptor have recently made this transition from agriculture into public health.

Acetylcholinesterase: The OPs and carbamates target acetylcholinesterase (AChE). Alterations in AChE in resistant insects result in a decreased sensitivity to insecticide inhibition of the enzyme (Hemingway and Georghiou, 1983). The OPs are converted to their oxon analogues, via the action of monooxygenases before acting as AChE inhibitors.

GABA Receptors: Resistance to dieldrin occurred in the 1950s, but the involvement of the GABA receptors in this resistance was not elucidated until 1990. The GABA receptor in insects is a widespread inhibitory neurotransmission channel in the central nervous system and in neuromuscular junctions (Bermudez et al., 1991). It is a site of action for pyrethroids and avermectins as well as cyclodienes (Kadous et al., 1983; Bloomquist, 1994).

Sodium Channels: The pharmacological effect of DDT and pyrethroids is to cause persistent activation of the sodium channels by delaying the normal voltage-dependent mechanism of inactivation (Soderlund and Bloomquist, 1989). In mosquitoes there have been many reports of suspected "*kdr*"-like resistance inferred from cross-resistance between DDT and pyrethroids, which act on the same site within the sodium channel. These reports have been validated by electrophysiological measurements in *Ae. aegypti* and *An. stephensi* (Hemingway et al., 1989; Vatandoost et al., 1996).

The Molecular Biology of Resistance

Mutations in Structural Genes

Resistance to malathion is caused by a single Trp^{251}-Leu substitution within the E3 esterase of *Lucilia cuprina* (Campbell et al., 1998). A similar phenotype has been observed in malathion-resistant *Anopheles* (Hemingway and Georghiou, 1983). A second Gly^{137}-Asp substitution in E3 confers broad cross-resistance to many OPs, but not to malathion (Newcomb et al., 1997).

Non-silent point mutations within structural genes are the cause of target site resistance. The mutations reduce insecticide binding without causing a loss of primary function of the target site. The number of possible amino acid substitutions is limited and identical resistance-associated mutations are found across divergent taxa. The degree to which function is impaired by the mutations is reflected in the fitness of resistant individuals in the absence of insecticide selection. This fitness cost is important in the persistence of resistance in the field.

An alanine to serine substitution in the channel-lining domain of the GABA receptor confers resistance to cyclodienes (ffrench-Constant et al., 1998). The mutation occurs in a broad range of dieldrin-resistant insects (Thompson et al., 1993), occasionally in an alanine to glycine form. Despite the widespread switch away from cyclodienes for agricultural and public health use, the resistance allele is still found at relatively high frequencies in insect field populations (Aronstein et al., 1995).

A reduction in the sensitivity of the voltage gated sodium channel to insecticide binding causes the *kdr* resistance phenotype. *Kdr* mutants are more variable than those in the GABA receptors, but are still limited to a small number of regions on this large channel protein. The first mutation to be characterized in *kdr* insects was a leucine to phenylalanine mutation in the S6 transmembrane segment of domain II in the sodium channel sequence (Martinez-Torres et al., 1998) that produces 10- to 20-fold resistance to DDT and pyrethroids. In "*super-kdr*" houseflies, this mutation is combined with a second methionine to threonine substitution further upstream in the same domain resulting in >500-fold resistance (Williamson et al., 1996). A PCR-based diagnostic discriminates between homozygous-susceptible, homozygous-resistant, and heterozygotes with the Leu to Phe mutation (Martinez-Torres et al., 1998). Since *kdr* is partially recessive the ability to detect heterozygotes is of paramount importance in the early detection and management of resistance in the field.

The number of changes may be constrained by the possible modifications that can influence pyrethroid/DDT binding to the sodium channels. However, a note of caution is needed, as there is a tendency to investigate pyrethroid-resistant insects with a PCR approach confined to regions where a *kdr* mutation has already been seen. Hence changes in other parts of the sodium channel gene could be missed. A different approach to isolating *kdr*-type mutants has been used in *Drosophila*, utilizing the relative ease with which large numbers of mutants in the para sodium channel gene can be isolated based on their temperature sensitivity. Two classes of these mutations are in positions equivalent to the *kdr* and *super-kdr* mutations in different domains. The third class is in a novel position (ffrench-Constant et al., 1998).

A range of different amino acid substitutions in the acetylcholinesterase *Ace* genes of *Drosophila* and the housefly *M. domestica* cause resistance (Feyereisen, 1995). Many of these mutations lie close to or within the active site gorge. Five point mutations associated with OP and carbamate resistance have been identified in *D. melanogaster*. AChE and site directed mutagenesis of the sex-linked AChE from *Ae. aegypti* have demonstrated that these same mutations also confer resistance in the mosquito enzyme, but none of these mutations have been identified in field-collected insects.

Gene Amplification

In three *Culex* species an *estβ* gene is amplified in resistant insects (Vaughan et al., 1995; Whyard et al., 1995; Karunaratne et al., 1998). The commonest amplified esterase-based mechanism involves the co-amplification of two esterases, *est$\alpha 2^1$* and *est$\beta 2^1$* in *C. quinquefasciatus* and other members of the *C. pipiens* complex (Vaughan et al., 1997). Other strains of *Culex* have amplified *estα3* and *estβ1* co-amplified (DeSilva et al., 1997), while the TEM-R strain has amplified *estβ1* alone (Mouches et al., 1986).

The *estα* and *estβ* genes have arisen as the result of an ancient gene duplication. The genes are in a head-to-head arrangement approximately 1.7 kb apart in susceptible insects (Vaughan et al., 1997). In resistant insects the amplified *est$\alpha 2^1$/est$\beta 2^1$* genes are 2.7 kb apart; the difference is accounted for by expansion with three indels in the intergenic spacer (Vaughan et al., 1997), which have introduced further gene regulators (Hemingway et al., 1998). Amplification of these alleles has occurred once and spread worldwide by migration (Raymond et al., 1991).

Transcriptional Regulation

Amplified esterases are expressed at different levels. For example, there is four-fold more estβ than estα in resistant *C. quinquefasciatus*, although the genes are present in a 1:1 ratio. This difference in expression is reflected at the protein and mRNA level (Karunaratne et al., 1995).

GSTs metabolize DDT and OPs (Hemingway et al., 1985) and moderate the toxic effects of pyrethroid-generated radicals (Vontas et al., 2001). GST-based DDT resistance is common in *Anopheles*, reflecting decades of heavy use of DDT for malaria control. Molecular characterization of GSTs is most developed in *An. gambiae* and *An. dirus* (Hemingway et al., 1998; Prapanthadara et al., 1998). Three classes of insect GSTs are important in insecticide metabolism in insects. *Aedes aegypti* GST-2, is overexpressed in

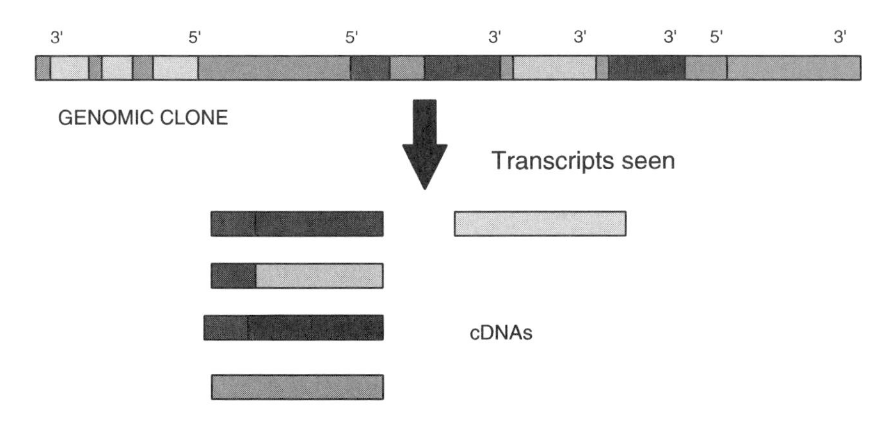

FIGURE 3-1 The class I and class III glutathione S-transferase family of *Anopheles gambiae*, which include an intronless gene aggst1-2, an alternatively spliced gene aggst1α with four distinct viable transcripts, and the aggst1β gene with two introns.

a DDT-resistant GG strain, where the resistance mutation leads to disruption of a trans-acting repressor (Grant and Hammock, 1992).

In *An. gambiae* multiple class I and class III GST genes are clustered in separate single locations. One gene, aggst1α, is alternatively spliced to produce four distinct mRNA transcipts each of which shares a common 5' exon but differing 3' exons (see Figure 3-1) (Ranson et al., 1998). The organizations of the class I GST gene family in insecticide-resistant and -susceptible *An. gambiae* are similar.

Insect P^{450}s belong to six families. Increased transcription of genes belonging to the CYP4, CYP6, and CYP9 families occurs in insecticide-resistant strains. It is not known which enzymes are responsible for insecticide metabolism in mosquitoes. *Helicoverpa armigera* has different resistance-associated P^{450}s between strains; CYP6B2 is overexpressed in a pyrethroid-resistant strain (Xiao-Ping and Hobbs, 1995), whereas CYP4G8 is overexpressed in another (Pittendrigh et al., 1997).

P^{450}-based resistance in *M. domestica* (housefly) and *D. melanogaster* is mediated by mutations in *trans*-acting regulatory genes. CYP6A8 is highly expressed in the DDT-resistant 91-R strain of *D. melanogaster* but not detectable in the uninduced 91-C susceptible strain (Maitra et al., 1996; Dombrowski et al., 1998). Hybrids between the two strains show low levels of expression suggesting that the 91-C strain carries a repressor that suppresses transcription of CYP6A8 (Liu and Scott, 1997).

Management of Insecticide-Resistant Vector Populations

The use of an insecticide until resistance becomes a limiting factor is rapidly eroding the number of suitable insecticides for insect control. Rotations, mosaics, and mixtures have all been proposed as resistance management tools. Numerous mathematical models have been produced to estimate how these tools should be optimally used (Tabashnik, 1989). However, these models have rarely been tested under field conditions due to the practical difficulties in estimating changes in resistance gene frequencies in large samples of insects (Hemingway et al., 1997). With the advent of different biochemical and molecular techniques for resistance gene frequency estimation, field trials of resistance management strategies have become more feasible. A large-scale trial of the use of rotations or mosaics of insecticides compared to single use of DDT or a pyrethroid is currently under way in Mexico (Penilla et al., 1998). Changes in resistance gene frequencies in *An. albimanus* are being monitored over a four-year period. Information resulting from such large-scale trials may allow us to establish rational strategies for long-term insecticide use. As our ability to manipulate the insect genome improves and our understanding of the regulation of insecticide resistance mechanisms increases, new strategies should be devised for incorporation into these control programs.

MANAGING THE EMERGENCE OF PESTICIDE RESISTANCE IN VECTORS

William G. Brogdon, Ph.D.

Centers for Disease Control and Prevention, Atlanta, GA

A linked four-stage process, involving investment, surveillance, interpretation, and remediation, is described for management of insecticide resistance in vectors. Insecticide resistance has been a problem in all insect groups that serve as vectors of emerging diseases. Although mechanisms by which insecticides become less effective are similar across all vector taxa, each resistance problem is potentially unique and may involve a complex pattern of resistance foci. The main defense against resistance is close surveillance of the susceptibility of vector populations. This requires the investment of programs in surveillance. Once surveillance data have been gathered, it is crucial that the results be interpreted practically, in terms of control efficacy. Only then can strategies for remediation be undertaken.

There are fundamental differences between the management of pesticide and that of antimicrobial resistance. Rapid generation times in microbes can lead to rapid selection of highly resistant populations, even in the course of a single infection. Generation times in vectors are significantly longer, resulting in more gradual selection of resistance. Among the more rapid emergences of insecticide resistance we have observed was the appearance and intensification of fenitrothion resistance over a three-month period at one location in Haiti following an insecticide spray cycle (Brogdon et al., 1988).

The focus of antibiotic resistance management is on infections in individual patients or in specific institutions. The focus of insecticide resistance management is on vector populations in a geographic control area. The use of antibiotics follows similar principles throughout the world. The application strategies for insecticides are radically different around the world. For control of malaria, wall spraying and the use of insecticide-impregnated bednets are the most used methods of control. In the United States, ground and aerial application of ultra-low volumes of insecticide are widely used.

Changes in antibiotic use have little environmental impact. Changes in insecticide use can have significant environmental impact. Collection, culture, and testing of resistant microbe strains is not technically difficult or expensive. Collection, culture, and testing of resistant insects can be both difficult and expensive. Generally, teams of individuals must go into the field and collect through the night, sometimes for days, to obtain an adequate number of insects for resistance testing. Collections may include adults, larvae, or eggs of vectors.

Control failure in antibiotic use can have immediate fatal consequences for the patient. Insecticide control failure may have less obvious impact on disease control. The continued survival of a vector species may be less noticeable against a background of pest species that have been controlled, giving the illusion of adequate vector control. For example, good control of pest species of mosquitoes in Florida gave the impression that control with a particular insecticide was adequate. Further testing revealed that *Culex nigripalpus*, the principal vector species, did not respond to that insecticide (Brogdon, unpublished data).

The most significant feature shared by antimicrobial and insecticide resistance management is that the choice of new chemical options is dangerously limited. It is crucial that legislators and health officials make the *investment* necessary to manage resistance. Funding allows resistance problems to be detected and assessed through the use of resistance *surveillance*. Going through the motions of resistance surveillance is a waste of resources unless the data obtained are subjected to professional and timely *interpretation*. Only after the problem has been adequately detected and interpreted can the program develop a strategy for *remediation* of the problem.

Investment in Resistance Management

The investment that is being applied to antimicrobial resistance becomes obvious if one simply does an Internet search with the keywords "antimicrobial resistance." Key sites that are immediately located include those established by WHO, the European Antimicrobial Resistance Surveillance System, and the Centers for Disease Control and Prevention (CDC). These sites provide timely data on the detection, assessment, and distribution of antimicrobial resistance throughout the world.

Corresponding sites dedicated to insecticide resistance are not found. The extent of the problem was revealed by a fortunate investment under the Emerging Infections Program at CDC that funded an Insecticide Resistance Surveillance Laboratory. Through collaborative work with over 20 states, it became clear that insecticide resistance is widespread, though highly focal in the United States (Brogdon, unpublished data). More troubling is the observation that knowledge of insecticide resistance status is virtually nonexistent in vector control programs. Similar difficulties apply overseas. In general, insecticide susceptibility testing is the last activity funded in control programs. If funded, it is the first activity cut. A serious commitment to resistance management is not made. Though there are exceptions, these observations are generally applicable.

Reversing the trend regarding investment in insecticide resistance testing will require training of the appropriate health officials in the techniques that may be used to detect and assess resistance problems. This may be done through training courses or through training-oriented websites. One such website for insecticide resistance testing has been produced at the CDC (http://www.cdc.gov/ncidod/wbt/resistance/).

Insecticide Resistance Surveillance

The most fundamental feature of insecticide resistance problems may be that each such problem is potentially unique, given the broad variety of resistance mechanisms available to the insect and the great disparity in insecticide use history and thus selection pressure on natural populations of vectors. Given the diversity of problem types and the focal nature of resistance, it becomes the primary goal of resistance surveillance to measure resistance as it exists, at a particular place, at a particular time. Fortunately, an array of bioassay, biochemical assay, and molecular methods already exist (and many others are under active development) to facilitate detection and assessment of resistance problems.

The first line of defense (and the most cost-effective) is a bioassay method, such as the bottle bioassay developed at the CDC (Brogdon and

McAllister, 1998a). Using this technique, the specific formulation of insecticide(s) used in a program may be used in a simple test of susceptibility of the vector species. A discriminating insecticide dosage is empirically determined, a resistance threshold (upper range limit of time of survival of a susceptible population) is established, and testing can proceed to rapidly characterize populations in the control area. Use of insecticide resistance enzyme inhibitors (synergists) can provide information on the mechanism of insecticide resistance in bottle assays, but, typically, the most detailed information on resistance mechanisms comes through application of biochemical resistance assays, generally conducted in microtiter plates. Knowledge of the mechanism allows a program to make an informed decision on how to combat the problem. For example, some mechanisms may be rendered ineffective through the judicious use of synergists. In other cases, it becomes necessary to switch insecticides. Knowing the resistance mechanism protects the program from falling prey to cross-resistance, where resistance to the insecticide used also crosses to insecticides that have not been used, but that are susceptible to the same resistance mechanism.

Biochemical microplate assays are available for the oxidase, esterase, glutathione S-transferase, and insensitive acetylcholinesterase resistance mechanisms. These assays give clear evidence of resistance mechanisms, provided their results are carefully correlated to bioassay data from the same vector populations. One drawback of these techniques is that the insects to be tested must be fresh or frozen at dry ice (–80°C or better) temperatures. This becomes a real problem in field situations, particularly in the tropics. Moreover, no biochemical assay yet exists (though one is under development) for the target site resistance mechanism (*kdr*) that afflicts pyrethroid use.

Biochemical data are interpreted similarly to bioassays, in that an upper range limit for resistance enzyme activity is established as a threshold, allowing individuals with higher than normal activities to be classified as less susceptible (given corroborative bioassay data). The biochemical data should account for a similar proportion of a vector population above the resistance threshold as bioassay tests on the same population. An advantage of biochemical assays is that they may be conducted as a complete panel or battery of tests, generally conducted in triplicate, on each insect. Data from multiple tests may be plotted on the same graph, clearly revealing instances of cross-resistance.

Increasing understanding of insect molecular biology is transforming the field of resistance detection, through direct sequencing of resistance genes and the applied use of both qualitative and quantitative PCR and RTPCR. Advanced techniques such as fluorescence PCR are allowing efficient detection of resistance gene copy number (multiple esterase copies are a frequent cause of resistance), level of gene expression (important in the increased expression of oxidase genes), and the efficient detection of point mutations in insecticide target genes (Brogdon and McAllister, 1998b).

There are two huge advantages to the use of molecular resistance detection techniques. First, preserved (in alcohol or desiccated) specimens may now be used in the analysis, allowing much easier logistics in the collection and transport of collected vector insects. Also, molecular analysis allows the use of insects collected as pools. Collection of vector samples is expensive in both time and personnel. It would be invaluable if the same pools of insects collected for routine viral surveillance, for example, could also be used for identification of species (and their relative number), measurement of resistance mechanism indices, and correlation of resistance-positive and disease-positive pools. This exciting scenario should be within reach of current molecular technology.

Given investment in surveillance, we now have the technology to provide the necessary raw data for us to manage insecticide resistance. These techniques are making it possible to deal with the greatest emerging problem in resistance surveillance, that of multiple resistance. Multiple resistance is the resistance to an insecticide through multiple resistance mechanisms. Additional resistance mechanisms may enhance, reduce, or modify the insecticide specificity of the resistance based upon a single mechanism. Such complex problems make proper interpretation of data a critical factor in resistance management.

Interpretation of Resistance Data

It is an unfortunate part of the history of vector control that so much routine resistance surveillance data was detected in the absence of subsequent informed analysis. Frequently such testing was done as a routine, with the methods carefully followed, but with the data filed away uninterpreted. It is the most frequent failing in the process of conducting resistance management.

One particular problem that arises is that field personnel do not know how to cope with interpretation when they lack access to an established susceptible strain of the insect being tested. All that is required is for the program to establish a susceptibility baseline using the current target population. These data are interpreted though evaluation of the level of current control success on that population. The mission then becomes to monitor for changes in resistance baseline and in control success. The presence of even high levels of insecticide resistance may or may not be relevant to vector control. If the efficacy of control is not being concurrently assessed, it serves no purpose to conduct resistance susceptibility testing. Even if resistance is "detected," its significance will remain unknown. All successful control programs carefully assess the efficacy of their program, whether by plotting incidence of disease cases or by counting adult or larval collections at informative sites. These data must be integrated with the resistance surveillance data for effective remediation of problems to be contemplated.

Remediation of Resistance

Just as every resistance problem may be unique, every solution is potentially unique. Management schemes take one of two forms. The simplest is surveillance-response. The most inexpensive strategy, it involves establishment of susceptibility baselines, periodic susceptibility testing, correlation of changes with control efficacy, and change of control strategy when the data indicate the necessity of doing so. Response choices are to switch chemicals, to apply chemicals focally, or where chemicals are ineffective, to use source reduction or concentrate on personal protection.

The more complicated and expensive strategy, integrated pest management (IPM), presupposes a deeper understanding of the disease and vector. Strategies for IPM include rotations of chemicals, timed application of chemicals, use of mixtures, and the provision of refugia (mosaic application of insecticides) for resistance genes. Thus far, the best example of a resistance management program in a disease vector is the Onchocerciasis Control Program in Africa. There, 11 countries *invested* (through the assistance of 80 development partners) in resistance *surveillance*, *interpretation*, and *remediation* in an area where 35 million people are at risk for the disease (WHO, 1997). Where there has been success in one program lies the potential for success in others.

WHAT IS THE ROLE OF INSECTICIDE RESISTANCE IN THE RE-EMERGENCE OF MAJOR ARTHROPOD-BORNE DISEASES?

Donald R. Roberts, Ph.D.[*]

Department of Preventive Medicine and Biometrics
Uniformed Services University of the Health Sciences, Bethesda, MD

Paul B. Hshieh, Ph.D.

Office of Biostatistics and Epidemiology, Center for Biologics Evaluation and Research
Food and Drug Administration, Rockville, MD

Twenty years of spectacular and continual growth in cases (see Figure 3-2) and geographical spread of human malaria (Roberts et al., 1997) and dengue fever (Gubler, 1998) in the Americas should send a resounding message that something is horribly wrong in modern approaches to disease control. Within the last few months dengue has spread to Hawaii and Easter Island, and an outbreak is occurring in Argentina. In fact, outbreaks are occurring commonly throughout the Americas (ProMED-mail, 2002). *Aedes aegypti* is the primary vector of dengue. This vector has re-invaded and proliferated in almost all areas of the New World where it had previously been eliminated. Modern vector control methods have not measurably slowed re-conquest of the Americas by this important vector of dengue and yellow fever viruses.

The insecticide and methods previously used to exert decades of control over malaria and to eliminate *Ae. aegypti* are no longer (or rarely) used. Malaria and dengue were controlled in different ways; but the insecticide (DDT) was the same for both. The environmental movement has forced the move away from proven methods of disease control. Environmental activists have campaigned to stop use of DDT and other insecticides in public health (Amato, 1993; World Wildlife Fund [WWF], 1999). Claims that resistance neutralized the effectiveness of insecticides have been part of the environmental campaign, as illustrated in the claim that "DDT resistance has been a factor in the failure of many national malaria eradication programs." (WWF, 1999).

*Disclaimer: The opinions and assertions contained in this article are not to be considered as official or as reflecting the views of the Department of Defense or the Uniformed Services University of the Health Sciences.

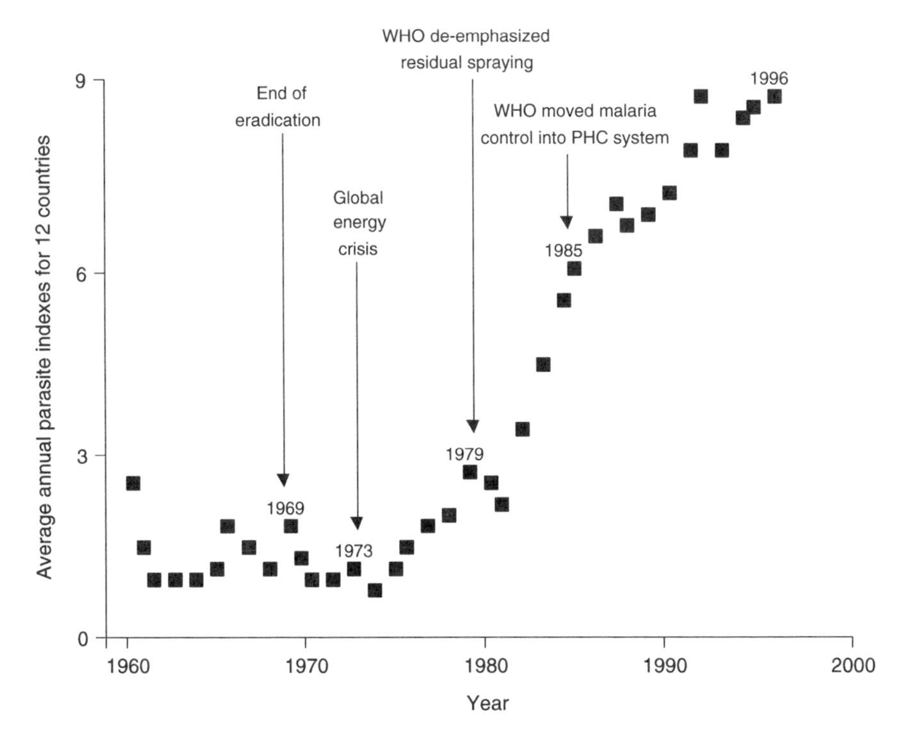

FIGURE 3-2 Growth in standardized malaria indexes from 1960 to 1996. The pattern of growth in malaria cases represents index values that have been standardized on the basis of annual blood examination rates across 12 countries of the Americas (Belize, Bolivia, Brazil, Colombia, Costa Rica, Ecuador, Guatemala, Guyana, Mexico, Panama, Peru, and Venezuela).

Decades of research have been employed to reduce the complex phenomena of insecticide resistance in disease vectors into simpler subsystems. As comprehensively reviewed by Hemingway and Ranson (2000), resistance has been studied in many vector species, especially in vectors of malaria and dengue viruses, and at many levels, to include its molecular basis. This reductive approach has not led to accurate models and predictive theories that are broadly applicable to disease control operations. As recently shown with insecticide-treated nets, resistance does not necessarily counter the benefits of insecticide use (Sina and Aultman, 2001). The same has been shown for the continuing effectiveness of sprayed houses in controlling malaria, even when the vectors are resistant to the insecticide that is being used (Roberts and Andre, 1994).

Failure of predictive accuracy has occurred because research has focused almost completely on toxicological resistance, which, in turn, is based on the erroneous premise that insecticides control disease transmission by killing insects. No example of this fundamental error is more revealing than in the resistance of malaria vector mosquitoes to DDT.

A recent probability model (Roberts et al., 2000) quantifies DDT's mode of action in controlling malaria transmission inside houses. The model shows that greatest impact of DDT residues stems from a repellent action. A contact irritant action is next in order of importance. The model was tested against field data for important malaria vectors in the Americas, Africa, and Asia. The results showed that mortality accounted for less than 10 percent of the total impact of DDT residues against two vectors, from 10 percent to about 36.2 percent against a third vector, and 18.3 percent against a fourth vector. In a separate study, the model was field validated in experimental hut studies against a fifth vector species in southern Belize (Grieco et al., 2000). This model represents the first use of stochastic methods to elucidate actual functions of DDT residues, but it was certainly not the first demonstration of DDT's powerful repellent and irritant actions.

From the very beginning of DDT's use, it was known as a slow-acting poison (Metcalf et al., 1951) that strongly influenced insect behavior. In 1947 Kennedy published a paper (Kennedy, 1947) entitled "The Excitant and Repellent Effects on Mosquitoes of Sub-Lethal Contacts with DDT." This paper warrants careful consideration because its 1947 publication date means that the research was actually conducted before wide-scale use of DDT in malaria control (which started in 1946). Kennedy's experiments demonstrated repellent and irritant actions of DDT against a vector of malaria (*Anopheles maculipennis atroparvus*) and *Ae. aegypti*. Kennedy's work was published five years before the first report of DDT resistance in a malaria vector mosquito.

Kennedy introduced his paper as follows:

> During the war it was necessary to concentrate on the practical development of DDT as an insecticide without waiting for studies of its mode of action. Working assumptions had to be made, especially with regard to the possible repellency of DDT deposits. Buxton (1945) sums up what has been the accepted opinion on this subject, as follows: "DDT does not act as a repellent to any insect, so far as is known" (Kennedy, 1947).

He went on to say that ". . . the existence of contact repellency has been firmly established." Buxton (1945) mentioned "restlessness" as an early symptom of DDT poisoning. This has been described under semi-field conditions by Gahan and others (1945) and by Metcalf and others (1945), who observed also that mosquitoes excited by contact with DDT no longer stayed in dark corners but made for the windows.

However, such repellency has been discounted as of no practical significance because, in Buxton's (1945) words: "So far as is known, once visible symptoms develop, death follows: recovery from an early stage of poisoning does not occur."

"This idea is perhaps even more widespread than the idea that DDT is not repellent" (Kennedy, 1947).

Kennedy ended his introductory paragraph with the statement that "Our laboratory observations did not bear out these statements" (Kennedy, 1947).

Kennedy then reported on a series of laboratory experiments showing that mosquitoes were strongly repelled by DDT residues (for example, see Figure 3-3), and that the test specimens often recovered completely after showing preliminary symptoms of poisoning. With this documentation he concluded that "DDT must be regarded as acting in two contradictory ways simultaneously. It acts as a lethal agent on the one hand, and as an excitant and thereby sometimes a repellent on the other" (Kennedy, 1947).

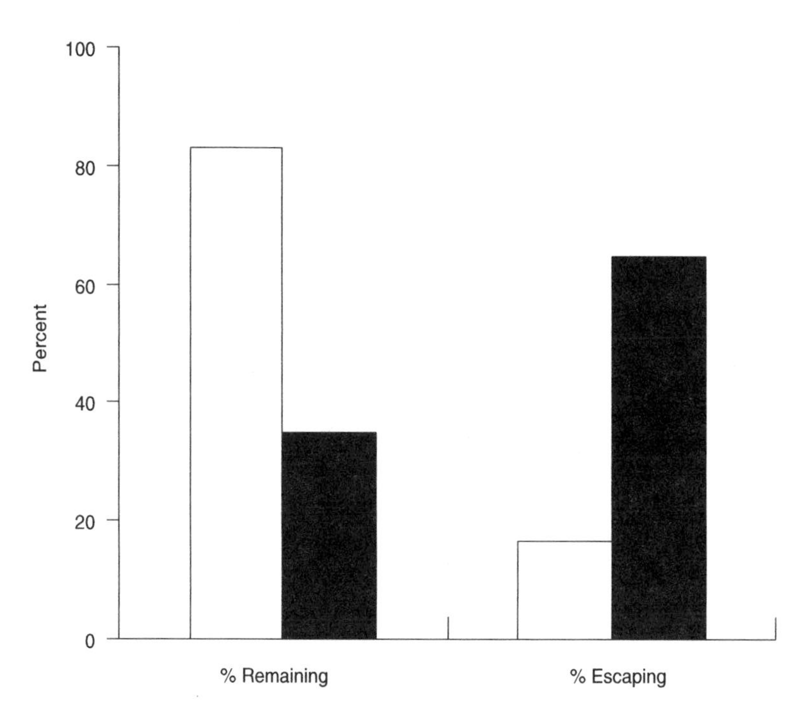

FIGURE 3-3 Percent of *Anopheles maculipennis atroparvus* females escaping from DDT-treated and untreated chambers in just three minutes post-exposure. Black bars represent data for DDT-treated chambers; white bars are for control chambers. Percent remaining accounts for those that did not immediately escape from the exposure chamber. SOURCE: Kennedy, 1947.

Kennedy's work was conducted at a time when Professor George Macdonald was establishing the mathematical foundations of malaria control. Kennedy commented on Macdonald's views:

> Macdonald (in discussion on Buxton, 1945, p. 394) was convinced that the reduction in anopheline infestation of sprayed rooms was due to actual destruction of mosquitoes and "not due to repellent effect, a point of extreme importance." His evidence was the presence of dead mosquitoes and the lack of any increase in the infestation of adjoining, untreated rooms. Nevertheless he remarked that there was no evidence of any reduction in such untreated rooms for which, as he said, "one might legitimately hope" in view of the passage of mosquitoes from room to room. The solution of this puzzle is surely that there was both destruction and repulsion of the mosquitoes (Kennedy, 1947).

Six years later, in 1953, Macdonald and Davidson published what became the founding principles for using insecticides in malaria control. Their analyses were based on field studies from 1947 to 1952. They did not cite Kennedy's paper and chemical actions favoring mosquito survival were characterized as undesirable. Macdonald and Davidson struggled valiantly to reconcile DDT's slow killing power with its spectacular ability to reduce malaria.

The authors knew of DDT's complex influence on vector behavior, as revealed in assessments that:

- "DDT was the most irritant of the three insecticides (DDT, BHC, and Dieldrin), and a very large proportion of the mosquitoes escaped its action."
- "The marked irritant properties of DDT were evident in all these treatments, the greater proportion, and sometimes as much as 90 per cent, of the mosquitoes being caught in the window traps."
- "The marked irritant effect of DDT on mosquitoes makes adequate dosage . . . imperative" (Macdonald and Davidson, 1953).

In the end, Macdonald and Davidson concluded that the answer to DDT's "irritant" action was to increase dosage so that mosquitoes would absorb a lethal dose before chemical repulsion. A surprising conclusion considering that Kennedy (1947) reported that ". . . excitation appears quickly, often in a matter of seconds after the insects are brought into contact with DDT . . ." (Kennedy, 1947).

One might wonder how Macdonald and Davidson, with their comprehensive knowledge of malaria, could so seriously err in understanding DDT's mode of action? In their defense, key elements of field data were missing, as revealed in their assessment that "In most, if not all, . . . entomological assessment of the efficiency of the insecticides has been based on records of the reduction in numbers of the daytime-resting population of treated shelters. No account has been taken of mosquitoes entering and leaving the shelters during the night" (Macdonald and Davidson, 1953).

Macdonald and Davidson stated that, of their tentative conclusions, "the one most clearly brought to light is that a considerable expansion of our knowledge is urgently needed—an expansion in the fields of basic theory, anopheline habits, the physical chemistry of insecticides, and their mode of action" (Macdonald and Davidson, 1953).

Unfortunately, rapid acceptance of their model virtually guaranteed that research and expansion of knowledge, particularly regarding chemical mode of action, would not occur. Macdonald and Davidson allowed that DDT killed mosquitoes that entered houses and reduced longevity of malaria vector populations below what is needed to maintain malaria transmission. Acceptance of this concept ended debate and support for research on DDT's mode of action. With preeminence of the idea that DDT reduced vector population longevity, Kennedy's research, and that of many others, was relegated to obscurity. The facts that DDT was a powerful repellent, a functional irritant, and only a slow-acting poison were ignored. Those facts have now been resurrected in the probability model, described above.

To fully appreciate the probability model, it is important to understand that insects have extraordinary abilities to detect and respond to chemicals; for example, certain species are capable of detecting a single molecule in 10^{17} molecules of air. Insects have developed these abilities as an adaptation to secondary chemicals that occur in nature. Plants and animals produce the so-called "secondary" chemicals to repel, deter, irritate, or poison herbivores, predators, and parasites (Schoonhoven, 1985). DDT is an organohalogen compound, and organohalogens are produced as secondary chemicals in nature (Gribble, 1999). The similarity of DDT to natural organohalogens is suggested by the finding that males of a species of euglossine bee are attracted to DDT and will travel to houses and collect DDT from sprayed walls (Roberts et al., 1982). The bees store (relative to their size) large amounts of DDT in hind tibial pouches and, remarkably, are not harmed. It is also worth noting that we now know that some natural organohalogens are persistent in the environment, are lipophilic, bioaccumulate, and may be present in greater abundance than synthetic compounds like DDT (Vetter et al., 2001). As a final point, winged adult insects can easily and rapidly move away from a poison (given that the chemical is not useful to the insect) and avoid the biological cost of premature death or metabolic detoxification.

When a malaria vector is inside a house it is exposed to human hosts, outdoors it is exposed to a variety of hosts. Thus, it is generally understood that malaria transmission becomes most efficient when vectors and humans come together inside the confined spaces of homes. When the vector is outside, it only has access to indirect human host stimuli emanating from inside the house. Once the vector is indoors, host proximity and unobstructed "view" of the human host (no intervening wall) alters the balance between factors that inhibit versus factors that stimulate a vector to bite. These factors and host availability influence probabilities of disease transmission.

By definition, a repellent action occurs when the mosquito is repelled without making physical contact with the chemical. In contrast, a mosquito is irritated only after making physical contact with a sprayed surface. Physical contact that results in an irritant response (escape response) can occur after very brief physical contact (as shown by Kennedy, 1947). A toxic action requires more prolonged physical contact with a sprayed surface (Roberts and Andre, 1994). The vector's actions, for example, moving to a house, entering the house, resting on walls, and biting, can be aligned sequentially with repellent actions that prevent house entering; irritant actions that promote premature exiting and prevent biting indoors; and toxic actions that produce mortality (Roberts et al., 2000).

We used the following notations to simulate interactions of repellent, irritant, and toxic actions of insecticides:

T: treatment house.
C: control house.
p_e: probability a mosquito will enter the house.
$p_{b|e}$: probability a mosquito will bite, given that it enters the house.
p_{be}: probability a mosquito will enter the house and bite indoors.
$p_{s|be}$: probability a mosquito survives, given that it entered the house and took a blood meal indoors.
p_{sbe}: probability a mosquito will enter the house, bite indoors, and survive.

Applying the multiplication law of probability (Rosner, 1995), we have the following equations

$$p_{be} = p_{b|e} \times p_e \quad (1)$$
$$p_{sbe} = p_{s|be} \times p_{b|e} \times p_e \quad (2)$$

As stated above, we assume that probabilities for different vector activities in the control house each equate to unity. This assumption leads to the relationship of $p_e^c = p_{b|e}^c = p_{s|be}^c = 1$ and implies that $p_e^c = p_{be}^c = p_{sbe}^c = 1$; see equations (1) and (2). The influence of insecticide on mosquito activities can be described as the probability difference between control and treatment for entering, biting, and surviving. For the act of entering the house, the probability difference is $1-p_e^t$; and for the biting and surviving, $1-p_{be}^t$

and, $1-p^t_{sbe}$ respectively. Actually, based on conditional probabilities, $1-p^t_e$ is the cumulative effect due to insecticide repellency, $1-p^t_{be}$ is the cumulative effect due to repellency plus irritancy, and $1-p^t_{sbe}$ is the cumulative effect due to repellency, irritancy, and toxicity. The probability of entering, p^t_e, can be estimated by

$$p^t_e = \frac{\text{Number entered sprayed house}}{\text{Number entered control house}}$$

Using comparative data from the control house, $p_{b|e}$ can be estimated by the observed proportion of mosquitoes that bite or become blood engorged within the treated house, and $p_{s|be}$ can be estimated by the observed proportion of mosquitoes that survived after they entered and fed in the treated house. To model field data, we would further adjust probabilities to account for natural differences in numbers collected in houses as a result of location differences.

Our simulations (formulas not presented) partitioned the total impact of a sprayed house by the percent of effect that can be attributed to each chemical action. Overall, the combined effects of repellent and irritant actions ($1-p^t_{be}$) did not drop below a cumulative level of 50 percent effectiveness until probabilities of entering and biting indoors were very high, p^t_e=> 0.7 and p^t_{be}=> 0.7 (i.e., almost no repellent or irritant action).

In experimental hut studies the repellent actions of DDT residues can function at levels above 90 percent compared to unsprayed huts (Grieco et al., 2000; Roberts et al., 2000). No repellent action was detected in a deltamethrin-sprayed hut, but a pronounced irritant action drove mosquitoes out of the deltamethrin-sprayed hut several hours before they exited the control hut. The combined message from model simulations and experimental hut studies is that DDT functions as a repellent, secondarily as an irritant, and lastly as a poison. In contrast, deltamethrin seems to function as an irritant and secondarily as a poison. These findings highlight a simple truth, an insecticide is just one more chemical in the mosquito's chemical world. The mosquito can detect and respond to an insecticide in many ways, perhaps the least likely being physical contact and death.

We have shown that repellent and irritant actions of DDT did not suddenly surface after decades of DDT use; but were actually recognized as major actions of DDT residues from the very start of DDT's use as a public health insecticide. In conclusion, funding agencies should formally recognize behavioral actions of vectors to insecticides as a priority area for future support.

REFERENCES

Amato I. 1993. The crusade against chlorine. *Science* 261:152–154.

Aronstein K, Ode P, ffrench-Constant RH. 1995. PCR based monitoring of specific *Drosophila (Diptera: Drosophilidae)* cyclodiene resistance alleles in the presence and absence of selection. *Bulletin of Entomological Research* 85:5–9.

Bermudez I, Hawkins CA, Taylor AM, Beadle DJ. 1991. Actions of insecticides on the insect GABA receptor complex. *Journal of Receptor Research* 11:221–232.

Bloomquist JR. 1994. Cyclodiene resistance at the insect GABA receptor chloride channel complex confers broad cross-resistance to convulsants and experimental phenylpyrazole insecticides. *Archives of Insect Biochemistry and Physiology* 26:69–79.

Brogdon WG and McAllister JC. 1998a. Simplification of adult mosquito bioassays through use of time-mortality determinations in glass bottles. *Journal of the American Mosquito Control Association* 14:159–164.

Brogdon WG and McAllister JC. 1998b. Insecticide resistance and vector control. *Emerging Infectious Diseases* 4:605–613.

Brogdon WG, Hobbs JH, St. Jean Y, Jacques JR, Charles LB. 1988. Microplate assay analysis of reduced fenitrothion susceptibility in Haitian *Anopheles albimanus. Journal of the American Mosquito Control Association* 4:152–158.

Brown AWA. 1986. Insecticide resistance in mosquitoes: a pragmatic review. *Journal of the American Mosquito Control Association* 2:123–140.

Brown AWA and Pal R. 1971. Insecticide resistance in arthropods. *WHO Monograph Series* 38.

Campbell PM, Newcomb RD, Russell RJ, Oakeshott JG. 1998. Two different amino acid substitutions in the ali-esterase, E3, confer alternative types of organophosphorus insecticide resistance in the sheep blowfly, *Lucilia cuprina. Insect Biochemistry and Molecular Biology* 28:139–150.

Chandre F, Darriet F, Darder M, Cuany A, Doannio JMC, Pasteur N, Guillet P. 1998. Pyrethroid resistance in *Culex quinquefasciatus* from West Africa. *Medical and Veterinary Entomology* 12:359–366.

Chosidow O, Chastang C, Brue C, Bouvet E, Izri M, Monteny N, Bastuji-Garin S, Rousset JJ, Revuz J. 1994. Controlled study of malathion and *d*-phenothrin lotions for *Pediculus humanus* var *capitis*-infested schoolchildren. *Lancet* 344:1724–1727.

Clark AG and Shamaan NA. 1984. Evidence that DDT-dehydrochlorinase from the house fly is a glutathione S-transferase. *Pesticide Biochemistry and Physiology* 22:249–261.

Clark AG, Dick GL, Martindale SM, Smith JN. 1985. Glutathione S-transferases from the New Zealand grass grub, *Costelytra zealandica. Insect Biochemistry* 15:35–44.

Clark AG, Shamaan NA, Dauterman WC, Hayaoka T. 1984. Characterization of multiple glutathione transferases from the housefly, *Musca domestica (L). Pesticide Biochemistry and Physiology* 22:51–59.

DeSilva D, Hemingway J, Ranson H, Vaughan A. 1997. Resistance to insecticides in insect vectors of disease: Estα3, a novel amplified esterase associated with estβ1s from insecticide resistant strains of the mosquito *Culex quinquefasciatus. Experimental Parasitology* 87:253–259.

Dombrowski SM, Krishnan R, Witte M, Maitra S, Diesing C, Waters LC, Ganguly R. 1998. Constitutive and barbital-induced expression of the CYP6A2 allele of a high producer strain of CYP6A2 in the genetic background of a low producer strain. *Gene* 221:69–77.

El-Sayed S, Hemingway J, Lane RP. 1989. Susceptibility baselines for DDT metabolism and related enzyme systems in the sandfly *Phlebotomus papatasi (Scopoli) (Diptera: Psychodidae). Bulletin of Entomological Research* 79:679–684.

Feyereisen R. 1995. Molecular biology of insecticide resistance. *Toxicology Letters* 82:83–90.

ffrench-Constant RH, Pittendrigh B, Vaughan A, Anthony N. 1998. Why are there so few resistance-associated mutations in insecticide target genes? *Philosophical Transactions of the Royal Society of London. Series B: Biological Sciences* 353:1685–1693.

Fine BC. 1963. The present status of resistance to pyrethroid insecticides. *Pyrethrum Post* 7:18–21.

Grant DF and Hammock BD. 1992. Genetic and molecular evidence for a trans-acting regulatory locus controlling glutathione S-transferase-2 expression in *Aedes aegypti. Molecular and General Genetics* 234:169–176.

Grant DF and Matsumura F. 1989. Glutathione S-transferase 1 and 2 in susceptible and insecticide resistant *Aedes aegypti. Pesticide Biochemistry and Physiology* 33:132–143.

Gribble GW. 1999. Chlorine—element from hell or gift from God? The scientific side of the chlorine story. *Technology* 6:193–201.

Grieco JP, Achee NL, Andre RG, Roberts DR. 2000. A comparison study of house entering and exiting behavior of *Anopheles vestitipennis (Diptera: Culicidae)* using experimental huts sprayed with DDT or deltamethrin in the southern district of Toledo, Belize, C.A. *Journal of Vector Ecology* 25:62–73.

Gubler DJ. 1998. Resurgent vector-borne diseases as a global health problem. *Emerging Infectious Diseases* 4:442–450.

Hemingway J. 1982. The biochemical nature of malathion resistance in *Anopheles stephensi* from Pakistan. *Pesticide Biochemistry and Physiology* 17:149–155.

Hemingway J. 1983. Biochemical studies on malathion resistance in *Anopheles arabiensis* from Sudan. *Transactions of the Royal Society of Tropical Medicine and Hygiene* 77:477–480.

Hemingway J. 1985. Malathion carboxylesterase enzymes in *Anopheles arabiensis* from Sudan. *Pesticide Biochemistry and Physiology* 23:309–313.

Hemingway J and Georghiou GP. 1983. Studies on the acetylcholinesterase of *Anopheles albimanus* resistant and susceptible to organophosphate and carbamate insecticides. *Pesticide Biochemistry and Physiology* 19:167–171.

Hemingway J and Karunaratne SH. 1998. Mosquito carboxylesterases: a review of the molecular biology and biochemistry of a major insecticide resistance mechanism. *Medical and Veterinary Entomology* 12:1–12.

Hemingway J and Ranson H. 2000. Insecticide resistance in insect vectors of human disease. *Annual Review of Entomology* 45:371–391.

Hemingway J, Boddington RG, Harris J, Dunbar SJ. 1989. Mechanisms of insecticide resistance in *Aedes aegypti (L.) (Diptera: Culicidae)* from Puerto Rico. *Bulletin of Entomological Research* 79:123–130.

Hemingway J, Callaghan A, Kurtak DC. 1991. Biochemical characterization of chlorphoxim resistance in adults and larvae of the *Simulium damnosum* complex (*Diptera: Simulidae*). *Bulletin of Entomological Research* 81:401–406.

Hemingway J, Hawkes N, Prapanthadara L, Jayawardena KG, Ranson H. 1998. The role of gene splicing, gene amplification and regulation in mosquito insecticide resistance. *Philosophical Transactions of the Royal Society of London. Series B: Biological Sciences* 353:1695–1699.

Hemingway J, Malcolm CA, Kissoon KE, Boddington RG, Curtis CF, Hill N. 1985. The biochemistry of insecticide resistance in *Anopheles sacharovi*: comparative studies with a range of insecticide susceptible and resistant *Anopheles* and *Culex* species. *Pesticide Biochemistry and Physiology* 24:68–76.

Hemingway J, Penilla RP, Rodriguez AD, James BM, Edge W, Rogers H, Rodriguez MH. 1997. Resistance management strategies in malaria vector mosquito control. A large scale field trial in Southern Mexico. *Pesticide Science* 51:375–382.

Herath PR, Hemingway J, Weerasinghe IS, Jayawardena KG. 1987. The detection and characterization of malathion resistance in field populations of *Anopheles culicifacies* B in Sri Lanka. *Pesticide Biochemistry and Physiology* 29:157–162.

Kadous AA, Ghiasuddin SM, Matsumura F, Scott JG, Tanaka K. 1983. Difference in the picrotoxinin receptor between the cyclodiene-resistant and susceptible strains of the German cockroach. *Pesticide Biochemistry and Physiology* 19:157–166.

Karunaratne SH, Hemingway J, Jayawardena KG, Dassanayaka V, Vaughan A. 1995. Kinetic and molecular differences in the amplified and non-amplified esterases from insecticide-resistant and susceptible *Culex quinquefasciatus* mosquitoes. *Journal of Biological Chemistry* 270:31124–31128.

Karunaratne SH, Vaughan A, Paton MG, Hemingway J. 1998. Amplification of a serine esterase gene is involved in insecticide resistance in Sri Lankan *Culex tritaeniorhynchus*. *Insect Molecular Biology* 7:307–315.

Kasai S, Weerasinghe IS, Shono T. 1998. P^{450} Monooxygenases are an important mechanism of permethrin resistance in *Culex quinquefasciatus* say larvae. *Archives of Insect Biochemistry and Physiology* 37:47–56.

Kennedy JS. 1947. The excitant and repellent effects on mosquitoes of sub-lethal contacts with DDT. *Bulletin of Entomological Research* 37:593–607.

Liu N and Scott JG. 1997. Inheritance of CYP6D1-mediated pyrethroid resistance in house fly (*Diptera: Muscidae*). *Journal of Economic Entomology* 90:1478–1481.

Macdonald G and Davidson G. 1953. Dose and cycle of insecticide applications in the control of malaria. *Bulletin of the World Health Organization* 9:785–812.

Maitra S, Dombrowski SM, Waters LC, Gunguly R. 1996. Three second chromosome-linked clustered CYP6 genes show differential constitutive and barbital-induced expression in DDT-resistant and susceptible strains *of Drosophila melanogaster*. *Gene* 180:165–171.

Malcolm CA and Boddington RG. 1989. Malathion resistance conferred by a carboxylesterase in *Anopheles culicifacies* Giles (Species B) (*Diptera: Culicidae*). *Bulletin of Entomological Research* 79:193–199.

Martinez-Torres D, Chandre F, Williamson MS, Darriet F, Berge JB, Devonshire AL, Guillet P, Pasteur N, Pauron D. 1998. Molecular characterization of pyrethroid knockdown resistance (*kdr*) in the major malaria vector *Anopheles gambiae s.s. Insect Molecular Biology* 7:179–184.

Metcalf CL, Flint WP, Metcalf RL. 1951. *Destructive and Useful Insects: Their Habits and Control*. New York: McGraw-Hill Book Company. P. 289.

Mouches C, Pasteur N, Berge JB, Hyrien O, Raymond M, de Saint Vincent BR, de Silvestri M, Georghiou GP. 1986. Amplification of an esterase gene is responsible for insecticide resistance in a Californian *Culex* mosquito. *Science* 233:778–780.

Mourya DT, Hemingway J, Leake CJ. 1993. Changes in enzyme titres with age in four geographical strains of *Aedes aegypti* and their association with insecticide resistance. *Medical and Veterinary Entomology* 7:11–16.

Mumcuoglu KY, Miller J, Uspensky I, Hemingway J, Klaus S, Ben-Ishai F, Galun R. 1995. Pyrethroid resistance in the head louse *Pediculus humanus capitis* from Israel. *Medical and Veterinary Entomology* 9:427–432.

Newcomb RD, Campbell PM, Russell RJ, Oakeshott JG. 1997. cDNA cloning, baculovirus-expression and kinetic properties of the esterase, E3, involved in organophosphorus resistance in *Lucilia cuprina*. *Insect Biochemistry and Molecular Biology* 27:15–25.

Penilla RP, Rodriguez AD, Hemingway J, Torres JL, Arredondo-Jimenez JI, Rodriguez MH. 1998. Resistance management strategies in malaria vector mosquito control. Baseline data for large scale field trial against *Anopheles albimanus* in Mexico. *Medical and Veterinary Entomology* 12:217–233.

Pittendrigh B, Aronstein K, Zinkovsky E, Andreev O, Campbell BC, Daly J, Trowell S, ffrench-Constant RH. 1997. Cytochrome P^{450} genes from *Helicoverpa armigera*: expression in a pyrethroid-susceptible and -resistant strain. *Insect Biochemistry and Molecular Biology* 27:507–512.

Prapanthadara L, Hemingway J, Ketterman AJ. 1993. Partial purification and characterization of glutathione S-transferase involved in DDT resistance from the mosquito *Anopheles gambiae. Pesticide Biochemistry and Physiology* 47:119–133.

Prapanthadara LA, Ranson H, Somboon P, Hemingway J. 1998. Cloning, expression and characterization of an insect class I glutathione S-transferase from *Anopheles dirus* species B. *Insect Biochemistry and Molecular Biology* 28:321–329.

ProMED-mail. 2002. *Dengue/DHF Update (13): 5 Apr 2002.* [Online]. Available: http://www.promedmail.org/pls/askus/wwv_flow.accept [accessed July 26, 2002].

Ranson H, Collins FH, Hemingway J. 1998. The role of alternative mRNA splicing in generating heterogeneity within the *Anopheles gambiae* class I glutathione S-transferase family. *Proceedings of the National Academy of Sciences* 95:14284–14289.

Raymond M, Callaghan A, Fort P, Pasteur N. 1991. Worldwide migration of amplified insecticide resistance genes in mosquitoes. *Nature* 350:151–153.

Roberts DR and Andre RG. 1994. Insecticide resistance issues in vector-borne disease control. *American Journal of Tropical Medicine and Hygiene* 50 (6 Suppl):21–34.

Roberts DR, Alecrim WD, Heller JM, Ehrhardt SR, Lima JB. 1982. Male *Eufriesia purpurata*, a DDT-collecting uglossine bee in Brazil. *Nature* 297:62–63.

Roberts DR, Alecrim WD, Hshieh P, Grieco JP, Bangs M, Andre RG, Chareonviriphap T. 2000. A probability model of vector behavior: effects of DDT repellency, irritancy, and toxicity in malaria control. *Journal of Vector Ecology* 25:48–61.

Roberts DR, Laughlin LL, Hshieh P, Legters LJ. 1997. DDT, global strategies, and a malaria control crisis in South America. *Emerging Infectious Diseases* 3:295–302.

Rosner B. 1995. *Fundamentals of Biostatistics.* Belmont, CA: Duxbury Press. P. 56.

Rupes V, Moravec J, Chmela J, Ledvidka J, Zelenkova J. 1994. A resistance of head lice (*Pediculus capitis*) to permethrin in Czech Republic. *Central European Journal of Public Health* 3:30–32.

Schoonhoven LM. 1985. Insects in a chemical world. In: Morgan ED, Mandava NB, eds. *Handbook of Natural Pesticides: Volume VI: Insect Attractants and Repellents.* Boca Raton, FL: CRC Press. Pp. 1–21.

Sina BJ and Aultman K. 2001. Resisting resistance. *Trends in Parasitology* 17:305–306.

Soderlund DM and Bloomquist JR. 1989. Neurotoxic action of pyrethroid insecticides. *Annual Review of Entomology* 34:77–96.

Tabashnik BE. 1989. Managing resistance with multiple pesticide tactics: theory, evidence and recommendations. *Journal of Economic Entomology* 82:1263–1269.

Thompson M, Shotkoski F, ffrench-Constant RH. 1993. Cloning and sequencing of the cyclodiene insecticide resistance gene from the yellow fever mosquito *Aedes aegypti. FEBS* 325:187–190.

Toung YS, Hsieh T, Tu CD. 1990. *Drosophila* glutathione S-transferase 1-1 shares a region of sequence homology with maize glutathione S-transferase III. *Proceedings of the National Academy of Sciences* 87:31–35.

Vatandoost H, McCaffery AR, Townson H. 1996. An electrophysiological investigation of target site insensitivity mechanisms in permethrin-resistant and susceptible strains of *Anopheles stephensi. Transactions of the Royal Society of Tropical Medicine and Hygiene* 90:216.

Vaughan A and Hemingway J. 1995. Mosquito carboxylesterase Est$\alpha 2^1$ (A2). Cloning and sequence of the full length cDNA for a major insecticide resistance gene worldwide in the mosquito *Culex quinquefasciatus. Journal of Biological Chemistry* 270:17044–17049.

Vaughan A, Hawkes N, Hemingway J. 1997. Co-amplification explains linkage disequilibrium of two mosquito esterase genes in insecticide-resistant *Culex quinquefasciatus*. *Biochemical Journal* 325:359–365.

Vaughan A, Rodriguez M, Hemingway J. 1995. The independent gene amplification of indistinguishable esterase B electromorphs from the insecticide resistant mosquito *Culex quinquefasciatus*. *Biochemical Journal* 305:651–658.

Vetter W, Scholz E, Gaus C, Muller JF, Haynes D. 2001. Anthropogenic and natural organohalogen compounds in blubber of dolphins and dugongs (*Dugong dugon*) from northeastern Australia. *Archives of Environmental Contamination and Toxicology* 41:221–231.

Vontas JG, Small GJ, Hemingway J. 2001. Glutathione S-transferases as antioxidant defence agents confer pyrethroid resistance in *Nilaparvata lugens*. *Biochemical Journal* 357:65–72.

Vulule JM, Beach RF, Atieli FK, Roberts JM, Mount DL, Mwangi RW. 1994. Reduced susceptibility of *Anopheles gambiae* to permethrin associated with the use of permethrin-impregnated bednets and curtains in Kenya. *Medical and Veterinary Entomology* 8:71–75.

WHO (World Health Organization). 1992. Vector resistance to pesticides. Fifteenth report of the Expert Committee on Vector Biology and Control. In: *WHO Technical Report Series* 818.

WHO. 1997. Onchocerciasis Control Programme in West Africa (OCP). [Online]. Available: http://www.who.int/ocp/ocp002.htm.

Whyard S, Downe AE, Walker VK. 1995. Characterization of a novel esterase conferring insecticide resistance in the mosquito *Culex tarsalis*. *Archives of Insect Biochemistry and Physiology* 29:329–342.

Williamson MS, Martinez-Torres D, Hick CA, Devonshire AL. 1996. Identification of mutations in the housefly para-type sodium channel gene associated with knockdown resistance (kdr) to pyrethroid insecticides. *Molecular and General Genetics* 252:51–60.

WWF (World Wildlife Fund). 1999. *Disease Vector Management for Public Health and Conservation*. Washington, DC: WWF. Pp. 1–10.

Xiao-Ping W and Hobbs AA. 1995. Isolation and sequence analysis of a cDNA clone for a pyrethroid inducible P450 from *Helicoverpa amrigera*. *Insect Biochemistry and Molecular Biology* 25:1001–1009.

4

The Economics of Resistance

OVERVIEW

Microbes that are resistant to therapeutic agents arise and proliferate at a rate that is far faster than is socially desirable because individuals, as well as governments and institutions, make choices that fail to recognize the cost that use of such agents (including their overuse and misuse) exacts on society. Cost and choice, of course, are the coins of the realm in economics. The focus of this session of the workshop was to examine how economics can help in developing innovative responses to the problem of antimicrobial resistance. Participants identified several important roles for economic analysis.

First, economics can provide purely descriptive analysis, quantifying the phenomena which are of interest, such as national expenditure on health care and how much antimicrobial resistance costs individual hospitals. This is the most basic level of analysis, but nonetheless important in providing foundational information on which further analysis is based, as well as providing information on the consequence of choices that have already been made.

In this regard, various economic analyses indicate that antimicrobial resistance greatly increases the cost of health care, in a variety of ways. For example, treating individuals with alternative drugs is nearly always much more expensive than conventional treatment with generic drugs. Also, patients infected with resistant microorganisms may require extra investigations and treatment, and for some patients a cascade of drugs will be tried before one is successful in eradicating the infection. The end result is longer and more expensive hospital stays. For the United States as a whole, the American Society for Microbiology estimated in 1995 that health care costs associated with treatment of resistant infections amounted to more than $4 billion annually. And this figure significantly underestimates the actual cost of resistance, since it includes only direct health care costs and excludes an array of other costs, such as lost lives and lost workdays. Moreover, these costs are expected to increase considerably given increasing rates of antimicrobial resistance.

In addition, economics can be used predictively to identify how changes in the health care system might affect the use of antimicrobial agents—and hence the emergence and spread of antimicrobial resistance. These analyses make use of descriptive data, together with conceptual models, to guide choices that are yet to be made.

Economics also can prove vital in developing specific strategies and policies to contain antimicrobial resistance. Key among current available strategies are regulation; charges (taxes) on the use of antimicrobials; and rights to trade (permits, licenses, or marketable property rights), which often are used in an attempt to combine the ease of regulation with the flexibility and efficiency of charges. To fill this role, however, the single biggest problem is lack of a comprehensive economic model for fully assessing the impact of antimicrobial resistance, as well as the cost and effectiveness of interventions to reduce the emergence and transmission of such resistance. Efforts are now under way to develop such a model. And while scientific and epidemiological development is vital, additional support also is required to advance understanding of the economics of resistance.

WHAT DOES ECONOMICS HAVE TO OFFER IN THE WAR AGAINST ANTIMICROBIAL RESISTANCE?

Richard D. Smith, M.Sc.

School of Medicine, Health Policy & Practice
University of East Anglia, Norwich, United Kingdom

"We may look back at the antibiotic era as just a passing phase in the history of medicine, an era when a great natural resource was squandered, and the bugs proved smarter than the scientists" (Cannon, 1995).

We begin the 21st century in a position of retreat against infectious disease, with the latter half of the 20th century in danger of being consigned to the history books as the time when a valuable new resource in this battle was both discovered and squandered.

"Superbugs," micro-organisms that have become resistant to the major therapies used to treat them, present a major threat to current and future medical advances (Neu, 1992; Murray, 1994; Tomasz, 1994). Resistant bacteria causing global concern include multi-drug-resistant *Mycobacterium tuberculosis*, penicillin-resistant *Streptococcus pneumoniae*, and methicillin-resistant *Staphylococcus aureus* (Neu, 1992; Tomasz, 1994; Cox et al., 1995). The effects of antimicrobial resistance (AMR) are documented in developed and developing nations alike, although arguably with greater potential for harm in the developing world, where many of the second- and third-line therapies for drug-resistant infections are unavailable, and many of the narrow spectrum antimicrobials available in the developed world are not affordable (Fasehun, 1999; Smith, 1999). However, despite increasing awareness, across both the medical (Levy, 2002) and lay communities (Cannon, 1995), of the rising prevalence of resistance, there is little evidence that the use of antimicrobials is changing.

The potential impact of this increasing antimicrobial resistance on health care expenditure and population morbidity and mortality is causing professional, government, and public concern (House of Lords Select Committee on Science and Technology, 1998; Standing Medical Advisory Committee Sub-Group on Antimicrobial Resistance, 1998; American Society for Microbiology, 1995; OTA, 1995; World Health Organization [WHO], 2001). Indeed, the United States considers the potentially destabilizing economic and social effects of antimicrobial resistance, as well as its potential in biological warfare, sufficient to classify antimicrobial resistance as a national security risk (Kaldec et al., 1997; CIA, 2000; World Bank, 2001).

The Discipline of Economics "in a Nutshell"

Economics is based on the fundamental premise that our resources (goods, services, time, raw materials, and all else that we use to make something else) are limited compared to what we want from them (which is virtually unlimited). On a personal level this means that one's time and wealth are limited compared to what we would like to be able to do. Nationally, this also applies, with national resources limited compared to what they could be used for. At all levels this means that choices have to be made. As individuals we have to choose whether to have a new car or holiday, or spend time working or playing golf. Nationally, we have to decide whether to have more health care, more education, more defense, or more consumer items. Economics then is fundamentally the study of *choice*.

However, there are other disciplines that study choice, such as psychology and sociology, so what makes economics special? The "angle" of economics is that choice is studied from the perspective of *efficiency*. That is, that economists study choices that can be (have been) made with a view to assessing whether the most benefit will be (was) gained from the resources used. What economics is fundamentally about then is quite simple: it is about assessing ways and means by which our choices, as individuals and nations, will lead to that allocation of resources amongst alternatives that will yield the most overall benefit. There are broader concerns than this of course, such as the equity of this resource allocation, but for the purposes of this paper, this simple definition provides the most important background to discussion.

Another important element of background to economics generally is the empirical manner in which economists approach the study of choice. Here there are three important categories of empirical activity, each of which will be considered in the paper with respect to the economic analysis of AMR.

First, economics may provide purely "descriptive" analysis, quantifying the phenomena which are of interest, such as national expenditure on health care, how much AMR costs a hospital, and so on. This is the most basic level of analysis, but nonetheless an important one in providing foundational information on which further analysis is based, as well as providing information on the consequence of choices that have already been made.

Second, economics may be used "predictively," identifying the impact of a change. For example, if health care expenditure rises, what will happen to physician income? How will user-charges for pharmaceuticals affect their use? These analyses make use of descriptive data, together with conceptual models, to guide choices that are yet to be made.

Third, economics may be used "evaluatively," suggesting whether one situation is "preferable," more efficient, to another; for example, whether national health insurance is better than private health insurance, competition between health care suppliers is more efficient or prevention is better than cure. Here, prediction is taken further to provide an assessment of what should be done if efficiency is to be maximized.

Economic Conceptualization of AMR

The use of antimicrobials can result in the unwanted "side effect" of the development of resistance. Economists conceptualize this side effect as a negative "externality" resulting from the consumption of antimicrobials. A negative externality refers to a situation where a cost is imposed on others not directly involved in the decision to produce or consume the commodity causing the pollution. A classic example of a negative externality is pollution, such as acid rain.

Antimicrobial resistance is an externality associated with the consumption of antimicrobials (as part of the production of health), and is a **negative** externality because it has adverse consequences for society as a whole (Phelps, 1989).

The form of the externality may be specified as:

$$E^R_t = f(A_t, X^i_t)$$

where E^R_t is the extent of the (negative) externality in time t, A_t is the quantity of antimicrobials consumed in time t, and X^i_t is a vector of other factors (e.g., background level of resistance, population mobility, and population density) which may determine the level of resistance in a community (Coast et al., 1998).

However, antimicrobials also have a positive impact, not just upon treated individuals, but also upon those individuals who would, in the absence of antimicrobials, have been infected by the treated individual. Thus, benefits from consumption include an improved outcome for the patient, reduced transmission of pathogens which would lead to disease in others, and a reduction in morbidity associated with sub-clinical infections which would otherwise be "accidentally" treated. The latter two benefits comprise a **positive** externality which results from taking antimicrobials. The format of this externality is:

$$E^P_t = f(A_t, E^R_t, X^i_t)$$

where E^P_t is the positive externality associated with reduced transmission and treatment of sub-clinical infections during time t, A_t is the quantity of antimicrobials used in time t, E^R_t (as before) is the extent of resistance in time t, and X^i_t is a vector of exogenous factors which might influence the positive externality. It is important to note the presence of E^R_t in this equation. This represents the fact that, as time progresses and resistance increases, the positive externality associated with reduced transmission may in itself be reduced.

Thus, the net benefit from antimicrobial usage in any period would therefore be:

$$NB^A_t = f(B_t, E^P_t, C_t, S_t, D_t, E^R_t, A_t, X^i_t)$$

where NB^A_t is the net benefit resulting from antimicrobial usage in time t, E^P_t, E^R_t, A_t, and X^i_t are defined as previously, B_t is the direct benefit to the patient of taking the antimicrobial, C_t is the drug plus administration cost, S_t is the cost associated with side effects, and D_t represents problems caused by difficulties in diagnosis.

There are several important implications arising from this conceptualization. First, the balance between costs and benefits, and negative and positive externalities, means that we are not seeking the eradication of AMR, but rather the *containment* of AMR to an "optimal" level. Important here is the balance struck between securing the best interests of the individual patient presenting with an infection, versus the global need for sustainable antimicrobial use to ensure that benefits of these drugs are available for others.

Second is the importance of this optimization over time. The negative externality of AMR occurs in time $t + 1$ as a result of the consumption of antimicrobials in time t. This time period may vary from days, to months, to years, to decades. However, it is undoubtedly the case that many of the major effects of resistance are likely to be incurred by future generations, and policy decisions will therefore have to weigh current costs and benefits against those occurring to future generations.

Third, there is the obvious implication that one needs to assess all the relevant costs and benefits (direct and externality) of antimicrobial use, and thus strategies to contain AMR, as well as other strategies not primarily aimed at AMR, but which will impact upon AMR. For example, changes in user charges or reimbursement systems may impact levels of AMR.

Applications of Economics to AMR

There are several areas where economics may be, or have been, applied in the context of AMR. Most significantly, these include:

1. Assessment of the cost of AMR, by country, institution (e.g., hospital), and disease;
2. Assessment of the cost-effectiveness of strategies to contain AMR, including new and existing antimicrobial therapies;
3. Assessment of the value of the (cost and) benefit of AMR containment over time; and
4. Development of specific economic strategies/policies to contain AMR.

Work in these areas is summarized briefly here.

Assessment of the Cost of AMR

It is relatively easy to point to some of the likely consequences of AMR (Smith et al., 1996). Patients infected with a resistant microorganism are less likely than those infected with a sensitive microorganism to recover from infection with the first antimicrobial used in treatment. Patients with resistant microorganisms may require extra investigations and treatment (usually more expensive), and for some patients a cascade of antimicrobial drugs will be tried before one is successful in eradicating the infection. This may result in longer hospital stays and longer periods of time away from work. Most seriously, of course, is that AMR will result in a greater likelihood of premature death. However, there has been little empirical research in this area, and estimates of the cost impact of AMR are therefore few and, inevitably, relatively crude.

For example, estimates of the cost of AMR by *country* have been largely limited to work in the United States. The American Society for Microbiology (1995) have estimated the annual health care costs associated with treatment of resistant infections in the United States at over $4 billion (equivalent to approximately 0.5 percent of U.S. health care costs). More recent estimates suggest that, for the United States, the continued rise in use of antimicrobials has resulted in current costs of more than $7 billion annually, with up to $4 billion used for the treatment of nosocomial infections due to AMR bacteria (John and Fishman, 1997).

Estimates by *institution* have also been few. For example, in the United Kingdom in 1989 a five-week outbreak of MRSA was estimated to have cost £12,935 (Mehtar et al., 1989), excluding the costs of additional or lost bed days. In 1995, the cost of containing an MRSA outbreak in a district general hospital was estimated to be greater than £400,000 (Cox et al., 1995).

Estimates by *disease* are similarly limited. For example, recent work in the area of multi-drug-resistant tuberculosis has suggested that resistance effectively doubles the cost of standard treatment for sensitive tuberculosis, from around $13,000 to $30,000 (Wilton et al., 2001).

However, it is likely that these costs are an underestimate of the total current costs of resistance (as they include only health care costs) and that such costs will increase considerably in the future. Further, although AMR has a significant impact on current health care expenditure and health of the population, it is the potential long-term impact that resistance, and, specifically, failure to tackle resistance, will have which is arguably of greatest concern.

Assessment of the Cost-Effectiveness of Strategies to Contain AMR

There are a variety of strategies which may address resistance, that may be categorized according to two dimensions.

First, in terms of their focus—whether the strategy aims to decrease the *transmission* of resistance among organisms, individuals, and the environment (e.g., hand-washing, restriction on travel) or whether it aims to prevent or reduce the emergence of resistance, largely focused upon the appropriate use, and reduction in the level of use, of antimicrobials (e.g., cycling of drugs in the hospital).

Second, in terms of the level at which the strategy is focused—whether the strategy focuses on the "micro" level of an individual institution, for example, a "closed" environment such as a hospital, or whether it is a "macro" strategy focused at the broader community level.

A recent systematic literature review of studies assessing the cost and/or effectiveness of interventions specifically aimed at reducing the emergence and transmission of AMR, found only 127 studies of moderate to good quality, of which 68 were effectiveness studies, 10 economic evaluations, 2 cost studies, and 2 modeling studies (Smith et al., 2001; Wilton et al., 2002). The main conclusions of this study were that most studies:

- are of poor methodological quality (i.e., at high risk of bias), which means that we cannot be confident of their results;
- are from developed nations (principally the United States), although this could be a function of the search strategy which was restricted to papers published in English, or of research funding;
- do not measure the impact on AMR in terms of costs, although this is not surprising as effectiveness studies always outnumber cost or cost-effectiveness studies;
- are micro (institution) not macro (community) strategies, which may be because the strategy is more "contained" and the costs and effects are more observable, compared with the more diffuse impacts of the macro interventions focused on the community, and also because often hospitals and other institutions have financial incentives to try to control resistance; and
- are concerned with transmission not emergence of AMR.

Assessment of the Value of the (Cost and) Benefit of AMR Containment over Time

The critical problem identified above is that although (macro) policies to contain emergence are likely to be optimal in the long term, (micro) policies to contain transmission are more likely to be rigorously evaluated. This is due to the problems caused by attempting to assess the costs and benefits of something which occurs now (i.e., reduced transmission has immediate and obvious effects) versus something which will occur in the future (i.e., reduced emergence has effects that will not be seen until sometime hence). This time-lag with containing emergence causes two main problems: (i) uncertainty with respect to effects occurring in the future; and (ii) discounting of costs and benefits in the future may result in such benefits being given lower weight than equivalent benefits now. This means that there is a potential bias both against evaluating strategies aimed at emergence and in the cost-effectiveness result (Coast et al., 1996; Coast et al., 2002).

The issue of uncertainty can be addressed through the use of modeling, but really needs improved clinical and epidemiological evidence for the relevant relationships over time. The issue of discounting and time preference might be dealt with either through use of a zero discount rate, or perhaps through direct assessment of "option value." That is, people may be willing to trade increases in morbidity, inconvenience, and cost incurred through reducing consumption of antimicrobials now in return for the option to consume them in the future. That is, maintain the effectiveness of treatment in case it is required in the future, at the expense of reduced use now, even if they do not in practice use them. Thus there may be a value attached to maintaining the option to benefit from antimicrobials in the future which would not be captured by valuations of the health impacts of different policies alone.

Development of Specific Economic Strategies/Policies to Contain AMR

The conceptualization of AMR as a negative externality allows the consideration of economic strategies (i.e., strategies designed to change incentive structures) developed to deal with similar instances of negative externalities in other areas. Key among these strategies are regulation, charges, and rights to trade. Each of these has been outlined in detail elsewhere (Coast et al., 1998; Smith and Coast, 1998), but a summary is provided below.

Regulation is the most obvious means of controlling the production of a negative externality, through control of the quantity produced (Turner et al., 1994; Hodge, 1995). However, although it is relatively easy to introduce and administer, it is less efficient than policies relying on price-based incentives, with evidence that regulation imposes considerable excess costs over these other policies (Tietenberg, 1990). In terms of AMR, the focus would be either on limiting the use of antimicrobials for particular types of patients or, alternatively, limiting the total supply of antimicrobials available to doctors for prescription to their patients. Issues arising in this would include heterogeneity of patients, enforcement (e.g., ensuring physicians were following the explicit rules about who should, and who should not, receive antimicrobial treatment), and cost of enforcement.

Charges, or taxes, on use of antimicrobials should, on the basis of economic theory, provide an efficient means of containing AMR, whereby the charge equates to the marginal external cost imposed. However, in practice, this is difficult to achieve because government would need information about this marginal external cost (Pearce and Turner, 1990). Application of charges on the basis of levels of AMR would almost certainly be impractical, and would be more likely to be levied on the consumption of antimicrobials, as a proxy for the generation of AMR. These products are easily identifiable, and the application of a charge relating to each antimicrobial would be relatively simple. The key issue then is who will pay this charge—the patient, the prescriber, or the manufacturer? In each case there would be implications for the effectiveness of the policy and equity of impact of any system of charges.

Rights to trade (permits, licenses, or marketable property rights) are used to try to combine the ease of regulation and flexibility and efficiency of charges. Here the total quantity is limited, but each consumer/producer may utilize any quantity up to that limit through the trade of that limited quantity. Thus, it uses regulation to set the overall level, and then the price mechanism to distribute that total most efficiently. This is a common method in the environment, such as for trading sulfur dioxide pollution (Winebrake et al., 1995) or fishery quotas (Turner et al., 1994), and has been proposed in the area of AMR (Smith and Coast, 1998).

What Does Economics Have to Offer in the War Against AMR?

As alluded to in this short paper, economics as a discipline has much to offer under three broad classifications.

Conceptualization of Problem

The economic conceptualization of AMR as a negative externality was highlighted. By concentrating upon efficiency—maximizing benefits for given resources—economists seek to determine the optimal rate at which resistance should be allowed to develop, balancing the costs and benefits of antimicrobial usage over time. This approach stresses, first, the importance of *optimization* and balance in the use of antimicrobial products, and thus in the level of AMR which exists, rather than eradication of AMR, and, second, the importance of this optimization and balance being one to be struck over *time*: that the balance is really against the (costs and benefits of) use of antimicrobial treatments now and their continued availability for use in the future.

Informing the policy options for the containment of AMR will thus require information relevant to these issues. The assessment of costs and benefits is discussed below, but the assessment of balance over time requires information about the development of new and/or alternative products to those currently being used, which is largely outside the sphere of economics, but also the perceptions of the public on their willingness to trade current use and future availability. This is important, as it is the public who will be asked to forego some beneficial treatment if we are to constrain use of these treatments. There is much work to be done, therefore, on the assessment of "time preference" and discount rates used in economic analysis.

Technical Analysis

Economics can also assist with the development of an explicit basis for policy, through not only assessment of time preference rates, but also assessment of costs and benefits, and use of modeling to analyze the impact of a variety of policy options across various time periods.

A comprehensive economic model enabling assessment of the potential cost and impact of AMR containment strategies, and interventions upon antimicrobial use and AMR, is vital to the long-term management of antimicrobial use in two ways. First, it will enable estimates of the costs of resistance to be incorporated into economic evaluations of new antimicrobials, or other interventions, affecting AMR. In the absence of such information, current economic evaluations are mis-specifying the true cost of antimicrobial usage. Second, a model assessing the optimal use of antimicrobial drugs is essential for evaluating viable policy alternatives and prioritizing resource allocation between them.

However, the single biggest problem faced in the assessment of the economic impact of AMR, and the assessment of the cost and effectiveness of interventions to reduce the emergence and transmission of AMR, is the lack of a coherent and comprehensive economic model of AMR, although, together with colleagues, the author is currently seeking to develop one.

Strategies

Medical literature and research tends to focus on physical methods of reducing the transmission or emergence of resistance, such as through improved hygiene (for example, hand washing) or the cycling of antimicrobial treatments. Within economics, the focus tends to be upon developing policy responses which "internalize" the externality of resistance. In relation to antimicrobial resistance, this would mean, for example, providing incentives for consumers, prescribers, and/or producers to take account of the possible "externality" costs of the consumption of antimicrobials to society. Although work in this area has, to date, been relatively limited, there has been some discussion of policy instruments such as taxation and transferable permit markets, and a more extensive assessment of how such a permits system might operate in the United Kingdom (Smith and Coast, 1998).

A further consideration is the containment of AMR, on a global level, and the increasing interconnectedness of AMR meaning that no one country is likely to provide an effective policy response without considering the actions of neighboring countries. This has been considered from an economics perspective both within the "WHO Global Strategy for the Containment of AMR," and more specifically with respect to the concept of "Global Public Goods" for health (Smith and Coast, 2001; 2002; in press).

Conclusion

Although further developments are undoubtedly required, economics can assist in clarifying the basis for policy development, can identify and develop policy options and, through the assessment of the cost and benefits of alternative options, can help to recognize optimal policy solutions. Although scientific and epidemiological development is vital, support is also required for development of the economics of resistance.

ECONOMIC INSTRUMENTS FOR THE CONTROL OF ANTIMICROBIAL RESISTANCE

William Jack, D.Phil.

Department of Economics, Georgetown University, Washington, DC

The mechanisms that govern the evolution of resistance of pathogens are subtle and complicated, depending on the individual- and population-level characteristics of the organisms and the interventions. These mechanisms can be studied, understood, and hopefully improved through scientific analysis. There is widespread agreement however, that a further determinant of the evolution of resistance is the behavior of the human host. Microeconomics—the study of the way people choose amongst alternatives—can provide a vehicle for understanding the behavior of people in disease environments, and hopefully (again) lead to suitable interventions to help control resistance.

A first question that can be posed is what outcome, in terms of drug resistance, is desired in a particular circumstance. Using economic language, it is possible to think of an existing drug as a capital asset—one that provides a flow of services over time, like a machine. Machines tend to run down as they are used more, and if they are used unwisely. Of course, one way of keeping a machine in good condition is to leave it unused. The extent to which one would want to allow depreciation of the physical asset depends crucially on how easy it is to replace it, or to innovate and make a better one.

Similarly, drugs can become less effective as they are used more, and if they are used unwisely. And drug resistance can be halted by discontinuing all drug therapy. Where to make the trade-off depends, as with a capital asset, on how easy it is to replace the drug, and on how likely a more effective intervention is to become available.

This qualitative similarity between physical equipment and drugs can help rationalize public interventions aimed at affecting drug use. The underlying reason that there is a potential role for government aimed at controlling drug use is that, while we expect individuals to have appropriate incentives to "wisely use" their physical assets, there are reasons to expect them to (rationally) overuse drug therapies. The simple reason is that the costs of overuse by one person are borne by all other individuals who might one day need the drug, while the costs of running a machine into the ground are borne primarily by the owner of that machine. Another way of saying this is that an effective drug has some of the characteristics of what economists call a public good, incentives for the maintenance of which might be attenuated at the individual level.

Societies respond to public good problems by sometimes agreeing to limit the use of a resource. Thus, numerous international agreements concerning, for example, fisheries, aim to limit the amount each nation will exploit a reserve, given that individually rational behavior would lead to depletion that is too rapid. Economists also like to rely on the price mechanism (as opposed to quotas) to implement such contractions in use, for example by levying a tax on use. In international settings, deciding which body collects (and keeps) the revenue from such taxes is politically dicey, and quotas are often employed instead.[1]

When dealing with a large population of individuals using drugs, the price mechanism seems to have important advantages over quotas. For one thing, many individuals will not need to use the drug, so allocating a fixed number of units to them, and the same number to an individual in dire need, is inefficient. On the other hand, trying to pick the right number to allocate to each person as a function of his/her health status could quickly become hopelessly complicated. "Getting the price right" is a potentially more fruitful approach.

That, at least, is the theory. The problem with this story is that it assumes that resistance is caused simply by overuse. However, there are two margins on which decisions are made by individuals (and their doctors) regarding drug use: the number of treatments (e.g., the number of prescriptions filled), and the extent to which the treatment is completed. In richer

[1]For a formal model of the trade-off between using prices and quotas, see Weitzman (1974).

countries, drug resistance is blamed in part on excessive prescribing behavior, but in poorer parts of the world, incomplete treatment and/or inappropriate self-medication with readily available, cheap, but often ineffective generic old-line therapies is often identified as the culprit.

Decisions on both of these margins could be controlled if it were possible to charge a certain price for a prescription, and a separate price for use of the drug. Other things being equal, we would want to set the first price on the high side, so as to reduce the number of prescriptions, and the second price on the low side, so as to encourage completion of the course. However, if only a single price instrument is available (e.g., the prescription charge), then raising it will tend to reduce both the number of prescriptions (which is good for controlling use and resistance), *and* the likelihood that an individual will complete a course (which is bad for controlling resistance). The reason that increasing the prescription price may reduce completion rates is that individuals who expect to contract the illness again will have an incentive to save some of the medication as a contingency against such an event. The higher the price of getting a new prescription in the future, the greater this incentive will be.

The net effect of a price increase on resistance is thus ambiguous. Indeed, it is possible that *reducing* the prescription charge could reduce the rate at which the drug became ineffective. If the two effects happen to offset each other exactly, the optimum tax would be zero. That is, it might be best to leave the price unchanged.

The impact of prescription charges on completion rates is likely to be more prevalent in environments where the likelihood of reinfection is higher, and for drugs that are more easily storable. One interesting implication of this is that it might be desirable to design therapies that depreciate quickly once a course is begun, thus lowering the value of saving some of the medication for future use. The trouble with such a policy is that it might also reduce the shelf-life of the drug before treatment, thus making it difficult for clinics and hospitals to manage their pharmaceutical stocks. These concerns would seem to be particularly relevant in developing countries, where, also, the chance of reinfection is typically higher.

Instead of relying on price instruments alone, WHO has addressed the problem of incomplete treatment of tuberculosis by developing and advocating the use of the DOTS (directly observed treatment [short course]) protocol. Individuals are induced to complete the course of medication not by being charged a low price per pill (conditional on obtaining a prescription), but by being directly monitored and encouraged by an outside agent. This kind of intervention is expensive, however, in terms of the labor costs incurred by the monitoring agent.

Finally, the issue of equity must be addressed in the context of contemplating price increases. To a first approximation, in order to correct a market imperfection associated with overuse, the same price increase should apply to all individuals, simply because it is aggregate use that affects resistance and needs to be controlled, not use by say the rich or the poor.[2] Policies that relate charges to income exist in other cases however: for example, in some countries (e.g., Sweden), speeding tickets, which presumably are meant to reduce the amount of speeding, are sometimes proportional to an individual's income.[3]

This prescription of uniform pricing is appropriate either if the distribution of income and well-being in society is of little concern to policy makers, or if that distribution can be improved through direct income transfers and other poverty alleviation programs. The institutional capacity to implement such transfers and programs in poor countries may be sufficiently weak however, that exempting the poor from higher prices may be attractive. Of course, such an exemption policy in itself will require a level of institutional capacity and targeting capability that may be beyond the reach of some countries. Applying different taxes to drug sales in urban and rural areas might represent a very blunt instrument to effect an appropriate targeting policy, but the possibility of resale and trade between rural and urban centers would weaken the implementability of such a scheme.

ECONOMIC RESPONSES TO THE PROBLEM OF DRUG RESISTANCE

*Ramanan Laxminarayan, Ph.D., M.P.H.**

Resources for the Future, Washington, DC

The increasing resistance of bacteria to antibiotics is a consequence of selection pressure placed by the use of antibiotics on susceptible organisms to the benefit of resistant organisms. Addressed as a behavioral problem, resistance is, at least in part, a consequence of missing economic incentives. Resistant bacteria arise and proliferate at a rate faster than is socially desirable because individuals fail to recognize the cost imposed by their use

---

[2]This argument might need to be adjusted when resistance follows a spatial pattern, and when the rich and the poor tend to live in separate areas. However, the tax is related to income in such cases only because of the correlation between the size of the distortion and income, not because income per se determines the appropriate price increase.

[3]Although this may appear efficient (because it takes a higher fine to stop a rich person speeding than to stop a poor person), if the objective is to reduce total speeding, and not any particular person's, it would be better to levy a fee independent of income.

*This paper is based on Laxminarayan, 2002, where the interested reader will find a more complete discussion and references.

or misuse of antibiotics on the rest of society. For this reason, economists are often asked what they bring to the table in terms of innovative responses to the problem of resistance. Broadly speaking, there are two fronts along which we can consider strategies to counter drug resistance, and economics can help on both. First, we can manage our existing arsenal of drugs and antibiotics carefully so as to maximize the value derived from their use by intervening on the demand side of the antibiotics market. Second, we can develop (or encourage the development of) new drugs and pesticides that could replace old products that resistance has rendered ineffective by intervening on the supply side.[4]

On the demand side, measures to encourage more efficient antibiotic use include both price and non-price measures. Price measures involve increasing the cost of antibiotics for patients to discourage their use. Non-price measures include patient counseling on the societal effects of antibiotic use, physician education, and so forth. These could also include measures to encourage the use of an economically efficient variety of drugs.

On the supply side, measures to address the resistance problem would include incentives that not only encourage drug firms to develop new antibiotics, but also give them a greater incentive to care about the impact of drug resistance. We discuss each of these measures in turn.

Intervening on the Demand Side

Price Measures

The most reliable axiom in economics is that as the price of any commodity goes up, the quantity of that commodity that people will consume declines, all else being equal. Therefore, if our objective is to reduce the use of antibiotics, then the most reliable way of doing so without second-guessing physicians' decision-making is by raising the cost of using antibiotics to the patient. One solution might be to impose a tax on antibiotics. However, a tax may be undesirable for two reasons. First, a tax may not discourage antibiotic use if insurance coverage shields many patients from drug costs and physicians are relatively insensitive to these costs. Second, the burden of a tax may be disproportionately borne by poorer patients

---

[4]These two strategies are linked in a very intricate way. Our efforts to better manage resistance to existing products could reduce the returns to investment in new products. So, paradoxically, the evolution of resistance may create a demand for new products, which in turn leads to greater investment in research and development. Conversely, the greater availability of new products may increase variety of products that we have available and this may help us make better use of existing products.

who are less likely to have health insurance to cover the cost of antibiotic prescriptions.

A logical alternative would be to mandate an increase in the extent of cost-sharing for antibiotics. This could be accomplished by increasing co-payments for antibiotic prescriptions for certain conditions where a regulatory or scientific body believes that antibiotics are overprescribed (such as for the treatment of ear infections).[5] Such a measure would not hurt the majority of economically disadvantaged patients who currently lack prescription drug coverage, but would effectively tax antibiotic use. Figure 4-1 shows how an increase in the cost-share borne by patients would decrease the quantity of antibiotics consumed from Q_1 to Q_2.

Empirical evidence on the effect of cost-sharing on antibiotic use is limited but consistent. For instance, a large randomized study conducted in 1985 showed that people who received free medical care used 85 percent more antibiotics than those required to pay for at least some portion of their medical care (Foxman et al., 1987). However, the same study found that cost-sharing was likely to equally reduce both appropriate as well as inappropriate antibiotic use.

To be sure, a price-based policy intervention is a blunt instrument, and may, in some instances, discourage the use of antibiotics even when their use is justified. However, targeted cost-sharing efforts aimed at certain diagnoses may be preferable to an across-the-board increase in mandatory cost-sharing for all antibiotics. Increased cost-sharing for antibiotics, or other methods of raising the cost of antibiotics to the patient may not be popular. However, short of direct case-by-case oversight of antibiotic prescriptions, there are few other alternative strategies that can effectively lower antibiotic use. Policy makers in the antibiotic resistance arena would do well to learn from the use of tobacco taxes in the United States. The tremendous success of higher tobacco taxes on lowering smoking in this and other countries is self-evident.

Non-Price Measures

While price measures could be effective in lowering antibiotic use, their effectiveness may be enhanced when used in combination with non-price measures as part of an overall strategy to fight resistance. Increasing patient awareness of the drawbacks of antibiotic use and improving physician education could promote judicious antibiotic use; much has been written

---

[5]Some economists have proposed tradable permits for resistance that would work in much the same way as tradable permits for pollution. While these may be economically efficient, they may be difficult to implement in a largely private health care system such as the one in the United States.

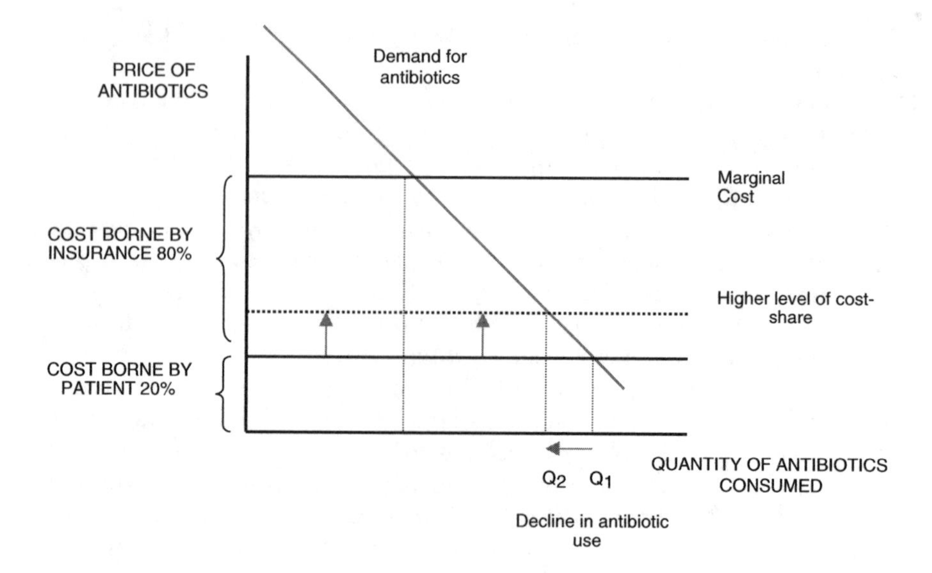

FIGURE 4-1 Increasing share of costs borne by patients decreases the quantity of antibiotics consumed from Q_1 to Q_2.

about these interventions and therefore these topics are not covered in this paper. Non-price measures could also include other innovative strategies, such as increasing treatment heterogeneity, that have received relatively less attention from the public health and medical communities. Treatment heterogeneity refers to the policy option of treating different patients afflicted with the same disease with antibiotics that have unrelated modes of action.

The rationale for treatment heterogeneity follows from the notion that the likelihood that bacteria will develop resistance to any single antibiotic can be reduced by treating fewer patients with that antibiotic. This is achieved by using a larger variety of antibiotics (Laxminarayan and Weitzman, 2002). Variety reduces the selection pressure for resistance to evolve to any single drug class. However, one is struck by the degree of homogeneity in antibiotic treatment, a fact that is attributable to industry concentration, uniform treatment guidelines, and to some extent, emphasis on providing the safest, and most cost-effective treatment to all patients. For instance, in 1997, nearly 60 percent of all cases of acute otitis media in the United States were treated with amoxicillin (Laxminarayan et al., 1998).[6] In fact, an earlier study found that in 1992, amoxicillin accounted

[6]This level of market concentration is remarkable considering the $240 million market for antibiotics for this condition alone.

for 39 percent of *all* antibiotics prescribed in the United States, and the five most commonly used antibiotics accounted for 80 percent of *all* antibiotics prescribed (McCaig and Hughes, 1995). The degree of treatment uniformity is even more striking in infectious disease treatment in the developing world. In most African countries, chloroquine has been the most commonly used drug to treat malaria for more than five decades.

To the extent that most patients in a region or country are treated with the same drug for a given infectious disease, the use of a single drug places excessively high selection pressure on organisms that are susceptible to that particular drug and increases the likelihood that a resistant strain will evolve and proliferate. As resistance to the recommended first-line drug builds up, that drug is replaced by an alternative that is used until resistance to this second drug also increases, and so on in succession. Therefore, the optimal solution may be to use not just a *single* drug throughout the population as first-line agent, but to prescribe a variety of drugs, randomized over patients, to ensure that inordinate selection pressure is not placed on any single drug, or class of drugs.

The notion that there is a single cost-effective treatment for an infectious disease fails to consider the effect of homogenous drug use on the evolution of resistance. Consequently, the standard cost-effectiveness method may lead to flawed conclusions in the case of drugs such as antibiotics and anti-malarials since it has no way of capturing the notion that using the same drug on all patients may be undesirable from a societal perspective. Encouraging treatment heterogeneity may not require any specific policy beyond issuing treatment guidelines that recognize this aspect of infectious disease treatment. There may be sufficient heterogeneity in physicians' preferences and patients' willingness to pay that will bring about sufficient variation in drug choice. However, treatment heterogeneity necessarily requires the availability of a variety of drugs, and this may require regulatory intervention.

Supply Side

While increasing treatment heterogeneity and lowering the demand for unnecessary antibiotics through both price and non-price measures comprise one side of the solution, the other side deals with increasing incentives for pharmaceutical firms to increase research spending on new antibiotics as well as to care about resistance to existing drugs.

The fundamental policy objective is not just to increase incentives for firms to develop and introduce *any* new antibiotics, but to specifically develop new products or classes of antibiotics that are significantly different from existing ones in their mechanisms of action. This minimizes the common property problem that arises when different firms make products with similar modes of action and, consequently, no single firm has sufficient incentive to care about declining product effectiveness. If one were to use the analogy of thinking about product effectiveness as a resource, like oil for instance, then an optimal policy would encourage drug firms to search for new "wells" of effectiveness against bacteria, rather than to drill new wells to extract existing reserves, thereby competing with other producers. Given this latter criterion, standard policy solutions such as research investment tax credits, and longer-duration patents may not solve the problem of incentives.

One policy option that may address this problem is to extend patent breadth (or scope) for antibiotics as a way of encouraging innovation. To be sure, this is a more difficult policy to implement. While patent lengths can be easily extended by legislative action or administrative fiat, patent breadths are more difficult to change. Patent offices are reluctant to alter the rules that guide their decisions. However, one might argue that there are few, if any, innovations that are in need of such alterations to patent breadth. Under this proposed policy, the scope of antibiotics patents could be increased so they cover an entire class of compounds and preempt "me too" antibiotics that increase competition for the same mechanism of action. This may be a good idea for three reasons.

First, increasing patent scope gives firms an incentive to care about the evolution of resistance since the firm owning the patent would have nearly complete control over the stock of effectiveness. The common property problem arises with antibiotics because different firms sell similar antibiotics with similar modes of action, and no firm bears the full resistance cost of its production decisions. Indeed, the quantity of antibiotics sold is only one factor, albeit an important one, that influences the growth of resistance. For instance, the care that a drug firm might take in selecting the indications that an antibiotic will be marketed for can play an important role in influencing the growth in resistance. These and other strategies to reduce resistance are more likely to be employed by a firm if it has a broader patent on the antibiotic, and is likely to reap the benefits of sustained effectiveness to a greater extent.

Second, increasing breadth would dramatically increase the returns from investing in new compounds rather than just tinkering with existing compounds. The returns from new discoveries would dramatically increase since the innovator will have broad rights over the newly innovated class of antibiotics rather than just the narrow chemical entity. The third reason for increasing patent breadth is that we attain the basic objective of focusing new drug research on increasing the variety of modes of action of antibiotics. Variety has social value that is not fully compensated for in the current market for antibiotics, and increasing patent breadths would encourage variety (Ellison and Hellerstein, 1999).

There are drawbacks of broader patent scope for antibiotics that would need to be considered as well. First, increasing the allowable breadth of antibiotics patents increases the social welfare costs associated with greater imperfect competition. Second, broader patents may discourage potentially valuable innovations such as new drugs that are closely related to existing antibiotics, but which are easier to administer and have fewer side-effects. These drawbacks should be addressed by other policies where possible, and balanced against the benefits of broader patents.

Recommendations

- The problem of reducing inappropriate antibiotic use calls for a combination of price and non-price measures. The appropriate mix will have to be tailored to the particular cultural and medical context. Patient and physician education, better surveillance data, increasing antibiotic heterogeneity, providing warning labels on antibiotics are all part of the policy response mix. However, they are likely to be ineffective without a compelling economic incentive for patients and physicians to face the cost they impose on the rest of society in the form of resistance when they use or misuse antibiotics.
- While lowering the demand for antibiotics is one part of the solution, further research should also look at incentives faced by pharmaceutical firms with respect to research and development expenditure on new classes of antibiotics, as well as resistance to existing products.

REFERENCES

American Society for Microbiology. 1995. Report of the ASM task force on antibiotic resistance. *Antimicrobial Agents and Chemotherapy* Supplement:1–23.

Cannon G. 1995. *Superbug. Nature's revenge*. London: Virgin Publishing. P. 189.

CIA (Central Intelligence Agency). 2000. *The Global Infectious Disease Threat and Its Implications for the United States*. [Online]. Available: http://www.odci.gov/nic/graphics/infectiousdiseases.pdf.

Coast J and Smith RD. 2001. Antimicrobial resistance: can economics help? *Eurohealth* 7:32–33.

Coast J, Smith RD, Karcher AM, Wilton P, Millar M. 2002. Superbugs II: How should economic evaluation be conducted for interventions which aim to reduce antimicrobial resistance? *Health Economics* 11:637–647.

Coast J, Smith R, Millar MR. 1996. Superbugs: should antimicrobial resistance be included as a cost in economic evaluation? *Health Economics* 5:217–226.

Coast J, Smith RD, Millar MR. 1998. An economic perspective on policy antimicrobial resistance. *Social Science and Medicine* 46:29–38.

Cox RA, Conquest C, Mallaghan C, Marples RR. 1995. A major outbreak of methicillin-resistant *Staphylococcus aureus* caused by a new phage-type (EMRSA-16). *Journal of Hospital Infection* 29:87–106.

Ellison SF and Hellerstein J. 1999. The economics of antibiotics: an exploratory study. In: Triplett JE, ed. *Measuring the Prices of Medical Treatment*. Washington, DC: Brookings Institution Press. Pp. 118–151.

Fasehun F. 1999. The antibacterial paradox: essential drugs, effectiveness and cost. *Bulletin of the World Health Organization* 77:211–216.

Foxman B, Valdez RB, Lohr KN, Goldberg GA, Newhouse JP, Brook RH. 1987. The effect of cost sharing on the use of antibiotics in ambulatory care: results from a population-based randomized controlled trial. *Journal of Chronic Diseases* 40:429–437.

Hodge I. 1995. *Environmental Economics*. Basingstoke, UK: MacMillan.

House of Lords Select Committee on Science and Technology. 1998. *Seventh Report*. [Online]. Available: http://www.parliament.the-stationery-office.co.uk/pa/ld199798/ldselect/ldsctech/081vii/st0701.htm.

John J and Fishman NO. 1997. Programmatic role of the infectious diseases physician in controlling antimicrobial costs in the hospital. *Clinical Infectious Diseases* 24:471–485.

Kaldec R, Zelicoff A, Vrtis A. 1997. Biological weapons control: prospects and implications for the future. *Journal of the American Medical Association* 278:351–356.

Laxminarayan R, ed. 2002. *Battling Resistance to Antibiotics and Pesticides: An Economic Approach*. Washington, DC: Resources for the Future Press.

Laxminarayan R and Weitzman ML. 2002. On the implications of endogenous resistance to medications. *Journal of Health Economics* 21:709–718.

Laxminarayan R, Jernigan DB, et al. 1998. *Using Antibiotic Resistance Surveillance Data in the Optimal Treatment of Acute Otitis Media*. Paper presented at the Infectious Diseases Society of America 36th Annual Meeting, Denver.

Levy S. 2002. *The Antibiotic Paradox. How the Misuse of Antibiotics Destroys Their Curative Powers*. Cambridge, MA: Perseus Publishing.

McCaig LF and Hughes JM. 1995. Trends in antimicrobial drug prescribing among office-based physicians in the United States. *Journal of the American Medical Association* 273:214–219.

Mehtar S, Drabu YJ, Mayet F. 1989. Expenses incurred during a 5-week epidemic methicillin-resistant *Staphylococcus aureus* outbreak. *Journal of Hospital Infection* 13(2):199–200.

Murray BE. 1994. Can antibiotic resistance be controlled? *New England Journal of Medicine* 330:1229–1230.

Neu HC. 1992. The crisis in antibiotic resistance. *Science* 257:1064–1073.

OTA (Office of Technology Assessment). 1995. *Impacts of Antibiotic-Resistant Bacteria*. OTA-H-629. Washington, DC: OTA.

Pearce D and Turner R. 1990. *Economics of Natural Resources and the Environment*. London: Harvester Wheatsheaf.

Phelps C. 1989. Bug-drug resistance. *Medical Care* 27:194–203.

Smith RD. 1999. Antimicrobial resistance: the importance of developing long term policy. *Bulletin of the World Health Organization* 77:862.

Smith RD and Coast J. 1998. Controlling antimicrobial resistance: a proposed transferable permit market. *Health Policy* 43:219–232.

Smith RD and Coast J. 2001. *Global Responses to the Growing Threat of Antimicrobial Resistance*. Working Paper prepared for Commission on Macroeconomics and Health, WHO. [Online]. Available: http://www3.who.int/whosis/cmh/cmh_papers/e/pdf/wg2_paper16.pdf.

Smith RD and Coast J. 2002. Antimicrobial resistance: a global response. *Bulletin of the World Health Organization* 80:126–133.

Smith RD and Coast J. In press. Antimicrobial resistance and global public goods for health. In: Smith RD, Beaglehole R, Drager N, eds. *Global Public Goods for Health: A Health Economic and Public Health Perspective*. Oxford: Oxford University Press.

Smith RD, Coast J, Millar MR. 1996. Over-the-counter antimicrobials: the hidden costs of resistance. *Journal of Antimicrobial Chemotherapy* 37:1031–1032.

Smith RD, Coast J, Millar MR, Wilton P, Karcher A-M. 2001. *Interventions Against Anti-Microbial Resistance: a Review of the Literature and Exploration of Modelling Cost-Effectiveness. Report to: Global Forum for Health Research.* Geneva: World Health Organization.

Standing Medical Advisory Committee Sub-Group on Antimicrobial Resistance. 1998. *The Path of Least Resistance.* [Online]. Available: http://www.doh.gov.uk/smac1.htm.

Tietenberg T. 1990. Economic instruments for environmental regulation. *Oxford Review of Economic Policy* 6:17–33.

Tomasz A. 1994. Multiple-antibiotic resistant pathogenic bacteria. A report on the Rockefeller University workshop. *New England Journal of Medicine* 330:1247–1251.

Turner R, Pearce D, Bateman I. 1994. *Environmental Economics. An Elementary Introduction.* London: Harvester Wheatsheaf.

Weitzman M. 1974. Prices versus quantities. *Review of Economic Studies* 41:477–491.

WHO (World Health Organization). 2001. *Global Strategy for the Containment of Antimicrobial Resistance.* WHO/CDS/CSR/DRS/2001.2. Geneva: WHO.

Wilton P, Smith RD, Coast J, Millar M. 2002. Strategies to contain the emergence of antimicrobial resistance: a systematic review of effectiveness and cost-effectiveness. *Journal of Health Services Research and Policy* 7:111–117.

Wilton P, Smith RD, Coast J, Millar M, Karcher A. 2001. Directly observed therapy for multi-drug resistant tuberculosis: an economic evaluation in the United States of America and South Africa. *The International Journal of Tuberculosis and Lung Disease* 5:1137–1142.

Winebrake J, Farrell A, Bernstein M. 1995. The Clean Air Act's sulfur dioxide emissions market: estimating the costs of regulatory and legislative intervention. *Resource and Energy Economics* 17:239–260.

World Bank. 2001. *World Development Report 2000/01.* New York: Oxford University Press.

5

Factors Contributing to the Emergence of Resistance

OVERVIEW

Although microbial resistance results primarily as a consequence of selection pressure placed on susceptible microbes by the use of therapeutic agents, a variety of social and administrative factors also contribute to the emergence and spread of resistance. The focus of this session of the workshop was to examine these factors and to describe potential ways to minimize their role in promoting antimicrobial resistance.

In the United States and other developed countries, one leading factor is the over-prescription by physicians of antimicrobials, particularly antibiotics, even in the absence of appropriate indications. Such inappropriate physician practices are often fostered by diagnostic uncertainty, lack of opportunity for patient follow-up, lack of knowledge regarding optimal therapies, and patient demand. In many developing countries, problems typically arise because antimicrobial agents are readily available and can be purchased as a commodity without the advice or prescription of a physician or other trained health care provider.

Some common types of human behavior also play a role in promoting resistance. Of particular importance, for example, are patient self-medication and noncompliance with recommended treatments. Noncompliance occurs when individuals forget to take medication, prematurely discontinue the medication as they begin to feel better, or cannot afford a full course of therapy. Self-medication almost always involves unnecessary, inadequate, and ill-timed dosing. In some countries, problems of noncompliance and self-medication are magnified because significant amounts of the available antimicrobials are poorly manufactured, counterfeit, or have exceeded their effective lifetimes.

Various practices common in hospitals contribute to the resistance problem as well. Indeed, hospitals are especially fertile grounds for breeding resistant microbes. They deal regularly with large numbers of patients (many with suppressed immune systems) in relatively close proximity to each other, and they frequently treat their patients with intensive and prolonged antimicrobial therapy. Large hospitals and teaching hospitals generally experience more problems with drug-resistant microbes, probably because they treat greater numbers of the sickest patients and those at highest risk of becoming infected. Transmission of drug-resistant organisms among patients may be airborne, from a point source (such as contaminated equipment), or by direct or indirect contact with a contaminated environment or the contaminated hands of staff. Failure of health care workers to practice simple control measures (e.g., hand washing and changing gloves after examining a patient) is a leading contributor to the spread of infection in hospitals.

Hospitals typically rely on two major forms of intervention to minimize resistance problems. One approach involves limiting antimicrobial use as much as possible; the other involves implementing intensive infection-control programs. Important components of these programs include surveillance; outbreak investigation and control; sterilization and disinfection of equipment; and implementation of such patient-care practices as handwashing, isolation, and barriers between infected patients.

Although much is known about how hospitals can minimize the spread of infection, research is still needed to fill some important gaps in knowledge. One need is for development of rapid, reliable diagnostic methods for identifying the presence of infection, the specific infecting organism, and the susceptibility of the microbe to various therapeutic agents. Diagnostic precision is the key to effectively modifying the current approach of widespread empiric antimicrobial use in ill patients with suspected infections. A further need is to develop materials for use in medical devices, such as catheters, that are resistant to colonization by microorganisms. In addition, continuing development of new antimicrobial agents remains a priority.

Another factor that is widely believed to contribute to resistance problems is the use of various antimicrobial agents in animals raised commercially for food, such as poultry, pigs, and cows. Participants debated just what contribution such agricultural use makes to the spread of antimicrobial resistance among human pathogens. While some participants maintained that the problem is minimal and being effectively managed by various public and private programs, others described a greater level of risk. They expressed concern that use of antimicrobials in animals, either for therapeutic use or to promote growth, can lead to the development of drug-resistant microbes (largely bacteria, such as salmonella and campylobacter) that subsequently are transmitted to humans, usually through food products.

In response to the workshop presentation, "The Use of Antimicrobials in Food-Producing Animals," a paper was prepared to address the public health consequences of antimicrobials in agriculture and can be found in Appendix A.

ANTIBIOTIC USE AND RESISTANCE IN DEVELOPING COUNTRIES

Iruka N. Okeke, Ph.D.

Department of Biology, Haverford College, Haverford, PA

> "The ways and means for putting medicine in order must take account of the conditions of life and work among the people whom it must serve."
> Walton H. Hamilton, 1932

Antimicrobial resistance adversely affects the outcome of community- and hospital-acquired infections in developing countries. For example, mortality in recent cholera and dysentery epidemics has been significantly increased by antibiotic resistance (Goma Epidemiology Group, 1995; Sengupta et al., 2000; Okeke et al., 2001). Other cases in point include tuberculosis, respiratory tract infections, infectious diarrhea, sexually transmitted diseases, and malaria. These conditions account for most of the illness in the developing world. In these countries, the infectious disease burden is typically high, whereas the options available to prescribers are few—often limited to older, cheaper, and non-patent protected drugs. Studies that have monitored resistance rates over time have documented a rising prevalence of resistance to these commonly used antimicrobials (see Figure 5-1) (Hoge et al., 1998; Okeke et al., 2000; Hsueh et al., 2002). Drugs that have been rendered ineffective or for which there are serious concerns include the broad-spectrum antibacterials tetracycline, ampicillin, trimethoprim-sulfamethoxazole chloramphenicol and streptomycin, anti-tuberculosis drugs as well as the antimalarial chloroquine. Resistance to these drugs has promoted an upsurge in the use of previously second-line, more expensive agents that are, in many cases, agents of last resort. The fluoroquinolones and sulfadoxine-pyrimethamine are two such examples, and with both, an upward trend in the proportion of resistant strains has already been identified (Okeke et al., 2000; Winstanley, 2001; Mwansa et al., 2002). Although there are other agents, currently in routine use in

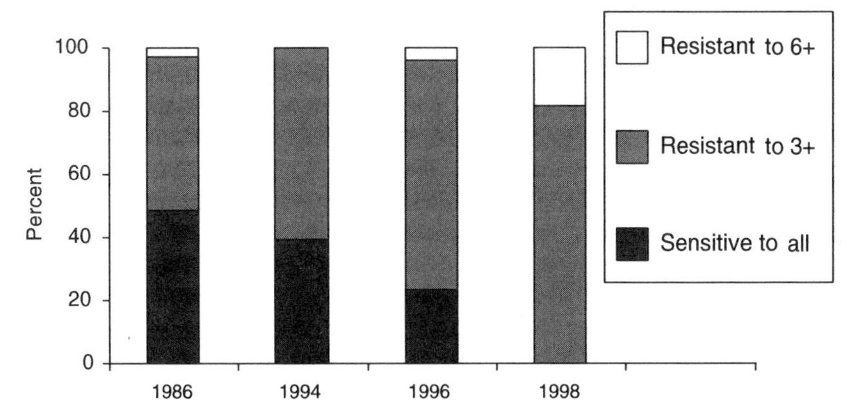

FIGURE 5-1 Trends in the proportion of *Escherichia coli* from healthy subjects resistant to three or more and six or more of seven antibacterial drugs. SOURCE: Okeke et al., 2000.

industrialized countries, the cost of these precludes their use by poor patients in the developing world. The extent and determinants of microbial resistance vary considerably from one geographic area to another but the current globalization trend means that the consequences transcend geographical borders (Okeke and Edelman, 2001). In some developing countries, unprescribed antibiotic use is relatively uncommon so that antibiotic use and resistance patterns may mirror what is seen in the industrialized world (O'Connor et al., 2001). In others, regulations that would encourage appropriate antibiotic use are in place but the infrastructure or the will to enforce them is not (Djimde et al., 1998; Chuc and Tomson, 1999; Okeke et al., 1999; Chatterjee, 2001; Siringi, 2001). Although there are many generalizations in this report, it must be emphasized that it is impossible to paint a picture of the current situation or draw a model for intervention that would fit every developing country. Examples are taken from different countries, but the principal focus here is on sub-Saharan Africa where the burden of infectious disease is highest and antibiotic use is commonly under-regulated (Djimde et al., 1998; Siringi, 2001).

Emergence of Resistance

Studies conducted in industrialized countries have correlated antibiotic consumption with the prevalence of antibiotic resistance. Per capita expenditure on antibiotics is lower in developing countries in spite of a greater burden of infectious disease, and microbial resistance is often highly prevalent. Some of the reasons for this are that cheaper agents are used, agricultural and veterinary consumption is often lower, and alternative (or no) therapy is common. However, a significant reason for high selection pressure in the face of modest antimicrobial expenditure is inappropriate antibiotic use.

Antibiotic Prescription by Health Professionals

Some of the types of antibiotic misuse in clinical practice include unjustified prescription (in such conditions as diarrhea and the common cold), under-prescription (for example, in urinary tract infections and sexually transmitted diseases), under-dosing, and short duration (Calva, 1996; Nizami et al., 1996; Paredes et al., 1996; Bartoloni et al., 1998). Antimicrobial prescription in many developing countries is almost entirely empirical and based on surveillance data obtained from locations or at a time that it is unlikely to be relevant to the ensuing situation. Broad-spectrum agents are frequently employed because susceptibility data is unavailable. In addition, the rising number of HIV-positive people increases selective pressure for resistant organisms by increasing the need for prophylactic and curative antimicrobial use.

As in industrialized countries, prescribers are subjected to pressure from patients (Paredes et al., 1996). In addition, health professionals rarely have the opportunity to review cases and are often dealing with life-threatening disease. Hence, antibiotics are often prescribed when unnecessary. Advocates of appropriate antibiotic use advise the prescriber to weigh the benefits to the individual against the risk to public health. This presents a dilemma even to those health professionals that are aware of the long-term consequences of antibiotic abuse. This is because many of the benefits to the individual actually impact public health. For example, the untreated, or improperly treated, but surviving, patient serves as a reservoir of resistant pathogens. Secondly, treatment failures in health centers will lead to lowered confidence by patients and consequent upsurge of visits to unorthodox practitioners, encouraging unsanctioned antibiotic distribution. Since health professionals frequently have only one opportunity to administer therapy, there is the inclination to use broad-spectrum therapy to increase the chances of successful treatment. These factors serve to dissuade health professionals who are aware of the consequences of inappropriate antimicrobial use from putting their knowledge into practice (Larsson et al., 2000). The dilemmas faced by prescribers are further complicated by the practices of patients in developing countries, who are more likely to fail to complete a prescribed course of antibiotics or to admit to reserving part of it for future use (Calva, 1996; Pechere, 2001).

Multiplicity of Sources

Patients in many developing countries will often seek care for the same ailment from multiple sources, a practice that prevents follow-up and confuses case history (Needham et al., 2001). This is a function of the wide variety of sources for antimicrobial drugs and the fact that many of these sources will dispense antibiotics without prescription (Chuc and Tomson, 1999; Wachter et al., 1999). Djimde et al. classified the sources of antimalarials in Malian villages as including sanctioned (physicians, pharmacists, nurses, pharmacy sellers, and midwives) and unsanctioned (stall keepers, itinerant vendors, and tradesmen dealing in clothing, confectionary, cosmetics, and motorcycle parts) (Djimde et al., 1998). The situation is similar in many other developing countries, and pharmacy premises, although sanctioned, often serve as an outlet for unprescribed antibiotics because of the competitive pressure from unsanctioned providers (Chuc and Tomson, 1999; Okeke et al., 1999). Unsanctioned providers tend to have shabbier premises and a smaller range of medicines but they flourish because they are often cheaper due to lower overheads. They are more accessible to the majority of the population than doctors and nurses and will accept a non-physiologic cause of disease. Unfortunately, they may supply poor quality medicines (but these are often dispensed by sanctioned providers) and could serve as an outlet for illicitly sourced drugs. As they often lack basic training on drug handling, they are often unaware or incapable of storing their wares appropriately. They have been known to ignore or are unaware of expiry dates and to mix batches, brands, and even different drugs. They also have limited (if any) clinical training and therefore offer diagnosis and prescription that may be incorrect (Wachter et al., 1999). Antibiotic choice is based on experience, folklore, or customer preference usually in complete disregard of the long-term consequences of antibiotic misuse. These providers supply antimicrobials to a varied but significant proportion of the populaces they serve. They are therefore a crucial target group for optimizing antibiotic use. Antibiotic policies directed at medical services alone will only affect a minority of treatments when unsanctioned persons are major providers. It is however difficult to integrate unsanctioned providers into official policies because they are often technically illegal.

Another category of health providers that must be taken into account is the traditional medicine practitioners. In a Malian study 23 percent of rural antimalarial consumers preferred herbs or traditional medicines (Djimde et al., 1998). Indeed, many herbal remedies have demonstrated some antimicrobial activity in vitro, and traditional medicine represents a potential alternative to antibiotic therapy, which could reduce selective pressure to orthodox antibiotics. To date, very few of these natural products have been subjected to scientific or clinical evaluation. The majority remain unevaluated and recipes are often held as family secrets akin to a trade secret (Sofowora, 1982). Traditional practitioners receive years or decades of apprenticeship in traditional medicine and herbs but have no training in Western clinical methods. Importantly, one traditional practitioner recently admitted adulterating his concoctions with antibiotics, and the extent to which this practice occurs is not known (Okeke et al., 1999). If traditional practitioners are using Western medicines, there is a need to ensure that they receive appropriate training in diagnosis, treatment, and undesirable effects, including antibiotic resistance.

In some developing countries, patients prefer to seek care from sanctioned providers, even though it is available from other sources (O'Connor et al., 2001). In many other countries, unsanctioned and traditional providers are more commonly frequented by the unwell. We have sought to identify reasons why patients seek care from unorthodox sources. In a study designed to determine the health-seeking practices of educated Nigerians, a cohort of university undergraduates was followed for one year. The students were all entitled to free medical care provided by physicians at the University Health Center and drug supply from an attached pharmacy. Within the year, of 43 students who had diarrhea, only 16 percent sought treatment at the health center. Twelve percent did not seek treatment at all but 72 percent resorted to self-medication, at their own expense, even though they could obtain medical care at no cost. Furthermore, 80 percent of the self-medicators took at least one antibacterial medicine and 45 percent took more than one antimicrobial (see Table 5-1). Clearly, factors other than cost and health care availability influence antibiotic misuse. Another relatively affluent population we studied were West Africans resident in Nigeria that had traveled by air to another country. Most of the travelers had visited Europe or North America. Of the 424 travelers to

TABLE 5-1 Use of Unprescribed Antibiotics by Students with Diarrhea

Antibiotic or combination	No. (%) of self-medicated cases
Tetracycline alone	7 (22.6)
Metronidazole alone	7 (22.6)
Pthalyl sulphathiazole alone	3 (9.7)
Tetracycline + Metronidazole	10 (32.3)
Tetracycline + Pthalyl sulphathiazole	3 (9.7)
Tetracycline + Metronidazole + Pthalyl sulphathiazole	1 (3.2)
Total taking at least one unprescribed antibiotic	25 (80.6)
Loperamide	1 (3.2)
Herbals	3 (9.7)

whom a questionnaire was administered, 52.4 percent traveled with at least one antimalarial and 30.4 percent with at least one antibacterial drug. Only 19.8 percent said that they would visit a doctor or clinic if they fell ill during their travels. The rest preferred to take medicines they had brought with them or obtain medicines from friends (Okeke et al., in press). These findings appear to suggest that the reasons why antibiotics are abused in sub-Saharan Africa are not entirely economic. Working in Zambia, Needham et al. (2001) have identified barriers to tuberculosis diagnosis, which give some insight of factors that lead patients to self-medicate or obtain treatment from unorthodox sources. Significant factors they identified included female sex ($p < 0.02$) and education ($p < 0.04$), but not economic or health factors. There was considerable delay in diagnosis if a patient made prior health seeking encounters, particularly to unsanctioned and traditional providers ($p < 0.001$).

Sub-Standard Medicines

Even when antibiotic prescription and use is optimal, sub-therapeutic dosing and consequent resistant selection can arise from poor quality antibiotic preparations. A recent survey of tablets claiming to contain the antimalarial Artesunate from Cambodia, Laos, Myanmar, Thailand, and Vietnam found that as many as 38 percent of the samples did not contain the drug (Newton et al., 2001). Multiple reports have described the dispensing of medicines in Nigeria that contain as little as half of their label content (Okeke and Lamikanra, 1995, 2001; Taylor et al., 2001). Some of the medicines are counterfeit—they were intentionally formulated with less than the stated content (Chatterjee, 2001; Newton et al., 2001), but significant proportions contain degraded drugs (Okeke and Lamikanra, 1995, 2001). Degradation of heat- and moisture-labile antibiotics occurs very readily in tropical developing countries where ambient temperatures may approach 40°C and humidity is high enough to distort capsule shells and soften tablets. The packaging of many pharmaceuticals may be insufficient to protect them in tropical developing countries, and in some cases it may be desirable to reformulate them for this environment or modify shelf life recommendations. One rationale for employing uniform shelf lives in temperate and tropical countries is that labels indicate that medicines are to be stored under controlled conditions. Indeed, local regulations usually stipulate that pharmacy premises in the tropics must be air-conditioned. In reality, frequent power cuts may mean that the air is only intermittently conditioned, warehouses and unsanctioned premises are almost never air-conditioned, and imported drugs may languish for many months at ports.

Dissemination

The warm moist climate and close proximity of non-human vectors in tropical countries increase the likelihood that pathogenic and commensal bacteria will survive in the environment and be transmitted to humans (Rosas et al., 1997). In many developing countries, these factors combine with poor sanitation and shortfalls in infection control to create havens for the amplification and dissemination of resistant strains in the community (Graczyk et al., 2001). Overcrowding, a direct consequence of urban migration, increases the chance that this dissemination will occur. The world's fastest-growing cities are in developing countries, many of which cannot provide potable water or safe sanitation for a majority of their residents (McMichael, 2000). Antibiotic misuse also tends to be more common in crowded areas and may be a feature of urban social change (Bojalil and Calva, 1994; Chuc and Tomson, 1999). Separate studies have suggested that cities serve as havens for the exchange of pathogenic and antibiotic-resistant organisms. In contrast to a Dutch study, which found that there was very little difference in the carriage of *E. coli* resistant to antibiotics in a rural and an urban area (Bonten et al., 1992), studies in Nigeria and Nepal have demonstrated that urban residents are more likely to harbor resistant bacteria than people residing in rural or provincial areas (Lamikanra and Okeke, 1997; Walson et al., 2001).

The capacity of laboratories in developing countries to conduct susceptibility testing and to diagnose infections needs to be strengthened. Not only is resistance surveillance insufficient or lacking, the ability to diagnose many infections and thereby prescribe appropriate and timely treatment is hampered by inadequate laboratory support. In many localities, the extent of the antibiotic resistance problem is not known and empirical antibiotic prescription is akin to guesswork. Similarly, evidence about resistance is of necessity commonly anecdotal. Even if interceptive strategies to control resistance are implemented, there are no local means of measuring the success or otherwise of such policies.

Conclusion

This report attempts to highlight a number of factors that predispose the emergence and spread of antibiotic resistant organisms in developing countries. Implementation of the World Health Organization's (WHO) *Global Strategy for Containment of Antimicrobial Resistance* will potentially address all of these issues (WHO, 2001). Priority should be given to education, directed at distributors and consumers as well as prescribers of antibiotics, infection control to prevent the dissemination of resistant strains, quality assurance of antibiotics and other medicines, and the institution of functional and sustainable laboratories for antibiotic resistance surveillance. The real challenge however will be implementing this strategy on a country- and sub-country-specific basis, taking the special features of each developing country into account to ensure sustainability. For example, in some countries, targeting educational intervention at physicians may reduce inappropriate use (O'Connor et al., 2001). In particular, it would be desirable to present incentives for prudent antibiotic use in order to address the gaps between knowledge and practice seen in health professionals and lay-people. In other areas, the approach must be different because of the extensive prescription of antibiotics by unsanctioned providers and patients themselves; antibiotic policies that target orthodox clinical practitioners and premises will have only limited impact. In these cases, policies and interventions that reach unconventional distributors and the patients themselves are more likely to have a broad and sustained effect. Most importantly, interventions will have to be tailored to specific countries and communities since the factors that determine their success will be to a large extent cultural.

HEALTHCARE-ACQUIRED INFECTIONS: HOSPITALS AS A BREEDING GROUND FOR ANTIMICROBIAL RESISTANCE

Lindsay E. Nicolle, M.D., F.R.C.P.C.

Department of Internal Medicine and Medical Microbiology
University of Manitoba, Winnipeg, Manitoba, Canada

Hospitalized populations are more likely to be colonized or infected with resistant microorganisms compared with community populations (Datta, 1969; McGowan et al., 1974). This association of acute care hospitalization with antimicrobial resistance was recognized soon after the introduction of antimicrobial therapy (McGowan et al., 1975). Widespread outbreaks of penicillin-resistant *Staphylococcus aureus* in the late 1950s reinforced this observation (LaForce, 1993). Repeatedly, review articles from 20–30 years ago identified the problem and the association of resistance with widespread empiric antimicrobial use (Jackson, 1979; Weinstein and Kabins, 1981; McGowan, 1983).

While antimicrobial resistance is more frequent in acute care hospitals, the prevalence of resistance across hospitals is highly variable. Some of this variability mirrors geographic variation in prevalence of resistant organisms. Large hospitals providing tertiary care and teaching hospitals have a higher prevalence of resistance than smaller community hospitals and have repeatedly been the site where new resistance is first described. This is the experience of methicillin-resistant *Staphylococcus aureus* (MRSA) emergence in U.S. hospitals (Haley et al., 1982), and was repeated in the 1990s with the emergence of vancomycin resistant enterococci (VRE) (Fridkin et al., 2001).

Determinants of Resistance

The high prevalence of antimicrobial resistance in acute care facilities, and repeated emergence of new resistance, is attributable to both patient and facility characteristics (see Table 5-2). Persons at highest risk of acquiring infection are found in hospitals. These include patients at extremes of age with biologically impaired immune systems, such as premature neonates and the very old. Other patients have acquired immunodeficiency, which is often therapeutically induced. These include the increasing numbers of solid organ and bone marrow transplant patients and profoundly neutropenic patients, as well as patients with severe trauma or extensive burns. These highest risk patients are primarily cared for in large, tertiary care, teaching hospitals. Hospitalized patients experience repeated interventions for monitoring or therapy which further impair normal host defenses and increase the risk of infection. Indwelling urethral catheters, central vascular lines, endotracheal tubes, and surgical wounds permit access of microorganisms to normally sterile body sites. Recent evolution in health care delivery with shortened hospital stay and increased patient acuity means patients now hospitalized are at even greater risk for infection.

TABLE 5-2 Variables Which Promote the Emergence and High Prevalence of Resistant Organisms in Acute Care Facilities

Patient variables	Inherent immunocompromised status e.g., neonate, very old Acquired immunocompromised status e.g., transplant patients, profound neutropenia, extensive burns Therapeutic interventions which compromise normal defenses e.g., indwelling urethral catheters, central lines, endotracheal tubes, surgical procedures
Intense antimicrobial use	Systemic: 30–50% of patients • Therapeutic • Prophylactic Topical use
Institutionalization	Increased opportunities for transmission • Shared equipment • Shared staff • Airborne

Intense antimicrobial use in acute care facilities ensures that infections, when they occur, are likely to be with an organism of increased resistance. From 30 to 50 percent or more of patients admitted to an acute care facility receive prophylactic or therapeutic systemic antimicrobials. In very high risk populations, such as intensive care unit patients or bone marrow or solid organ transplant units, virtually all patients receive antimicrobial therapy which is usually broad-spectrum and often more than one agent. There is also substantial topical antimicrobial use for burns and other skin lesions, although use of topical agents is not well described. The intensity of antimicrobial use has been repeatedly correlated with the emergence and prevalence of antimicrobial resistant organisms in the individual patient, and within the hospital unit or facility as a whole (McGowan, 1983; Fridkin et al., 2001).

Institutionalization increases the frequency of transmission of organisms among patients through a shared environment, equipment, and staff. Transmission may be airborne, as in the case of multiply drug resistant tuberculosis, from a point source such as contaminated equipment, or by direct or indirect contact through a contaminated environment or on the hands of staff. The likelihood of a patient acquiring a resistant organism correlates with the prevalence of resistant organisms in other patients in the unit or facility (Bonten et al., 1998). The frequency of antimicrobial resistance is highest in special care units such as intensive care units, burn units, or transplant units where severely ill patients, multiple invasive devices, intense antimicrobial use, and close spatial clustering combine.

Acquisition of Antimicrobial Resistance

An antimicrobial resistant organism may be acquired by emergence of resistance in endogenous flora, or by acquisition from other patients and the environment. Emergence from endogenous flora has been frequently reported among gram-negative organisms with inducible beta-lactamases and in *Pseudomonas aeruginosa*. A recent important example is the emergence of glycopeptide intermediate MRSA (GISA). These strains have usually developed in patients with persistent or relapsing MRSA infection associated with foreign bodies such as hemodialysis catheters which have not been removed, and after prolonged vancomycin therapy.

An organism may be transmitted from another patient in an outbreak setting where an increased number of cases is observed, or as endemic transmission where a continuing, stable, number of cases occur. A patient may also acquire a resistant organism, such as an aminoglycoside resistant *S. marcescens*, and the genetic resistance elements may be transferred to other colonizing flora resulting in resistance in other species such as *K. pneumoniae* or *E. coli* (McGowan, 1983; Alford and Hall, 1987).

There is overlap between these two types of acquisition. Once a patient develops endogenous resistance, the strain may be transmissible to other patients, leading to an outbreak or endemic colonization or infection with the resistant organism. Organisms which may initially cause outbreaks, such as MRSA and VRE, may subsequently become endemic in the facility.

Impact of Antimicrobial Resistance

Studies repeatedly report that acquisition of an antimicrobial resistant infection is associated with negative outcomes for the patient and the facility (Holmberg et al., 1987). These include increased mortality, increased morbidity, increased length of stay, and increased costs due, at least partly, to the need for more costly alternative antimicrobial therapy and infection control interventions.

While the conclusion that antimicrobial resistance in acute care facilities has negative impacts is valid, there are some methodologic concerns with studies measuring outcomes. Antimicrobial resistant organisms are not usually of greater virulence, so increased morbidity or mortality will result only if initial antimicrobial therapy not effective for the infecting organism is given. Where empiric therapy is effective for the resistant organism, excess morbidity or mortality would not occur. This concern certainly drives increasing use of broader spectrum empiric antimicrobial therapy, which is costly, but this practice also means that morbidity and mortality due to resistant organisms in acute care facilities in developed countries remains limited.

Patient colonization or infection with a resistant organism is not random. Patients from whom resistant organisms are isolated are characterized by a greater risk of infection due to underlying disease and immunosuppression, have received more antimicrobial therapy, and have longer hospital stays because of their illness or complications of therapy. These same characteristics identify patients with a greater likelihood of mortality, morbidity, prolonged length of stay, and cost of hospitalization irrespective of the presence of an antimicrobial resistant organism. Thus, there are substantial potential biases in any study of outcomes attributable to antimicrobial resistance. This partially explains the wide variation in impacts of resistant organisms reported in different studies. For case-control studies, differences in outcomes between patients with and without infections with antimicrobial resistant organisms become less marked as matching of case and control patients becomes more rigorous (Howard et al., 2001).

The major negative impact of antimicrobial resistance is, in fact, only a potential risk. With increasing acquisition of resistance, an organism not susceptible to any available antimicrobial therapy will evolve. This is of greatest concern for common, virulent, organisms such as *S. aureus* and *E.*

coli, which are important bacterial pathogens in both hospitals and the community. The likelihood, time course, and costs of such a development cannot currently be estimated.

Containment of Antimicrobial Resistance

Concerns about antimicrobial resistance have been repeatedly raised over many decades, and recommendations to limit progression have been made (McGowan, 1983; Goldman et al., 1996; Schlaes et al., 1997). The two major interventions are infection control to prevent transmission, and limitation of antimicrobial use. A recent consensus statement notes that all previous efforts have failed, and views this as a failure of leadership by both administration and medical staff who have not taken ownership of the problem (Goldman et al., 1996).

Infection Control

Infection control programs are effective in preventing hospital infections (Scheckler et al., 1998). These programs are essential for safe patient care and risk management in acute care facilities, regardless of the presence of antimicrobial resistance. Important activities include surveillance, outbreak investigation and control, patient care practices such as isolation, handwashing and barriers, and sterilization and disinfection of equipment. Hospital infection control activity should also decrease antimicrobial resistant infections and colonization.

Perhaps the evidence most strongly supporting efficacy of infection control in controlling antimicrobial resistance is found in reports of control of outbreaks of antimicrobial resistant strains. Over 200 such outbreaks have been reported since 1970 (Nicolle, 2001). The organisms most frequently described are MRSA, aminoglycoside resistant or extended spectrum beta-lactamase (ESBL) producing enterobacteriaceae, VRE, and Acinetobacter spp. Outbreak investigation and control was reported to eradicate or control infections and colonization with the outbreak strain in 80 to 90 percent of episodes. A common theme, however, is that initial infection control interventions of education, intensified handwashing, and barrier precautions did not achieve control. Further measures such as cohorting, closing units to new admissions, antiseptic handwashing, and either antimicrobial restriction or specific intensified antimicrobial use were required to achieve control.

While this experience is compelling evidence for the effectiveness of infection control, there are limitations to acknowledge. A substantial publication bias is likely, as reports describing a successful outcome will more often be submitted for publication. The majority of reports originate from academic tertiary care centers, where there may be increased resources and expertise for infection control. The durability of a successful outcome is usually not known. Many facilities may have initial success with eradicating MRSA and VRE, but subsequently have re-emergence with endemic transmission established. Studies are also noncomparative, and describe multiple interventions. Thus, the effectiveness of a specific intervention cannot be evaluated. A final observation is that the antimicrobial resistant phenotype is a unique marker for organism identification which facilitates early outbreak recognition. Seen from this perspective, antimicrobial resistance may make infection control interventions more effective.

The efficacy of infection control interventions in limiting endemic antimicrobial resistance is less clear. The most convincing reports supporting efficacy are from Europe, where some facilities have only recently changed practice from a hygienic model of infection control to one based on infection surveillance. When multifaceted control programs including screening, staff education, intensified barrier precautions, and intensified handwashing have been newly implemented in intensive care units with a high prevalence of resistance, decreased prevalence and incidence of infection and colonization with MRSA and ESBL producing organisms has been reported (Cosseron-Zerbib et al., 1998; Harbath et al., 2000; Souwein et al., 2000). These approaches, however, have been standard practice for most North American facilities. An increasing prevalence of MRSA and VRE has been observed despite appropriate continuing infection control practice (Goetz and Muder, 1992; Brooks et al., 1998). Infection control interventions may have delayed and limited resistance expansion, but cannot prevent establishment or progression altogether.

Another element of infection control practice is antimicrobial use to prevent infection. There is a trade-off, however, between prevention of infection, and the induction of even more antimicrobial resistance, especially among colonizing organisms (Flynn et al., 1987; Terpstra et al., 1999). This trade off is usually considered acceptable where valid clinical trials have documented improved patient outcomes. This is the case for appropriate prophylactic antimicrobial use for selected clean and clean-contaminated surgical procedures. More problematic is the widespread use of topical mupirocin for eradication of MRSA colonization. Widespread mupirocin use for preventing MRSA colonization has repeatedly been followed by emergence of mupirocin-resistant MRSA strains (Miller et al., 1996). Use of prophylactic antimicrobials, even when appropriate, contributes to the larger problem of antimicrobial resistant organisms within acute care facilities.

Finally, despite development of multifaceted national guidelines for control of selected high profile resistant organisms, the prevalence of these antimicrobial resistant organisms has continued to increase. The ongoing

MRSA outbreak in Britain (Austin and Anderson, 1999) and the continuing spread of VRE in the United States (CDC, 1999) are examples. While incomplete application of national recommendations at the institutional level may explain this failure, it must be appreciated that there are limitations in what infection control interventions, by themselves, may achieve in limiting emergence and dissemination of important resistant organisms in acute care facilities.

Antimicrobial Use Strategies

Throughout the United States in the 1970s and early 1980s tertiary care institutions repeatedly reported large, continuing outbreaks with aminoglycoside resistant gram-negative organisms (McGowan, 1983; Alford and Hall, 1987). Enterobacteriaceae and *Pseudomonas aeruginosa* were the most common organisms, and burn units were often identified as the source. Intensification of infection control measures had partial success in controlling this resistance in some facilities, but other institutions reported no improvement despite repeated and varied interventions (Alford and Hall, 1987). From the mid-1980s, however, these organisms were no longer identified as a significant problem in acute care facilities. This apparent spontaneous disappearance of widespread, important resistance likely resulted from changes in antimicrobial use with introduction of alternate gram-negative agents, and burn wound management with more rapid covering of the burn wound surface. Most important, however, was likely discontinuing the widespread use of topical aminoglycosides for burn wound prophylaxis. This is an example of how modifications in antimicrobial use may be a powerful determinant in limiting even widespread resistance.

Several activities to optimize antimicrobial use have been suggested (see Table 5-3) (Marr et al., 1988; Goldman et al., 1996; Schlaes et al., 1997). Despite the prominence of the concerns with antimicrobial resistance and continuing attention to this issue, there is limited systematic comparative evaluation of the efficacy of the proposed interventions. Educational strategies have, in fact, repeatedly been shown to have little long-term impact. Even optimal antimicrobial use in an acute care facility may not limit antimicrobial resistance given the large numbers of patients, especially in high risk units, who require antimicrobial therapy for legitimate clinical indications. The continuing approach to management of antimicrobial resistant organisms within acute care facilities is, in fact, ever-intensified use of broad-spectrum antimicrobials to "cover" ever-expanding antimicrobial resistance.

One study relevant to antimicrobial use and restriction described an outbreak of *Klebsiella aerogenes* in a neurosurgical unit in Britain from

TABLE 5-3 Recommendations Suggested for Optimizing Antimicrobial Use in Acute Care Facilities

- restrictive formulary
- automatic stop orders
- automatic substitution
- guidelines for antimicrobial use
- optimal surgical prophylaxis
- education
- academic detailing
- required consultation/approval
- antimicrobial resistance reports

1966 to 1968 (Price and Sleigh, 1970). Patients on this unit routinely received prophylactic cloxacillin for a continuing outbreak of penicillin-resistant *S. aureus*, and prophylactic ampicillin to prevent meningitis with cerebrospinal fluid leaks. Widespread colonization and infection with *K. aerogenes* emerged, including uniformly fatal cases of meningitis. The initial response to controlling this outbreak was intensification of infection control interventions including cohorting or placing patients in private rooms, and high dose colistin therapy to prevent and eradicate colonization. These strategies had minimal impact, and deaths from *K. aerogenes* meningitis continued. The draconian intervention of removal of all antimicrobial agents for either prophylaxis or therapy was then undertaken. There was a prompt and sustained disappearance of the outbreak strain, and during the subsequent four months while no antimicrobials were used there were no further cases of meningitis. Complete withdrawal of antimicrobial therapy is, of course, an intervention of the last resort and not an option which could currently be entertained for most acute care units. However, this study is intriguing in suggesting aggressive antimicrobial control may have profound and unpredicted impacts.

Research Needs

Antimicrobial resistance in acute care facilities is a large and complex issue. Despite identification of this problem immediately after antimicrobial use became widespread, and continuous attention, the problem is greater today than ever. This is, in part, the price for the remarkable advances in antimicrobial agents, which have allowed prevention and treatment of infections in highly compromised patients, leading to even more vulnerable populations. To address the problem now, interventions known to be effective must be rigorously applied, and continuing, targeted, systematic evaluation of potential effective interventions must be pursued. Some issues for further research and evaluation have been identified in the previous discussion of infection control and antimicrobial use. There are several other approaches that require intensive study.

Knowledge of the basic science of nosocomial transmission and pathogens is incomplete. Some strains of MRSA disseminate widely and rapidly, whereas other strains in the same environment are not transmitted among patients. Organism characteristics determining transmission in a facility are not known. The "big four" nosocomial infections of urinary tract, surgical site, ventilator-associated pneumonia, and central line are all primarily associated with foreign materials. A more complete understanding of interactions between the organism, the device, and the host will be essential to understand these infections, and associated resistance development.

Another need is development of rapid, reliable diagnosis to identify the presence of infection, the specific infecting organism, and antimicrobial susceptibilities. Diagnostic precision is the key to effectively modifying the current approach of widespread empiric antimicrobial use in ill patients with suspected infections. Without this improved diagnostic capability, it is not realistic to expect to modify current antimicrobial practices. A further need is development of materials resistant to colonization by organisms to limit infection and colonization with antimicrobial resistant organisms on medical devices. Given the prominent role of these devices in nosocomial infection, technological development of medical devices resistant to colonization by microorganisms is a priority.

Comprehensive strategies addressing the problem of antimicrobial resistance consistently identify a need for continuing development of antimicrobials as a priority. New antimicrobials will certainly be needed for patients in acute care facilities, where new resistance is always most likely to emerge. Development of additional antimicrobials, however, is unlikely to alter the paradigm of antimicrobial resistance in acute care facilities. This will remain a spiral of ever increasing resistance and empiric antimicrobial use until alternative effective approaches to prevention and management of nosocomial infections are developed.

THE USE OF ANTIMICROBIALS IN FOOD-PRODUCING ANIMALS

Thomas R. Shryock, Ph.D.

Elanco Animal Health, Greenfield, IN

The ultimate goal of food animal production is to deliver a safe, affordable, nutritious high-quality food product to the consumer. In the United

States in 2000, the food animal population totals were 8.4 billion chickens, 97 million cattle, and 98 million pigs. In order to raise this quantity of animals in today's commercial livestock and poultry operations, efficiencies of scale include grouping hundreds to tens of thousands of animals together on a single farm. This necessitates the application of herd health measures, applied on a population basis, to maintain a high level of herd (or flock) health status, since an epidemic disease outbreak would decimate the population. Measures such as vaccination, limited commingling, adequate ventilation and temperature controls for minimizing environmental extremes, biosecurity, appropriate nutrition and housing, and producer quality assurance programs and practices are currently used in modern agriculture. However, these measures are not always sufficient to prevent or control disease. The use of antimicrobial agents as a strategic tool to maintain animal health remains an essential component of today's food animal production system.

Antimicrobial agents are used in food animal production to prevent disease in high-risk animals and to control or treat disease; or to improve the ability of the animal to convert feed to muscle. Unlike the situation in human medicine where individual patients can be treated, food animal medicine is often practiced on a population basis for reasons of animal welfare, logistics, and efficiency since it is impractical to individually treat each animal in a group that consists of hundreds to tens of thousands. Herd health medicine also relies heavily on preventive medicine strategies to control or prevent disease in high risk populations. Addition of antimicrobial agents to feedstuffs, or by water, or parenteral administration to groups of animals by injection to prevent or control disease progression is done strategically when certain criteria are met. These criteria include prior experience of a disease outbreak associated with animal movement or weather extremes, or a noticeable increase in clinical signs of disease in a few animals in the group. This early therapeutic administration to the entire group is warranted, since many animals will have been exposed to the index cases and are now "incubating" the pathogens. Left untreated, as time elapses, more animals will "break" with clinical signs. Strategic application of an antimicrobial agent at the right time can minimize the pathogen load within a sufficient number of animals in the group (by allowing the host immune defenses to control the infection) and ultimately restore the group to an acceptable health status. Thus, preventive medicine, as a part of a herd health program, is in some cases the best way to maintain healthy animals. It is not appropriate to allow the majority of animals to suffer or die unnecessarily before beginning treatment (which is likely to fail at that late stage of the disease course). Many critics of this well-established practice incorrectly refer to the administration of "subtherapeutic" doses of antimicrobial agents in this instance, when in fact, the doses were developed to be therapeutic for those animals exhibiting signs of disease and are sufficient to benefit those animals that are incubating the pathogen and would soon break with disease. Routine administration of antimicrobials to healthy animals, with the intention of doing so as "insurance" or to "cover" poor management or hygiene is not a practice used by the leading production companies because it would be expensive, unsuccessful, and an unsustainable method of animal production. The administration of antimicrobials to enhance performance or growth of the animals may reflect the intention of the producer, but frequently the antimicrobial agents are in reality controlling an unrecognized subclinical disease exposure in the animals.

With respect to specific animal species, the use of antimicrobial agents is quite diverse (GAO, 1999; NRC, 1999; Prescott et al., 2000; Muirhead, 2001). Most poultry production requires the use of ionophores to prevent coccidia (intestinal parasites) infections, which otherwise would devastate a flock. Some antibiotics are administered at hatching, to reduce the prevalence and/or severity of infections that occur in day-old chicks due to vaccination stress on the immature immune system. In poultry house situations, rapid onset of respiratory or enteric diseases requires that antimicrobial agents be administered at the earliest opportunity to prevent significant morbidity and mortality in the flock. For the most part, poultry are medicated via feed or water because it would be impractical to individually treat thousands or tens of thousands of birds. Swine production can be divided into several stages from gestation, to farrowing, to nursery, to grower and finisher. Each stage has its own unique needs for antimicrobial usage, but in particular respiratory disease and enteric disease can frequently spread rapidly throughout a herd and require antimicrobial intervention. Thus strategically timed oral medications in groups of high risk pigs to prevent disease at times of movement, high stress, or waning maternal antibody may be needed. Injectable products are used when needed for therapy to individual sick sentinel pigs of the herd, that is, those showing the most and earliest clinical signs. Beef cattle that are affected by respiratory disease are usually treated with injectable antibiotics. Liver abscesses, coccidiosis and metabolic diseases are also common in feedlot cattle and are prevented or controlled by administration of antimicrobial agents in feed (Nagaraja et al., 1996; McGuffey et al., 2001; Muirhead, 2001). Infections in dairy cattle are usually cases of mastitis which are treated in acute cases or at "dry off" by intramammary infusion of antimicrobial agents. The use of antimicrobial agents in aquaculture is minimal (only tetracycline and a sulfa are approved), with applications done only in certain situations via medicated feed.

The antimicrobial agents that are used in food animal production are similar to those used in human medicine, but with several key exceptions (GAO, 1999). The Food and Drug Administration (FDA) or their equivalent in other countries has approved all of these products for use after a thorough review of the drug manufacturers' data that demonstrate efficacy, safety, and quality of the medicinal product. The common classes of antibiotics used in both humans and animals are: beta-lactams (including cephalosporins), tetracyclines, macrolides, aminoglycosides, lincosamides, sulfonamides, streptogramins, and fluoroquinolones. Examples of compounds not used (or minimally used) in humans, but important in food animals include: ionophores, avilamycin, bacitracin, carbadox, flavomycin, and pleuormutilins. It should be noted that some antimicrobial agents such as chloramphenicol and vancomycin are banned from use in food animals in the United States and other countries (Payne et al., 1999). Some of the antimicrobial agents used in food animals are approved for delivery by both a parenteral and an oral route, but in many cases only a feed administration route is approved and/or feasible for a variety of reasons. A detailed compendium of the technical aspects of feed additives is available (Muirhead, 2001). The actual amount of antimicrobials distributed by manufacturers in the U.S. animal sector has been reported (but doesn't include the amount of generic products distributed) (Muirhead, 2002). Of the total amount of 10,936 tons of active antimicrobials reported sold in 2001, 35 percent was classified as ionophore/arsenical, 33 percent was tetracycline, and 18 tons (<1 percent) was fluoroquinolone. Overall, 83 percent of the total was used for disease and 17 percent used for performance improvement. A separate estimation of U.S. usage, based on many assumptions, was calculated to be 12,300 tons just for a non-traditionally defined designation of "non-therapeutic" uses (Mellon et al., 2001).

Antimicrobial use in food animals has been a subject of discussion for over 30 years. A large number of reports, conferences, meetings, research studies and other communications have been produced. It is outside the scope of this short paper to review all of the key literature on this subject; however, a number of recent reviews and reports are provided for further information (IOM, 1998; Bezoen et al., 1999; Commonwealth of Australia Government, 1999; GAO, 1999; Barton, 2000). The primary concern has been that the use of antimicrobial agents in food animals will select for resistance to those agents in intestinal bacteria, and via foodborne transmission, an infection in humans will develop that is untreatable. A newer variation on this theme has been that foodborne commensal bacteria might transfer their resistance genes to existing susceptible normal human flora, and thereby set the stage for a non-treatable infection at a later time in the person's life. The bacteria at issue are limited to salmonella, campylobacter and enterococci, and vary with the animal species. Additional areas of concern include environmental contamination with excreted antimicrobials or their metabolites; residue concentrations of antimicrobials in edible tissues; and direct zoonotic transmission.

Some antimicrobial classes and routes of administration generate more concern than others. For example fluoroquinolone water medication use in poultry has resulted in a Notice of Opportunity for Hearing for the sponsor from the FDA, but the use of an injectable fluoroquinolone in cattle has not. In Europe, use of fluoroquinolones in animals is not considered to put human health at undue risk, but should be monitored (WHO, 1998; CVMP, 2001). Feed additive uses for efficiency claims and disease prevention have also come under scrutiny by some government officials, physicians, microbiologists, and others. The antimicrobial agents involved primarily include tetracyclines, beta-lactams, sulfonamides, macrolides, lincosamides, streptogramins, and bacitracin. The European Union Commission has legislatively removed the efficiency claim authorizations of several antimicrobial agents, and plans to remove the authorizations for the remaining agents in a few years. In the United States, the Center for Veterinary Medicine (CVM) is conducting a risk assessment on *E. faecium* and virginiamycin use.

Since foodborne bacterial transmission is an essential component of the issue, it represents a critical control point for ensuring food safety from all pathogens, not just those with antibiotic resistance genes. If one looked at a short list of the chain of events that are needed to "go wrong" in order for an antibiotic-resistant foodborne disease to result in an adverse outcome for a typical patient, it would include the following:

1. Antibiotic-resistant bacteria are present in a particular group of animals.
2. Selection of pre-existing strain with resistance gene(s) or a resistance mutation in the presence of an antibiotic.
3. Strain maintains itself in the presence of other gut flora until slaughter (with or without continued antibiotic selection pressure).
4. Fecal contamination of the carcass occurs during processing leaving bacteria on the meat.
5. Carcass decontamination measures are ineffective or incomplete.
6. Food product processing, shipment, or storage may result in the growth of the contaminating bacteria.
7. Cooking at an inadequate temperature and duration fails to kill the bacteria or the food is recontaminated after cooking by improper handling.
8. Human consumption of food results in resistant bacterial colonization or infection.
9. Infection severity requires physician care or hospitalization; antibiotic prescribed that is of the same class as was used on the farm.
10. Clinical resolution of infection may not be as rapid or complete as with a susceptible strain; culture and susceptibility testing in lab compel change in antibiotic.

11. Outcome is that the treatment period is prolonged or the patient may possibly die.

It should be obvious that not all foodborne bacteria are antibiotic-resistant. Each stage of the chain of events represents a decrease in the total number of "chances" for something to "go wrong" in the subsequent stage. For example, at step 7 only improperly cooked or recontaminated food is likely to result in cases of foodborne disease. Of the fraction of people exposed in step 7, not all will get sick in step 8. In essence, this is the type of rationale that comprises a risk assessment. One could use this approach to identify key steps to direct interventions to minimize bacterial transfer or impact from all foodborne pathogens, not just those with antibiotic resistance genes.

Thus the central issue is *not* whether antibiotic use in food animals can select for resistance in particular types of bacteria which can then cause foodborne disease in people that is more difficult to treat. *The real issue is what is the frequency at which this occurs and to what extent should resources be used to intervene?* In other words, should 50 percent of the available resources be directed to the use of antibiotics in food animals if the "resistance contribution" is 5 percent?

Many intervention recommendations have already been made (and are currently in the implementation phase) to minimize the contribution of food animal antibiotic use to the overall concern in human medicine. Additional reports with such guidance are cited here for reference (WHO, 2000; OIE, 2001; Torrence, 2001; U.S. Government, 2001; FDA, 2002a; FDA, 2002b). In general, the following themes can be found across these reports:

Risk assessment. This approach seeks to objectively evaluate the likelihood of an adverse effect through hazard identification, hazard characterization, exposure assessment, and risk characterization; and could potentially be used predictively to evaluate the effect of proposed intervention strategies as a part of the risk management phase.

Reduction in antibiotic usage. This approach seeks to reduce the need to use antibiotics by emphasizing improved hygiene, vaccination, housing, etc., in an effort to avoid disease outbreaks in the first place. In some recommendations, elimination of certain antibiotics or uses is advocated.

Rational or responsible antibiotic use. The development and implementation of a series of guidelines to veterinarians and other animal care specialists on the proper use of antibiotics is strongly advocated. Indeed, many veterinary organizations have already done so and producers are now incorporating them into their quality assurance programs.

Regulatory reform to address resistance. Regulatory reform is ongoing in the United States, the European Union, Australia, and many other countries with respect to the requirements that antibiotic manufacturers will have to meet in order to maintain their products or have new ones approved.

Resistance and usage monitoring. Monitoring of foodborne pathogens, principally campylobacter, salmonella and *E. coli*, and the "indicator" *E. faecium* for changes in antibiotic susceptibility patterns is ongoing in many countries, although test methods, isolate collection schemes, etc., are not optimal or consistent. Monitoring of the quantities of drug usage to assess reduction in antibiotice use is done in several small countries, and is being done on a self-reporting basis by the veterinary pharmaceutical industry in the United States and the European Union.

In conclusion, the use of antibiotics in food animals is essential to maintain a consistent supply of healthy animals entering the food chain. Although some antibiotic-resistant foodborne bacteria do make their way through the food chain to cause disease in consumers, the magnitude and clinical impact of that event remains unclear. In the larger context of human antibiotic resistance, antibiotic-resistant foodborne bacteria are a minor component compared to hospital- and community-acquired infections and antibiotic use. Nevertheless, the food animal production sector is doing its part to minimize antibiotic resistance by participating in the five activities above while continuing to deliver a safe, abundant food supply to the nation.

In response to this paper, "The Use of Antimicrobials in Food-Producing Animals," a paper was prepared to address the public health consequences of antimicrobials in agriculture and can be found in Appendix A.

REFERENCES

Alford RH and Hall A. 1987. Epidemiology of infections caused by gentamicin-resistant Enterobacteriaeceae and *Pseudomonas aeruginosa* over 15 years at the Nashville Veteran's Administration Medical Center. *Reviews of Infectious Diseases* 9:1079–1086.

Austin DJ and Anderson RM. 1999. Transmission dynamics of epidemic methicillin-resistant *Staphylococcus aureus* and vancomycin resistant Enterococcus in England and Wales. *Journal of Infectious Diseases* 179:883–891.

Bartoloni A, Cutts F, Leoni S, Austin CC, Mantella A, Guglielmetti P, Roselli M, Salazar E, Paradisi F. 1998. Patterns of antimicrobial use and antimicrobial resistance among healthy children in Bolivia. *Tropical Medicine and International Health* 3:116–123.

Barton MD. 2000. Antibiotic use in animal feed and its impact on human health. *Nutrition Research Reviews* 13:279–299.

Bezoen A, van Haren W, Hanekamp JC. 1999. *Emergence of a Debate: AGPs and Public Health Human Health and Antibiotic Growth Promoters (AGPs): Reassessing the Risk.* [Online]. Available: http://www.euronet.nl/~ssf/hanagp1.html.

Bojalil R and Calva JJ. 1994. Antibiotic misuse in diarrhea. A household survey in a Mexican community. *Journal of Clinical Epidemiology* 47:147–156.

Bonten MJM, Slaughter S, Ambergen AW, van Voorhis J, Nathan C, Weinstein RA. 1998. The role of "colonization pressure" in the spread of vancomycin-resistant enterococci. *Archives of Internal Medicine* 158:1127–1132.

Bonten M, Stobberingh E, Philips J, Houben A. 1992. Antibiotic resistance of *Escherichia coli* in fecal samples of healthy people in two different areas in an industrialized country. *Infection* 20:258–262.

Brooks S, Khan A, Stoica D, Griffith J, Friedman L, Mukherji R, Hameed R, Schupf N. 1998. Reduction in vancomycin-resistant Enterococcus and *Clostridium difficile* infections following change to tympanic thermometers. *Infection Control and Hospital Epidemiology* 19:333–336.

Calva J. 1996. Antibiotic use in a periurban community in Mexico: a household and drugstore survey. *Social Science and Medicine* 42:1121–1128.

CDC (Centers for Disease Control and Prevention). 1999. National Nosocomial Infections Surveillance (NNIS) System report, data summary from January 1990–May 1999, issued June 1999. *American Journal of Infection Control* 27:520–532.

Chatterjee P. 2001. India's trade in fake drugs—bringing the counterfeiters to book. *The Lancet* 357:1776.

Chuc NT and Tomson G. 1999. "Doi moi" and private pharmacies: a case study on dispensing and financial issues in Hanoi, Vietnam. *European Journal of Clinical Pharmacology* 55:325–332.

Commonwealth of Australia Government. 1999. *The Use of Antibiotics in Food-Producing Animals: Antibiotic-Resistant Bacteria in Animals and Humans: Report of the Joint Expert Technical Advisory Committee on Antibiotic Resistance (JETACAR)*. [Online]. Available: http://www.health.gov.au/pubs/jetacar.pdf.

Cosseron-Zerbib M, Roque Afonso AM, Naas T, Durand P, Meyer L, Costa Y, El Helali N, Huault G, Nordmann P. 1998. A control programme for MRSA containment in a paediatric intensive care unit: evaluation and impact on infections caused by other microorganisms. *Journal of Hospital Infection* 40:225–235.

CVMP (Committee for Veterinary Medicinal Products). 2001. Position Statement: Reflection by the CVMP within a European context on the intention of the FDA to withdraw the use of the fluoroquinolone enrofloxacin in poultry. [Online]. Available: http://www.emea.eu.int/pdfs/vet/press/pos/001401en.pdf.

Datta N. 1969. Drug resistance and R factors in the bowel bacteria of London patients before and after admission to hospital. *British Medical Journal* 2:407–411.

Djimde A, Plowe CV, Diop S, Dicko A, Wellems TE, Doumbo O. 1998. Use of antimalarial drugs in Mali: policy versus reality. *American Journal of Tropical Medicine and Hygiene* 59:376–379.

FDA (Food and Drug Administration). 2002a. *Center for Veterinary Medicine and Judicious Use of Antimicrobials*. [Online]. Available: http://www.fda.gov/cvm/fsi/JudUse.htm.

FDA. 2002b. *CVM Antimicrobial Activities: Surveillance, Research, Education, and International Coordination*. [Online]. Available: http://www.fda.gov/cvm/antimicrobial/AR2002Rpt.pdf.

Flynn DM, Weinstein RA, Nathan C, Gaston MA, Kabins SA. 1987. Patients' endogenous flora as the source of "nosocomial" Enterobacter in cardiac surgery. *Journal of Infectious Diseases* 156:363–368.

Fridkin SK, Edwards JR, Courval JM, Hill H, Tenover FC, Lawton R, Gaynes RP, McGowen JE Jr. 2001. The effect of vancomycin and third-generation cephalosporins on prevalence of vancomycin-resistant enterococci in 126 US adult intensive care units. *Annals of Internal Medicine* 135:175–183.

GAO (General Accounting Office). 1999. *Food Safety: The Agricultural Use of Antibiotics and Its Implications for Human Health*. GAO/RCED-99-74. Washington, DC: GAO.

Goetz AM and Muder RR. 1992. The problem of methicillin-resistant *Staphylococcus aureus*: A critical appraisal of the efficacy of infection control procedures with a suggested approach for infection control programs. *American Journal of Infection Control* 20:80–84.

Goldman DA, Weinstein RA, Wenzel RP, Tablan OC, Duma RJ, Gaynes RP, Schlosser J, Martone WJ. 1996. Strategies to prevent and control the emergence and spread of antimicrobial-resistant micro-organisms in hospitals: A challenge to hospital leadership. *Journal of the American Medical Association* 275:234–240.

Goma Epidemiology Group. 1995. Public health impact of Rwandan refugee crisis: what happened in Goma, Zaire, in July, 1994. *The Lancet* 345:339–344.

Graczyk TK, Knight R, Gilman RH, Cranfield MR. 2001. The role of non-biting flies in the epidemiology of human infectious diseases. *Microbes and Infection* 3:231–235.

Haley RW, Hightown AW, Khabbaz RF, Thornsberry C, Martone WJ, Allen JR, Hughes JM. 1982. The emergence of methicillin-resistant *Staphylococcus aureus* infections in United States hospitals: Possible role of the house staff-patient transfer circuit. *Annals of Internal Medicine* 97:297–308.

Harbarth S, Martin Y, Robner P, Henry N, Auckenthaler R, Pittet D. 2000. Effect of delayed infection control measures on a hospital outbreak of methicillin-resistant *Staphylococcus aureus*. *Journal of Hospital Infection* 46:43–49.

Hoge CW, Gambel JM, Srijan A, Pitarangsi C, Echeverria, P. 1998. Trends in antibiotic resistance among diarrheal pathogens isolated in Thailand over 15 years. *Clinical Infectious Diseases* 26:341–345.

Holmberg SD, Solomon SL, Blake PA. 1987. Health and economic impacts of antimicrobial resistance. *Reviews of Infectious Diseases* 9:1065–1078.

Howard D, Cordell R, McGowan JE Jr, Packard RM, Scott RD II, Solomon SL. 2001. Measuring the economic costs of antimicrobial resistance in hospital settings: Summary of the Centers for Disease Control and Prevention—Emory Workshop. *Clinical Infectious Diseases* 33:1573–1578.

Hsueh PR, Chen ML, Sun CC, Chen WH, Pan HJ, Yang LS, Chang SC, Ho SW, Lee CY, Hsieh WC, Luh KT. 2002. Antimicrobial drug resistance in pathogens causing nosocomial infections at a university hospital in Taiwan, 1981–1999. *Emerging Infectious Diseases* 8:63–68.

IOM (Institute of Medicine). 1998. *Antimicrobial Resistance: Issues and Options*. Washington, DC: National Academy Press.

Jackson GG. 1979. Antibiotic policies, practices and pressures. *Journal of Antimicrobial Chemotherapy* 5:1–4.

LaForce FM. 1993. The control of infections in hospitals: 1750 to 1950. In: Wenzel RP, ed. *Prevention and Control of Nosocomial Infections*. 2nd ed. Baltimore, MD: Williams and Wilkins. Pp. 1–12.

Lamikanra A and Okeke IN. 1997. A study of the effect of the urban/rural divide on the incidence of antibiotic resistance in *Escherichia coli*. *Biomedical Letters*. 55:91–97.

Larsson M, Kronvall G, Chuc NT, Karlsson I, Lager F, Hanh HD, Tomson G, Falkenberg T. 2000. Antibiotic medication and bacterial resistance to antibiotics: a survey of children in a Vietnamese community. *Tropical Medicine and International Health* 5:711–721.

Marr JJ, Moffet HL, Kunin CM. 1988. Guidelines for improving the use of antimicrobial agents in hospitals: a statement by the Infectious Diseases Society of America. *Journal of Infectious Diseases* 157:869–876.

McGowan JE Jr. 1983. Antimicrobial resistance in hospital organisms and its relation to antibiotic use. *Reviews of Infectious Diseases* 5:1033–1048.

McGowan JE Jr, Barnes MW, Finland M. 1975. Bacteremia at Boston City Hospital, occurrence and mortality during 12 selected years (1935–1972) with special reference to hospital-acquired cases. *Journal of Infectious Diseases* 132:316–335.

McGowan JE Jr, Garner C, Wilcox C, Finland M. 1974. Antibiotic susceptibilities of gram-negative bacilli isolated from blood cultures: Results of tests with 35 agents and strains from 169 patients at Boston City Hospital during 1972. *American Journal of Medicine* 57:225–238.

McGuffey RK, Richardson LF, Wilkinson JID. 2001. Ionophores for dairy cattle: Current status and future outlook. *Journal of Dairy Science* 84(Suppl.):E194–E203.

McMichael AJ. 2000. The urban environment and health in a world of increasing globalization: issues for developing countries. *Bulletin of the World Health Organization* 78:1117–1126.

Mellon M, Benbrook C, Benbrook KL. 2001. *Hogging It: Estimates of Antimicrobial Abuse in Livestock*. [Online]. Available: http://www.ucsusa.org/index.html.

Miller MA, Dascal A, Portnoy J, Mendelson J. 1996. Development of mupirocin resistance among methicillin-resistant *Staphylococcus aureus* after widespread use of nasal mupirocin ointment. *Infection Control and Hospital Epidemiology* 17:811–813.

Muirhead S, ed. 2001. *2002 Feed Additive Compendium*. Minnetonka, MN: Miller Publishing.

Muirhead S. 2002. Survey shows drop in antibiotic use. *Feedstuffs* 74:1, 3.

Mwansa J, Mutela K, Zulu I, Amadi B, Kelly P. 2002. Antimicrobial sensitivity in enterobacteria from AIDS patients, Zambia. *Emerging Infectious Diseases* 8:92–93.

Nagaraja TG, Laudert SB, Parrott JC. 1996. Liver abscesses in feedlot cattle. Part II. Incidence, economic importance, and prevention. *The Compendium* S264–S273.

Needham DM, Foster SD, Tomlinson G, Godfrey-Faussett P. 2001. Socio-economic, gender and health services factors affecting diagnostic delay for tuberculosis patients in urban Zambia. *Tropical Medicine and International Health* 6:256–259.

Newton P, Proux S, Green M, Smithuis F, Rozendaal J, Prakongpan S, Chotivanich K, Mayxay M, Looareesuwan S, Farrar J, Nosten F, White, NJ. 2001. Fake artesunate in southeast Asia. *The Lancet* 357:1948–1950.

Nicolle LE. 2001. *Infection Control Programmes to Control Antimicrobial Resistance*. Geneva: WHO.

Nizami SQ, Khan IA, Bhutta ZA. 1996. Drug prescribing practices of general practitioners and paediatricians for childhood diarrhoea in Karachi, Pakistan. *Social Science and Medicine* 42:1133–1139.

NRC (National Research Council). 1999. *The Use of Drugs in Food Animals: Benefits and Risks*. Washington, DC: National Academy Press.

O'Connor S, Rifkin D, Yang YH, Wang JF, Levine OS, Dowell SF. 2001. Physician control of pediatric antimicrobial use in Beijing, China, and its rural environs. *Pediatric Infectious Disease Journal* 20:679–684.

OIE (Office International des Epizooties). 2001 (October 2–4). *OIE Guidelines*. Paper resulting from the 2nd OIE International Conference on Antimicrobial Resistance: Use of Antimicrobials and Protection of Public Health, Paris, France. [Online]. Available: http://www.anmv.afssa.fr/oiecc/conference/guidelines.htm.

Okeke IN and Edelman R. 2001. Dissemination of antibiotic-resistant bacteria across geographic borders. *Clinical Infectious Diseases* 33:364–369.

Okeke IN and Lamikanra A. 1995. Quality and bioavailability of tetracycline capsules in a Nigerian semi-urban community. *International Journal of Antimicrobial Agents* 5:245–250.

Okeke IN and Lamikanra A. 2001. Quality and bioavailability of ampicillin capsules in a Nigerian semi-urban community. *African Journal of Medicine and Medical Sciences* 30:47–51.

Okeke IN and Lamikanra A. In press. Export of antimicrobial drugs by West African travelers. *Journal of Travel Medicine.*

Okeke IN, Abudu AB, Lamikanra A. 2001. Microbiological investigation of an outbreak of acute gastroenteritis in Niger State, Nigeria. *Clinical Microbiology and Infection* 7:514–516.

Okeke IN, Fayinka ST, Lamikanra A. 2000. Antibiotic resistance trends in *Escherichia coli* from apparently healthy Nigerian students (1986–1998). *Emerging Infectious Diseases* 6:393–396.

Okeke IN, Lamikanra A, Edelman R. 1999. Socioeconomic and behavioral factors leading to acquired bacterial resistance to antibiotics in developing countries. *Emerging Infectious Diseases* 5:18–27.

Paredes P, de la Pena M, Flores-Guerra E, Diaz J, Trostle J. 1996. Factors influencing physicians' prescribing behaviour in the treatment of childhood diarrhoea: knowledge may not be the clue. *Social Science and Medicine* 42:1141–1153.

Payne MA, Baynes RE, Sundlof SE, Craigmill A, Webb AI, Riviere JE. 1999. Drugs prohibited from extralabel use in food animals. *Journal of the American Veterinary Medical Association* 215:28–32.

Pechere JC. 2001. Patients' interviews and misuse of antibiotics. *Clinical Infectious Diseases* 33:S170–173.

Prescott JF, Baggot JD, Walker RD, eds. 2000. *Antimicrobial Therapy in Veterinary Medicine.* 3rd ed. Ames, IA: Iowa State University Press.

Price DJ and Sleigh JD. 1970. Control of infection due to *Klebsiella aerogenes* in a neurosurgical unit by withdrawal of all antibiotics. *Lancet* 2:1213–1215.

Rosas I, Salinas E, Yela A, Calva E, Eslava C, Cravioto A. 1997. *Escherichia coli* in settled-dust and air samples collected in residential environments in Mexico City. *Applied and Environmental Microbiology* 63:4093–4095.

Scheckler WE, Brimhall D, Buck AS, Farr BM, Friedman C, Garibaldi RA, Gross PA, Harris JA, Hierholzer WJ, Martone WJ, McDonald LL, Solomon SL. 1998. Requirements for infrastructure and essential activities of infection control and epidemiology in hospitals: A consensus panel report. *Infection Control and Hospital Epidemiology* 19:114–124.

Schlaes DM, Gerding DN, John JF Jr, Craig WA, Bornstein DL, Duncan RA, Eckman MR, Farrer WE, Greene WH, Lorian V, Levy S, McGowan JE Jr, Paul SM, Riskin J, Tenover FC, Watanakunakorn C. 1997. Society for Healthcare Epidemiology of America and Infectious Diseases Society of America Joint Committee on the Prevention of Antimicrobial Resistance: Guidelines for the prevention of antimicrobial resistance in hospitals. *Infection Control and Hospital Epidemiology* 18:275–291.

Sengupta PG, Niyogi SK, Bhattacharya SK. 2000. An outbreak of Eltor cholera in Aizwal town of Mizoram, India. *Journal of Communicable Diseases* 32:207–211.

Siringi S. 2001. Over-the-counter sale of antimalarial drugs stalls Kenyan disease strategy. *The Lancet* 357:1862.

Sofowora A. 1982. *Medicinal Plants and Traditional Medicine in Africa.* Chinchester: John Wiley and Sons.

Souwein B, Traore O, Aublet-Cuvelier B, Bret L, Sirot L, Laveran H, Deteix P. 2000. Role of infection control measures in limiting morbidity associated with multi-resistant organisms in critically ill patients. *Journal of Hospital Infection* 45:107–116.

Taylor RB, Shakoor O, Behrens RH, Everard M, Low AS, Wangboonskul J, Reid RG, Kolawole JA. 2001. Pharmacopoeial quality of drugs supplied by Nigerian pharmacies. *The Lancet* 357:1933–1936.

Terpstra S, Noordhoek GT, Voerten HGJ, Hendriks B, Degener JE. 1999. Rapid emergence of resistant coagulase negative staphylococci on the skin after antibiotic prophylaxis. *Journal of Hospital Infection* 43:195–202.

Torrence, ME. 2001. Activities to address antimicrobial resistance in the United States. *Preventive Veterinary Medicine* 51:37–49.

U.S. Government. 2001. *A Public Health Action Plan to Combat Antimicrobial Resistance.* [Online]. Available: http://www.cdc.gov/drugresistance/actionplan.

Wachter DA, Joshi MP, Rimal B. 1999. Antibiotic dispensing by drug retailers in Kathmandu, Nepal. *Tropical Medicine and International Health* 4:782–788.

Walson JL, Marshall B, Pokhrel BM, Kafle KK, Levy SB. 2001. Carriage of antibiotic-resistant fecal bacteria in Nepal reflects proximity to Kathmandu. *Journal of Infectious Diseases* 184:1163–1169.

Weinstein RA and Kabins SA. 1981. Strategies for prevention and control of multiple drug-resistant nosocomial infection. *American Journal of Medicine* 70:449–454.

WHO (World Health Organization). 1998. *Use of Quinolones in Food Animals and Potential Impact on Human Health.* [Online]. Available: http://www.who.int/emc-documents/zoonoses/whoemczdi9810c.html.

WHO. 2000. *WHO Global Principles for the Containment of Antimicrobial Resistance in Animals Intended for Food. Report of a WHO Consultation with the Participation of the Food and Agriculture Organization of the United Nations and the Office International des Epizooties. Geneva, Switzerland 5–9 June 2000.* [Online]. Available: http://www.who.int/emc/diseases/zoo/who_global_principles.html.

WHO. 2001. *WHO Global Strategy for Containment of Antibiotic Resistance.* Geneva: WHO.

Winstanley P. 2001. Modern chemotherapeutic options for malaria. *The Lancet Infectious Diseases* 1:242–250.

6

Emerging Tools and Technology for Countering Resistance

OVERVIEW

Most efforts to overcome problems resulting from microbial resistance have been aimed at either extending the useful life of current drugs or developing new drugs. But the first approach, which has typically involved developing slightly different chemical derivatives, has provided only marginal gains, and the second approach has in recent decades produced only a single new chemical class of antibiotics. And while many observers suggest that the genomics revolution may be opening promising new avenues for exploration, it has yet to populate the pharmaceutical development pipeline with new classes of compounds.

The focus of this session of the workshop was on examining advances in our understanding of the genetics and biochemistry of a variety of pathogens, and on exploring how this knowledge might lead to novel approaches to developing new drugs and other tools and technologies to help counter the spread of antimicrobial resistance.

Among the antibiotics discussed was the important family of β-lactams, which include penicillin, methicillin, oxacillin, and the newer cephalosporins. Recent research has revealed at least four strategies by which bacteria develop resistance to these antibiotics. The most common tactic involves certain enzymes, called β–lactamases, that break apart critical components of the drugs. Knowing the details of these mechanisms may provide scientists with new targets to attack in designing drugs that can circumvent a microbe's natural defenses.

Another research group is taking a radically different approach to drug design. Since most bacteria enter humans at a mucous membrane site, such as the upper and lower respiratory tract or the intestines, these locations act as reservoirs for many pathogens. However, there currently are no drugs that can kill pathogens on mucous membranes without killing surrounding normal bacteria as well, and physicians therefore must wait for infection to occur systemically before treating the patient. If it were possible to safely deplete this disease reservoir on mucous membranes, then it might be possible to markedly lower the incidence of infections. Toward this end, the scientists have developed a new type of reagent, called lytic enzymes, that can prevent infection by specifically destroying pathogenic bacteria on mucous membranes. The enzymes might prove especially useful in hospitals, nursing homes, daycare centers, and other locations where bacterial infections often run rampant.

Participants also examined how the current regulatory approval process for moving new drug candidates to market might be modified to help reduce problems of antimicrobial resistance. Drug developers now must conduct extensive clinical trials to evaluate whether their agent achieves a clinical cure; that is, whether it frees recipients of symptoms. But this marker may not show whether the drug actually killed all of the pathogens—an important requirement for minimizing the emergence of resistance. One suggestion is to examine the pharmacokinetics and pharmacodynamics of new drugs as a complementary part of the approval process. This technical approach, known as PK/PD, is built on taking regular cultures from a person receiving a therapeutic agent and determining when pathogenic microbes are no longer present. In this way, the technology offers a direct measure of the agent's ability not only to cure the patient but also to completely eliminate the pathogen.

EVOLUTION OF MULTIPLE MECHANISMS OF RESISTANCE TO β-LACTAM ANTIBIOTICS

Dasantila Golemi-Kotra, Ph.D., Sergei Vakulenko, M.D., Ph.D., and Shahriar Mobashery, Ph.D.

Departments of Chemistry, Pharmacology and
Biochemistry and Molecular Biology
Institute for Drug Design, Wayne State University, Detroit, MI

Major discoveries in antibiotics were made in succession from the 1950s through the 1970s, an era that has come to be known as the "Golden Age of Antibiotics." These accomplishments created a sense of euphoria in the medical community as it perceived that bacterial infections were curable.

Victory over bacteria was declared and financial resources were redirected toward more pressing scientific questions. By the late 1980s to the early 1990s, many pharmaceutical companies stopped research for discovery and development of new types of antibiotics, a trend that was shadowed by federal agencies such as the National Institutes of Health that showed more inclination to support studies of non-microbial systems during that period.

Meanwhile, liberal use of antibiotics in the clinics, in agriculture, in aquaculture, and in animal husbandry was facilitating a quiet revolution in microbial populations. These events resulted in antibiotic-resistant organisms that were perfectly treatable a decade or two earlier. These organisms were included among those defined as re-emerging infectious agents (IOM, 1992; Heymann and Rodier, 2001). While this trend was progressing steadily over the past decades, previously unknown infectious agents were also being discovered (WHO, 1996; Desselberger, 2000).

Acquired resistance to antibiotics can develop rapidly. As depicted in Figure 6-1, it takes typically a mere one to four years for clinical resistance to emerge for any antibiotic. The beginning of each arrow in Figure 6-1 indicates the time point when the given antibiotic was introduced to the clinic and the tip of the arrow indicates when resistance to it emerged.

Whereas the data of Figure 6-1 speak for themselves, three examples are worthy of a brief comment. The arrow is in reverse for penicillin G, since the first case of resistance to penicillin was reported two years prior to the first large-scale clinical use of penicillin in 1942 (Abraham and Chain, 1940). The resistant organism harbored a β-lactamase, an enzyme that to the present day is the major cause of resistance to β-lactam antibiotics. Figure 6-1 would seem to indicate that resistance to nalidixic acid took roughly 20 years to develop. This is true in part due to the antibiotic glut in the late 1950s into the 1960s. There were so many effective antibiotics that nalidixic acid was not used. Indeed, when quinolone and fluoroquinolone antibiotics, the structural descendants of nalidixic acid, were introduced to the clinic in earnest in the middle to late 1980s, resistance to them developed very rapidly.

The example of the first clinically used oxazolidinone, linezolid (Zyvox; Pharmacia, Inc.), is noteworthy. Linezolid was approved for clinical use in the United States in April 2000. It is an especially active antibiotic against infections caused by multi-drug-resistant gram-positive bacteria, including methicillin-resistant *Staphylococcus aureus* (MRSA), vancomycin-resistant enterococci (VRE) and penicillin-resistant *Streptococcus pneumonia* (Fung et al., 2001). Linezolid binds the bacterial ribosome reversibly and inhibits initiation of protein biosynthesis by preventing the formation of a ternary complex among $tRNA^{fMet}$, mRNA, and the ribosome (Swaney et al., 1998). The propensity of emergence of resistance to linezolid in *S. aureus* and *S.*

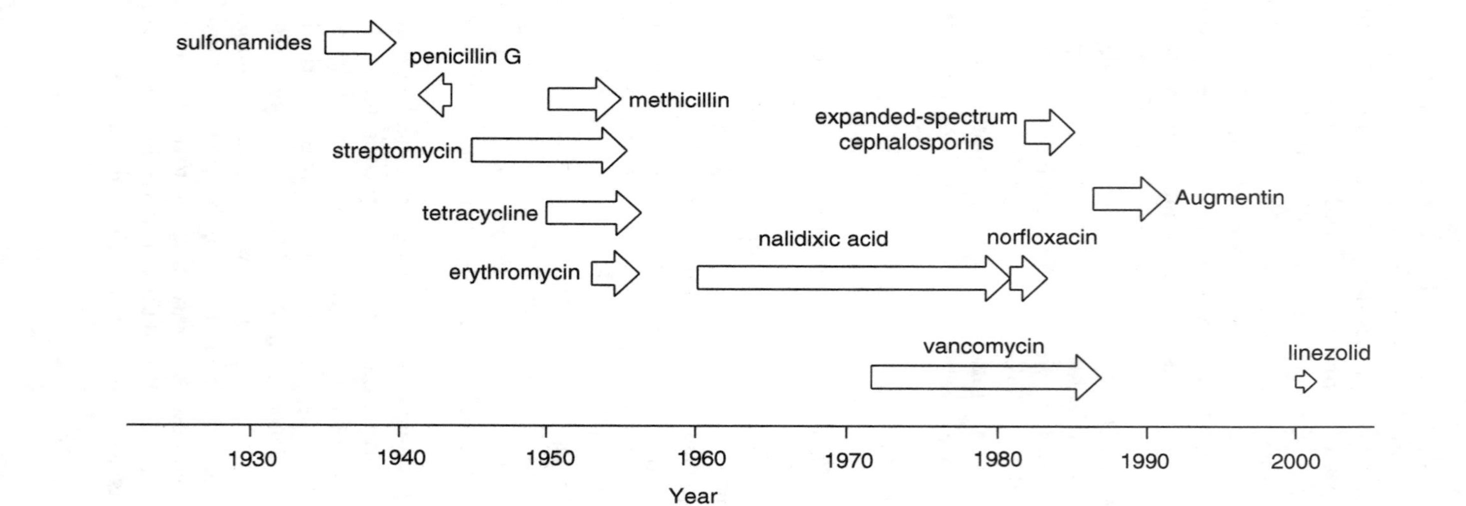

FIGURE 6-1 Resistance to antibiotics develops rapidly. The beginning of the arrow is when a given antibiotic was introduced to the clinic and the tip of the arrow is when the first clinical case of resistance to it was reported. Adopted and expanded from Wong and Pompliano, 1998.

epidermis is less than 10^{-9} (Kaatz and Seo, 1996). Studies have revealed that single-point mutations clustered in the DNA region encoding the central loop of the domain V of 23S rRNA cause resistance (Swaney et al., 1998; Gonzales et al., 2001; Prystowsky et al., 2001; Tsiodras et al., 2001). Because of the critical importance of the ribosome for survival of any organism, there exists redundancy in the genes for the ribosomal RNA to ensure that mutations in any one gene would not prove fatal. It would appear that mutation of one to three of these genes is necessary for manifestation of resistance to linezolid, and this indeed has happened. Clinical resistance to linezolid emerged in a mere seven months after its introduction to the clinic (Fung et al., 2001).

In principle, the genes that would confer resistance to an antibiotic could be acquired or could evolve. Gene acquisitions could take place as DNA sequences are shared among organisms by conjugation, transformation, and transduction or by classical recombination and transposition (Bennett, 1999). However, the issue of evolution of a resistance determinant is less commonly appreciated (Mobashery and Azucena, 2002). Many stretches of genes encode proteins that serve adventitious functions in addition to their physiological ones. These genes may be duplicated, and the fates of the copies could take them in disparate evolutionary tangents. One would encode the protein for the physiological function and the other may evolve to confer resistance to the antibiotic. Despite the fact that bacteria have enzymes for repair of genetic damage, random mutations do occur in bacteria and the rate is typically 10^{-10}. Considering the fact that the sizes of bacterial genomes are large (e.g., *Escherichia coli* K-12 has 4.6×10^6 base pairs) and that population sizes of bacteria in infections can also be very large (10^7 cells/ml for infections of blood and 10^9 cells/ml for infections of tissues), the opportunities for emergence of mutant variants are plentiful. These three factors taken together would indicate that there may be as many as 10^5 to 10^6 mutations per milliliter of bacteria growth, hence these populations are not homogeneous (Mobashery and Azucena, 2002).

These mutations occur at random throughout the genome. Some are silent, others are lethal, yet many may cause an incremental change in the organism that would not result in undue survival hardship to the organism. In the face of the challenge by a given antibiotic, should one or more of these mutant variants be better fit to survive, it would be selected at the expense of the susceptible organisms. The given selected gene for the protein that confers resistance may continue to evolve as a resistance determinant from that point on. For all members of the seven major classes of antibiotics (i.e., β-lactams, aminoglycosides, fluorquinolones, glycopeptides, macrolides, tetracyclines, and sulfonamides) there are documented mechanisms for resistance. Often, there are multiple known mechanisms for resistance to each.

A full discussion of the various mechanisms of resistance to all known antibiotics is outside the scope of this report, although such reviews have appeared in the literature (Kotra et al., 2000; Walsh, 2000; Poole, 2001; Golemi-Kotra and Mobashery, 2002; Mobashery and Azucena, 2002). In this report we concentrate on the case of the mechanisms of resistance to β-lactam antibiotics (i.e., penicillins, cephalosporins, carbapenems, etc.). As will be presented below, this has been a fertile field for evolution of resistance, which represents a well-studied microcosm of diversity that must also exist in the microbial world for other antibiotics that await discovery.

There are at least four documented mechanisms for resistance to β-lactam antibiotics (see Table 6-1). The first and the most common mechanism is the occurrence of β-lactamases, enzymes that hydrolyze and destroy β-lactam antibiotics. The reaction of β-lactamases with a penicillin is given in Figure 6-2. Over 340 distinct β-lactamases have been identified in bacteria (Bush and Mobashery, 1998; Bush, 1999). These enzymes fall into four classes: A to D. Enzymes of class B are zinc-dependent, and the remaining three classes are enzymes that depend on a catalytic serine in their mechanisms of action. These serine-dependent enzymes experience acylation at the serine by the substrate, and the acyl-enzyme species subsequently undergoes an enzyme-promoted deacylation that liberates the enzyme for additional catalytic cycles and releases the product of the reaction (Bush and Mobashery, 1998; Massova and Mobashery, 1998).

The three classes of β-lactamases that pursue this strategy all share the acylation event but differ significantly in the deacylation steps. The differences include the direction of the approach of the hydrolytic water and the mechanism of the enzyme-promoted step. In the case of class A enzymes, a glutamate (Glu-166) promotes the hydrolytic water from one face of the acyl-enzyme species (Strynadka et al., 1992; Miyashita et al., 1995; Maveyraud et al., 1998; Mourey et al., 1998). The class C enzymes pro-

TABLE 6-1 Four Known Mechanisms of Resistance to β-lactam Antibiotics

1. The catalytic function of β-lactamases (gram-positive and gram-negative)
2. DD-Transpeptidases that resist acylation by β-lactam antibiotics (gram-positive; MRSA)
3. Loss of porins or their alteration to reduce penetration into periplasm (gram-negative)
4. Selection of the LD-transpeptidase activity (documented only for *E. faecium*)

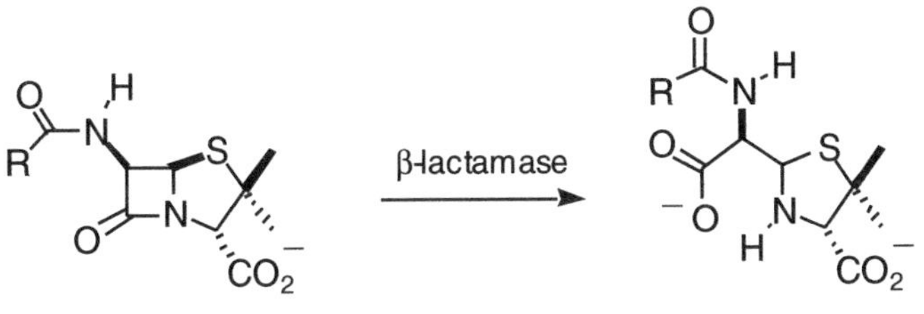

FIGURE 6-2 Hydrolytic reaction of β-lactamases results in products that lack antibacterial activity.

mote the hydrolytic water from the opposite face and they use a different residue (a tyrosine) along the substrate amine as the basic entities (Bulychev et al., 1995, 1997; Patera et al., 2000). Class D enzymes are different yet. These enzymes, in contrast to the cases of enzymes of classes A and C, pursue a symmetric mechanism for the two-step reaction by having a highly unusual carbamylated lysine that serves the role of a base for both steps of catalysis (Maveyraud et al., 2000; Golemi et al., 2001; Maveyraud et al., 2002). These observations argue for independent evolutions for all four classes of β-lactamases (Massova and Mobashery, 1998). Structural evidence argues that the family of penicillin-binding proteins (PBPs) is related to that of β-lactamases (Kelly et al., 1998; Massova and Mobashery, 1998). A sequence alignment of all known classes of β-lactamases and PBPs has supported the mechanistic assertion for independent evolution of each β-lactamase. It indicated that evolution of β-lactamases took place relatively recently on the evolutionary time scale and it did so at branching points for diversification of the biosynthetic PBPs (Massova and Mobashery, 1998).

These enzymes are extremely effective at what they do. It has been shown that class A and class C β-lactamases have reached catalytic perfection in that they operate at the diffusion limit (Hardy and Kirsch, 1984; Bulychev and Mobashery, 1999). Many others also function at or near the diffusion limit. We have shown that the class D OXA-10 β-lactamase from *Pseudomonas aeruginosa* is present in the periplasmic space of clinical strains in concentrations of 4–15 μM (Golemi et al., 2001). This will amount to as many as 1,200 molecules of the enzyme per bacterium. Considering the fact that each molecule of the enzyme turns over 1,500 molecules of cloxacillin (a penicillin) per second, each organism destroys 1.8 million molecules of the drug per second.

The second mechanism for resistance to β-lactam antibiotics is seen in gram-positive bacteria. The case of methicillin-resistant *Staphylococcus aureus* (MRSA) exemplifies this category. *S. aureus* has acquired a penicillin-binding protein (PBP 2a) that has the ability to carry out the functions of the other four PBPs that are normally present in this organism (Pinho et al.,

2001a). However, this PBP resists the inhibitory properties of all clinically used β-lactam antibiotics. Hence, MRSA survives the treatment by these commonly used antibiotics (Roychoudhury et al., 1994; Pinho et al., 2001b). In light of the fact that MRSA has become resistant to many other classes of antibiotics, it is currently a serious clinical problem. There are a number of projects in the pharmaceutical industry for development of specific cephalosporins that bind to PBP 2a of *S. aureus* (Chamberland et al., 2001; Hebeisen et al., 2001; Johnson et al., 2002; Wootton et al., 2002).

Antibiotics must penetrate the bacterial envelope to reach their targets. The protective effect of the gram-negative envelope is more than that of the gram-positive organisms in light of the presence of the outer membrane in the former. The outer membrane is a bilayer sheath that encloses the entire organism. Nutrients penetrate this membrane by traversing the porin channels. Porins are integral outer-membrane proteins that create water-filled channels through the outer membrane. β-lactam antibiotics also need to go through these channels, which set an upper limit of 700–1000 Da for the antibiotic size. It has been known that some organisms may eliminate certain porins or may acquire alterations to the structure of a specific type of porin to limit penetration of the antibiotic into the periplasmic space. This mechanism has been shown to be operative against certain carbapenem antibiotics (Martinez-Martinez et al., 2000; Ochs et al., 2000). It is not very common because the loss of porins or their structural alteration would have implications for potential survival of the organism as well.

The fourth mechanism of resistance to β-lactam antibiotics is seen only in *Enterococcus faecium*. Bacteria are required to cross-link the peptidoglycan strands of their cell wall in order to be viable. The cross-linking reaction is carried out by some PBPs referred to as DD-transpeptidases, because the enzymes link one strand of the peptidoglycan to the site of the acyl-D-Ala-D-Ala of the second strand. These enzymes recognize the unusual D-Ala-D-Ala entity of the peptidoglycan structure in their substrates. It would appear that *E. faceium* has evolved an entirely new PBP that is referred to as LD-transpeptidase. This enzyme attaches the first peptidoglycan strand to the L-amino acid adjacent to the D-Ala-D-Ala moiety, hence it is referred to as the LD-transpeptidase (Mainardi et al., 2000). This is essentially a bypass mechanism, since the LD-transpeptidase is insensitive to β-lactam antibiotics.

Concluding Remarks

We have disclosed in this report that nature has devised at least four strategies for resistance to β-lactam antibiotics in bacteria. Of these, the most prevalent is the occurrence of β-lactamases. Four distinct and independent mechanisms have evolved for the catalytic functions of these enzymes. Individually, these enzymes have undergone additional diversification. For example, a total of 102 variants of the TEM-1 β-lactamases from *E. coli* have been reported as of January 2002. These observations provide strong evidence that random mutation and selection would lead along a different evolutionary tangent depending on when the event takes place, in what organism, and what resources were available to the organism.

USING PHAGE LYTIC ENZYMES TO CONTROL ANTIBIOTIC-RESISTANT PATHOGENIC BACTERIA ON MUCOUS MEMBRANES

*Vincent A. Fischetti, Ph.D.**

Rockefeller University, New York, NY

Nearly all bacteria infect at a mucous membrane site (upper and lower respiratory, intestinal, urogenital, and ocular). In addition, the human mucous membranes are a reservoir for many pathogenic bacteria found in the environment (e.g., pneumococci, staphylococci, streptococci) some of which are resistant to antibiotics. In most instances, it is this reservoir that is the focus of infection in the population (Coello et al., 1994; de Lencastre et al., 1999; Eiff et al., 2001). To date, except for polysporin and mupirocin ointments, there are no anti-infectives that are designed to control pathogenic bacteria on mucous membranes; we must first wait for infection to occur before treating. Because of the fear of developing resistance, antibiotics are not indicated to control the carrier state of disease bacteria. It is clear, however, that by reducing or eliminating this human reservoir, the incidence of disease in the community will be markedly reduced. Our laboratory has developed enzymes that are designed to prevent infection by safely and specifically destroying disease bacteria on mucous membranes. For example, enzymes specific for *S. pneumoniae* and *S. aureus* may be used nasally to control these organisms in day care centers, hospitals, and nursing homes to prevent or markedly reduce both transmission and serious infections caused by these bacteria.

We accomplish this by capitalizing on the efficient system developed by bacteriophage to kill bacteria. When bacteriophage infect their host bacteria to produce progeny virus particles, they are faced with a problem: to release the progeny phage particles trapped in the bacterium at the end of the replicative cycle. They solve this problem by producing an efficient

---

*Acknowledgment: Supported by a grant from the Defense Advance Research Project Agency (DARPA).

enzyme termed lysin that rapidly degrades the cell walls of the infected bacteria to release the phage progeny (Young, 1992).

We have identified and purified these phage-encoded enzymes and found that when applied externally to gram-positive bacteria, the bacteria are killed seconds after contact (Loeffler et al., 2001; Nelson et al., 2001). For example, 10^7 group A streptococci could be reduced to an undetectable level ten seconds after enzyme addition. To date, except for chemical agents, there is no biological compound known that can kill bacteria this quickly. Such phage lytic enzymes are the culmination of billions of years of development by the bacteriophage during their association with bacteria.

Enzyme Structure

A feature of those phage lytic enzymes that have been characterized so far is their two-domain structure (Diaz et al., 1990; Garcia et al., 1990). Generally, the N-terminal domain contains the catalytic activity of the enzyme that will cleave one of the four major bonds in the peptidoglycan of the bacterial cell wall. This activity may be an endo-beta-N-acetylglucosaminidase or N-acetylmuramidase (lysozyme), both of which act on the sugar moiety, an endopeptidase which acts on the peptide cross bridge, or an N-acetylmuramyl-L-alanine amidase (or amidase) which hydrolyzes the amide bond connecting the sugar and peptide moieties (Young, 1992). Of the phage lytic enzymes that have been reported thus far, the great majority are amidases. The C-terminal domain of phage lytic enzymes has specificity for a cell wall substrate (Garcia et al., 1988; Lopez et al., 1992, 1997). Thus, unless the binding domain binds to its wall substrate the catalytic domain will not cleave, offering specificity to the enzyme. The reason for this specificity was not apparent at first, since it seemed counterintuitive that the phage would specifically design an enzyme that was lethal for its host organism. However, as we learned more about how these enzymes function, the possible reason for this specificity became apparent (see below, Resistance).

Mode of Action

By thin section electron microscopy of phage enzyme-treated bacteria, it appears that the enzymes exert their lethal effects by digesting the peptidoglycan, forming holes in the cell wall. This results in extrusion of the cytoplasmic membrane and, ultimately, hypotonic lysis (see Figure 6-3). Isolated cell walls treated with lysin are cut into pieces (see Figures 6-4 and 6-5), verifying the results seen with intact bacteria.

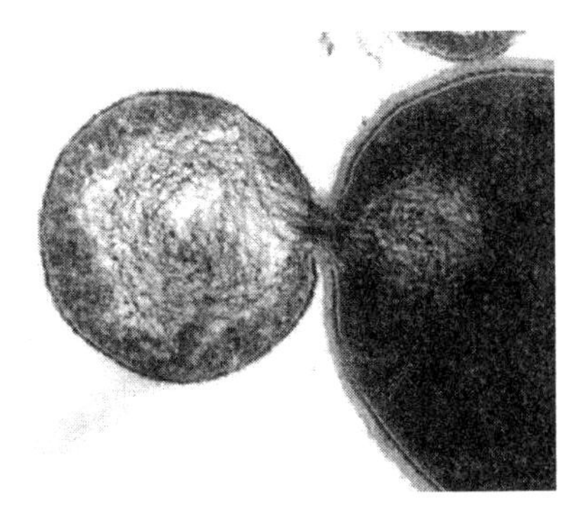

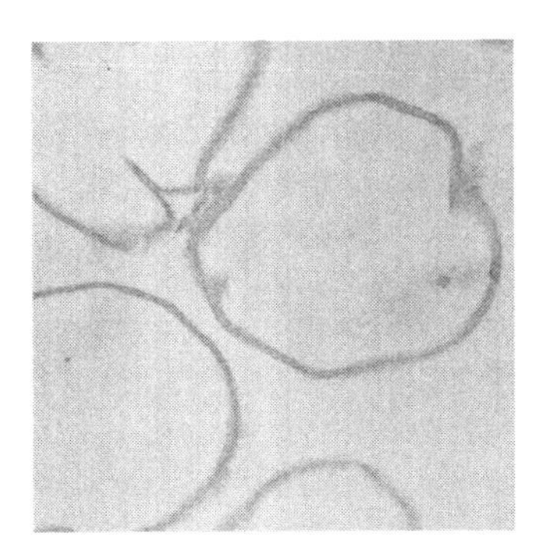

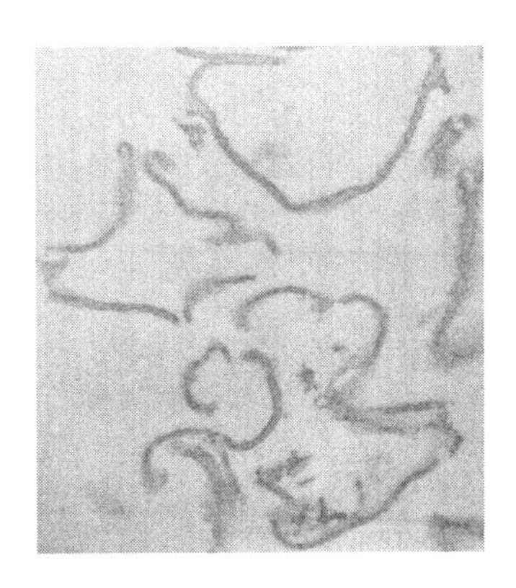

FIGURES 6-3–6-5 Effects of lysin on whole bacteria and cell walls. (Fig 6-3) Thin section electron micrographs of whole group A streptococci treated with C1 phage lytic enzyme for 15 seconds. A bacterium is seen in which a hole has been digested in the cell wall allowing the cytoplasmic membrane to become externalized resulting in osmotic lysis and death. Isolated group A streptococcal cell walls pre (Fig 6-4) and post (Fig 6-5) treatment with phage enzyme. Enzyme-treated cells exhibit pieces of wall in this thin section indicating that holes have been digested in the structure.

Targeted Killing

An interesting feature of these enzymes is that they kill the species of bacteria from which they were produced. For instance, enzymes produced from streptococcal bacteriophage kill streptococci, and enzymes produced by pneumococcal bacteriophage kill pneumococci (Loeffler et al., 2001; Nelson et al., 2001). Specifically, the group A streptococcal lysin will kill group A streptococci efficiently, and has a small effect on groups C and G streptococci, but essentially no effect on normal oral streptococci (see Figure 6-6).

Similar results are seen with a pneumococcal-specific lysine; however, in this case, the enzyme was also tested against strains of pneumococci that were resistant to penicillin and the killing efficiency was the same. Unlike antibiotics, which are usually more broad in their spectrum and kill many different bacteria found in the human body, some of which are beneficial, the phage enzymes kill only the disease bacteria with little to no effect on the normal human bacterial flora. Thus, the phage enzymes are molecules

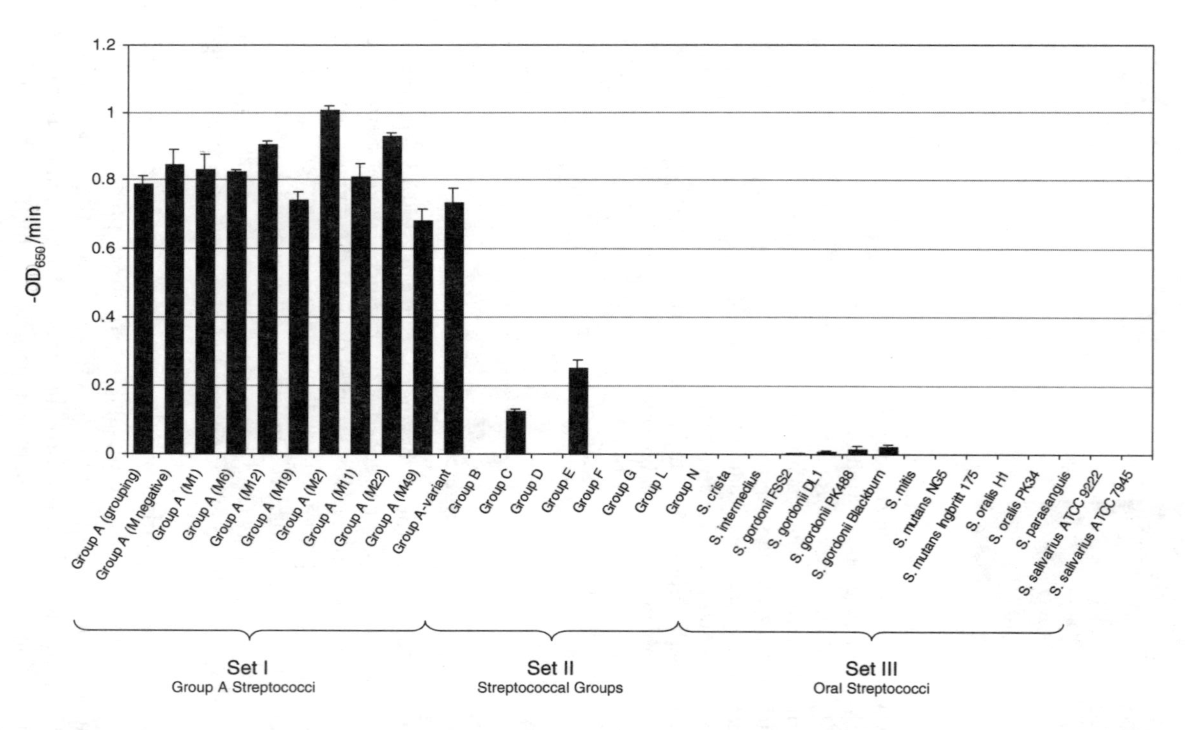

FIGURE 6-6 Representative streptococcal strains were exposed to 250 U of purified lysin and the OD_{650} was monitored. The activity of lysin for each strain was reported as the initial velocity of lysis, in $-OD_{650}$/min, based on the time it took to decrease the starting OD by half (i.e., from an OD_{650} of 1.0 to 0.5). All assays were performed in triplicate and the data are expressed as means ± standard deviations. As can be seen, the enzyme specifically kills group A streptococci, and groups C and G slightly, and has no effect on oral streptococci.

that enable targeted killing of pathogenic bacteria with little effect on the surrounding normal flora. The group A streptococcal enzyme was tested for safety in two animal model systems, one mucosal and the other skin. When enzyme was added to these surfaces daily for 7 days, and the tissues examined both visually and histologically, nothing unusual was observed. This was not surprising since the bonds cleaved by the phage enzymes are only found in bacteria and not mammalian tissues. Thus, it is anticipated that these enzymes will be well tolerated by the human mucous membranes.

In Vivo Experiments

Two in vivo animal models of mucosal colonization were developed to test the capacity for the lysins to kill organisms on these surfaces. An oral colonization model was developed for group A streptococci and a nasal model was developed for pneumococci (Loeffler et al., 2001; Nelson et al., 2001). In both cases, when the animals were colonized with their respective bacteria and treated with a small amount of lysin specific for the colonizing organism, the animals were found to be free of colonizing bacteria two to five hours after lysin treatment (see Figures 6-7 and 6-8). In the group A streptococcal experiment, animals were also swabbed 24 and 48 hours after lysin treatment. During that time most animals remained negative for streptococci but one animal had died and two others showed positive colonies

Mouse	10^7 Strep	Day 1	Day 2	Day 3	Day 4	Lysin	(2 hr) Day 4	(24 hr) Day 5	(48 hr) Day 6
•		>300	>300	>300	>300		0	0	200
•		>300	>300	>300	>300		0	50	0
•		>300	>300	>300	>300		0	0	0
•		>300	>300	>300	>300		0	0	0
•		>300	>300	>300	>300		0	Dead	Dead
•		>300	>300	>300	>300		0	ND	0
•		>300	>300	>300	>300		0	ND	0
•		>300	>300	>300	>300		0	ND	0
•		>300	>300	>300	>300		0	ND	0
	Total	9/9	9/9	9/9	9/9		0/9	2/5	2/9

FIGURE 6-7 Elimination of group A streptococci from the mucosal surface of colonized mice. Mice were colonized with streptococci orally followed by oral swab for 4 days. At this time they were treated orally with phage lysin and swabbed 2, 24, and 48 hours later. Figures are colony-forming units of streptococci recovered. ND = not determined.

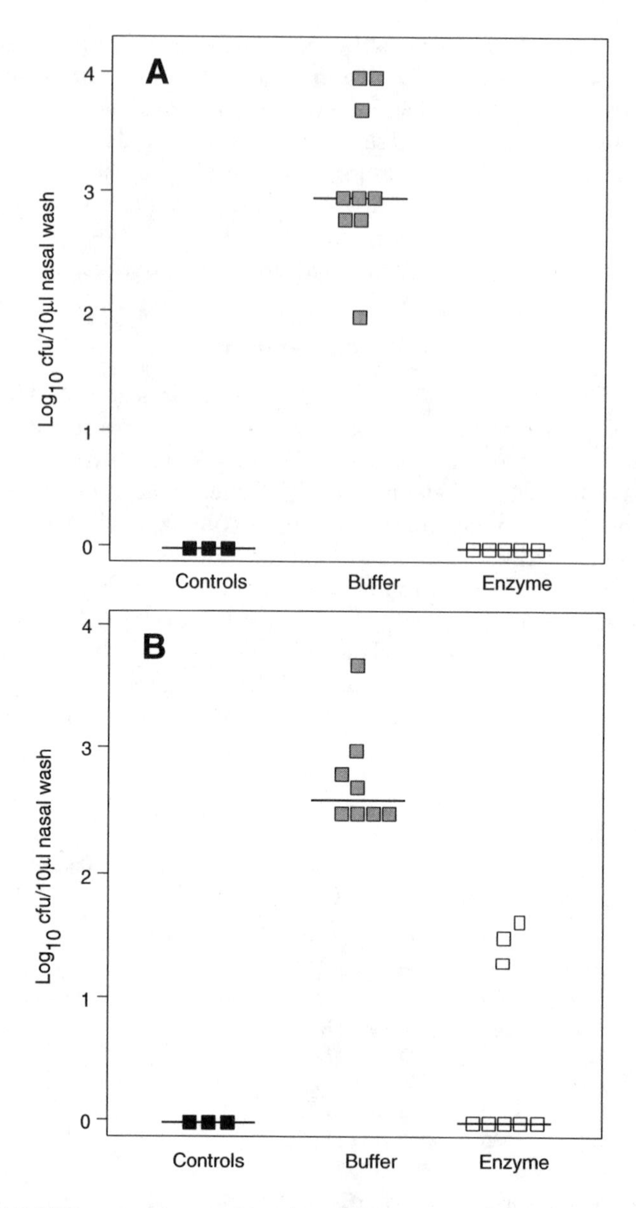

FIGURE 6-8 Killing pneumococci in vivo. Elimination of *S. pneumoniae* serotype 14 in the mouse model of nasopharyngeal carriage. (A) After nasal and pharyngeal treatment with a total of 1,400 µg of Pal enzyme, no pneumococci were retrieved in the nasal wash, compared to buffer-treated colonized mice ($p < 0.001$). No pneumococci were isolated from non-colonized control mice (controls). (B) After treatment with a total of 700 µg of Pal enzyme, pneumococci were completely eliminated in 5 of 8 colonized mice ($p < 0.001$) and overall significantly reduced.

(see Figure 6-7). We interpret these results to mean that the positive animals became infected during the first four days of colonization where some organisms became intracellular. Thus, while the lysin is able to clear organisms found on the surface, it was unable to kill organisms that had initiated an infection. We ruled out the possibility that the organisms that appeared in 24 and 48 hours did so because they became resistant to the lysin by assessing them for their sensitivity to the lysin.

Killing Biowarfare Bacteria

Because phage enzymes are so efficient in killing pathogenic bacteria, they may be a valuable tool in controlling biowarfare bacteria. To determine the feasibility of the approach we identified a lytic enzyme from the gamma phage that is specific for *Bacillus anthracis* (Watanabe et al., 1975). By cloning the gamma lysin we identified a ~700 bp ORF in the phage genome encoding a 26 kDa product very similar in size and features to a variety of *Bacillus*, *Listeria*, and *Mycobacteria* phage lysins. The gamma lysin, referred to as PlyG, was then purified to homogeneity by a two-step chromatographic procedure and tested for its lethal action on gamma phage sensitive bacilli. Three seconds after contact, as little as 100 units of PlyG (10 μg) mediated a 5,000-fold decrease in viable counts of a ~10^7 *Bacillus* culture (Schuch et al., 2002). This lethal activity was observed in growth media, phosphate buffer, and even human blood. When the enzyme was then tested against five mutant *B. anthracis* strains and ten different virulent *B. anthracis* strains isolated worldwide, it was found to be lethal for them all (Schuch et al., 2002). Although PlyG has no effect on bacillus spores, we discovered that by heat shocking at 60°C and the addition of the germinant L-alanine results in rapid generation of spores which are sensitive to the action of the PlyG enzyme. For example, 10^8 spores heat-activated for 5 minutes and treated with L-alanine for 5 minutes were reduced in viability by 4-logs after a 5-minute treatment with PlyG.

When 10^6 bacilli were administered intraperitoneally (IP) to 15 mice all of the animals died of rapidly fatal septicemia within four hours. When a second set of 13 mice was also challenged IP with bacilli but given only 150 μg of PlyG 15 minutes later by the same route, 77 percent of the animals recovered fully, and the remaining died within 6–21 hours (Schuch et al., 2002). We anticipate that higher doses or repeated treatment of enzyme will result in nearly 100 percent protection.

Resistance to Enzymes

Repeated exposure of bacteria grown on agar plates to low concentrations of lysin did not lead to the recovery of resistant strains. Nor were we able to identify resistant bacteria after several cycles of exposure to low concentrations of enzyme in liquid medium (Loeffler et al., 2001). This may be explained by the fact that the cell wall receptor for the pneumococcal lysin is choline (Garcia et al., 1983), a molecule that is necessary for pneumococcal viability. For group A streptococci, we find that polyrhamnose, a cell wall component of the bacteria, is necessary for lysin binding (Nelson and Fischetti, unpublished data), and polyrhamnose has also been shown to be important for streptococcal growth. While not yet proven, it is possible that during a phage's association with bacteria over the millennia, to avoid becoming trapped inside the host, the binding domain of their lytic enzymes has evolved to target a unique and essential molecule in the cell wall, making resistance to these enzymes a rare event.

Concluding Remarks

Phage lytic enzymes are new agents for the control of bacterial pathogens. Since this capability has not been previously available, its acceptance may take a while. For the first time we are able to specifically kill pathogens without affecting the surrounding normal bacteria. Whenever there is a need to kill bacteria, and contact can be made with the organism, phage enzymes may be freely utilized. They may not only be used to control pathogenic bacteria on human mucous membranes, but may find utility in the food industry to control disease bacteria without the extensive use of antibiotics in feed or harsh agents to decontaminate. Because of the serious problems of antibiotic-resistant bacteria in hospitals, day care centers, and nursing homes, particularly staphylococci and pneumococci, such enzymes will be of immediate benefit in these environments. The enzymes isolated thus far are remarkably heat stable (up to 60°C) and are very easy to produce in a purified state, resulting in pennies a dose to manufacture. Thus, we may add phage enzymes to our armamentarium against pathogenic bacteria. They are molecules that have been in development for millions of years by bacteriophage in their battle to survive within bacteria. All we have done is exploit them.

ROLES FOR PHARMACOKINETICS AND PHARMACODYNAMICS IN DRUG DEVELOPMENT FOR RESISTANT PATHOGENS

Jerome J. Schentag, Pharm.D. and Alan Forrest, Pharm.D.

University at Buffalo School of Pharmacy, Buffalo, NY

Antimicrobial resistance is a troubling problem, but not all patients have it, and some appear to overcome it even without new antibiotics. As a consequence, newly marketed antibiotics that cost more are placed on the reserve list, not to be used unless their price either drops to the level of the older generics, or unless an individual patient is failing to respond to other therapies. These issues have made an impact on antibiotic development. When there is no profit from the use of the new antibiotics, the incentive to develop them disappears. It was pointed out that a number of large pharmaceutical companies had either recently exited the antibiotic development business, or were openly contemplating this move in the near future. Disaster loomed large in the audience, because the only solution to the resistance problem that enjoyed unanimous support was a robust pipeline of new antibiotics and many companies involved in their development.

Stakeholders (industry, the Food and Drug Administration [FDA], and academia) need to gather and decide as a group what improvements can be made in the drug development process for antibiotics. The industry needs regulatory assistance to lower antibiotic development costs, and in return they must produce a pipeline containing a wider variety of new chemical or biological entities that deserve use (but only) when they are needed. We cannot expect a wide variety of choices of many chemical classes, unless many companies stay in the hunt for new antibiotics. We believe there are a number of issues that can be addressed in the course of human trials that will lower costs and speed time to approval.

Current and Alternative Means of Developing Antibiotics

The typical New Drug Application (NDA) contains data on antibiotic efficacy and safety in 3,000–5,000 patients. By study design, these NDAs contain no patients with organisms resistant to either the new drug or to existing agents, because under current design specifications for equivalence trials, all patients with an organism resistant to either the new drug or the comparator are excluded from the trials before data analysis. Equivalence cannot be served, after all, if some of the patients on conventional therapy would be expected to fail. The logic of this design has persisted since the 1970s, when marketing an antibiotic required only safety and efficacy equivalent to what was already on the market. The legacy of equivalence models is a large number of closely related compounds with marginal differences, and the need for aggressive sales and marketing efforts to differentiate them after marketing.

The links between strategy and resistance go well beyond the equivalence model. For example, it is widely believed that antibiotics must have only a one-dosage regimen for all patients. This is considered a strategic advantage, because if one is successful in demonstrating efficacy and safety equivalent to the older comparators, one dosage regimen fosters widespread use. Unfortunately, the fixed dose may under- or over-expose some bacterial pathogens, and this situation in the face of monopolistic use creates maximal opportunities for selection pressure. This combination of factors can bring about a speedy end to the drug because of selection of resistant strains (Schentag, 1995). We shall return to this particular problem using the example of the fluoroquinolones (FQ) in pneumococcal pneumonia (Schentag et al., 2001a; 2001b) later in this paper.

Obviously, the equivalence model is useless if the question is to establish superiority on the basis of greater action against resistant organisms. If the development plan for the new antibiotic calls for replacement of an older one that is losing effectiveness because of resistance, forcing this new antibiotic to become equivalent to this older antibiotic places the new antibiotic at a competitive disadvantage. Patients who would contribute to superiority arguments are usually excluded from consideration in equivalence models, since both comparators must be active in order to retain the patient in the trial database used to determine equivalence.

The alternative study design for this new antibiotic is a superiority trial. When the goal is to show the new antibiotic as being better for the treatment of resistant pathogens, this should become the standard model. Industry suspects that demonstration of clear superiority would result in low usage during the time when most pathogens are at least somewhat susceptible to the older antibiotics. Low use results in low profit, and a longer time to recover the investment in the antibiotic development and marketing. But it appears that equivalence also results in low use in some cases. We encounter this dilemma with the newer gram-positive antibiotics. Clinicians only use the newer gram-positive antibiotics in situations where there is clinical failure of vancomycin, or when bacterial pathogens are resistant to vancomycin (Moise and Schentag, 2000; Schentag, 2001). With equivalence in trials as their only argument, there is low use of the replacement antibiotics because of their high selling price.

So why do a superiority trial, given the risks of use only when needed? Quite simply, if the new agent has any safety problems at all, equivalence to old but widely used antibiotics will no longer be sufficient reason to allow it on the market, especially if the existing market is largely satisfied by the conventional antibiotics. Recently, it is clear that new agents must be superior just to reach the market in the first place.

So how does industry best manage antibiotic regulatory risk in the next few years, assuming they do not withdraw from antibiotic development? Let us first discuss the setting of an antibiotic for community infections, with wide potential to be a "blockbuster" product. Here it seems most prudent to gather antibiotic experience data *both* for equivalence (i.e., 3,000–5,000 patients) on safety and efficacy *and* to perform some targeted superiority studies to establish medical need, just in case there might be safety problems of nearly any degree. Demonstration of the safety of a new agent will ordinarily be a sufficient justification to collect the large numbers, and equivalence might be the goal here on efficacy, so that may be affirmation of the currently accepted procedure. The additional challenge is to manage the targeted superiority trials, which need to be submitted at the time of the NDA. These studies either can be performed on a subset of the safety population or they can be added on to subsets of the equivalence population. A third possibility, in the event that neither of the above will work, is to conduct the superiority trial as a free-standing study. If conducted late, after safety problems arise, the superiority trial must certainly be done free-standing.

What about the antibiotic that is clearly superior, but the market is a niche? The good news on superiority is that if the new antibiotic is truly superior, it does not require large numbers of patients to prove it, especially if you use a microbiological response. If the patient is failing conventional therapy with a resistant organism, and you change to an antibiotic effective against that pathogen, you should be rewarded by a cure (both microbiologically and clinically). This mentality is pervasive in the real world, but is just coming to the attention of the regulatory debates that occur in advisory committee meetings focused on equivalence design and equivalence-based statistical modeling.

The problem we typically encounter is that superiority is only rarely as black and white as the same dose of one drug always being superior to the same dose of the other. Most antibiotics perform differently as the minimum inhibitory concentration (MIC) of the pathogen varies and as you change the dose of the drug (Schentag et al., 1991, 1996, 1997, 1998, 2001b; Schentag, 1999a, 2001). The "one dose for all" strategy (Schentag, 1998) offers many opportunities for low exposure (i.e., low area under the inhibitory time curve [AUIC]) and failure, and for high exposure (renal failure with high blood levels) and resulting toxicity. Therefore, we see a major role for pharmacokinetics/pharmacodynamics [PK/PD] and time to bacterial eradication endpoints in the study of superior responses in failing patients, as well as in the study of antimicrobial resistance selection. The benefits of incorporating PK/PD measurements into superiority trials are clear. Demonstrations of superiority are possible on small numbers of patients ($N = 20$ per group can yield statistical significance). This does illustrate that for most antibiotics, it is not one dose for all, it is one dose for each. PK/PD will only rarely allow the conclusion of equivalence (i.e., allow defeat); one antibiotic is always better than the other when you have enough information to decide.

Pharmacokinetics and Pharmacodynamics (PK/PD)

When we discuss PK/PD, we typically use the serum AUC measured in the patient being treated versus the MIC of the organism infecting that particular patient. The diagram in Figure 6-9 illustrates the various PK/PD parameters that can be used to describe the interactions between concentration and MIC. We prefer the use of the simple ratio termed AUIC, because it encompasses all the exposure parameters, and has the advantage of being independent of the oscillations created by different divisions of the same 24-hour dose (Schentag et al., 1996, 1997; Schentag, 1999b). The power of considering individual patient response as a direct function of PK as AUC, and PD as the concentration that will kill the organism, becomes apparent in the statistical treatment of superiority. Every regimen has its own unique PK/PD predicted outcome, and very little of the overall clinical or microbiological outcomes is left as "random noise." This is most clearly apparent when PK/PD is linked to bacterial outcome in bacterially dependent conditions like nosocomial pneumonia (Schentag, 1999b), but it also works if you target the organism rather than the clinical symptoms in mild infections such as acute exacerbation of chronic bronchitis (AECB) (Forrest et al., 1997).

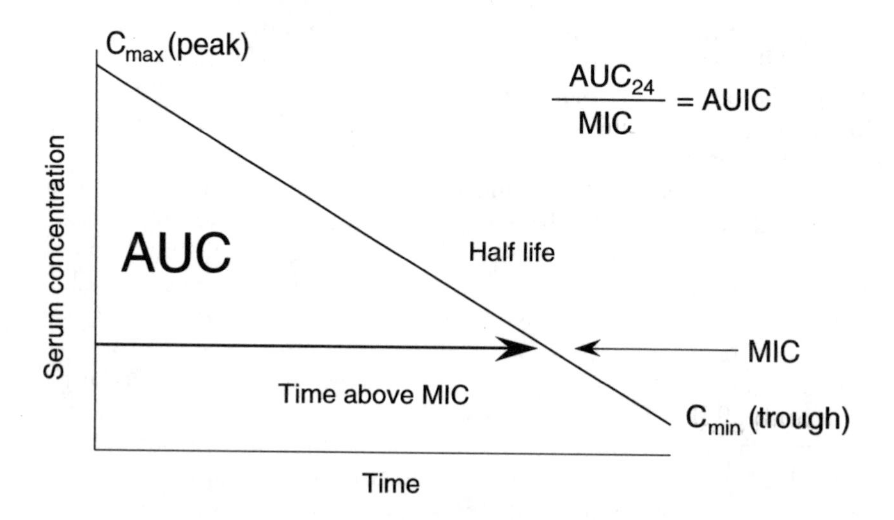

FIGURE 6-9 Diagram illustrating the relationships between antibiotic serum concentrations and MIC. Shown are area under the curve (AUC), peak to MIC, and time above MIC and AUIC, which is the ratio of AUC over 24 hours to MIC. SOURCE: Schentag et al., 2001a.

The most important feature of PK/PD is the use of serial culture to target outcomes such as the rate (speed) of bacterial killing in the individual patient. When expressing individual patient PK/PD as AUIC, it is possible to account for over 80 percent of the variability in (clinical and microbiological) outcomes in a logistic regression model, as well as to determine how fast the organism dies in the patient, as was shown for ciprofloxacin in nosocomial pneumonia in Figure 6-10 (Forrest et al., 1993).

If you collect the data, it becomes possible to use PK/PD to explain selection of a resistant strain when one emerges during therapy, as shown in Figure 6-11 (Thomas et al., 1998). In this study we modeled the day of resistance emergence versus the initial exposure profile (described by AUIC) of the antibiotic regimen (Thomas et al., 1998). Clearly, data of this type explain clinical failure as a failure to eradicate the organism, and link that

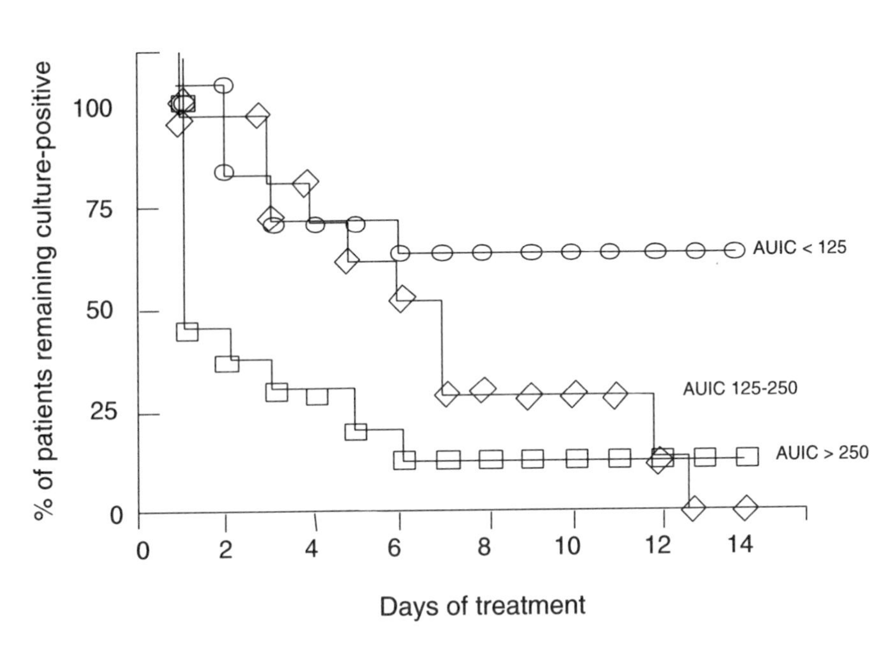

FIGURE 6-10 Relationships between AUIC values and time to bacterial eradication in 74 patients treated with ciprofloxacin for nosocomial lower respiratory tract infection. Each patient had daily tracheal aspirate cultures and the three groups differed significantly from each other. AUIC values >250 produced over 60 percent of the patients culture negative on the first day of treatment. AUIC values of 125–250 required 6 days to convert 60 percent of the cultures to negative, and AUIC values <125 never eradicated the organism in 70 percent of the patients. These data illustrate concentration-dependent microbial killing in humans. SOURCE: Forrest et al., 1993.

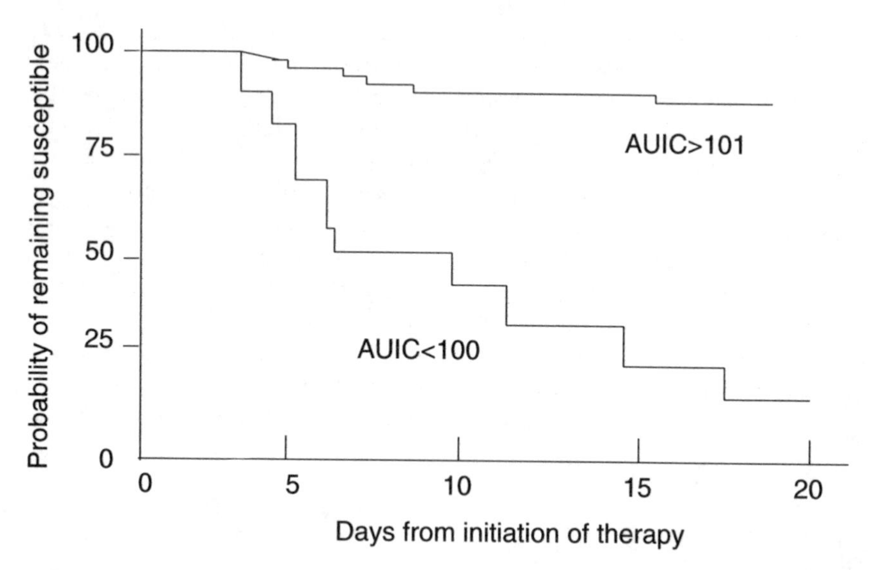

FIGURE 6-11 Relationships between the time cultures remain positive and the initial AUIC value of a group of 127 patients who initially were infected with susceptible organisms. Each patient was followed with serial cultures. Those patients with AUIC <100 demonstrated selection of resistance and overgrowth of these strains progressively over the monitoring period, and most required changes in antimicrobial regimen. If the initial AUIC exceeded 101, only 8 percent of the patients had overgrowth of selected strains resistant to the initial antimicrobial regimen. These data illustrate that it is most dangerous from a resistance selection perspective to have too low an AUIC for too long. SOURCE: Thomas et al., 1998.

occurrence to a low AUIC. The data were among the first to establish a predictability to emergence of resistance caused by selection pressure.

Considering Resistance in Antibiotic Development

If the focus of a new antibiotic becomes superiority to existing alternatives, it is necessary to focus on the microbe that fails conventional antibiotics. Clinical evidence of failure is also important, but you can receive confusing information from failure defined in the absence of knowledge regarding the impact of the antibiotic on the microbe. This is because the impact of antibiotics is on the organism itself, not necessarily the clinical symptoms.

There are many conditions that cause clinical symptoms besides the bacterial pathogen, and there are many things that ablate clinical signs and symptoms of infection besides successful eradication of the organism. Witness the simple treatment of fever with an antipyretic, as an example of why it is necessary to focus on the antimicrobial effect of the antibiotic. In patients who are severely ill from bacterial infection, it is relatively easy to measure superiority if an antibiotic works better than a comparator that is less active. But more often than not, NDAs powered for equivalence exclude these types of patients, because the organism must be susceptible to both the newer and the older antibiotics to remain in the evaluable population.

The impact of the underlying host defense and its potential to confuse the cause of clinical cure are greatest in modestly ill patients. Host response (in modestly ill outpatients) is more than sufficient to overcome failure of the antibiotic to eradicate a pathogen and even selection of resistance. Many of these patients will not show clinical failure patterns even if they have selected a resistant pathogen from low AUICs.

Measuring AUIC and Correlations with Selection Pressure Resistance

One means of achieving equivalence even though you may have a superior antibiotic is to develop and market it at a marginally low dose. We would like to offer an example of an antibiotic developed at low dosing using equivalence design, now widely used in the community, where the selection pressure resulting from low AUICs is rapidly leading to resistance to the entire class it represents. The example is FQ-resistant *Streptococcus pneumoniae*, and the antibiotic cited by virtue of frequency is levofloxacin.

The current party line is that there are no resistance problems with older FQs such as ciprofloxacin and levofloxacin regarding *S. pneumoniae* (Sahm et al., 2000, 2001). Even if this is considered to be a problem, it is argued that all members of the class are the cause, not one compound. The core counter-argument is that if one uses a laboratory breakpoint of 8.0 mcg/ml as a definition of resistance to levofloxacin, resistance went from 0.6 percent to 1.2 percent in the United States in 2000–2001 (Whitney et al., 2000; Doern et al., 2001). Most labs in the United States do not even test levofloxacin against *S. pneumoniae* unless requested by clinicians who are treating a clinical failure (Thornsberry et al., 2001; Davidson et al., 2002). Fluoroquinolone resistance is widely underappreciated in the laboratories. Testing practices are likely to change quite soon, in the face of a rapidly growing number of case reports of clinical failures worldwide (Ho et al., 1997, 1999a, 1999b, 2001; Davidson et al., 2000; Empey et al., 2001; Schentag et al., 2001b; Urban et al., 2001; Weiss et al., 2001; Davidson et al., 2002; Kays et al., 2002). Our thesis is that this "low" incidence of lab-defined resistance is a product of three problems:

1. The use of a breakpoint of 8.0 mcg/ml, which is well above the peak concentration of the drug in serum; indeed, a false sense of security under the circumstances.

2. Microbiology laboratories seldom test levofloxacin against *S. pneumoniae* isolates, and even when they do test MICs, the test misses the single step mutants because hetero-resistant MICs of 1–2 mcg/ml are still below the breakpoint of 8.0 mcg/ml (Richardson et al., 2001).

3. Every time levofloxacin is used in patients at its current low dose, its AUIC is below 100, which is the root cause of widespread selection pressure in the community (Schentag et al., 2001a), and MICs continue to rise under the breakpoint of 8.0 mcg/ml.

I should like to briefly illustrate this low AUIC question, focusing on Figure 6-12 (Schentag et al., 2001a; 2001b). First of all, the AUC of levofloxacin (in a volunteer given a dose of 500 mg) is approximately 48

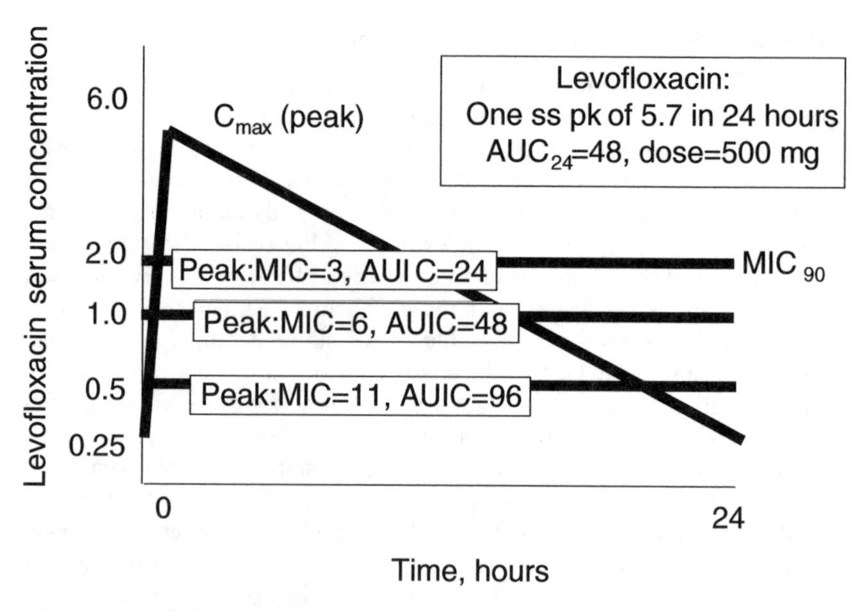

FIGURE 6-12 Relationship between levofloxacin pharmacokinetics and organism MICs of "susceptible" strains. In each case, the AUC of levofloxacin is chosen to be 48, the value typical of normal volunteers and patients with normal renal function. When the MIC is 0.5 mcg/ml (approximately 10 percent of strains in 2001), the AUIC is 96. When the MIC is 1.0 mcg/ml (40–50 percent of strains), the resulting AUIC is 48, and when the MIC is 2.0 mcg/ml (the usual MIC_{90}) for this drug, the AUIC is 24. These calculations illustrate that the AUIC is below 100 in nearly all patients treated with levofloxacin, and illustrate a high risk for selection pressure against *S. pneumoniae*. SOURCE: Schentag et al., 2001a.

mcg × hr/ml. The MIC_{90} of *Streptococcus pneumoniae* to levofloxacin was ~0.5 mcg/ml in 1995 when the drug was marketed, with an initial AUIC of 96. So at the time of marketing, exposure usually resulted in a borderline but probably acceptable AUIC, and assisted by the good host defense in outpatients, the drug appeared to work. The only patients who would be expected to select resistance in the early days were those infected with a strain having an occasional MIC higher than 0.5 mcg/ml or the occasional AUC below 48. Thus, the at-risk population would be younger patients with good renal function or patients who had already been treated with prior levofloxacin and had selected an organism.

As the organism MIC rose from widespread use, extreme selection pressure, and the introduction of one step mutants into the "susceptible" population, all the organisms progressed to intermediately susceptible strains with MICs of 1.0–2.0 mcg/ml. The four-fold loss of activity was not compensated for by increasing the levofloxacin dose four-fold. As the dose remained 500 mg once daily throughout the rise in MICs, all the AUICs became 24–48 (see Figure 6-12) unless the patient had some renal failure, in which case they may have been above 100 on this dose (Ambrose et al., 2001; Drusano et al., 2001; Nicolau and Ambrose, 2001; Owens et al., 2001). The consequences of continued and steady selection pressure include more resistance and eventually clinical failure of a sufficient frequency as to abandon this and other fluoroquinolones in community infections. If we wait until all of the organisms out there are resistant to levofloxacin, we will also lose the rest of the FQs, since most of the double mutants (MICs $\geq$ 8.0 mcg/ml) selected by levofloxacin are resistant to all of the members of this antimicrobial class, even the newest ones (Urban et al., 2001).

Superiority trials of antibiotics that are active against this newly mutated *S. pneumoniae*, such as telithromycin or linezolid, ought to be easy to carry out. As the clinicians abandon levofloxacin and the FQs, there will be widespread use of these newer agents for clinical failures of FQs in community-acquired pneumonia.

The first task before contemplating a superiority trial versus *S. pneumoniae* is to analyze why equivalence trial design did not reveal the differences that are becoming so clearly apparent in retrospect. We believe there are a number of reasons:

1. The organism is changing rapidly in response to widespread use at low AUIC, but this event followed the marketing of levofloxacin for penicillin-resistant *S. pneumoniae*. The clinical trials themselves did not create enough selection pressure, because use was not monopolistic at that early time.
2. Equivalence design studies which brought the drug to market used cephalosporin comparators, which would logically exclude penicillin-resis-

tant *S. pneumoniae* from the study population used to establish equivalence, and would prevent superiority from being discovered. In fact, one study did conclude superiority (File et al., 1997).

3. Widespread monopolistic use upon marketing, catalyzed by formularies and managed care practices trying to save money, lead to increasing selection pressure in communities with at-risk, reservoir populations.

4. Equivalence designs only measure outcomes at times approximately 14 days post-cessation of the antibiotics. This obscures the other natural phenomenon found when antibiotics begin to fail, which is slower and slower rate of bacterial killing (see Figure 6-13). Two antibiotics which differ as dramatically as A and B in Figure 6-13 are equivalent if your endpoint measurement is taken after host response produces resolution in the case of antibiotic B.

So what could a superiority trial model offer a new antibiotic in this situation, assuming it was highly active against FQ-resistant pneumococci? Certainly, you could not establish superiority in a relatively healthy popula-

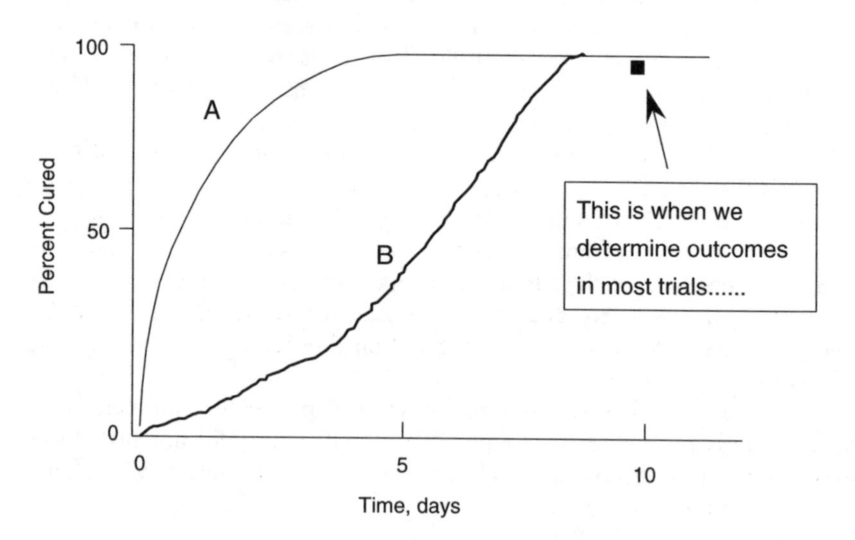

FIGURE 6-13 Illustration of the relationships between speed of cure on two different antibiotics (A vs. B) and the time that clinical assessment is made in typical clinical trials. This illustrates why equivalence studies are unlikely to show differences between two antibiotics that illustrate different rates of killing, such as a concentration-dependent FQ versus a time-dependent macrolide or beta-lactam. Serial cultures will clarify these early and more rapid cure patterns and illustrate differences between the antibiotics. Adapted with permission from Dr. C.H. Nightingale, Hartford, CT.

tion with host defense if your trial endpoint was test of cure at 10–14 days post-treatment. If the patient population has good host defense and/or signs and symptoms of infection are modest, you show no differences.

However, if you would collect serial assessments of organism viability (serial cultures) and if you have serial assessments of infection signs and symptoms early in therapy, and if you can accurately characterize PK/PD of each patient, superiority is possible with as few as 20 patients per group with an active drug. Furthermore, with AUICs and serial cultures on all patients, you could "probably" differentiate the contribution of the host defense from that of the antibiotic, and could easily separate time-dependent killing from concentration-dependent killing in the infected patient, provided that differences are apparent in vitro.

Endpoints

Killing or inhibiting growth of the bacteria is the only measurable effect of an antibiotic. To further increase the power of discrimination with bacterial killing endpoints, measure how fast bacteria are killed, or how many are killed per unit of time. This technique works in vitro, in animal models and in humans. Furthermore, all three testing models are progressively coming to consensus on the PK/PD characteristics necessary for prediction of outcome.

Any other endpoints, including clinical cure, non-culture proven "micro cure," and resolution of infection signs and symptoms, are surrogate markers of the results from either presumed or proven bacterial killing. How accurately or successfully the surrogates perform depends on whether the bacteria originally caused the signs and symptoms used to define the disease and its cure.

On the basis of endpoints, it is logical to change the clinical trial endpoint from clinical cure to microbiological eradication. We can further enhance the discriminatory powers of anti-infective trials by using the microbiological results to define parameters like time to eradication (to handle bacteriostatic versus bactericidal, and time-dependent versus concentration-dependent killing in vivo). In addition, resistance can be linked to MICs and achieved serum concentrations and AUICs. This allows prospective definition of when combination therapy is needed, and which antibiotic combinations will be most successful.

Perhaps the most important benefit of expressing antibiotic action as microbiological eradication is that fewer patients are needed for statistical significance in superiority trials, which yields a substantial lowering of drug development costs and produces faster time to NDA approval.

Sample Size, Delta, and Statistical Power on a Dichotomous versus Continuous Endpoint; Tests of Equivalence versus Superiority, and Why Such Large Numbers for Cure versus Failure?

The primary statistical problem of equivalence design and equivalence doctrine is that a large portion of the data in a cure-failure clinical trial are non-contributory to the goal of discriminating the best regimens. All of the following conditions discourage differentiation and force large numbers just to conclude equivalence (Powers et al., 2002):

- Patients with symptoms but not caused by bacterial pathogens,
- Patients with self-limiting disease not dependent for cure on antimicrobial actions, and
- Infected patients where the antimicrobial itself is barely active or inadequate, but there is still some activity of this comparator plus host defense. You conclude clinical cure in these settings regardless of what condition or drug produced it.

The current trend is how many patients do we need to study in order to conclude two antibiotics are equivalent, and yet the new drug is *better* than placebo, which has led recently to the tightening of the delta to $\leq$ 10 percent for some infections (Powers et al., 2002). Delta is a measure of statistical differentiation, useful in setting sample size in non-crossover clinical trial designs. As might be surmised, a tighter delta increases the size of the study. A tighter delta does not yield a beneficial return if the goal is to differentiate and the model is superiority, as shown in Table 6-2. However, tighter deltas do not cause an increase in the already small numbers of patients who will show superiority in a well-conducted PK/PD trial (see Table 6-2).

Is Compromise Possible Between PK/PD/Micro Superiority and the Clinical Cure-Based Equivalence Models?

In reality, antibiotics are never equivalent, one is always better. Given the diversity in MICs among bacterial populations, the right endpoint can differentiate almost any antibiotic from any other, with only small numbers of patients. And on the surface, it would seem that both trial designs (equivalence and superiority) have some merit. We have compared the two designs in Table 6-2, extracting some information from recent literature on the topic of delta (Shlaes and Moellering, 2002). The comparison shows that the best features of each can be merged into a development plan that should be less expensive to all concerned.

By way of example, start out with the usual two proof of claim studies

TABLE 6-2 Delta, Power, and Sample Size on a Dichotomous versus Continuous Endpoint

	Dichotomous (cure/failure)	Continuous (T to Erad versus AUIC)
Power	90%	90%
Delta	10%	± 1 day
Variability: Type I two tailed error	-	SD = 20–40%
Cure Rate (%)	85–90% (clinical)	80% (MicroErad) at median Terad 3d
# pts per group to conclude A=B	1532	< 10 to ~ 90
# pts per group to conclude A>>B	inf	< 10 to ~ 90

per indication in Table 6-2. In the new mode, these two studies no longer would both be the same design, changing only the comparators but keeping the equivalence mode. Rather, one of the two is equivalence, designed for the therapeutic indication, with a delta even as tight as 10 percent acceptable, since the first study is to gather numbers of patients for safety. You typically want 1,000 per claim and 4 claims is average. The second is designed around the PK/PD and targets superiority for efficacy against microbes (~10 patients per bacteria plus comparator differences at delta 10 percent). The superiority study has a total patient population as few as 40 and as many as 250 patients, depending on how many individual organisms seeking superiority claims.

Beyond the compromise forged between the statistical equivalence and superiority models, the merging of the two types of trials in the same NDA would accomplish some other goals of those who use antibiotics on sick patients. These include data on situations such as:

- Rare and less encountered indications can be studied with these PK/PD models (e.g., endocarditis, meningitis, pediatric infections).
- Labeling for unusual or resistant bacteria could be obtained with 10–20 patients per organism if PK/PD targets are used.
- For antibiotics where there is no active comparator, studies of individual patient AUICs versus the standard AUIC target of 100 could be

carried out. These superiority models (based on speed of bacterial killing or time to eradication) would yield labeling in cases where there is no labeled or active comparator, such as vancomycin-resistant *Enterococcus faecium* (VREF).

- We could, early on, vigorously pursue combination regimens with PK/PD; combination therapies are the real world and antibiotic development needs to address this topic very soon.
- Begin to build these superiority models and study designs into phase II-III rather than waiting for phase IV, since they could lead to claims and will certainly guide use of the new antibiotic in the post-marketing period.

Clearly, if a new drug is better than the old, there is some advantage to proving that for patients using PK/PD. Of course, if it does not differ from the old, it may be better to remove it from trials early, before scarce resources are consumed that are better applied to a follow-on compound.

So what happens if the industry sticks with the equivalence model, and the tighter delta is applied to the community infection models like AECB, sinusitis, otitis media, and others? The prospect is not good, since even with equivalence proven at a now considerably higher clinical trial cost, you might get FDA approval if you show safety, but you still cannot sell the new antibiotic for more. Of course, such cure-failure studies in equivalence populations are primarily valuable for safety, regardless of the statistical treatment. However, if your design will not show a new FQ or a new beta-lactam to be better than an old and largely inactive antibiotic (e.g., cefaclor) in outpatients (Gotfried and Ellison, 1992; Bandak et al., 1999), then you are using the wrong disease and clinical cure is the wrong endpoint. Unfortunately, no improvements in statistical methodology will fix that problem. Somewhere in every antibiotic NDA, there will need to be a demonstration of superiority and medical need, especially to offset any side effects that develop in the course of the trials, and to offset any plans to charge more for the drug when it reaches the market.

Order Out of Chaos?

The current antibiotics development, regulatory, promotion, and clinical use pattern is illogical; the resulting selection pressure from aggressive equivalence-based marketing causes great ecological harm. We advocate changes in the drug development process for antibiotics, so as to achieve the following benefits:

1. A return to a focus on the true target of effect, the bacteria, would greatly improve this situation.

2. New antibiotics should be rapidly developed and marketed precisely for their intended infections, using superiority trials as a basis.

3. Local surveillance could drive use patterns against locally resistant organisms, as well as become the basis for logical dosing and applications of AUIC at the bedside.

4. Public health and microbiology laboratories could gain new relevance in our resistant microbe-enriched world, since resistance is continually evolving in response to local antibiotic use practices.

5. We could finally tackle the important questions of microbial population ecology and evolutionary biology, such as the proper dose and duration to lessen selection pressure.

6. Antibiotics could be developed for use against organisms, or groups of organisms, and health care professionals could be taught to use them when diseases are caused by bacteria, which would finally permit appropriate diagnosis (we could even bring back the bedside gram stain).

7. Industry could run direct to consumer ads teaching patients about the differences between bacteria and viruses, and the rationale for treatment of specific pathogens with effective antibiotics labeled for that purpose.

In summary, we are certain that antibiotic development compromises can be made, and that they should be made. Compromises will speed the development of superior new antibiotics and lower the costs of development and marketing. Absence of compromise will raise antimicrobial development costs and likely aggravate resistance by fostering aggressive marketing and monopolistic use. All of the strategy outlined can be implemented relatively quickly, and further testing of the underlying principles would occur as the superiority trial designs achieve wider use. It is clear there are major problems ahead if we follow the current path. While the new pathways are not free of confrontations and problems, the promise for the future more than outweighs the short-term challenges.

REFERENCES

Abraham EP and Chain E. 1940. An enzyme from bacteria able to destroy penicillin. *Nature* 146:837–840.

Ambrose PG, Grasela DM, Grasela TH, Passarell J, Mayer HB, Pierce PF. 2001. Pharmacodynamics of fluoroquinolones against *Streptococcus pneumoniae* in patients with community-acquired respiratory tract infections. *Antimicrobial Agents and Chemotherapy* 45:2793–2797.

Bandak SI, Bolzon LD, Turnak MR, Johns D, Henle SK, Allen BS. 1999. Cefaclor af versus amoxycillin/clavulanate in acute bacterial exacerbations of chronic bronchitis: a randomised multicentre study. *International Journal of Clinical Practice* 53:578–583.

Bennett PM. 1999. Integrons and gene cassettes: a genetic construction kit for bacteria. *Journal of Antimicrobial Chemotherapy* 43:1–4.

Bulychev A and Mobashery S. 1999. Class C β-lactamases operate at the diffusion limit for turnover of their preferred cephalosporin substrates. *Antimicrobial Agents and Chemotherapy* 43:1743–1746.

Bulychev A, Massova I, Lerner SA, Mobashery S. 1995. Penem BRL 42715: an effective inactivator for β-lactamases. *Journal of the American Chemical Society* 117:4797–4800.

Bulychev A, Massova I, Miyashita K, Mobashery S. 1997. Nuances of mechanisms and their implications for evolution of the versatile β-lactamase activity: from biosynthetic enzymes to drug resistance factors. *Journal of the American Chemical Society* 119:7619–7625.

Bush K. 1999. β-lactamases of increasing clinical importance. *Current Pharmaceutical Design* 5:839–845.

Bush K and Mobashery S. 1998. How β-lactamases have driven pharmaceutical drug discovery: from mechanistic knowledge to clinical circumvention. *Advances in Experimental Medicine and Biology* 456:71–98.

Chamberland S, Blais J, Hoang M, Dinh C, Cotter D, Bond E, Gannon C, Park C, Malouin F, Dudley MN. 2001. In vitro activities of RWJ-54428 (MC-02,479) against multiresistant gram-positive bacteria. *Antimicrobial Agents and Chemotherapy* 45:1422–1430.

Coello R, Jimenez J, Garcia M, Arroyo P, Minguez D, Fernandez C, Cruzet F, Gaspar C. 1994. Prospective study of infection, colonization and carriage of methicillin-resistant *Staphylococcus aureus* in an outbreak affecting 990 patients. *European Journal of Clinical Microbiology and Infectious Diseases* 13:74–81.

Davidson R, Cavalcanti R, Brunton JL, Bast DJ, de Azavedo JC, Kibsey P, Fleming C, Low DE. 2002. Resistance to levofloxacin and failure of treatment of pneumococcal pneumonia. *New England Journal of Medicine* 346:747–750.

Davidson R, de Azavedo J, Bast D, Arbique J, Bethune R, Duncan K, McGeer A, Low DE. 2000. Levofloxacin treatment failure of pneumococcal pneumonia and development of resistance during therapy. Abstract 2103. In: Abstracts of the 40th Interscience Conference on Antimicrobial Agents and Chemotherapy, Toronto, September 17–20, 2000.

de Lencastre H, Kristinsson KG, Brito-Avo A, Sanches IS, Sa-Leao R, Saldanha J, Sigvaldadottir E, Karlsson S, Oliveira D, Mato R, de Sousa MA, Tomasz A. 1999. Carriage of respiratory tract pathogens and molecular epidemiology of *Streptococcus pneumoniae* colonization in healthy children attending day care centers in Lisbon, Portugal. *Microbial Drug Resistance* 5:19–29.

Desselberger U. 2000. Emerging and re-emerging infectious diseases. *Journal of Infectious Diseases* 40:3–15.

Diaz E, Lopez R, Garcia JL. 1990. Chimeric phage-bacterial enzymes: a clue to the modular evolution of genes. *Proceedings of the National Academy of Sciences* 87:8125–8129.

Doern GV, Heilmann KP, Huynh HK, Rhomberg PR, Coffman SL, Brueggemann AB. 2001. Antimicrobial resistance among clinical isolates of *Streptococcus pneumoniae* in the United States during 1999–2000, including a comparison of resistance rates since 1994–1995. *Antimicrobial Agents and Chemotherapy* 45:1721–1729.

Drusano GL, Preston SL, Owens RC Jr, Ambrose PG. 2001. Fluoroquinolone pharmacodynamics. *Clinical Infectious Diseases* 33:2091–2096.

Eiff CV, Becker K, Machka K, Stammer H, Peters G. 2001. Nasal carriage as a source of *Staphylococcus aureus* bacteremia. *New England Journal of Medicine* 344:11–16.

Empey PE, Jennings HR, Thornton AC, Rapp RP, Evans ME. 2001. Levofloxacin failure in a patient with pneumococcal pneumonia. *Annals of Pharmacotherapy* 35:687–690.

File TM Jr, Segreti J, Dunbar L, Player R, Kohler R, Williams RR, Kojak C, Rubin A. 1997. A multicenter, randomized study comparing the efficacy and safety of intravenous and/or oral levofloxacin versus ceftriaxone and/or cefuroxime axetil in treatment of adults with community-acquired pneumonia. *Antimicrobial Agents and Chemotherapy* 41:1965–1972.

Forrest A, Chodosh S, Amantea MA, Collins DA, Schentag JJ. 1997. Pharmacokinetics and pharmacodynamics of oral grepafloxacin in patients with acute bacterial exacerbations of chronic bronchitis. *Journal of Antimicrobial Chemotherapy* 40 Suppl A:45–57.

Forrest A, Nix DE, Ballow CH, Goss TF, Birmingham MC, Schentag JJ. 1993. Pharmacodynamics of intravenous ciprofloxacin in seriously ill patients. *Antimicrobial Agents and Chemotherapy* 37:1073–1081.

Fung HB, Kirschenbaum HL, Ojofeitimi BO. 2001. Linezolid: an oxazolidinone antimicrobial agent. *Clinical Therapeutics* 23:356–391.

Garcia E, Garcia JL, Arraras A, Sanchez-Puelles JM, Lopez R. 1988. Molecular evolution of lytic enzymes of *Streptococcus pneumoniae* and its bacteriophages. *Proceeding of the National Academy of Sciences* 85:914–918.

Garcia P, Garcia E, Ronda C, Tomasz A, Lopez R. 1983. Inhibition of lysis by antibody against phage-associated lysin and requirement of choline residues in the cell wall for progeny phage release in *Streptococcus pneumoniae. Current Microbiology* 8:137–140.

Garcia P, Garcia JL, Sanchez-Puelles JM, Lopez R. 1990. Modular organization of the lytic enzymes of *Streptococcus pneumoniae* and its bacteriophages. *Gene* 86:81–88.

Golemi D, Maveyraud L, Vakulenko S, Samama JP, Mobashery S. 2001. Critical involvement of a carbamylated lysine in catalytic function of class D β-lactamases. *Proceedings of the National Academy of Sciences* 98:14280–14285.

Golemi-Kotra D and Mobashery S. 2002. Antibiotic resistance. In: *Kirk-Othmer Encyclopedia of Chemical Technology* (4th ed.). New York: John Wiley. [Online]. Available: http://www.mrw.interscience.wiley.com/kirk/.

Gonzales RD, Schrekenberger P, Graham C, Kelkar S, DenBesten K, Quinn JP. 2001. Infections due to vancomycin-resistant *Enterococcus faecium* resistant to linezolid. *Lancet* 357:1179–1185.

Gotfried MH and Ellison WT. 1992. Safety and efficacy of lomefloxacin versus cefaclor in the treatment of acute exacerbations of chronic bronchitis. *American Journal of Medicine* 92(4A):108S–113S.

Hardy LW and Kirsch JF. 1984. Diffusion-limited component of reactions catalyzed by *bacillus cereus* β-lactamase I. *Biochemistry* 23:1275-1282.

Hebeisen P, Heinze-Krauss I, Angehrn P, Hohl P, Page MG, Then RL. 2001. In vitro and in vivo properties of Ro 63-9141, a novel broad-spectrum cephalosporin with activity against methicillin-resistant staphylococci. *Antimicrobial Agents and Chemotherapy* 45:825–836.

Heymann DL and Rodier GR. 2001. Hot spots in a wired world: WHO surveillance of emerging and re-emerging infectious diseases. *Lancet Infectious Diseases* 5:345–353.

Ho A, Leung R, Lai CK, Chan TH, Chan CH. 1997. Hospitalized patients with community-acquired pneumonia in Hong Kong: a randomized study comparing imipenem/cilastatin and ceftazidime [published erratum appears in *Respiration* 1997; 64(4):303]. *Respiration* 64(3):224–228.

Ho PL, Que TL, Tsang DN, Ng TK, Chow KH, Seto WH. 1999a. Emergence of fluoroquinolone resistance among multiply resistant strains of *Streptococcus pneumoniae* in Hong Kong. *Antimicrobial Agents and Chemotherapy* 43:1310–1313.

Ho PL, Que TL, Tsang DN, Ng TK, Seto WH. 1999b. Characterization of fluoroquinolone-resistant *Streptococcus pneumoniae* in Hong Kong. Abstract 818. In: Abstracts of the 39th Interscience Conference on Antimicrobial Agents and Chemotherapy, San Francisco, September 26–29, 1999.

Ho PL, Tse WS, Tsang KW, Kwok TK, Ng TK, Cheng VC, Chan RM. 2001. Risk factors for acquisition of levofloxacin-resistant *Streptococcus pneumoniae*: a case-control study. *Clinical Infectious Diseases* 32:701–707.

IOM (Institute of Medicine). 1992. Lederberg J and Shope RE (eds). *Emerging Infections: Microbial Threats to Health in the United States.* Washington, DC: National Academy Press.

Johnson AP, Warner M, Carter M, Livermore DM. 2002. In vitro activity of cephalosporin RWJ-54428 (MC-02479) against multidrug-resistant gram-positive cocci. *Antimicrobial Agents and Chemotherapy* 46:321–326.

Kaatz GW and Seo SM. 1996. In vitro activities of oxazolidinone compounds U100592 and U100766 against *Staphylococcus aureus* and *Staphylococcus epidermidis. Antimicrobial Agents and Chemotherapy* 40:799–801.

Kays MB, Smith DW, Wack ME, Denys GA. 2002. Levofloxacin treatment failure in a patient with fluoroquinolone-resistant *Streptococcus pneumoniae* pneumonia. *Pharmacotherapy* 22:395–399.

Kelly JA, Kuzin AP, Charlier P, Fonze E. 1998. X-ray studies of enzymes that interact with penicillins. *Cellular and Molecular Life Sciences* 54:353–358.

Kotra LP, Golemi D, Vakulenko S, Mobashery S. 2000. Bacteria fight back. *Chemistry and Industry* 341–344.

Loeffler JM, Nelson D, Fischetti VA. 2001. Rapid killing of *Streptococcus pneumoniae* with a bacteriophage cell wall hydrolase. *Science* 294:2170–2172.

Lopez R, Garcia E, Garcia P, Garcia JL. 1997. The pneumococcal cell wall degrading enzymes: a modular design to create new lysins? *Microbial Drug Resistance* 3:199–211.

Lopez R, Garcia JL, Garcia E, Ronda C, Garcia P. 1992. Structural analysis and biological significance of the cell wall lytic enzymes of *Streptococcus pneumoniae* and its bacteriophage. *FEMS Microbiology Letters* 79:439–447.

Mainardi JL, Legrand R, Arthur M, Schoot B, Van Heijenoort J, Gutmann L. 2000. Novel mechanism of β-lactam resistance due to bypass of DD-transpeptidation in *Enterococcus faecium. Journal of Biological Chemistry* 275:16490–16496.

Martinez-Martinez L, Conejo MC, Pascual A, Hernandez-Alles S, Ballesta S, Ramirez de Arellano-Ramos A, Benedi VJ, Perea EJ. 2000. Activities of imipenem and cephalosporins against clonally related strains of *Escherichia coli* hyperproducing chromosomal β-lactamase and showing altered porin profiles. *Antimicrobial Agents and Chemotherapy* 44:2534–2536.

Massova I and Mobashery S. 1998. Kinship and diversification of bacterial penicillin-binding proteins and β-lactamases. *Antimicrobial Agents and Chemotherapy* 42:1–17.

Maveyraud L, Golemi D, Ishiwata A, Meroueh, O, Mobashery S, Samama JP. 2002. High-resolution X-ray structure of an acyl-enzyme species for the class D OXA-10 β-lactamase. *Journal of the American Chemical Society* 124:2461–2465.

Maveyraud L, Golemi D, Kotra LP, Tranier S, Vakulenko S, Mobashery S, Samama JP. 2000. Insights into class D β-lactamases are revealed by the crystal structure of the Oxa10 enzyme from *Pseudomonas aeruginosa. Structure* 8:1289–1298.

Maveyraud L, Mourey L, Kotra LP, Pedelacq JD, Guillet V, Mobashery S, Samama JP. 1998. Structural basis for clinical longevity of carbapenem antibiotics in the face of challenge by the common class A β-lactamases from the antibiotic-resistant bacteria. *Journal of the American Chemical Society* 120:9748–9752.

Miyashita K, Massova I, Taibi P, Mobashery S. 1995. Design, synthesis and evaluation of a potent mechanism-based inhibitor for the TEM β-lactamase with implications for the enzyme mechanism. *Journal of the American Chemical Society* 117:11055-11062.

Mobashery S and Azucena E. 2002. Bacterial antibiotic resistance. In: *Encyclopedia of Life Sciences*. Vol. 2. London: Nature Publishing Group. Pp. 472–477.

Moise PA and Schentag JJ. 2000. Vancomycin treatment failures in *Staphylococcus aureus* lower respiratory tract infections. *International Journal of Antimicrobial Agents* 16 Suppl 1:S31–34.

Mourey L, Miyashita K, Swarén P, Bulychev A, Samama JP, Mobashery S. 1998. Inhibition of the NMC-A β-lactamase by a penicillanic acid derivative, and the structural bases for the increase in substrate profile of this antibiotic resistance enzyme. *Journal of the American Chemical Society* 120:9382.

Nelson D, Loomis L, Fischetti VA. 2001. Prevention and elimination of upper respiratory colonization of mice by group A streptococci by using a bacteriophage lytic enzyme. *Proceedings of the National Academy of Sciences* 98:4107–4112.

Nicolau DP and Ambrose PG. 2001. Pharmacodynamic profiling of levofloxacin and gatifloxacin using Monte Carlo simulation for community-acquired isolates of *Streptococcus pneumoniae. American Journal of Medicine* 111 Suppl 9A:13S–18S; discussion 36S–38S.

Ochs MM, Bains M, Hancock RE. 2000. Role of putative loops 2 and 3 in imipenem passage through the specific porin OprD of *Pseudomonas aeruginosa. Antimicrobial Agents and Chemotherapy* 7:1983–1985.

Owens RC Jr, Tessier P, Nightingale CH, Ambrose PG, Quintiliani R, Nicolau DP. 2001. Pharmacodynamics of ceftriaxone and cefixime against community-acquired respiratory tract pathogens. *International Journal of Antimicrobial Agents* 17:483–489.

Patera A, Blaszczak LC, Shoichet BK. 2000. Crystal structures of substrate and inhibitor complexes with AmpC β-lactamase: possible implications for substrate-assisted catalysis. *Journal of the American Chemical Society* 122:10504–10512.

Pinho MG, Filipe SR, de Lencastre H, Tomasz A. 2001a. Complementation of the essential peptidoglycan transpeptidase function of penicillin-binding protein 2 (PBP2) by the drug resistance protein PBP2A in *Staphylococcus aureus. Journal of Bacteriology* 183:6525–6531.

Pinho MG, de Lencastre H, Tomasz A. 2001b. An acquired and a native penicillin-binding protein cooperate in building the cell wall of drug-resistant staphylococci. *Proceedings of the National Academy of Sciences.* 98:10886–10891.

Poole K. 2001. Overcoming antimicrobial resistance by targeting resistance mechanisms. *Journal of Pharmacy and Pharmacology* 53:283–294.

Powers JH, Ross DB, Brittain E, Albrecht R, Goldberger MJ. 2002. The United States Food and Drug Administration and noninferiority margins in clinical trials of antimicrobial agents. *Clinical Infectious Diseases* 34:879–881.

Prystowsky J, Siddiqui F, Chosay J, Shinabarger DL, Millichap J, Peterson LR, Noskin GA. 2001. Resistance to linezolid: characterization of mutations in rRNA and comparison of their occurrences in vancomycin-resistant enterococci. *Antimicrobial Agents and Chemotherapy* 45:2154–2156.

Richardson DC, Bast D, McGeer A, Low DE. 2001. Evaluation of susceptibility testing to detect fluoroquinolone resistance mechanisms in *Streptococcus pneumoniae. Antimicrobial Agents and Chemotherapy* 45:1911–1914.

Roychoudhury S, Dotzlaf JE, Ghag S, Yeh WK. 1994. Purification, properties, and kinetics of enzymatic acylation with β-lactams of soluble penicillin-binding protein 2a. A major factor in methicillin-resistant *Staphylococcus aureus. Journal of Biological Chemistry* 269:12067–12073.

Sahm DF, Karlowsky JA, Kelly LJ, Critchley IA, Jones ME, Thornsberry C, Mauriz Y, Kahn J. 2001. Need for annual surveillance of antimicrobial resistance in *Streptococcus pneumoniae* in the United States: 2-year longitudinal analysis. *Antimicrobial Agents and Chemotherapy* 45:1037–1042.

Sahm DF, Peterson DE, Critchley IA, Thornsberry C. 2000. Analysis of ciprofloxacin activity against *Streptococcus pneumoniae* after 10 years of use in the United States. *Antimicrobial Agents and Chemotherapy* 44:2521–2524.

Schentag JJ. 1995. Understanding and managing microbial resistance in institutional settings. *American Journal of Health-System Pharmacy* 52(6 Suppl 2):S9–14.

Schentag JJ. 1998. Antibiotic dosing—does one size fit all? [editorial; comment]. *Journal of the American Medical Association* 279:159–160.

Schentag JJ. 1999a. Optimizing antimicrobial therapy in respiratory-tract infections: new agents, new strategies. Introduction. *American Journal of Health-System Pharmacy* 56(22 Suppl 3):S3.

Schentag JJ. 1999b. Antimicrobial action and pharmacokinetics/pharmacodynamics: the use of AUIC to improve efficacy and avoid resistance. *Journal of Chemotherapy* 11:426–439.

Schentag JJ. 2001. Antimicrobial management strategies for gram-positive bacterial resistance in the intensive care unit. *Critical Care Medicine* 29(4 Suppl):N100–107.

Schentag JJ, Birmingham MC, Paladino JA, Carr JR, Hyatt JM, Forrest A, Zimmer GS, Adelman MH, Cumbo TJ. 1997. In nosocomial pneumonia, optimizing antibiotics other than aminoglycosides is a more important determinant of successful clinical outcome, and a better means of avoiding resistance. *Seminars in Respiratory Infections* 12:278–293.

Schentag JJ, Gilliland KK, Paladino JA. 2001a. What have we learned from pharmacokinetic and pharmacodynamic theories? *Clinical Infectious Diseases* 32 Suppl 1:S39–46.

Schentag JJ, Gilliland KK, Paladino JA. 2001b. Reply. *Clinical Infectious Diseases* 33(12):2091–2096.

Schentag JJ, Nix DE, Adelman MH. 1991. Mathematical examination of dual individualization principles (I): Relationships between AUC above MIC and area under the inhibitory curve for cefmenoxime, ciprofloxacin, and tobramycin. *DICP: The Annals of Pharmacotherapy* 25:1050–1057.

Schentag JJ, Nix DE, Forrest A, Adelman MH. 1996. AUIC—the universal parameter within the constraint of a reasonable dosing interval [editorial; comment]. *Annals of Pharmacotherapy* 30:1029–1031.

Schentag JJ, Strenkoski-Nix LC, Nix DE, Forrest A. 1998. Pharmacodynamic interactions of antibiotics alone and in combination. *Clinical Infectious Diseases* 27:40–46.

Schuch R, Nelson D, Fischetti VA. 2002. A bacteriolytic agent that detects and kills *Bacillus anthracis*. *Nature* 418:884–889.

Shlaes DM and Moellering RC. 2002. The United States Food and Drug Administration and the end of antibiotics. *Clinical Infectious Diseases* 34:420–422.

Strynadka NC, Adachi H, Jensen SE, Johns K, Sielecki A, Betzel C, Sutoh K, James MN. 1992. Molecular structure of the acyl-enzyme intermediate in β-lactam hydrolysis at 1.7 A resolution. *Nature* 359:700–705.

Swaney SM, Aoki H, Ganoza MC, Shinabarger DL. 1998. The oxazolidinone linezolid inhibits initiation of protein synthesis in bacteria. *Antimicrobial Agents and Chemotherapy* 42:3251–3255.

Thomas JK, Forrest A, Bhavnani SM, Hyatt JM, Cheng A, Ballow CH, Schentag JJ. 1998. Pharmacodynamic evaluation of factors associated with the development of bacterial resistance in acutely ill patients during therapy. *Antimicrobial Agents and Chemotherapy* 42:521–527.

Thornsberry C, Karlowsky JA, Sahm DF, Jorgensen JH, Weigel LM, Swenson JM, Whitney CG, Tenover FC, Ferraro MJ. 2001. Levofloxacin-resistant *Streptococcus pneumoniae*: second look. *Antimicrobial Agents and Chemotherapy* 45:2183–2184.

Tsiodras S, Gold HS, Sakoulas G, Eliopoulos GM, Wennersten C, Vankataraman L, Moellering RC Jr, Ferraro MJ. 2001. Linezolid resistance in a clinical isolate of *Staphylococcus aureus*. *Lancet* 358:207–208.

Urban C, Rahman N, Zhao X, Mariano N, Segal-Maurer S, Drlica K, Rahal JJ. 2001. Fluoroquinolone-resistant *Streptococcus pneumoniae* associated with levofloxacin therapy. *Journal of Infectious Diseases* 184:794–798.

Walsh CT. 2000. Molecular mechanisms that confer antibacterial drug resistance. *Nature* 406:775–781.

Watanabe T, Morimoto A, Shiomi T. 1975. The fine structure and the protein composition of gamma phage of *Bacillus anthracis*. *Canadian Journal of Microbiology* 21:1889–1892.

Weiss K, Restieri C, Gauthier R, Laverdiere M, McGeer A, Davidson RJ, Kilburn L, Bast DJ, de Azavedo J, Low DE. 2001. A nosocomial outbreak of fluoroquinolone-resistant *Streptococcus pneumoniae*. *Clinical Infectious Diseases* 33:517–522.

Whitney CG, Farley MM, Hadler J, Harrison LH, Lexau C, Reingold A, Lefkowitz L, Cieslak PR, Cetron M, Zell ER, Jorgensen JH, Schuchat A. 2000. Increasing prevalence of multidrug-resistant *Streptococcus pneumoniae* in the United States. *New England Journal of Medicine* 343:1917–1924.

WHO (World Health Organization). 1996. *The World Health Report 1996: Fighting Disease, Fostering Development*. Geneva: WHO.

Wong KK and Pompliano DL. 1998. Peptidoglycan biosynthesis. Unexploited antibacterial targets within a familiar pathway. *Advances in Experimental Medicine and Biology* 456:197–217.

Wootton M, Bowker KE, Holt HA, MacGowan AP. 2002. BAL 9141, a new broad-spectrum pyrrolidinone cephalosporin: activity against clinically significant anaerobes in comparison with 10 other antimicrobials. *Journal of Antimicrobial Chemotherapy* 49:535–539.

Young R. 1992. Bacteriophage lysis: mechanism and regulation. *Microbiological Reviews* 56:430–481.

7

Strategies to Contain the Development and Consequences of Resistance

OVERVIEW

Managing the varied problems associated with antimicrobial resistance will require a coordinated response that includes participation by individuals, organizations, and governments at the local, state, national, and international levels. The focus of this session of the workshop was on examining current management efforts and highlighting additional steps needed to contain the development and consequences of resistance. In light of the increasing magnitude of the problem, participants universally agreed that implementing a comprehensive attack on antimicrobial resistance must proceed without further delay.

The primary blueprint for federal actions in the United States is the *Public Health Action Plan to Combat Antimicrobial Resistance*, issued in 2001 by a multiagency task force led by the Centers for Disease Control and Prevention (CDC), the Food and Drug Administration (FDA), and the National Institutes of Health (NIH). The plan has four focus areas: surveillance, prevention and control, research, and product development. Complete implementation of the plan will require adequate funding to support activities across a range of organizations.

Various public agencies and private organizations already are putting parts of the action plan into practice. The FDA is using its regulatory responsibility to ensure that drugs and other chemical agents used in both humans and animals do not pose unacceptable health risks, including risks that may arise as a result of antimicrobial resistance. In addition, the agency's Center for Drug Evaluation and Research is exploring ways to enhance available approaches for the development of new antibiotics. Such activities include fostering early communication between the FDA and pharmaceutical companies, using the agency's product labeling system to help educate physicians and other health care workers about antimicrobial resistance, and exploring methods for using data collected in clinical trials to make reliable inferences about a drug's potential to trigger antimicrobial resistance.

The CDC is implementing a variety of surveillance efforts and prevention and control activities, and is both undertaking and supporting applied research. In one effort, the agency has initiated the Campaign to Prevent Antimicrobial Resistance in Healthcare Settings, a nationwide program that targets clinicians, patient care partners, health care organizations, purchasers, and patients. The campaign centers around four basic strategies that front-line clinicians can use to prevent antimicrobial resistance. These strategies include preventing infections so as to directly reduce the need for antimicrobial exposure and the emergence and selection of resistant strains; diagnosing and treating infection properly, which will benefit patients and decrease the opportunity for development and selection of resistant microbes; using antimicrobials wisely, since optimal use will ensure proper patient care while avoiding overuse of broad-spectrum antimicrobials and unnecessary treatment; and preventing transmission of resistant organisms from one person to another.

At the international level, the World Health Organization (WHO) in 2001 issued the *WHO Global Strategy for Containment of Antimicrobial Resistance*. The plan details a comprehensive framework of interventions designed to reduce the disease burden and the spread of infection, improve access to and improve use of appropriate antimicrobial agents, strengthen health systems and their surveillance capabilities, introduce and enforce regulations and legislation, and encourage the development of new drugs and vaccines. In implementing the plan, special priority will be given to educating the distributors, prescribers, and consumers of antimicrobial agents; to infection control measures aimed at preventing the dissemination of resistant strains; to quality assurance programs for antibiotics and other medicines; and to the establishment of functional and sustainable laboratories for antibiotic resistance surveillance.

Much of the responsibility for implementing the WHO plan will fall on individual countries, and some of them—especially in the developing world—will need assistance. Toward this end, the Rational Pharmaceutical Management Plus Program, based at a nongovernmental organization, is helping to develop a systematic approach to designing national-level efforts to contain antimicrobial resistance. This approach will provide a framework by which various stakeholders, working with technical consultants when necessary, can assess policies, drug use, and levels of resistance in their countries, and then tailor a range of strategies for advocacy, policy development, and systems change. Although this approach is generic, its implementation likely will be country-specific and unfold in distinct ways, according to circumstances in each country.

DEVELOPMENT OF THE *PUBLIC HEALTH ACTION PLAN TO COMBAT ANTIMICROBIAL RESISTANCE* AND CDC ACTIVITIES RELATED TO ITS IMPLEMENTATION

David M. Bell, M.D.

Office of the Director, National Center for Infectious Diseases
Centers for Disease Control and Prevention, Atlanta, GA

The Public Health Action Plan to Combat Antimicrobial Resistance

To provide a blueprint for federal actions to address the emerging threat of antimicrobial resistance (AR), the *Public Health Action Plan to Combat Antimicrobial Resistance (Part I Domestic Issues)*, was developed by a Federal Interagency Task Force on Antimicrobial Resistance and released in January 2001 (http://www.cdc.gov/drugresistance/actionplan/index.htm). The Task Force had been formed in 1999, after hearings held by Senators Frist and Kennedy, in recognition of the fact that addressing the multifaceted problem of antimicrobial resistance (AR) required action by multiple agencies and departments. Co-chaired by CDC, FDA, and NIH, the Task Force also includes the Agency for Healthcare Research and Quality, the Centers for Medicare and Medicaid Services, the Health Resources and Services Administration, the Department of Agriculture, the Department of Defense, the Department of Veterans Affairs, the Environmental Protection Agency, and, since 2001, the U.S. Agency for International Development.

The plan was developed based on input from consultants from state and local health agencies, universities, professional societies, pharmaceutical companies, health care delivery organizations, agricultural producers, consumer groups, and other members of the public. It will be implemented incrementally, in collaboration with these and other partners, as resources become available. The plan has 4 focus areas: surveillance, prevention and control, research, and product development. Of 84 action items, 13 are designated top priority. Seven of the 13 are already underway, and 6 are planned to begin by 2003. Part I of the plan focuses on domestic issues; Part II, under development, will identify federal actions that more specifically address global AR issues in collaboration with the WHO and other partners. The Task Force is continuing to meet to monitor implementation of the plan and will release annual progress reports and seek additional input at public meetings.

CDC Activities

CDC activities in 2001–2002 primarily implement action items in the surveillance and prevention and control (which includes prevention research) sections. Of CDC's $25 million appropriation for AR in fiscal year 2001, about 75 percent was awarded extramurally, primarily to health departments and universities. This appropriation included approximately $12 million in new funds, of which $3.2 million was awarded through a new AR applied research grant program. CDC's 2002 appropriation for AR, also $25 million, will primarily be used to continue ongoing activities summarized below. More information on these activities is available at www.cdc.gov/drugresistance.

Surveillance

In the United States, disease reporting is mandated by state laws, but most states do not require reporting of drug susceptibility information and the completeness of reporting varies. In collaboration with state health departments and other partners, CDC monitors resistance for several pathogens of public health importance and collects limited data on antimicrobial drug prescribing. For example, resistance in invasive *S. pneumoniae* infections is monitored on a population basis in 9 states or portions thereof through the Emerging Infections Programs, health care-acquired infections (e.g., *S. aureus*, enterococci, gram-negative bacteria) in approximately 300 hospitals, and foodborne pathogens such as *Salmonella* in 27 states in a joint project with the FDA and Department of Agriculture. In this project, resistance in foodborne pathogens and commensal organisms is also monitored in animals (and, beginning in 2001, in retail meat products). CDC-supported projects monitor drug resistance for several other pathogens or infections, for example, community-onset *Staphylococcus aureus*, tuberculosis, gonorrhea, influenza, Group B streptococci, *Neisseria meningitidis*, *Helicobacter pylori*, HIV, and malaria.

These systems need enhancement using updated laboratory and informatics technologies, such as through the National Electronic Disease Surveillance System under development. The major problem, however, is that with the exception of tuberculosis, none provides even close to nationwide coverage. Most communities probably do not need sophisticated systems such as those that provide data to help develop and evaluate national prevention and control strategies. However, awareness of the extent to which resistance is present locally is helpful in guiding treatment decisions and in generating support for local public health interventions such as appropriate drug use and vaccine campaigns. To implement the action plan, CDC seeks to support coordinated national surveillance of drug resistance and use at two levels. One level would involve surveillance that could be done by most states, communities, and health care systems to meet local needs; the second level would consist of more specialized projects to address specific national needs in more detail and monitor emerging problems. Examples of new projects in 2001 include:

- Monitoring drug-resistant *Staphylococcus aureus* in the community in 5 states and a national population sample (the National Health and Nutrition Examination Survey).
- Increasing surveillance of enteric pathogens (through the National AR Monitoring System: Enteric Bacteria) from 17 to 25 states, characterizing and tracking resistance genes; monitoring drug-resistant bacteria in retail meat, and supporting new joint projects of state public health and veterinary laboratories.
- Monitoring resistance of influenza virus to newly licensed antiviral drugs.
- Beginning to develop a coordinated system to monitor antimicrobial drug use, through analyzing existing databases, identifying gaps, and exploring standardization of methods.
- Improving state, local, and health care system infrastructure to support development of local surveillance and enhance the capacity for electronic reporting.

Reliable surveillance information—as well as patient care and safety—requires that front-line clinical laboratories detect emerging drug resistance accurately. Faced with evidence from surveys that this is frequently not the case (CDC, 2000), CDC is working with partners such as the Association of Public Health Laboratories and the American Society for Microbiology to develop training and proficiency testing programs. For example, in 2001, a new website "MASTER" was introduced that includes discussions of difficult cases in diagnostic microbiology, recommendations and references, and opportunities to question CDC microbiologists (www.phppo.cdc.gov/dls/master/default.asp). In its first year of operation, this site has received approximately 33,000 hits from 20 countries. The need for constant updating of clinical laboratory proficiency offers an opportunity for state public health laboratories to provide important leadership and strengthen their linkages with clinical laboratories. Through the National Laboratory Training Network and other programs, CDC's goal is to work with partners to ensure training and proficiency in drug resistance testing and reporting for clinical laboratories in all states and territories.

Prevention and Control

Prevention and control of drug resistance primarily involve promoting appropriate use of antimicrobial drugs[1] to extend their useful life and preventing infection transmission (e.g., through appropriate infection control and vaccine use). Prevention and control programs do not obviate the need for a constantly flowing "pipeline" of new drugs, as current drugs will inevitably become less effective with time due to resistance. CDC has been working with a variety of partners to promote appropriate antimicrobial use in the community (outpatient prescribing), in health care settings, and in agriculture (Bell, 2001).

For acute infections in outpatients, a major objective is to reduce antimicrobial drug prescribing for illnesses for which these drugs offer no benefit (e.g., viral respiratory infections). In 1995, CDC launched a National Campaign for Appropriate Antibiotic Use that involves partnerships with state and local health departments, health care delivery organizations, health care purchasers and insurers, professional societies, consumer groups, and others. Often working through state-based coalitions, these partners implement coordinated educational and behavioral interventions directed to patients and clinicians, including public education programs, prescribing principles, clinical training materials, and aids (e.g., "viral prescription pads") to help clinicians avoid prescribing an antibiotic when not indicated (see Figures 7-1 and 7-2). Data from controlled trials indicate that these interventions can be effective in reducing inappropriate antibiotic prescribing for respiratory infections in the United States, as has been reported in other countries—although resistance rates of respiratory pathogens, having reached a certain level, may not necessarily decline thereafter (Gonzales et al., 1999; Belongia et al., 2001; Finkelstein et al., 2001; Hennessy et al., 2002).

Encouraging data from the National Ambulatory Medical Care Survey indicate that antibiotic prescribing rates for children seen in physician offices declined in the 1990s after having increased in the late 1980s (McCaig et al., 2002) (see Figure 7-3). Initially focused primarily on pediatrics, the

[1]In the action plan, appropriate antimicrobial drug use is defined as use that maximizes therapeutic impact while minimizing toxicity and the development of resistance. In practice, this means prescribing antimicrobial therapy when and only when beneficial to a patient, targeting therapy to the desired pathogens, and using the appropriate drug, dose, and duration.

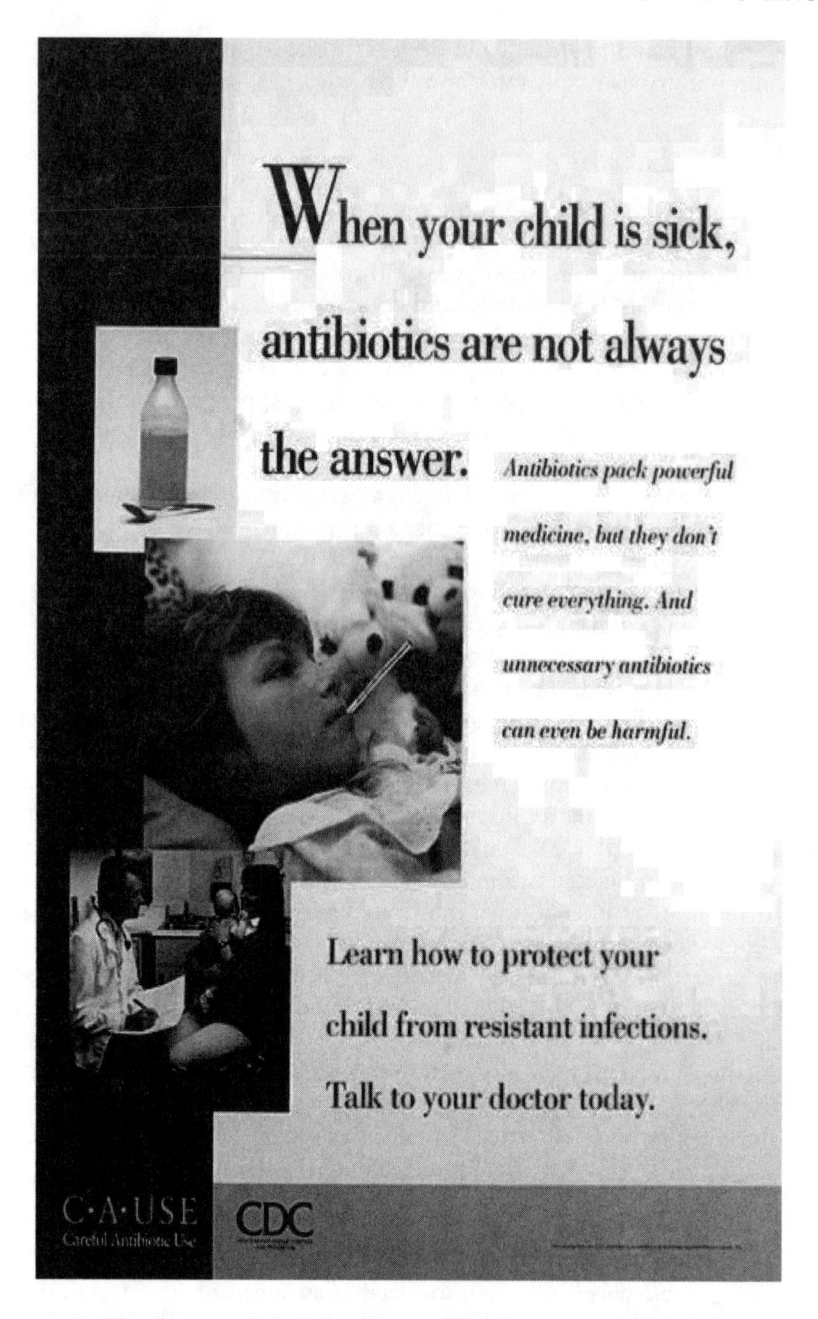

FIGURE 7-1 Example of a poster, used in public education campaigns, promoting appropriate use of antimicrobial drugs, developed by CDC in partnership with the American Society for Microbiology. SOURCE: CDC, 2002.

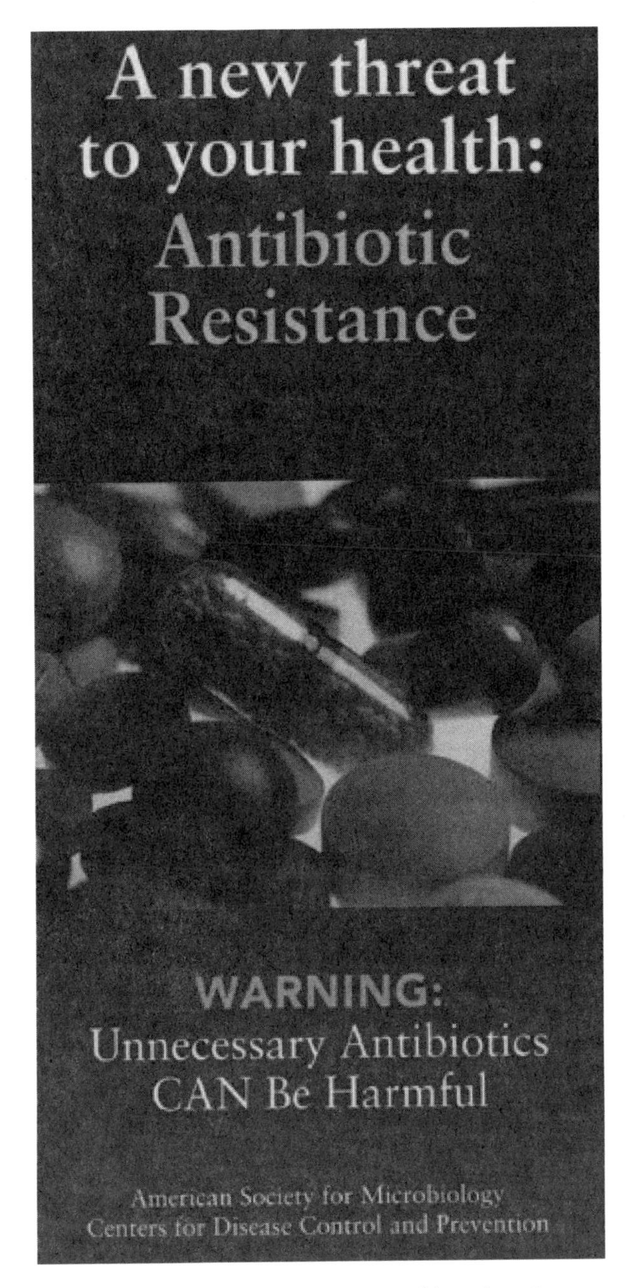
A new threat
to your health:
Antibiotic
Resistance
WARNING:
Unnecessary Antibiotics
CAN Be Harmful
American Society for Microbiology
Centers for Disease Control and Prevention

FIGURE 7-2 Example of a pamphlet, used in public education campaigns, promoting appropriate use of antimicrobial drugs, developed by CDC in partnership with the American Society for Microbiology. SOURCE: CDC, 2002.

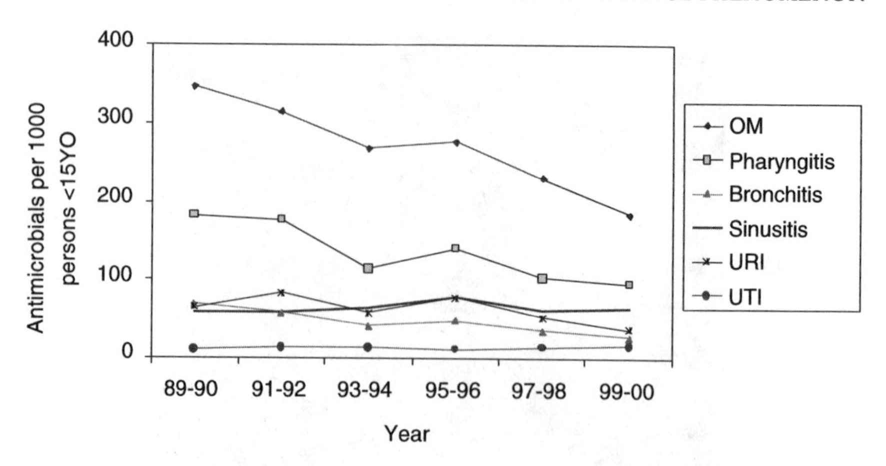

FIGURE 7-3 Trends in annual population-based rates of antimicrobial drug use at physician office visits for children under 15 years of age by selected infectious respiratory diseases and urinary tract infection: United States, 1989–2000. NOTE: Figures are based on 2-year averages. All trends shown are significant ($p < 0.001$), except sinusitis ($p = 0.61$) and UTI ($p = 0.19$). OM denotes otitis media. URI denotes upper respiratory infection. SOURCE: McCaig et al., 2002.

campaign was expanded in 2001 to target prescribing for adults (Gonzales et al., 2001), to increase to 18 the number of state health departments funded to develop coalitions and to develop a national advertising campaign, a model medical curriculum, and HEDIS measures (benchmarks for health plans) for appropriate prescribing. Future goals include expanding the campaign to all states and major health plans and implementing the national advertising campaign.

In health care settings, where infection with multi-drug-resistant organisms is a major patient safety issue, promoting appropriate antimicrobial drug prescribing is complicated by the higher stakes involved in treating sicker patients and the need to develop partnerships with a greater number of medical and surgical specialties involved in their care, as well as with other clinical staff and administrators. *Prevent Antimicrobial Resistance*, a campaign that emphasizes 12 evidence-based steps for diagnosis of infection, appropriate treatment, appropriate use of antibiotics, and preventing transmission, was launched by the CDC in March 2002, initially focusing on hospital care of adults. Future goals include implementing this campaign in other health care settings, for example, dialysis clinics and long-term care facilities, and for patients in all age groups, and evaluating and facilitating the appropriate use of new informatics technologies, for example, computerized decision support for online prescribing (Evans et al., 1998).

Promoting appropriate antimicrobial drug use in agriculture and veterinary medicine has been complicated by longstanding disagreement between public health and agricultural communities regarding the benefits and risks of these uses, which may have economic implications for major industries. The American Veterinary Medical Association has developed principles for judicious therapeutic use of antimicrobials in veterinary medicine with input from CDC and FDA. CDC has also awarded cooperative agreements to four schools of veterinary medicine to assess the impact of antibiotic use in swine and dairy cattle, develop alternatives to the use of antimicrobials as growth promoters, and evaluate new practices to reduce resistant bacteria in food animals. Finally, CDC strongly supports the FDA's proposals for a new framework to evaluate antimicrobial drugs used in food animal production and for withdrawal of approval for the use of fluoroquinolones in poultry as important steps toward protecting public health while ensuring the availability of antimicrobials needed for food-producing animals.

Preventing transmission of infections (e.g., through appropriate use of vaccines, infection control in health care, food safety) reduces disease incidence and drug prescribing (Fridkin et al., 1999; Neuzil et al., 2000; Whitney et al., 2001). In 2001 CDC supported projects to evaluate the impact of pneumococcal conjugate vaccine in reducing infections with drug-resistant pneumococci, demonstration programs evaluating comprehensive approaches to infection control in health care settings in Chicago and Pittsburgh, and infection prevention and control research and evaluation programs at seven university-based Centers of Excellence in Healthcare Epidemiology. Regional approaches are important, as illustrated by the early recognition and successful control of the spread of vancomycin-resistant enterococci (VRE) in acute and long-term care facilities in the tri-state area surrounding Sioux City, Iowa. With leadership from the Sioux City health department and support from the Iowa, South Dakota, and Nebraska state health departments and CDC, health care institutions rigorously implemented surveillance and prevention and control guidelines and communicated freely. As a result, they were able to eliminate VRE from hospitals and drastically reduce VRE rates in long-term care facilities, an unprecedented success (Ostrowsky et al., 2001). Greater support for comprehensive regional programs such as this is a top priority of the action plan.

Applied Research

In 2001, CDC initiated a new AR applied research grant program. Based on external peer review, four grants totaling $3.2 million were awarded to universities for investigator-initiated research projects addressing: 1) prevention and control of AR in rural settings, and 2) resistance mechanisms and the role of drug use in promoting the spread of resistance in hospitals and from food animals to humans. Future goals of this research program include addressing additional Action Plan items through peer-reviewed, investigator-initiated proposals, for example, on diagnostic testing, infection control, drug and vaccine use, monitoring spread of resistance genes, impact of drug use in agriculture, clinical and economic outcomes of AR, and novel interventions.

In summary, federal agencies now have a strategy and an action plan to address AR domestically—and a similar plan is being developed to address global resistance. Progress to date is encouraging, indicating that additional investments can be expected to pay dividends in converting AR from an urgent to a routine problem that does not compromise the availability of safe and effective therapy for patients today and in future generations.

ANTIBIOTIC RESISTANCE: ENCOURAGING THE DEVELOPMENT OF NEW THERAPIES, PRESERVING THE USEFULNESS OF CURRENT THERAPIES

Mark J. Goldberger, M.D., M.P.H.

Center for Drug Evaluation and Research
U.S. Food and Drug Administration, Rockville, MD

Antibiotic resistance in a broad range of microrganisms has been steadily increasing. This has affected many of the therapies commonly used to treat infections caused by these organisms. This problem is not limited to bacterial infections but also includes fungi, parasites, and viruses. The focus of the following issues will be largely on antibacterial drugs; however, the approaches and issues would also be applicable to therapies for these other organisms.

One obvious part of the solution to this problem is to develop new antimicrobials that are active against resistant organisms. There has already been progress in this area. Two new fluoroquinolone antibiotics, gatifloxacin (Bristol Myers Squibb, 1999) and moxifloxacin (Bayer, 1999), with increased activity against gram-positive bacteria have been recently approved. Members of three new classes of antimicrobials, the oxazolidinones (Pharmacia and Upjohn, 2000), streptogramins (Aventis, 1999), and ketolides (Ketek presented to advisory committee January 2003), have also either recently been approved or are far along in the drug development process. These are all examples of drugs that include some degree of activity against resistant organisms. Nonetheless, despite these advances serious concerns remain about our ability to successfully treat many infections due to either resistant gram-positive or gram-negative organisms. An ongoing focus in the coming months for staff in the Center for Drug Evaluation and

Research (CDER) is to continue to enhance the available approaches to the development of new antibiotics.

The development of new antimicrobials is no easy task, and trying to keep pace with increasing antimicrobial resistance only through the development of new drugs would be a daunting undertaking. It would be highly desirable to link increased development with approaches that preserve the usefulness of these new drugs as well as current antimicrobials. There is an inherent tension in these two approaches that must be reconciled as we move forward. This tension is particularly noteworthy for new antimicrobials that in addition to their activity against resistant organisms also possess broader activity against more susceptible organisms. As part of our efforts at FDA we would certainly also like to encourage the development of drugs whose primary focus would be the treatment of infections due to resistant organisms.

FDA already has a number of regulatory tools to facilitate the development of drugs for serious and life-threatening illness (FDA, 1998). These include our Subpart E and Subpart H regulations and fast track designation. These encourage early communication between FDA and firms, allow us to use data collected earlier in the drug development process as the basis for approval, and permit the use of surrogate markers to form the basis of approval. These approaches have the effect of accelerating drug development by improving the overall quality of the development program, allowing a reduced number of patients in the clinical program, and permitting the use of data collected from an ongoing trial to support approval. They have been used very effectively in the development of new antivirals and drugs for opportunistic infections in patients infected with HIV, as well as for therapies for cancer and other serious illness.

The above methods all have their limitations. Smaller clinical trial programs may leave greater uncertainty as to the efficacy of a product and they unquestionably limit conclusions that can be drawn about safety. Surrogate markers such as CD4 and viral load have been extraordinarily useful in the development of antiretroviral drugs; however, surrogate markers are not always predictive of the ultimate outcome in a clinical trial. In studies of the antiarrythmic drugs, ecanide and flecanide, suppression of ventricular premature depolarizations (the surrogate) was actually associated with a poorer longer-term outcome as measured by mortality (Echt et al., 1991).

Current legislation also provides several options that allow a company developing a product to obtain additional marketing exclusivity beyond that available from an existing patent. The Waxman Hatch Act permits an applicant to recover a portion of patent life that was used during development. This statute also provides for non-patent exclusivity when clinical studies are required for approval. Although not previously eligible, recent changes in legislation have made these benefits applicable to new antibiotic compounds. Products developed to treat or prevent infection for which the applicable U.S. patient population is less than 200,000 are eligible for Orphan Product exclusivity. This provides seven years of marketing exclusivity for the specific product regardless of whether there is existing patent protection.

Beyond the above it is appropriate to consider how we can improve our ability to make inferences from clinical trials conducted for resistance claims. This would be of particular value for products whose primary emphasis is treatment of resistant infections. In the study of a new agent for treatment of serious gram-positive infections such an approach could include a study of the new agent in smaller numbers of very well characterized patients with a predictable clinical course. Patients with bacterial endocarditis or related infections could be an example of this. Data from such a trial could be supported by a clinical trial in a more conventional situation such as pneumonia to collect additional efficacy and safety data. Collecting pharmacokinetic and pharmacodynamic (PK/PD) data in these settings might also increase our understanding of the product.

As part of these efforts some unresolved scientific and medical issues must also be explored. The definitions and significance of resistance are not always clear. In many circumstances, for instance, penicillins maintain clinically useful activity against penicillin-resistant pneumococci. In other situations pre-existing resistance does not appear to correlate with ultimate outcome.

There are a variety of approaches to studying antimicrobials in both in vitro and in vivo pre-clinical models. Such studies could be extremely useful in defining preliminary activity of a drug as well as providing useful information on dosing regimen. Ideally these approaches would be integrated with PK/PD studies with the overall goal of increasing the efficiency of the development process. There is currently considerable work being done in all these areas. Their ultimate usefulness in facilitating drug development in this area is not yet adequately defined.

It is important to recognize the limits of FDA authority. We cannot, for example, actually develop a drug even though we can facilitate its development by others. There must be some other entity willing and able to do this. Although as previously mentioned existing authority allows us to grant certain types of marketing exclusivity, we have no authority to grant so-called "wildcard exclusivity" that might, for example, apply to another drug of a firm's choosing in return for development of a drug with more limited economic value. Such authority would require new legislation.

We must recognize that it will not be an easy task to keep up with increasing rates of resistance in many pathogens even if we can improve our approach to the development of new antimicrobials. We must also consider ways to preserve the usefulness of these new products as well as those already available. There are a variety of approaches that may be of value.

At FDA the product label is the starting point for communicating information to physicians and patients. The information contained within this label is the basis for the promotional material prepared by companies and should also provide a basis for any FDA educational efforts. Our initial efforts with regard to providing additional information in product labeling will include reminders of the value of antimicrobial susceptibility information (when available) in choosing therapy and of the role of antimicrobials in bacterial as opposed to viral infections. These efforts are well under way. It is clear, however, that to effectively communicate information to patients and physicians will require a broad effort from the overall medical community.

Existing regulations provide FDA with the authority to approve drugs with restrictions for safe use (FDA, 1998). This has been done in limited instances, for example, thalidomide. A restricted distribution program can be quite flexible in implementation ranging from statements in labeling, reminding providers who should receive the drug, to programs mandating special testing and limited to certain providers and pharmacies. Such a program could be quite useful particularly for a product that has been approved with limited data on safety and efficacy. Many pharmaceutical firms have limited enthusiasm for such programs. The potential to use such a program may serve as a disincentive to product development. Implementing such a program would also be problematic for a drug that had demonstrated broad antimicrobial activity, including activity against resistant organisms, and for which a more substantial safety database was available.

Antimicrobial therapy is used in a wide variety of clinical situations. In severe infections its value versus no treatment is clearly established. In milder illness the benefits may be more difficult to quantify. In an effort to avoid unnecessary patient exposure to antibiotics and as part of our efforts to rethink our approach to the development of antimicrobial therapy we must, consider with the assistance of our advisory committees and stakeholders, approaches to trial design to deal with this issue.

We also believe that in our approach to product approval and labeling, current issues in medical practice should be considered. As an example, otitis media, an infection of the ear generally seen only in children, is usually caused by one of three bacterial species. It is uncommon however for physicians to routinely do the testing to determine the specific bacterial cause as this involves puncturing the eardrum—a potentially difficult and painful procedure. As a result children are treated empirically. Most drugs approved for this indication are active against the three major pathogens so that this does not pose a problem. However at least one product approved in the past had lower activity against one of the organisms. This problem was addressed by including such information in product labeling. Given that the physician will not know the actual cause of the infection for a given child it is not clear what he/she could do with such information. Should similar situations occur in the future we will need to reconsider whether an approach using labeling is the most appropriate solution.

There are areas of research that may contribute to better ways to preserve the usefulness of antimicrobial therapy. The availability of rapid diagnostic tests for bacterial and viral infections would allow practitioners to make more informed judgments regarding the need for antimicrobial therapy. Having available additional information on the relationship between dose, duration of therapy, and outcome including development of resistance would also be of value in developing more optimal treatment regimens.

In addition to antibacterial resistance, a worldwide problem, it is worth emphasizing that the broader problem of antimicrobial resistance is also a global one. Drug-resistant malaria and multi-drug-resistant tuberculosis are major health issues throughout much of the world. As the use of antiretroviral therapy increases throughout the world, issues of resistant HIV can be expected to become more widespread.

THE CENTERS FOR DISEASE CONTROL AND PREVENTION'S CAMPAIGN TO PREVENT ANTIMICROBIAL RESISTANCE IN HEALTH CARE SETTINGS

Julie L. Gerberding, M.D., M.P.H.

Centers for Disease Control and Prevention, Atlanta, GA

Each year in the United States, approximately 2 million patients acquire an infection while hospitalized, and about 90,000 of these patients die as a result of their infection (CDC, 1992). Many more people acquire infections in nursing homes and other health care facilities in which vulnerable patients receive care. More than 70 percent of the bacteria that cause hospital-onset infections are resistant to at least one of the drugs most commonly used to treat them (CDC, 1999). Patients infected with antimicrobial-resistant organisms are more likely to have longer hospital stays and require treatment with second- or third-choice drugs that may be less effective, more toxic, and/or more expensive.

The proportion of pathogens that cause hospital-onset infections and are resistant to drugs continues to increase. For example, data collected through the National Nosocomial Infections Surveillance (NNIS) system indicate that more than 50 percent of *Staphylococcus aureus* isolates causing infections in intensive care units were resistant to methicillin in 2000, compared to about 30 percent in 1989 (CDC, 2001). (In other hospital units, more than 40 percent of *S. aureus* isolates were resistant to methicillin in 2000, up from about 20 percent in 1989.) Vancomycin-resistant enterococci, which emerged in the late 1980s, are now endemic in many hospitals, and they accounted for more than 25 percent of enterococcal infections in 2000 (CDC, 2001).

Indeed, the rate of increased prevalence of resistance for some organisms is alarming. Data from NNIS indicate, for example, that fluoroquinolone resistance among *Pseudomonas* species increased by almost 50 percent between 1994 and 1999. The prevalence of both methicillin-resistant *S. aureus* and vancomycin-resistant enterococci increased by 40 percent over the same period (CDC, 2001).

Guidelines for preventing antimicrobial-resistant infections in health care settings exist; however, these guidelines often are not read by clinicians and adherence is not optimal. Most data indicate that guidelines alone are not effective in preventing antimicrobial resistance. New approaches are needed to help clinicians who treat patients with infections translate these guidelines into routine practice behaviors that will prevent antimicrobial resistance.

In response to this issue, the CDC has initiated the Campaign to Prevent Antimicrobial Resistance in Healthcare Settings. The campaign is a nationwide effort that targets front-line clinicians, patient care partners, health care organizations, purchasers, and patients. Its general goals include informing clinicians, patients, and other stakeholders about the escalating problem of antimicrobial resistance in health care settings; motivating interest in and acceptance of interventional programs to prevent resistance; and providing clinicians with tools to support needed practice changes. Targeting clinicians at the front end of care is an important step toward preventing the morbidity, mortality, and costs associated with drug resistance. The campaign was developed and is being implemented in collaboration with the CDC Foundation, corporate partners, professional societies, health care organizations, public health agencies, and expert consultants. Additional information about the campaign is available at http://www.cdc.gov/drugresistance/health care.

The campaign centers around four basic strategies that clinicians can use to prevent antimicrobial resistance. These strategies are:

- *Prevent infection.* Preventing infections in the first place will directly reduce the need for antimicrobial exposure and the emergence and selection of resistant strains.
- *Diagnose and treat infection effectively.* Proper diagnosis and treatment will benefit the patient and decrease the opportunity for development and selection of resistant microbes. This requires rapid diagnosis, identifi-

cation of the causative pathogen, and determination of its antimicrobial susceptibility.

- *Use antimicrobials wisely.* Optimal use will ensure proper patient care and at the same time avoid overuse of broad-spectrum antimicrobials and unnecessary treatment.
- *Prevent transmission.* Preventing transmission of resistant organisms from one person to another is critical to successful prevention efforts.

An integral component of the campaign is the development, dissemination, and implementation of a number of intervention programs for clinicians caring for targeted groups of high-risk patients. These programs, called "12 Steps to Prevent Antimicrobial Resistance," spell out actions that can be taken immediately to promote patient safety and prevent antimicrobial-resistant infections. The first 12-step program targets hospitalized adults; other programs are being developed for hospitalized children, geriatric patients and nursing home residents, obstetrical patients, critical-care patients, dialysis patients, and surgical patients. The programs are created in close partnership with professional societies and key opinion leaders in the relevant specialties, and all of the action steps are based on scientific evidence and/or published guidelines.

The 12 steps detailed in the programs are framed around the four strategies described above. Each step provides some key facts and background information that serve to buttress the importance of the actions recommended. The steps also include links to other Web-based resources that provide more detailed information.

In the program targeted at hospitalized adults, two steps address the importance of preventing infection. These steps are:

1. *Vaccinate.* Pre-discharge influenza and pneumococcal vaccination of at-risk hospital patients and influenza vaccination of health care personnel will prevent infections. These infections and their complications are a major cause of hospitalization and exposure to antimicrobials, and they create opportunities for emergence and spread of antimicrobial resistance.
2. *Get the catheters out.* Catheters and other invasive devices are the leading exogenous cause of hospital-onset infections. Catheters should be used only when essential to patient care, not for convenience or as a "routine" practice. Proper insertion and catheter care may decrease contamination and infection risk, and in some cases antimicrobial-impregnated catheters may be warranted to prevent infections.

Two steps focus on the need to diagnose and treat infection effectively:

3. *Target the pathogen.* Appropriate antimicrobial therapy saves lives.

When managing patients with known or suspected infection, cultures are almost always indicated. Empiric therapy should be selected to target likely pathogens and be consistent with local antimicrobial susceptibility data. Definitive therapy should target known pathogens once they are identified and their antimicrobial susceptibility test results are known.

4. *Access the experts.* Infectious diseases expert input improves the outcome of serious infections. Infectious disease specialists are one important resource for providing input, but many other professionals, such as health care epidemiologists, clinical pharmacologists, and surgical infection experts, also can contribute to optimal care for patients with infections. As with all patient safety endeavors, multidisciplinary collaboration is key.

Six steps address the importance of using antimicrobials wisely:

5. *Practice antimicrobial control.* Programs to improve antimicrobial use are effective. Methods to improve antimicrobial use include passive and interactive prescriber education; use of standardized antimicrobial order forms; formulary restrictions; prior approval to start or switch antimicrobials; multidisciplinary drug utilization evaluation; provider or unit feedback; and computerized decision support (including on-line ordering), which is likely to be the best long-term approach for improving antimicrobial use. Whatever options are available for improving antimicrobial use, the commitment and participation of the prescribing clinician and the institution are essential.

6. *Use local data.* The prevalence of resistance can vary by time, locale, patient population, hospital unit, and length of stay. Local antimicrobial susceptibility data are the most relevant for predicting the probability of resistance. Thus, clinicians should be fully informed about their local "antibiograms," which provide a summary picture of common organisms and their susceptibility to many antimicrobial drugs, as well as about the characteristics of their patient populations.

7. *Treat infection, not contamination.* A major cause of antimicrobial overuse is "treatment" of contaminated cultures. Contamination of blood cultures and other patient specimens is common, often leading to unnecessary antimicrobial use. Proper specimen collection and management is key to preventing contaminated cultures. Clinicians should use proper antisepsis for blood and other cultures; culture the blood, not the skin or catheter hub; and use proper methods to obtain and process all cultures.

8. *Treat infection, not colonization.* A major cause of antimicrobial overuse is treatment of colonization. Patients often become colonized with new bacterial flora while hospitalized, and when fever or other evidence of infection is mistakenly attributed to these colonizing organisms, unneces-

sary broad-spectrum antimicrobial therapy often ensues. Clinical criteria and additional laboratory data can help distinguish infection from colonization. Among specific actions, clinicians should treat pneumonia, not the tracheal aspirate; treat bacteremia, not the catheter tip or hub; and treat urinary tract infection, not the indwelling catheter.

9. *Know when to say "no" to vanco.* Vancomycin overuse promotes emergence, selection, and spread of resistant pathogens. Emergence of vancomycin resistance among gram-positive organisms is a major threat to patient safety in hospitals. Clinicians should recognize that fever in a patient with an intravenous catheter is not a routine indication for vancomycin. The CDC's Healthcare Infection Control Practices Advisory Committee has developed a set of guidelines that detail situations in which the use of vancomycin either is acceptable or should be discouraged (CDC, 1995).

10. *Stop treatment when infection is cured or unlikely.* Failure to stop unnecessary antimicrobial treatment contributes to overuse and resistance. Once antimicrobial therapy is started, it is often difficult to stop, even when there is no indication for ongoing treatment. However, unnecessary treatment adds to treatment costs and may, in some cases, actually harm patients. It is important that treatment be stopped when infection is cured, when cultures are negative and infection is unlikely, and/or when infection is not diagnosed.

The final two steps focus on preventing transmission of resistant organisms:

11. *Isolate the pathogen.* Patient-to-patient spread of pathogens can be prevented. Adherence to accepted measures to isolate antimicrobial-resistant organisms before they are transferred to other patients or become endemic in a facility is essential. Clinicians and facilities should use standard infection-control procedures and approved techniques for containing infectious body fluids. When in doubt about appropriate isolation procedures, consultation with an infection-control professional is indicated.

12. *Break the chain of contagion.* Healthcare personnel can spread antimicrobial-resistant pathogens from patient to patient. They also can transmit their own flora and infectious pathogens to patients. Thus, personnel should undertake a number of simple, common-sense measures to prevent the spread of pathogens. These measures include staying home when ill with an infection, covering the mouth when coughing or sneezing, and maintaining appropriate hand hygiene before and after patient contact. Clinicians also should set an example for students, trainees, and colleagues.

This program, and the other 12-step programs when they are ready, will be marketed widely, through Web presentations, "slide sets" detailing the steps, posters, pocket cards, and other media. CDC also will foster partnerships to implement campaign activities, and will support efforts to evaluate the effectiveness of these programs in preventing antimicrobial resistance in health care settings.

ANTIMICROBIAL RESISTANCE CONTAINMENT STRATEGIES OF THE RATIONAL PHARMACEUTICAL MANAGEMENT PLUS PROGRAM

Terry Green and Anthony Savelli

Rational Pharmaceutical Management Plus (RPM Plus) Program*
Management Sciences for Health, Arlington, VA

The use of antimicrobial agents has contributed to the significant decline in infectious diseases over the past half century. However, this achievement in controlling infectious diseases is being undermined by the rapidly growing problem of antimicrobial resistance. Resistance to antimicrobials is increasing, making many infectious diseases more difficult to treat, and raising levels of morbidity, mortality, and health care costs. Major infectious diseases like tuberculosis, gonorrhea, pneumonia, malaria, and dysentery are becoming increasingly difficult and expensive to treat, particularly in developing countries where resources are limited and infection rates are high. With international attention focused on HIV and its treatment, there is much concern about drug resistance and the possibility of future resistance to current antiretrovirals.

Antimicrobial resistance is a natural, progressive reaction that is tied directly to the use and misuse of antimicrobials in humans, animals, and agriculture. As more of the sensitive bacteria are eliminated by antimicrobials, resistant ones will survive and proliferate, transferring their resistance by genes to future generations of bacteria. With time, all antibiotics will encounter resistance development by various bacteria. Depending on the antimicrobial and the bacterium, the degree of resistance can be minimal to almost total.

*The Rational Pharmaceutical Management Plus (RPM Plus) Program is supported by the U.S. Agency for International Development under the terms of cooperative agreement number HRN-A-00-00-00016-00. The opinions expressed herein are those of the authors and do not necessarily reflect the views of the U.S. Agency for International Development.

How Severe Is the AMR Problem?

The increased morbidity, mortality, and treatment costs associated with resistant infections are complicating infectious disease prevention and control efforts worldwide, underscoring the need to preserve the effectiveness of existing antimicrobials. The increased costs for treating resistant infections and new infections that result from the failure of first-line antimicrobials are draining health resources in developing countries. Hospital-acquired infections, which account for thousands of deaths in countries yearly, are frequently caused by antimicrobial-resistant organisms.

A single treatment course for regular tuberculosis (TB) costs about $20, while treatment for multi-drug-resistant TB costs $2000 (WHO, 2000a). Multi-drug-resistant shigella requiring treatment with ciprofloxacin has occurred in 11 countries since 1989. While the cost of ciprofloxacin is high, of more critical importance is the fact that resistance is developing to ciprofloxacin, with no other effective treatment available at this time. Treatment failures due to resistant strains of gonorrhea are a driving force in the HIV epidemic (WHO, 2000b). Persons infected with gonorrhea are more susceptible to HIV infection, and once infected, shed HIV virus at nine times the rate of infected individuals without gonorrhea (WHO, 2000c). Increasing access to antiretroviral therapy for AIDS patients in developing countries should help to reduce opportunistic infections associated with high levels of resistance (i.e., gonorrhea, pneumonia, and TB). However, without proper case management, the benefit of the new drugs may be short-lived. Similar concerns exist for the increased availability of TB and malaria drugs that will occur under the Global Fund to Fight AIDS, Tuberculosis and Malaria. The AMR containment strategies discussed below will increase awareness about this issue and provide opportunities to reduce the risks associated with the Global Fund.

WHO Global Strategy for Containment of AMR

As a major step toward containing AMR, the WHO has recently published a comprehensive set of strategies. WHO recommends a number of interventions, including strategies for use by (1) patients and communities; (2) prescribers and dispensers; (3) hospitals; (4) growers of food-producing animals; (5) national governments and health systems; (6) drug and vaccine developers; (7) pharmaceutical companies and marketers; and (8) international organizations and partnerships concerned with containing AMR. Such a complex, diverse approach is critical in addressing the threats posed by AMR.

RPM Plus AMR Containment Strategies

RPM Plus is a five-year cooperative agreement with USAID to provide technical leadership, assistance, and training on pharmaceutical management in the developing world, and to foster coordination of donor groups to improve health commodity availability and appropriate use. RPM Plus has a portfolio of strategies aimed at managing AMR in various areas of the health care system. These include drug and therapeutics committees (DTC) training, infection-control quality-improvement programs (in the WHO Global Strategies, both are highly recommended for hospitals), national-level implementation strategies, research activities to guide drug use improvement, activities of the International Network for Rational Use of Drugs (INRUD) to provide education for providers/dispensers, and activities to support the national AMR program in Nepal. These strategies are summarized in the discussion below.

Developing and Implementing National AMR Strategies

The WHO global plan is comprehensive and complex, making it difficult to implement in many developing countries. A succinct methodology is needed for implementing the plan at the country level.

To improve the reach of the WHO global initiative, RPM Plus (and our partner the Alliance for Prudent Use of Antibiotics [APUA]), in collaboration with the Academy for Educational Development's CHANGE project and Boston University's Applied Research in Child Health (ARCH) project, is supporting the development of a systematic approach to guide the design of national-level efforts to contain AMR. This approach will provide a framework by which stakeholders, working with technical consultants when necessary, can assess policies, drug use, and AMR in their countries, using local data, and can then design strategies for advocacy, policy development, and systems change. For these efforts to succeed, many groups must have a role, including national governments, health care professionals and societies, consumers, non-governmental organizations (NGOs), and the pharmaceutical industry. Although the approach is generic, the implementation process will likely be country-specific and will unfold in distinct ways, according to circumstances in each country. Whatever its specific character, it is anticipated that the systematic approach will result in more active local health organizations, a higher level of awareness about AMR, and stronger policies and programs to monitor and contain the spread of resistance. Figure 7-4 represents the framework for implementing the country strategy for containment of AMR.

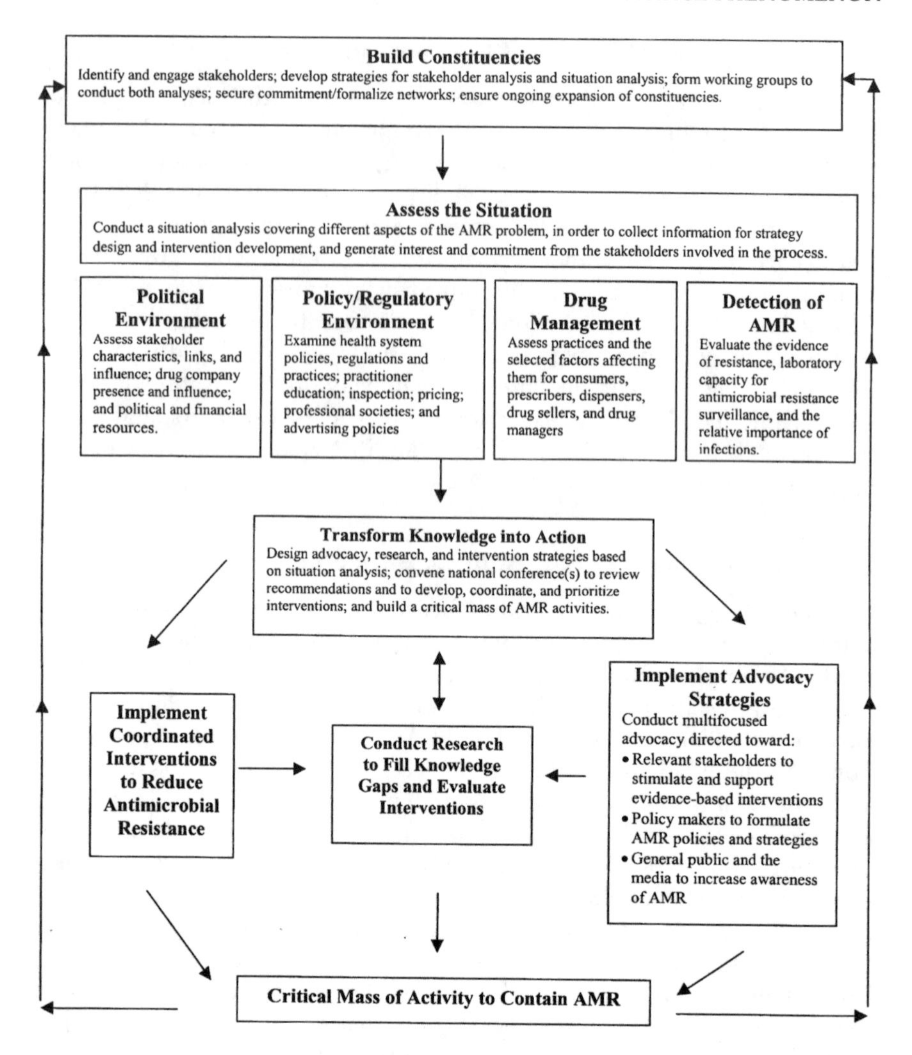

Build Constituencies
Identify and engage stakeholders; develop strategies for stakeholder analysis and situation analysis; form working groups to conduct both analyses; secure commitment/formalize networks; ensure ongoing expansion of constituencies.
Assess the Situation
Conduct a situation analysis covering different aspects of the AMR problem, in order to collect information for strategy design and intervention development, and generate interest and commitment from the stakeholders involved in the process.
Political Environment
Assess stakeholder characteristics, links, and influence; drug company presence and influence; and political and financial resources.
Policy/Regulatory Environment
Examine health system policies, regulations and practices; practitioner education; inspection; pricing; professional societies; and advertising policies
Drug Management
Assess practices and the selected factors affecting them for consumers, prescribers, dispensers, drug sellers, and drug managers
Detection of AMR
Evaluate the evidence of resistance, laboratory capacity for antimicrobial resistance surveillance, and the relative importance of infections.
Transform Knowledge into Action
Design advocacy, research, and intervention strategies based on situation analysis; convene national conference(s) to review recommendations and to develop, coordinate, and prioritize interventions; and build a critical mass of AMR activities.
Implement Coordinated Interventions to Reduce Antimicrobial Resistance
Conduct Research to Fill Knowledge Gaps and Evaluate Interventions
Implement Advocacy Strategies
Conduct multifocused advocacy directed toward:
• Relevant stakeholders to stimulate and support evidence-based interventions
• Policy makers to formulate AMR policies and strategies
• General public and the media to increase awareness of AMR
Critical Mass of Activity to Contain AMR

FIGURE 7-4 Outline of a systematic approach for containing antimicrobial resistance.

Establishing and Strengthening Drug and Therapeutics Committees

The DTC is a critical component of a health care organization's drug selection and use program. This committee evaluates the clinical use of drugs, develops policies for managing drug use and administration, and manages the formulary system.

Many countries spend 30 to 40 percent of their health care budgets on drugs, and much of that money is wasted on irrational drug use and inefficiencies in procurement and distribution. Other serious drug use problems faced by health care organizations include the overuse of antibiotics, increasing levels of AMR, and increasing rates of adverse drug reaction. DTCs can provide the leadership and structure to help ensure that appropriate drugs are selected for the formulary, rational drug use is promoted, and waste is reduced, thereby reducing costs.

The committee has broad responsibilities in determining what drugs will be available, at what cost, and how they will be used. Some of the important benefits of a functioning DTC are:

- Selection of effective, safe, high-quality, and cost-effective pharmaceuticals for the formulary
- Control and management of drug expenditures
- Identification of drug use problems
- Rational drug use, including improved antimicrobial utilization
- Improved drug procurement and inventory management
- Increased staff- and patient-education levels on matters related to drug use
- Decreased adverse drug reactions and medication errors.

The functions of a DTC are numerous and will vary with each country and with the size of each health facility. The most important functions are:

- Advising medical, administrative, and pharmacy departments on drug-related issues
- Developing drug policies and procedures
- Evaluating and selecting drugs for the formulary and providing information for its periodic revision
- Assessing drug use to identify potential problems
- Promoting and conducting effective interventions to improve drug use (including educational, managerial, and regulatory methods)
- Managing adverse drug reactions
- Managing medication errors.

RPM Plus DTC Training Courses

DTCs are weak or non-existent in developing countries and irrational drug use is a common problem. To improve the capacity of committees, RPM Plus (in collaboration with WHO) has developed training materials for a DTC course, which is designed to stimulate the creation of DTCs in hospitals, improve the functioning of existing committees, and train locally based staff to teach the course to others. The training series emphasizes the technical aspects of a DTC, including selecting drugs for the formulary, managing drug expenditures, identifying drug use problems, and implementing interventions to improve drug use.

An integral part of the DTC training is a field study where participants utilize skills learned in the course and apply them at local hospitals. The field study allows participants to see firsthand how a DTC would work in selecting drugs, identifying drug use problems, and implementing plans to improve drug use.

An important part of the course focuses on developing DTC work plans. The course assists participants in developing comprehensive plans for starting or improving their local DTCs. These plans are monitored by RPM Plus staff members, who also provide technical assistance to help participants complete the plans over the ensuing months.

DTC Website

The DTC Website seeks to encourage former course participants to use what they have learned and to track their progress on work plans. RPM Plus staff monitor the site and provide technical assistance to individuals and teams as necessary. The Website provides course announcements, links to information sources, and access to work plans developed during the courses. The website also provides a discussion board that allows participants and facilitators to keep in contact.

Achievements from DTC Courses

RPM Plus has trained 117 participants from 35 countries in eight training courses since February 2001. DTC course participants have subsequently been active in improving drug management at the local and national level. DTCs have been implemented and are now more effective than previous drug management systems in selecting appropriate drugs for the formulary. Formularies have been evaluated and inappropriate drugs deleted, making procurement activities more efficient and less expensive. Reporting systems for adverse drug reactions (ADRs) have been upgraded and DTCs are reviewing spontaneous reports. Drug use studies and standard treatment guidelines are in use and are guiding strategies to improve drug use. RPM Plus will continue to hold DTC training courses while it monitors the work of past course participants.

Promoting Infection Control Improvement

Hospital-acquired infections are a major cause of preventable morbidity and mortality in developing countries worldwide, putting both patients and health care workers at risk. These infections also impose a high financial cost by increasing the length of hospitalization and requiring the use of additional, expensive laboratory tests and broad-spectrum antibiotics. They are often caused by AMR organisms that have developed due to poor infection-control and prevention practices and the overuse of antibiotics.

There are many root causes of poor infection control and prevention in hospitals. There is a lack of both an infection-control infrastructure and training in basic infection control, and in many hospitals, basic hand hygiene and sanitation practices are substandard. The use of invasive devices and procedures, such as indwelling lines and catheters and implanted devices, can often be debilitating and even lethal when infection control practices are inadequate.

In addition to the substantial impact on morbidity, mortality, and health care costs, there are other compelling reasons to focus on developing practical strategies for improving infection control and decreasing the emergence of AMR in hospitals:

- Hospitals are major incubators for resistant bacteria, because antimicrobial agents are commonly prescribed
- Hospitals can amplify resistance, because resistant bacteria spread quickly among vulnerable patients in facilities that are understaffed, overcrowded, or lack basic infection control practices
- Patients who acquire resistant infections in hospitals have the potential to disseminate these bacteria in their homes and communities

RPM Plus is developing an infection-control quality improvement program (in collaboration with Harvard University) that will use local assessments, training, and intervention based on assessment results to improve infection control and decrease the rate of nosocomial infections at the hospital level. A distance-learning component will make it possible for many more institutions to take advantage of the program. The program's objectives are to provide for:

- Development and use of assessment instruments to identify priority areas for site-specific interventions
- Training in continuous quality improvement techniques and methodologies
- Comprehensive training in infection control for teams and other clinical and administrative hospital personnel, available on a multimedia CD-ROM
- Development of a stand-alone infection control program, using CD-ROM, e-mail, and the Web, to establish or improve infection control

systems by providing assessment instruments, training materials, coaching, and support to local team leaders.

Joint Research Initiative to Improve Use of Medicines in Developing Countries

RPM Plus is a partner with WHO, the Academy for Educational Development (AED), INRUD, and ARCH in the Joint Research Initiative to Improve Use of Medicines. The goal of the initiative is to build a body of evidence on effective drug use interventions in developing countries. Partners provide technical assistance to research groups in applying and testing interventions, as well as in pursuing publication of studies relevant to antimicrobial use.

Current research activities are divided into three categories (see Table 7-1). Phase I studies are nearing completion, and Phase II studies are in the development and funding stage. Phase III studies will begin in late 2002.

Other AMR Containment Support

RPM Plus has developed a manual on hospital antimicrobial indicators, designed to help hospital staff evaluate and improve antimicrobial use in their institutions. The manual is useful in making comparisons of antimicrobial drug use in one hospital over time or between use in two or more hospitals.

The RPM Plus portfolio also includes technical assistance activities for the Nepal national AMR program, which works to enhance AMR sentinel surveillance sites and improve drug management programs in the public and private sectors. Other AMR-related work includes support of INRUD activities including participation in Africa and Asia regional training courses on Promoting Rational Drug Use.

RPM Plus interventions are designed to improve drug selection, appro-

TABLE 7-1 Joint Research Initiative to Improve Use of Medicine

Phase I	Phase II	Phase III
Research focused on improving the prescribing and dispensing behavior of health professionals	Activities focused on improving the use of antimicrobials in communities and households	Studies to evaluate the impact of specific national, district, and local policies that affect drug use, including strategies for scaling up

priate use of drugs, and infection control practices at the local level, and to develop a process to implement these and other WHO global AMR containment strategies at the national level. With implementation of these key drug management programs, AMR containment strategies can be optimized.

ANTIMICROBIAL RESISTANCE AND FUTURE DIRECTIONS

Mary E. Torrence, D.V.M., Ph.D., D.A.C.V.P.M.

USDA, Cooperative State Research
Education and Extension Service, Washington, DC

There are several common themes from the last two days. Emerging and re-emerging infectious diseases will continue to occur. These diseases will necessitate the use of current and new antimicrobials for treatment and are an important component of health care. The most important theme is that antimicrobial resistance exists, will continue to exist, and cannot be prevented or stopped. Our goal, therefore, must be to slow down its emergence and continue to develop new antibiotics that will take the place of those drugs that become useless because of resistance.

No one would disagree that the public health action plan is a significant effort among various groups and represents a comprehensive strategy to address antimicrobial resistance (U.S. Government, 2001). However, one may wonder if this document will achieve the goals and action items outlined or whether the plan will remain just a comprehensive paper document. It is important that there is some measure of progress and a means of measuring the outcome or impact of the various actions and strategies. Continual feedback is needed so that revisions can be made and the plan remains responsive to the issues.

In the spirit of the public health action plan, I will make my suggestions within each of the four categories: surveillance, research, prevention and control, and product development.

Surveillance

As we all know, there are multiple, existing surveillance efforts. Some are specifically targeted toward a particular disease or niche, for example, the hospital infectious control program, while others are more general in order to collect data that is representative. The starting question for the design of the best surveillance system has to be, "What is the question that we are trying to answer?" The answer drives the design of the system, the population sampled, and the collection of the data.

The National Antimicrobial Resistance Monitoring System (NARMS) that began in 1996 provides a good framework for antimicrobial resistance surveillance (Tollefson et al., 1998). Would any of the other existing surveillance programs offer additional data? If so, how do we coordinate or integrate the programs or data? In the evaluation of NARMS, limitations must also be considered.

Sampling differs from year to year. For example, isolates from healthy animals are taken from ongoing research projects and from the National Animal Health Monitoring System (NAHMS). The NAHMS studies vary each year as to geographic region represented, the animal species, and the number sampled. Samples taken from slaughter facilities also vary each year. For example, in 1999, campylobacter samples were only taken for 3 months; in 2000, samples were taken the entire year; and for 2001, samples were taken for 10 months (Torrence, 2001). These sampling differences make it difficult to make generalizations about the data and possible trends.

There are currently two laboratories doing testing. Evaluations have been done so that the methods are standardized, and there is validity. If this system expands, standardization of methods is important. Expansion of laboratories may be necessary if this system is to provide quicker feedback of data. Currently results can lag more than a year behind.

Another question is whether there is a role for animal diagnostic laboratories and clinical samples in the surveillance of antimicrobial resistance. Some of the funding available for capacity building for epidemiology and laboratories in public health could be used for animal diagnostic laboratories and epidemiological expertise. This enhancement would be useful for both antimicrobial resistance and for bioterrorism. Funding and human resources are needed for antimicrobial resistance surveillance.

Research

A common response for future directions is the request for more infrastructure, in terms of both expertise and funding. The U.S. Department of Agriculture (USDA) in relation to the CDC and the National Institutes of Health is largely underfunded even though USDA provides the majority of funding for antimicrobial resistance research in agriculture. For example, USDA's Cooperative State Research Education and Extension Service funded $4 million in 1999 and $4.5 million in 2000. This funding came from food safety programs. The USDA's Agricultural Research Service continues to budget for research to develop alternatives to antimicrobials, such as competitive exclusion products. The aim of competitive exclusion is to take advantage of the protective effect of normal healthy flora. Competitive exclusion products contain normal healthy microorganisms that compete with and replace pathogenic microorganisms, consequently, lowering the pathogenic burden. Significant issues of confidentiality of the data and the coordination of research have not been addressed.

Specific Areas of Research

There are basic research projects on the genetics of antimicrobial resistance and whether it occurs through gene transfer (e.g., integrons, plasmids) or through chromosomal mutation. However, it is also important to focus on applied research in an attempt to understand what is occurring in the populations.

It is essential for intervention and mitigation strategies to identify critical control points along the continuum of food production. For example, management changes at the farm level will not prevent the transfer of pathogenic organisms if there is significant contamination at the processing or post-harvest level. Deboning and hide removal are two production steps that have potential for significant bacterial contamination.

The majority of research has been done on important foodborne organisms such as *E. coli* O157:H7, Salmonella, and Campylobacter. But research is needed to evaluate the role of commensals in the development, persistence, and transference of antimicrobial resistance. Other bacteria that are more difficult to culture, such as anaerobes, must also be studied.

Two primary questions in the study of antimicrobial resistance seem to be two of the simplest; yet, there seems to be no agreement on the answers. First, what is the unit of analysis? Is it the gene, bacterium, host, or population? Second, how do we measure antimicrobial resistance? Is it morbidity, the existence of a gene, or treatment failure? Determining the unit of analysis is also an issue if trying to evaluate drug usage in agriculture. Research is needed to determine which dosage, treatment regimen, or drug might be the most important in the development of resistance. Two recent drug use surveys reported different results because of disagreements in the measurement of drug use (Animal Health Institute, 2000; Lipsitch et al., 2002).

Although economic research has been mentioned, much more needs to be done both in the human and agricultural sectors. For example, what are the costs and the benefits for certain management strategies on the farm?

There has been an increased priority for doing risk assessments in food safety-related areas and in antimicrobial resistance but the methodologies are still primitive. This is particularly true in risk assessments of antimicrobial resistance because data are less available and the unit of measurement not determined.

Finally, as more intervention and mitigation strategies emerge, there needs to be measurement of the outcome or impact of these strategies. This information will help in decision-making about production practices. It is time to move beyond simple prevalence studies to more applied practical studies.

Prevention and Control

There is still a great need for more rapid diagnostic tests and more rapid, sensitive detection methods. These methods could be used in finished food products and even in fruits and vegetables.

Prudent use needs to be expanded to additional management strategies. There has been a large effort in the development of judicious use guidelines. But evidence of their dissemination and impact is lacking. If professionals have no interest or do not use them, then the existence of guidelines has no impact on antimicrobial resistance.

Within the agricultural and veterinary medical community, the educational efforts need to be more aggressive and creative. For example, there could be information disseminated to pet owners to educate them that viral diseases, such as kennel cough, do not require the use of antibiotics and that less use of antibiotics is better for their pets and themselves.

Educational research methodologies will help with the evaluation of the effect of current and future educational strategies as well as possible management and intervention approaches. There needs to be communication and feedback between education and research so there is continual improvement in both sectors.

Product Development

There are not the same financial incentives for veterinary drugs as human drugs so it is even less likely that new veterinary drugs will be developed or approved. Yet, new drug development for animal drugs may prove useful for human medicine in the common goal of finding new effective drugs. How can incentives be created? Currently most of the thinking is toward alternatives, alternative products and alternative management strategies. A significant effort in agriculture is toward alternative products such as competitive exclusion products, immune modulators, and vaccines. However, it is also important to concentrate on possible alternative management approaches. A more vigorous vaccination program or production design may decrease the amount of bacterial disease and the need for antimicrobials.

Conclusions

Antimicrobial resistance is not easily definable, which makes it more difficult to measure. A unit of analysis is needed. Antimicrobial resistance is not a product of one source and cannot be isolated in one niche of the world or the environment. It is the result of a confluence of humans, environment, microbes, and animals that are continually interacting with each other. These interactions fluctuate. Therefore, it is more important for researchers, professionals, and policy makers to work together to solve this problem rather than assign blame. Solutions in this area of resistance may come from previous experiences such as insecticide resistance.

There needs to be coordination of the state, local, and federal governments as well as other groups such as industry and professional organizations. How do we better coordinate government, industry, and academia? How do we build trust so we can collaborate? There are many studies in academia that would provide important data and even samples for government initiatives.

In conclusion, I think there are two final questions, "What is our ultimate goal regarding antimicrobial resistance?" Most importantly, "What are we willing to settle for?" I do not think we have answered these questions.

REFERENCES

Animal Health Institute. 2000. Survey indicates most antibiotics used in animals are used for treating and preventing disease. Press Release, February 14, 2000. [Online]. Available: http://www.ahi.org/news%20room/press%20release/2000/feb/antibiotic%20usage%20data.htm.

Aventis. September 21, 1999. Dalfopristin; quinupristin injectable (Synercid). U.S. Patents: no unexpired patents.

Bayer. December 10, 1999. Moxifloxacin tablet (Avelox). U.S. Patents 4,990,517, 5,607,942, 5,849,752.

Bell DM. 2001. Promoting appropriate antimicrobial drug use: perspective from the Centers for Disease Control and Prevention. *Clinical Infectious Diseases* 33 (Suppl 3):S245–S250.

Belongia EA, Sullivan BJ, Chyou PH, Madagame E, Reed KD, Schwartz B. 2001. A community intervention trial to promote judicious antibiotic use and reduce penicillin-resistant *Streptococcus pneumoniae* carriage in children. *Pediatrics* 108:575–583.

Bristol Myers Squibb. December 17, 1999. Gatifloxacin injectable (Tequin). U.S. Patents 4,980,470, 5,880,283.

CDC (Centers for Disease Control and Prevention). 1992. Public health focus: surveillance, prevention and control of nosocomial infections. *Morbidity and Mortality Weekly Report* 41:783–787.

CDC. 1995. Recommendations for preventing the spread of vancomycin resistance. Recommendations of the Hospital Infection Control Practices Advisory Committee (HICPAC). *MMWR Recommendations and Reports* 44(RR-12):1–13.

CDC. 1999. Antimicrobial resistance: a growing threat to public health. [Online]. Available: http://www.cdc.gov/ncidod/hip/Aresist/am_res.htm.

CDC. 2000. Laboratory capacity to detect antimicrobial resistance, 1998. *Morbidity and Mortality Weekly Report* 48:1167–1171.

CDC. 2001. National Nosocomial Infections Surveillance (NNIS) System Report, Data Summary from January 1992–June 2001, issued August 2001. *American Journal of Infection Control* 29:404–421.

CDC. 2002. Promoting Appropriate Antibiotic Use in the Community. [Online]. Available: http://www.cdc.gov/drugresistance/community/tools.htm.

Echt DS, Liebson PR, Mitchell LB, Peters RW, Obias-Manno D, Barker AH, Arensberg D, Baker A, Friedman L, Greene HL, et al. 1991. Mortality and morbidity in patients receiving encainide, flecainide, or placebo. The Cardiac Arrhythmia Suppression Trial. *New England Journal of Medicine* 324:781–788.

Evans RS, Pestotnik SL, Classen DC, Clemmer TP, Weaver LK, Orme JF Jr, Lloyd JF, Burke JP. 1998. A computer-assisted management program for antibiotics and other anti-infective agents. *New England Journal of Medicine* 338:232–238.

FDA (Food and Drug Administration). 1998. *Guidance for Industry: Fast Track Drug Development Programs—Designation, Development and Application Review*. [Online]. Available: http://www.fda.gov/cder/guidance/2112fnl.pdf.

Finkelstein JA, Davis RL, Dowell SF, Metlay JP, Soumerai SB, Rifas-Shiman SL, Higham M, Miller Z, Miroshnik I, Pedan A, Platt R. 2001. Reducing antibiotic use in children: a randomized trial in 12 practices. *Pediatrics* 108:1–7.

Fridkin SK, Edwards JR, Pichette SC, Pryor ER, McGowan JE Jr, Tenover FC, Culver DH, Gaynes RP. 1999. Determinants of vancomycin use in adult intensive care units in 41 United States hospitals. *Clinical Infectious Diseases* 28:1119–1125.

Gonzales R, Bartlett JG, Besser RE, Cooper RJ, Hickner JM, Hoffman JR, Sande MA. 2001. Principles of appropriate antibiotic use for treatment of acute respiratory infections in adults: Background, specific aims, and methods. *Annals of Internal Medicine* 134:479–486.

Gonzales R, Steiner JF, Lum A, Barrett PH Jr. 1999. Decreasing antibiotic use in ambulatory practice: impact of a multidimensional intervention on the treatment of uncomplicated acute bronchitis in adults. *Journal of the American Medical Association* 281:1512–1519.

Hennessy TW, Petersen KM, Bruden D, Parkinson AJ, Hurlburt D, Getty M, Schwartz B, Butler JC. 2002. Changes in antibiotic-prescribing practices and carriage of penicillin-resistant *Streptococcus pneumoniae:* A controlled intervention trial in rural Alaska. *Clinical Infectious Diseases* 34:1543–1550.

Lipsitch M, Singer RS, Levin BR. 2002. Antibiotics in agriculture: when is it time to close the barn door? *Proceedings of the National Academy of Sciences* 99:5752–5754.

McCaig LF, Besser RE, Hughes JM. 2002. Trends in antimicrobial prescribing rates for children and adolescents. *Journal of the American Medical Association* 287:3096–3102.

Neuzil KM, Mellen BG, Wright PF, Mitchel EF, Griffin MR. 2000. The effect of influenza on hospitalizations, outpatient visits, and courses of antibiotics in children. *New England Journal of Medicine* 342:225–231.

Ostrowsky BE, Trick WE, Sohn AH, Quirk SB, Holt S, Carson LA, Hill BC, Arduino MJ, Kuehnert MJ, Jarvis WR. 2001. Control of vancomycin-resistant enterococcus in health care facilities in a region. *New England Journal of Medicine* 344:1427–1433.

Pharmacia and Upjohn. April 18, 2000. Linezolid injectable (Zyvox). U.S. Patent: 5,688,792.

Tollefson L, Angulo FJ, Fedorka-Cray PJ. 1998. National surveillance for antibiotic resistance in zoonotic enteric pathogens. *Veterinary Clinics of North America: Food Animal Practice* 14:141–150.

Torrence M. 2001. Activities to address antimicrobial resistance in the United States. *Preventive Veterinary Medicine* 51:37–49.

U.S. Government. 2001. *A Public Health Action Plan to Combat Antimicrobial Resistance*. [Online]. Available: http://www.cdc.gov/drugresistance/actionplan.

Whitney CG, Farley MM, Hadler J, et al. 2001. Decline in invasive pneumococcal disease in the U.S. in 2000: an effect of pneumococcal conjugate vaccine? Abstract G-2041 In: Abstracts of the 41st Interscience Conference on Antimicrobial Agents and Chemotherapy, Chicago, December 16–19, 2001.

WHO. 2000a. Antimicrobial resistance: a global threat. *Essential Drugs Monitor* 28&29:1.

WHO. 2000b. Antimicrobial resistance: the facts. *Essential Drugs Monitor* 28&29:7.

WHO. 2000c. *World Health Report on Infectious Diseases 2000: Overcoming Antimicrobial Resistance*. WHO/CDS/2000.2. Geneva: WHO.

Appendix A

PUBLIC HEALTH CONSEQUENCES OF USE OF ANTIMICROBIAL AGENTS IN AGRICULTURE

Alicia D. Anderson, D.V.M., M.P.H.; Jennifer McClellan, M.P.H.; Shannon Rossiter, M.P.H.; and Frederick J. Angulo, D.V.M., Ph.D.

Foodborne and Diarrheal Diseases Branch
Division of Bacterial and Mycotic Diseases
Centers for Disease Control and Prevention, Atlanta, GA

Antimicrobial agents have been used in agriculture, including livestock and poultry, since the early 1950s to treat infections and improve growth and feed efficiency. The actual amount of antimicrobial agents used in agriculture is unknown; however, a substantial portion given to food animals is for subtherapeutic use (i.e., use in the absence of disease) for growth promotion, a practice that is becoming increasingly controversial. The agricultural use of antimicrobial agents that have a human analog increases the likelihood that human bacterial pathogens that have food animal reservoirs will develop cross-resistance to drugs approved for use in human medicine. The World Health Organization (WHO), following a series of consultations in 1997, 1999, and 2000, has recommended that the use of antimicrobial growth promoters that belong to an antimicrobial class used in humans be terminated in the absence of risk-based evaluations (WHO, 1997, 1999, 2000).

Several European countries have already taken steps toward this goal. In 1998, the European Union banned four growth promoters (tylosin, spiramycin, bacitracin, and virginiamycin) because of their structural relatedness to antimicrobial agents used in human medicine (European Commission, 1998). In that same year, chicken farmers and beef producers in Denmark voluntarily stopped using antimicrobial agents as growth promoters; swine farmers followed suit in 1999. This ban has reduced the total volume of antibiotics used in food animals in Denmark by 60 percent (from 206 to 81 tons) (DANMAP, 2000; Sorensen et al., 2002). Studies to investigate the influence of the ban have shown no negative consequence for farmers' profits or animal health in broiler chickens (Emborg et al., 2001). Similar conclusions were reported in fattening pigs, although diarrhea in weaned piglets has required other interventions, such as improved feeding and weaning procedures (Sorensen et al., 2002). In Sweden, all antibiotics were banned as growth promoters in 1986, decreasing their total antibiotic usage by 55 percent and demonstrating their ability to achieve competitive production results in the absence of growth promoters (Wierup, 1998; Greko, 1999). The effects of discontinuation of growth promoters in these countries have been a decrease in antibiotic resistance in animals, food products, and humans (Bager et al., 1999; Klare et al., 1999; Pantosti et al., 1999; DANMAP, 2000; van den Bogaard et al., 2000a; Aarestrup et al., 2001).

Clinicians should be aware that antimicrobial resistance is increasing in foodborne pathogens such as *Salmonella* and *Campylobacter* and that patients who are taking antimicrobial agents for any reason are at increased risk for acquiring antimicrobial-resistant foodborne infections. The increasing prevalence of antimicrobial resistance among these pathogens increases the potential for treatment failures and other adverse outcomes, including death. Appropriate use of antimicrobial agents in humans and food animals is necessary to maintain their effectiveness and reduce the potential for spread of resistant organisms. While therapeutic usage of antimicrobial agents in food animals is important to promote animal health and provide an affordable supply of meat, milk, and eggs, it is vital that the long-term effectiveness of antimicrobial agents used in human medicine be preserved. This report presents current surveillance information on the frequency of resistant foodborne infections in the United States, reviews scientific evidence linking antimicrobial agent usage in agriculture to resistant foodborne infections in humans, and makes recommendations for measures to protect public health.

Antimicrobial Use in Food Animals

At least 17 classes of antimicrobial agents are approved for growth promotion and feed efficiency in the United States, including tetracyclines, penicillins, macrolides, lincomycin (analog of clindamycin), and virginiamycin (analog of quinupristin/dalfopristin). To understand the human health consequences of the agricultural use of antimicrobial agents, it is important to evaluate the quantity of antimicrobials used in U.S. agriculture. Unfortunately, no reporting system exists for the quantity of antimicrobials used in food animals in the United States. The Animal Health Institute (AHI), which represents 80 percent of the companies that produce antimicrobials for animals in the United States, has estimated that their member companies produced 18 million pounds of antimicrobials for use in food animals in the United States in 1999 (AHI, 2000). An alternative estimate was provided by the Union of Concerned Scientists (UCS) in 2001 which calculated that 89 percent of the 35 million pounds of antimicrobial agents used annually in the United States are given to animals. Of the amount used in agriculture, 28 million pounds (93 percent) are used in the absence of disease (Mellon et al., 2001). Though more precise data on the quantity of antimicrobial agents used in food animals is needed, these initial estimates provide some perspective on the quantity.

As in human medicine, the use of antimicrobial agents in agriculture creates a selective pressure for the emergence and dissemination of antimicrobial-resistant bacteria including animal pathogens, human pathogens which have food animal reservoirs, and other bacteria which are present in food animals (Cohen and Tauxe, 1986; Levy, 1997; van den Bogaard and Stobberingh, 1999). These resistant bacteria may be transferred to humans either through the food supply or by direct contact with animals (Oosterom, 1991; Levy, 1997; Khachatourians, 1998; Witte, 1998). The transfer of resistant bacteria from food-producing animals to humans is most evident in human bacterial pathogens which have food animal sources, such as Campylobacter, which has a reservoir in chickens and turkeys (Tauxe, 1992; USDA, 1996; Altekruse et al., 1999), and Salmonella, which has reservoirs in cattle, chickens, pigs, and turkeys (Meng and Doyle, 1998; Angulo et al., 2000). To monitor antimicrobial resistance in foodborne enteric pathogens, the National Antimicrobial Resistance Monitoring System (NARMS) for Enteric Bacteria was launched in 1996.

NARMS is a collaboration among the Centers for Disease Control and Prevention (CDC), the Center for Veterinary Medicine at the Food and Drug Administration (FDA), the United States Department of Agriculture (USDA), and state and local health departments. In addition to NARMS, the Foodborne Diseases Active Surveillance Network (FoodNet) conducts population-based studies to estimate the burden and sources of specific foodborne diseases in nine states.

Campylobacter

NARMS has been used to monitor the prevalence of fluoroquinolone-resistant Campylobacter in the United States since 1997. The emergence of fluoroquinolone resistance among Campylobacter is an example of antimicrobial resistance resulting from the use of antimicrobial agents in food animals and the subsequent transfer via the food supply of resistant bacteria to humans. Fluoroquinolones were approved for human medicine in 1986. A national prospective study of reported Campylobacter cases between 1989–1990 found no Campylobacter isolates to be resistant to fluoroquinolones (CDC, 2000). The first fluoroquinolones approved for use in food animals in the United States were sarofloxacin in 1995 and enrofloxacin in 1996. These fluoroquinolones were approved for the treatment of respiratory disease in chickens and turkeys.

A study conducted in Minnesota reported that resistance of human *Campylobacter jejuni* infections to quinolones increased from 1 percent in 1992 to 10 percent in 1998. Resistant infections that were domestically acquired increased significantly from 1996 through 1998, a finding that was temporally associated with the licensure of fluoroquinolones for use in poultry in 1995. Molecular subtyping of human isolates and domestic chicken products from retail stores showed a significant association between resistant *Campylobacter jejuni* strains from chickens and domestically acquired infections in residents (Smith et al., 1999). Testing of 1997 NARMS *Campylobacter jejuni* isolates found fluoroquinolone resistance among 13 percent of the isolates; this figure has remained high at 14 percent of isolates in 2000 (CDC, 2000).

In a case-control study of fluoroquinolone-resistant Campylobacter infections conducted in the FoodNet sites, 58 percent of resistant infections were acquired domestically (Kassenborg et al., unpublished data). When domestically acquired fluoroquinolone-resistant Campylobacter cases were compared with well controls, cases were 10 times more likely to have eaten poultry cooked at a commercial establishment. Since chicken is not imported into the United States, this observation supports the conclusion that poultry is the dominant source of domestically acquired fluoroquinolone-resistant Campylobacter infections in the United States. In a recent risk assessment, FDA concluded that the use of fluoroquinolones in chickens in the United States has compromised the treatment with fluoroquinolones of almost 10,000 people a year; meaning that each year, thousands of people with Campylobacter infections seek medical care and are treated with fluoroquinolones, but their infection is already fluoroquinolone-resistant (FDA, 2000).

Salmonella

In addition to fluoroquinolone-resistant Campylobacter, there is also the potential for an emergence of domestically acquired fluoroquinolone-resistant Salmonella in the United States. Fluoroquinolones are the most commonly used antimicrobial for the treatment of invasive Salmonella infections in adults (Angulo et al., 2000). In 2000, 1.4 percent of Salmonella isolates collected by NARMS had a decreased susceptibility to fluoroquinolones (MIC $\geq$ 0.25 μg/ml), an increase from 0.4 percent in 1996 (CDC, 2000). This decreasing susceptibility to fluoroquinolones among Salmonella infections is of immediate concern as isolates with a MIC $\geq$ 0.25 μg/ml typically only require a single additional point mutation to become resistant (MIC $\geq$ 4 μg/ml), and therefore represent a potential reservoir for the emergence of resistant Salmonella should such isolates be exposed to continued selective pressure (Nakamura et al., 1993). Furthermore, patients infected with Salmonella strains with a decreased susceptibility to fluoroquinolones may respond poorly to treatment with fluoroquinolones and have been associated with apparent treatment failures (Molbak et al., 1999; Angulo et al., 2000).

Third-generation cephalosporins, such as ceftriaxone, are commonly used for treatment of invasive Salmonella infections in children because of their pharmacodynamic properties and low prevalence of resistance to these agents. There is therefore concern about the potential emergence of ceftriaxone-resistant Salmonella. The first reported case of domestically acquired ceftriaxone-resistant Salmonella was in a 12-year-old child in Nebraska (Fey et al., 2000). Investigation by public health officials revealed that the child lived on a farm and his father was a veterinarian. Before the child's illness, the father was treating several cattle herds for outbreaks due to culture-confirmed Salmonella infection.

Although no information was available regarding the use of antimicrobial agents among the infected herds, a third-generation cephalosporin, ceftiofur, is widely used in cattle. Ceftriaxone-susceptible and ceftriaxone-resistant Salmonella were isolated from ill cattle treated by the veterinarian. Both ceftriaxone-resistant and ceftriaxone-susceptible cattle isolates and the ceftriaxone-resistant isolate from the child had similar genetic structures as determined by pulsed-field gel electrophoresis (PFGE). These similar molecular "fingerprints" and their temporal isolation suggest that ceftriaxone resistance emerged in the cattle herds, probably following use of ceftiofur or other antibiotics that would have selected for and maintained the ceftriaxone-resistant determinant within the intestinal flora of the involved herds.

The Nebraska child's ceftriaxone-resistant infection was not an isolated event. The percentage of non-Typhi Salmonella isolates in NARMS resistant to ceftriaxone increased 13-fold from 0.1 percent in 1996 to 1.3 percent in 2000 (CDC, 2000). When patients from whom isolates were received in 1996–1998 were interviewed, few reported international travel, suggesting that most infections were domestically acquired (Fey et al., 2000). Furthermore, ceftriaxone resistance in most domestically acquired infections is due to a unique *Amp*C-type resistance gene (*CMY-2*), which resides on a plasmid. The finding of a similar molecular mechanism of resistance among different Salmonella strains supports horizontal dissemination of a resistance determinant (Dunne et al., 2000). A 1999 study at the University of Iowa found multi-drug-resistant, cephalosporin-resistant bovine, porcine, and human *Salmonella* isolates from the same geographic region. All human and animal resistant isolates encoded a *CMY-2 Amp*C-like gene (Winokur et al., 2000).

The emergence of multi-drug-resistant *Salmonella typhimurium* definitive type 104 (DT104) in the United States and the United Kingdom, which is resistant to ampicillin, chloramphenicol, streptomycin, sulfonamides, and tetracycline (ACSSuT), is an example of how a highly resistant clone of Salmonella has the ability to effectively spread among animals and then to humans. Described by Glynn et al. (1998), the emergence of *S. typhimurium* DT104 in the United States can be traced back to as early as 1985 (Glynn et al., 1998). The prevalence of Typhimurium isolates with the five-drug pattern of resistance increased from 0.6 percent in 1979–1980 to 34 percent in 1996 (Glynn et al., 1998). Among Typhimurium isolates submitted to NARMS, the prevalence of the ACSSuT resistance pattern was 28 percent in both 1999 and 2000 (CDC, 2000).

The highest frequency of ceftriaxone-resistant Salmonella among NARMS isolates is emerging in multi-drug-resistant (MDR) *Salmonella Newport*, which is defined as resistance to at least ampicillin, chloramphenicol, streptomycin, sulfamethoxazole, and tetracycline. Of all MDR *Salmonella Newport* isolates submitted to NARMS in 2000, a remarkable 50 percent are resistant to ceftriaxone (CDC, 2000).

Commensal Bacteria

Pathogenic bacteria, such as Campylobacter and Salmonella, are not the only concern when considering antimicrobial resistance in bacteria with food animal reservoirs. Commensal bacteria, which are naturally occurring host flora, constitute an enormous potential reservoir of resistance genes for pathogenic bacteria. The prevalence of antibiotic resistance in the commensal bacteria of humans and animals is considered to be a good indicator of the selective pressure of antibiotic usage and reflects the potential for resistance in future infections (Hummel et al., 1986; Lester et al., 1990; Murray, 1992; van den Bogaard et al., 2000b).

Most resistant bacteria have mobile genetic elements such as R-plasmids and transposons. As the reservoir of resistant commensal bacteria increases, the plasmid reservoir becomes larger and enables more frequent transfer of resistance to pathogenic bacteria including Salmonella and Shigella. *Escherichia coli*, which is the predominant isolate of aerobic fecal flora in humans and most animals, has demonstrated its ability to transfer resistance genes to other species, including pathogenic bacteria (Chaslus-Dancla et al., 1986; Hummel et al., 1986; Tauxe et al., 1989; Shoemaker et al., 1992; Nikolich et al., 1994; Berkowitz and Mechock, 1995; Winokur et al., 2001). Recent studies have shown an emerging resistance in *E. coli* to fluoroquinolones and third-generation cephalosporins. A study by Garau et al. (1999), demonstrated an increase in quinolone-resistant *E. coli* infections in Spain from 9 percent to 17 percent over the course of five years. This study also showed a high prevalence of quinolone-resistant *E. coli* in healthy children and adults (26 percent and 24 percent, respectively) which could not be explained by previous use of quinolones.

Animal testing from slaughterhouses in the area found a high rate of quinolone-resistant *E. coli* in swine and chickens (45 percent and 90 percent, respectively) (Garau et al., 1999). Winokur et al. (2001) found 16 percent of clinical *E. coli* isolates from cattle and swine and 1 percent of clinical human *E. coli* isolates collected in Iowa to be resistant to extended spectrum cephalosporins. This study also identified identical *CMY-2* genes in resistant isolates from both humans and animals, suggesting transfer of the resistance gene between food animals and humans.

Another example of potential animal-to-human transfer of resistant commensal bacteria is quinupristin/dalfopristin-resistant *Enterococcus faecium*. Quinupristin/dalfopristin (Synercid®) was approved for use in humans in 1999 for treatment of vancomycin-resistant *E. faecium* infections. However, virginiamycin, an analog of quinupristin/dalfopristin that is cross-resistant, has been used as a growth promoter in food animals in the United States since 1974 (Rende-Fournier et al., 1993; National Research Council, 1999). A study conducted by CDC in 1998–1999, before the approval of Synercid® use in humans, found quinupristin/dalfopristin-resistant *E. faecium* on 58 percent of chickens purchased in grocery stores from four different states. Additionally, quinupristin/dalfopristin-resistant *E. faecium* was found in 1 percent of the stools from non-hospitalized people who submitted a stool specimen to clinical laboratories (McDonald et al., 2001). Similar data in Europe led the European Union to ban the subtherapeutic use of virginiamycin in food animals in 1998 (Wegener et al., 1999). These findings suggest virginiamycin use in chickens has created a large reservoir of quinupristin/dalfopristin-resistant *E. faecium* to which humans are commonly exposed. The use of quinupristin/dalfopristin in humans for the treatment of vancomycin-resistant *E. faecium* and other serious infections may contribute additional selective pressure leading to an increased prevalence of quinupristin/dalfopristin resistance in humans.

Clinical Implications

Two human health consequences of increasing antimicrobial resistance in foodborne bacteria are an increase in foodborne illnesses and an increase in number of treatment failures. Increased human infections by resistant foodborne pathogens occur as the prevalence of resistance increases and as humans are exposed to antimicrobial agents. Taking an antimicrobial may lower the infectious dose for Salmonella and potentially other foodborne bacteria, if the pathogen is resistant to that antimicrobial (Ryan et al., 1985). Analyses of antimicrobial-resistant Salmonella outbreaks have demonstrated that previous exposure to antimicrobials can result in a larger number of cases than would have occurred if the outbreak had been caused by a sensitive strain (Cohen and Tauxe, 1986).

Bohnhoff et al., showed in the early 1960s that mice with an "undisturbed" normal intestinal flora have a Salmonella infectious dose of about 10^6 organisms (Bohnhoff aand Miller, 1962). When they "disturbed" the normal flora by administering streptomycin, the infectious dose for streptomycin-resistant Salmonella decreased to only 10 organisms. In Salmonella outbreaks, it has been observed that preceding, unrelated treatment with an antimicrobial can predispose humans to infection with resistant (Holmberg et al., 1984; Ryan et al., 1987; Spika et al., 1987) or susceptible Salmonella (Pavia et al., 1990). Similarly, in studies of sporadic salmonellosis, preceding treatment with an antimicrobial was a risk factor for a resistant infection, compared to susceptible infections (Riley et al., 1984; MacDonald et al., 1987; Lee et al., 1994). Physicians should be aware that as foodborne pathogens become increasingly resistant, treating patients with antimicrobials, regardless of the reason, increases the risk for that patient to develop a subsequent infection caused by resistant foodborne bacteria. The public health impact of this potentiation effect is more cases of illness and larger outbreaks.

In addition to causing more human illnesses, increasing antimicrobial resistance in foodborne pathogens may result in treatment failures if the foodborne pathogen is resistant to an antimicrobial used for treatment. As previously described, resistance is emerging to antimicrobials commonly used for treatment of serious Salmonella infections, that is, fluoroquinolones in adults and extended-spectrum cephalosporins in children. An example of probable treatment failures was recently described by researchers in Denmark, where a multi-drug-resistant *S. typhimurium* DT104 outbreak attributed to contaminated pork was traced back to a swine herd (Molbak et al., 1999). The Salmonella isolates from humans and pork samples had decreased susceptibility to fluoroquinolones, and two patients who were treated with fluoroquinolones died. An official review of these deaths concluded that decreased susceptibility to fluoroquinolones was a contributing factor.

Conclusion

Given that there is an increasing prevalence of antimicrobial resistance and that this resistance has clinical implications, there is a need for mitigation efforts. Such actions will require collaborative efforts by several partners, including the farming, veterinary, medical, and public health communities. Enhanced surveillance is essential for evaluating and directing these efforts. There is a particular need to establish surveillance of antimicrobial usage in animals.

In the United States, collaborative federal actions to address antimicrobial resistance in agriculture are outlined in the Public Health Action Plan to Combat Antimicrobial Resistance, released in 2001 by an interagency task force (U.S. Government, 2001). Action items in this plan include improved surveillance of antimicrobial drug use and resistance, research and education, and, as a top priority item, refining and implementing the FDA's Framework Document. This Framework Document proposes a modified approval process for antimicrobials used in animals (FDA, 1999). It intends to ensure the human safety of antimicrobials used in animals by prioritizing these drugs according to their importance in human medicine. Additionally, it proposes to establish required mitigation actions with increasing resistance and to account for resistance developing from specific animal uses. Education of veterinarians regarding appropriate use of antibiotics has been promoted by the American Veterinary Medical Association (AVMA) with published guidelines for the therapeutic use of antibiotics (AVMA, 1998).

The widespread use of antimicrobial agents in food animals is associated with increasing antimicrobial resistance in foodborne pathogens, which subsequently may be transferred to humans. The transfer of these resistant bacteria or the genetic determinants for resistance causes adverse health consequences in humans by increasing the number of foodborne illnesses and increasing the potential for treatment failures. To address this public health problem, overuse and misuse of antimicrobial agents in food animals and humans must be reduced. This will be accomplished by adherence to guidelines for therapeutic use of antimicrobial agents in food animals, and the discontinuation of use of antimicrobial agents with a human analog as growth promoters unless risk assessments have indicated their safety for public health. Several European countries have already demonstrated the feasibility of such measures and the effectiveness of these interventions to combat antimicrobial resistance and reduce public health risks.

REFERENCES

Aarestrup FM, Seyfarth AM, Emborg HD, Pedersen K, Hendriksen RS, Bager F. 2001. Effect of abolishment of the use of antimicrobial agents for growth promotion on occurrence of antimicrobial resistance in fecal enterococci from food animals in Denmark. *Antimicrobial Agents and Chemotherapy* 45:2054–2059.

AHI (Animal Health Institute). 2000. Survey indicates most antibiotics used in animals are used for treating and preventing disease. Press release. February 14. [Online]. Available: http://www.ahi.org/news%20room/press%20release/2000/feb/antibiotic%20usage%20 data.htm.

Altekruse S, Stern N, Fields P, Swerdlow D. 1999. *Campylobacter jejuni*—an emerging foodborne pathogen. *Emerging Infectious Diseases* 5:28–35.

Angulo FJ, Johnson KR, Tauxe RV, Cohen ML. 2000. Origins and consequences of antimicrobial-resistant nontyphoidal Salmonella: implications for the use of fluoroquinolones in food animals. *Microbial Drug Resistance* 6:77–83.

AVMA (American Veterinary Medical Association). 1998. Judicious Therapeutic Use of Antimicrobials. [Online]. Available: http://www.avma.org/scienact/jtua/jtua98.asp.

Bager F, Aarestrup FM, Madsen M, Wegener HC. 1999. Glycopeptide resistance in *Enterococcus faecium* from broilers and pigs following discontinued use of avoparcin. *Microbial Drug Resistance Mechanisms, Epidemiology and Disease* 5:53–56.

Berkowitz FE and Mechock B. 1995. Third generation cephalosporin-resistant gram-negative bacilli in the feces of hospitalized children. *Pediatric Infectious Disease Journal* 14:97–100.

Bohnhoff M and Miller CP. 1962. Enhanced susceptibility to Salmonella infection in streptomycin-treated mice. *Journal of Infectious Diseases* 111:117–127.

CDC (Centers for Disease Control and Prevention). 2000. *NARMS 2000 Annual Report.* [Online]. Available: http://www.cdc.gov/narms/annuals.htm.

Chaslus-Dancla E, Martel JL, Carlier C, Lafont JP, Courvalin P. 1986. Emergence of aminoglycoside 3-*N*-acetyltransferase IV in *Escherichia coli* and *Salmonella typhimurium* isolated from animals. *Antimicrobial Agents and Chemotherapy* 29:239–243.

Cohen ML and Tauxe RV. 1986. Drug-resistant Salmonella in the United States: an epidemiological perspective. *Science* 234:964–969.

DANMAP. 2000. *Consumption of Antimicrobial Agents and Resistance to Antimicrobial Agents in Bacteria from Food Animals, Food and Humans in Denmark.* Report from Statens Serum Institut, Danish Veterinary and Food Administration, Danish Medicines Agency and Danish Veterinary Institute. [Online]. Available: http://www.vetinst.dk/dk/Publikationer/Danmap/Danmap%202000.pdf.

Dunne EF, Fey PD, Kludt P, Reporter R, Mostashari F, Shillam P, Wicklund J, Miller C, Holland B, Stamey K, Barrett TJ, Rasheed JK, Tenover FC, Ribot EM, Angulo FJ. 2000. Emergence of domestically acquired ceftriaxone-resistant Salmonella infections associated with *ampC* beta-lactamase. *Journal of the American Medical Association* 284:3151–3156.

Emborg H, Ersboll AK, Heuer OE, Wegener HC. 2001. The effect of discontinuing the use of antimicrobial growth promoters on the productivity in the Danish broiler production. *Preventive Veterinary Medicine* 50:53–70.

European Commission. 1998. Commission regulation of amending council directive 70/524/EEC concerning additives in feeding stuffs as regards withdrawal of the authorization of certain antibiotics. Document No.: VI/7767/98. European Commission, Brussels.

FDA (Food and Drug Administration). 1999. *A Proposed Framework for Evaluating and Assuring the Human Safety of the Microbial Effects of Antimicrobial New Animal Drugs Intended for Use in Food-Producing Animals.* [Online]. Available: http://www.fda.gov/cvm/index/vmac/antimi18.html#statement.

FDA. 2000. *Human Health Impact Fluoroquinolone-Resistant Campylobacter Attributed to the Consumption of Chicken.* [Online]. Available: http://www.fda.gov/cvm/antimicrobial/Risk_asses.pdf.

Fey PD, Safranek TJ, Rupp ME, Dunne EF, Ribot E, Iwen PC, Bradford PA, Angulo FJ, Hinrichs SH. 2000. Ceftriaxone-resistant Salmonella infection acquired by a child from cattle. *New England Journal of Medicine* 342:1242–1249.

Garau J, Xercavins M, Rodriguez-Carballeira M, Gomez-Vera JR, Coll I, Vidal D, Llovet T, Ruiz-Bremon A. 1999. Emergence and dissemination of quinolone-resistant *Escherichia coli* in the community. *Antimicrobial Agents and Chemotherapy* 43:2736–2741.

Glynn MK, Bopp C, Dewitt W, Dabney P, Mokhtar M, Angulo FJ. 1998. Emergence of multidrug-resistant *Salmonella* enterica serotype *typhimurium* DT104 infections in the United States. *New England Journal of Medicine* 338:1333–1338.

Greko C. 1999. Antibiotics as growth promoters. *Acta Veterinaria Scandinavica* Suppl 92:87–100.

Holmberg SD, Osterholm MT, Senger KA, Cohen ML. 1984. Drug-resistant Salmonella from animals fed antimicrobials. *New England Journal of Medicine* 311:617–622.

Hummel R, Tschape H, Witte W. 1986. Spread of plasmid-mediated nourseothricin resistance due to antibiotic use in animal husbandry. *Journal of Basic Microbiology* 26:461–466.

Khachatourians GG. 1998. Agricultural use of antibiotics and the evolution and transfer of antibiotic-resistant bacteria. *Canadian Medical Association Journal* 159:1129–1136.

Klare I, Badstubner D, Konstabel C, Bohme G, Claus H, Witte W. 1999. Decreased incidence of VanA-type vancomycin-resistant enterococci isolated from poultry meat and fecal samples of humans in the community after discontinuation of avoparcin usage in animal husbandry. *Microbial Drug Resistance* 5:45–52.

Lee LA, Puhr ND, Maloney EK, Bean NH, Tauxe RV. 1994. Increase in antimicrobial-resistant Salmonella infections in the United States, 1989–1990. *Journal of Infectious Diseases* 170:128–134.

Lester SC, del Pilar Pla M, Wang F, Perez Schael I, Jiang H, O'Brien TF. 1990. The carriage of *Escherichia coli* resistant to antimicrobial agents by healthy children in Boston, in Caracas, Venezuela, and in Qin Pu, China. *New England Journal of Medicine* 323:285–289.

Levy SB. 1997. Antibiotic resistance: an ecological imbalance. In: Levy SB, Goode J, Chadwick DJ, eds. *Antibiotic Resistance: Origins, Evolution, Selection, and Spread.* New York: John Wiley & Sons. Pp. 1–9.

MacDonald KL, Cohen ML, Hargrett-Bean NT, Wells JG, Puhr ND, Collin SF, Blake PA. 1987. Changes in antimicrobial resistance of Salmonella isolated from humans in the United States. *Journal of the American Medical Association* 258:1496–1499.

McDonald LC, Rossiter S, Mackinson C, Wang YY, Johnson S, Sullivan M, Sokolow R, DeBess E, Gilbert L, Benson JA, Hill B, Angulo FJ. 2001. Quinupristin-dalfopristin-resistant *Enterococcus faecium* on chicken and in human stool specimens. *New England Journal of Medicine* 345:1155–1160.

Mellon M, Benbrook C, Benbrook K. 2001. *Hogging It: Estimates of Antimicrobial Abuse in Livestock*. Cambridge: Union of Concerned Scientists Publications.

Meng J and Doyle MP. 1998. Emerging and evolving microbial foodborne pathogens. *Bulletin de l'Institut Pasteur* 96:151–164.

Molbak K, Baggesen DL, Aarestrup FM, Ebbesen JM, Engberg J, Frydendahl K, Gerner-Smidt P, Petersen AM, Wegener HC. 1999. An outbreak of multi-drug resistant, quinolone-resistant *Salmonella* enterica serotype *typhimurium* DT104. *New England Journal of Medicine* 341:1420–1425.

Murray BE. 1992. Problems and dilemmas of antimicrobial resistance. *Pharmacotherapy* 12:86S–93S.

Nakamura S, Yoshida H, Bogaski M, Nakamura M, Kojima T. 1993. Quinolone resistance mutations in DNA gyrase. In: Andoh T, Ikeda H, Oguro M, eds. *Molecular Biology of DNA Topoisomerases and Its Application to Chemotherapy*. London: CDC Press. Pp. 135–143.

National Research Council. 1999. Committee on Drug Use in Food Animals, Panel on Animal Health, Food Safety, and Public Health, Board on Agriculture. *The Use of Drugs in Food Animals: Benefits and Risks*. Washington, DC: National Academy Press.

Nikolich MP, Hong G, Shoemaker NB, Salyers AA. 1994. Evidence for natural horizontal transfer of *tetQ* between bacteria that normally colonize humans and bacteria that normally colonize livestock. *Applied and Environmental Microbiology* 60:3255–3260.

Oosterom J. 1991. Epidemiological studies and proposed preventive measures in the fight against human salmonellosis. *International Journal of Food Microbiology* 12:41–51.

Pantosti A, Del Grosso M, Tagliabue S, Macri A, Caprioli A. 1999. Decrease of vancomycin-resistant enterococci in poultry meat after avoparcin ban. *Lancet* 354:741–742.

Pavia AT, Shipman LD, Wells JG, Puhr ND, Smith JD, McKinley TW, Tauxe RV. 1990. Epidemiologic evidence that prior antimicrobial exposure decreases resistance to infection by antimicrobial-sensitive Salmonella. *Journal of Infectious Diseases* 161:255–260.

Rende-Fournier R, Leclercq R, Galimand M, Duval J, Courvalin P. 1993. Identification of the *satA* gene encoding a streptogramin *A* acetyltransferase in *Enterococcus faecium* BM4145. *Antimicrobial Agents and Chemotherapy* 37:2119–2125.

Riley LW, Cohen ML, Seals JE, Blaser MJ, Birkness KA, Hargrett NT, Martin SM, Feldman RA. 1984. Importance of host factors in human salmonellosis caused by multiresistant strains of Salmonella. *Journal of Infectious Diseases* 149:878–883.

Ryan C, et al. 1985. Abstract. In: Abstracts of the 25th Interscience Conference on Antimicrobial Agents and Chemotherapy, Minneapolis, September 29–October 2, 1985.

Ryan CA, Nickels MK, Hargrett-Bean NT, Potter ME, Endo T, Mayer L, Langkop CW, Gibson C, McDonald RC, Kenney RT, et al. 1987. Massive outbreak of antimicrobial-resistant salmonellosis traced to pasteurized milk. *Journal of the American Medical Association* 258:3269–3274.

Shoemaker NB, Wang G, Salyers AA. 1992. Evidence for natural transfer of a tetracycline resistance gene between bacteria from the human colon and bacteria from the bovine rumen. *Applied and Environmental Microbiology* 58:1313–1320.

Smith KE, Besser JM, Hedberg CW, Leano FT, Bender JB, Wicklund JH, Johnson BP, Moore KA, Osterholm MT. 1999. Quinolone-resistant *Campylobacter jejuni* infections in Minnesota, 1992–1998. *New England Journal of Medicine* 340:1525–1532.

Sorensen TL, Wegener HC, Frimodt-Moller N. 2002. [Letter] Resistant bacteria in retail meats and antimicrobial use in animals. *New England Journal of Medicine* 346:777–779.

Spika JS, Waterman SH, Hoo GW, St Louis ME, Pacer RE, James SM, Bissett ML, Mayer LW, Chiu JY, Hall B, et al. 1987. Chloramphenicol-resistant *Salmonella Newport* traced through hamburger to dairy farms. *New England Journal of Medicine* 316:565–570.

Tauxe R. 1992. Epidemiology of *Campylobacter jejuni* infections in the United States and other industrialized nations. In: Nanchamkin I, Blaser MJ, Tompkins LS, eds. *Campylobacter jejuni: Current Status and Future Trends.* Washington, DC: American Society for Microbiology Press. Pp. 9–19.

Tauxe RV, Cavanagh TR, Cohen ML. 1989. Interspecies gene transfer in vivo producing an outbreak of multiply resistant shigellosis. *Journal of Infectious Diseases* 160:1067–1070.

USDA (United States Department of Agriculture). 1996. Nationwide Broiler Chicken Microbiological Baseline Data Collection Program, July 1994–June 1995. [Online]. Available: http://www.fsis.usda.gov/OPHS/baseline/contents.htm.

U.S. Government. Interagency Task Force on Antimicrobial Resistance. 2001. *A Public Health Action Plan to Combat Antimicrobial Resistance.* [Online]. Available: http://www.cdc.gov/drugresistance/actionplan.

van den Bogaard AE and Stobberingh EE. 1999. Antibiotic usage in animals: impact on bacterial resistance and public health. *Drugs* 58:589–607.

van den Bogaard AE, Bruinsma N, Stobberingh EE. 2000a. The effect of banning avoparcin on VRE carriage in the Netherlands. *Journal of Antimicrobial Chemotherapy* 46:146–147.

van den Bogaard AE, London N, Stobberingh EE. 2000b. Antimicrobial resistance in pig faecal samples from The Netherlands (five abattoirs) and Sweden. *Journal of Antimicrobial Chemotherapy* 45:663–671.

Wegener HC, Aarestrup FM, Jensen LB, Hammerum AM, Bager F. 1999. Use of antimicrobial growth promoters in food animals and *Enterococcus faecium* resistance to therapeutic antimicrobial drugs in Europe. *Emerging Infectious Diseases* 5:329–335.

WHO (World Health Organization). 1997. *The Medical Impact of the Use of Antimicrobials in Food Animals: Report and Proceedings of a WHO Meeting.* Berlin, October 13–17, 1997. Geneva: WHO.

WHO. 1999. *Containing Antimicrobial Resistance: Review of the Literature and Report of a WHO Workshop on the Development of a Global Strategy for the Containment of Antimicrobial Resistance.* Geneva, February 4–5, 1999. Geneva: WHO.

WHO. 2000. *WHO Global Principles for the Containment of Antimicrobial Resistance in Animals Intended for Food: Report of a WHO Consultation.* Geneva, Switzerland, June 5-9, 2000. Geneva: WHO.

Wierup M. 1998. Preventive methods replace antibiotic growth promoters: ten years experience from Sweden. *APUA Newsletter* 16:1–4.

Winokur PL, Brueggemann A, DeSalvo DL, Hoffmann L, Apley MD, Uhlenhopp EK, Pfaller MA, Doern GV. 2000. Animal and human multidrug-resistant, cephalosporin-resistant Salmonella isolates expressing a plasmid-mediated CMY-2 AmpC beta-lactamase. *Antimicrobial Agents and Chemotherapy* 44:2777–2783.

Winokur PL, Vonstein DL, Hoffman LJ, Uhlenhopp EK, Doern GV. 2001. Evidence for transfer of CMY-2 AmpC β-lactamase plasmids between *Escherichia coli* and Salmonella isolates from food animals and humans. *Antimicrobial Agents and Chemotherapy* 45:2716–2722.

Witte W. 1998. Medical consequences of antibiotic use in agriculture. *Science* 279:996–997.

Appendix B

Issues of Resistance: Microbes, Vectors, and the Host
February 6–7, 2002
Lecture Room
National Academy of Sciences
2101 Constitution Avenue, NW
Washington, DC 20418

AGENDA

WEDNESDAY, FEBRUARY 6, 2002

**** A PUBLIC DISSEMINATION PANEL DISCUSSION OF THE BIOLOGICAL THREATS REPORT will take place from 9:00–10:00 am. Breakfast will be served. ****

10:30 am **Welcome and Opening Remarks**
Adel Mahmoud, Chair, Forum on Emerging Infections
President, Merck Vaccines

10:45 **Arms Races with Evolving Diseases: Patterns, Costs and Containment**
Stephen Palumbi, Harvard University

Session I: Case Studies of Antimicrobial Resistance

Moderator: Carlos Lopez, Eli Lilly

11:15 **The Cost of Antimicrobial Resistance**
Richard Smith, University of East Anglia, United Kingdom

11:45 **Resistant Strains of Pneumococci, Staphylococci, and Enterococci**
Alexander Tomasz, Laboratory of Microbiology, Rockefeller University

12:15 pm **LUNCH**

1:30 **Resistance to HIV-1 Drug Therapies**
Robert Redfield, The Institute of Human Virology, University of Maryland

2:00 **Chloroquine-Resistant Malaria**
Thomas Wellems, National Institute for Allergy and Infectious Diseases, NIH

2:30 **Schistosomiasis and Antihelminth Resistance**
Charles King, Division of Geographic Medicine, Case Western Reserve University

3:00 **Epitope Escape Variants**
Robert Webster, St. Jude Children's Research Hospital and World Health Organization Collaborating Center for Studies on the Ecology of Influenza in Animals and Birds

Session II: Vector Resistance

Moderator: Barry Beaty, Colorado State University

3:30 **Pesticide Resistance: Implications for Disease Emergence and Control**
Janet Hemingway, Liverpool School of Tropical Medicine, United Kingdom

4:00 **Studies in Antibiotic Resistance and Insecticide Resistance: Commonalties, Differences, and New Directions**
Steven Peck, Zoology Department, Brigham Young University

4:30 **Managing the Emergence of Pesticide Resistance in Disease Vectors**
William Brogdon, Division of Parasitic Diseases, Centers for Disease Control and Prevention

Session III: Discussion Panel

Moderator: Carole Heilman, National Institute for Allergy and Infectious Diseases

5:00 **William Jack,** Georgetown University
Lynn Marks, GlaxoSmith Kline
Steve Brickner, Pfizer

6:00 **Adjournment of the first day**

6:15 **DINNER MEETING OF THE FORUM ON EMERGING INFECTIONS**

THURSDAY, FEBRUARY 7, 2002

8:30 am Continental Breakfast
9:00 **Opening Remarks / Summary of Day 1**
Stanley Lemon, Vice Chair, Forum on Emerging Infections
Dean of Medicine, The University of Texas Medical Branch, Galveston
9:15 **Antibiotic Resistance 1992–2002: A Decade's Journey**
Stuart Levy, School of Medicine, Tufts University

Session IV: Factors of Emergence

Moderator: Mary Wilson, Harvard University
9:45 **Patterns of Use for Antimicrobials in Developing Countries**
Iruka Okeke, University of Bradford, United Kingdom
10:15 **Health Care-Acquired Infections: Hospitals and Long-Term Care Facilities as Breeding Grounds for Antimicrobial Resistance**
Lindsay Nicolle, University of Manitoba, Canada
10:45 **The Use of Antimicrobials in Food-Producing Animals**
Thomas Shryock, Elanco Lilly Research
11:15 **Special Considerations: Anthrax, Large-Scale/Long-Term Prophylaxis or Therapy and the Emergence of Microbial Resistance**
Thomas Elliott, Armed Forces Radiobiology Research Institute, Uniformed Services University of the Health Sciences

Session V: Containing the Development of Resistance

Moderator: James Hughes, Centers for Disease Control and Prevention
11:45 **Emergence of Multiple Mechanisms of Resistance to Antibacterials**
Shahriar Mobashery, Department of Biochemistry, Wayne State University
12:15 pm **Emerging Technologies to Combat Resistance: Opportunities and Limitations**
Vincent Fischetti, Laboratory of Bacterial Pathogenesis, Rockefeller University
12:45 LUNCH

1:30 **Interagency Action Plan to Combat Antimicrobial Resistance**
David Bell, National Center for Infectious Diseases, Centers for Disease Control and Prevention
Murray Lumpkin, Office of the Commissioner, Food and Drug Administration

2:15 **Using Pharmacokinetics and Pharmacodynamics to Manage Resistance in the Hospital, at the Bedside, and in Drug Development**
Jerome Schentag, University at Buffalo School of Pharmacy

2:45 **FDA Regulatory Approaches to Controlling Antimicrobial Resistance**
Mark Goldberger, Center for Drug Evaluation and Research, Food and Drug Administration

3:15 **CDC's 12-Step Program to Address Antimicrobial Resistance**
Julie Gerberding, National Center for Infectious Diseases, Centers for Disease Control and Prevention

3:45 **The Challenges to Implementing Global Policy for the Control of Antimicrobial Resistance**
Anthony Savelli and Terry Green, Management Sciences for Health

4:15 **BREAK**

Session VI: Priorities for the Next Steps in Addressing Resistance

Moderator: Fredrick Sparling, University of North Carolina, Chapel Hill

4:30 With the backdrop of the previous days' presentations and discussion, Forum members, panel discussants, and the audience will comment on the issues and next steps that they would identify as priority areas for consideration within industry, academia, public health organizations, and other government sectors. The discussion of priorities will summarize the issues surrounding emerging opportunities for more effective collaboration as well as the remaining research and programmatic needs. The confounding issues of the major obstacles to preparing an optimal response, particularly as it relates to the complexities of interaction between private industry, research and public health agencies, regulatory agencies, policymakers, academic researchers, and the public will be explored with an eye toward innovative responses to such challenges.

Panel Discussants:

Ramanan Laxminarayan, Resources for the Future
Mary Torrence, U.S. Department of Agriculture, Cooperative State Research Education and Extension Service
Donald Roberts, Uniformed Services University of the Health Sciences

5:30 Adjourn

Appendix C

Information Resources

OVERVIEW

Brogdon WG, McAllister JC. 1998. Insecticide resistance and vector control. *Emerging Infectious Diseases* 4(4):605–613. Available at: http://www.cdc.gov/ncidod/EID/vol4no4/brogdon.htm.

Fidler DP. 1998. Legal issues associated with antimicrobial drug resistance. *Emerging Infectious Diseases* 4(2):169–177. Available at: http://www.cdc.gov/ncidod/eid/vol4no2/fidler.htm.

Jack W. 2001. The public economics of tuberculosis control. *Health Policy* 57(2):79–96.

Levy SB. 2001. Antibiotic resistance: consequences of inaction. *Clinical Infectious Diseases* 33 Suppl 3:S124–S149.

Levy SB. 2002. Factors impacting on the problem of antibiotic resistance. *Journal of Antimicrobial Chemotherapy* 49(1):25–30.

Molyneux DH. 2001. Vector-borne infections in the tropics and health policy issues in the twenty-first century. *Transactions of the Royal Society of Tropical Medicine and Hygiene* 95(3):233–238.

Palumbi SR. 2001. Humans as the world's greatest evolutionary force. *Science* 293(5536):1786–1790. Available at: http://www.sciencemag.org/cgi/content/full/293/5536/1786.

Schentag JJ. 1999. Antimicrobial action and pharmacokinetics/pharmacodynamics: the use of AUIC to improve efficacy and avoid resistance. *Journal of Chemotherapy* 11(6):426–439.

Stephenson I, Wiselka M. 2000. Drug treatment of tropical parasitic infections: recent achievements and developments. *Drugs* 60(5):985–995.

Wierup M. 2001. The Swedish experience of the 1986 year ban of antimicrobial growth promoters, with special reference to animal health, disease prevention, productivity, and usage of antimicrobials. *Microbial Drug Resistance* 7(2):183–190.

COST OF RESISTANCE

Coast J, Smith RD, Millar MR. 1998. An economic perspective on policy to reduce antimicrobial resistance. *Social Science and Medicine* 46(1):29–38.

Phillips M, Phillips-Howard PA. 1996. Economic implications of resistance to antimalarial drugs. *Pharmacoeconomics* 10(3):225–238.

Smith RD, Coast J, Millar MR. 1996. Over-the-counter antimicrobials: the hidden costs of resistance. *Journal of Antimicrobial Chemotherapy* 37(5):1031–1032.

BACTERIAL RESISTANCE

Arnadottir T. 2001. Tuberculosis: trends and the twenty-first century. *Scandinavian Journal of Infectious Diseases* 33(8):563–567.

Banatvala N, Peremitin GG. 1999. Tuberculosis, Russia, and the Holy Grail. *Lancet* 353(9157):999–1000.

Diwan VK, Thorson A. 1999. Sex, gender, and tuberculosis. *Lancet* 353(9157):1000–1001.

Gleissberg V. 1999. The threat of multidrug resistance: is tuberculosis ever untreatable or uncontrollable? *Lancet* 353(9157):998–999.

McCormick JB. 1998. Epidemiology of emerging/re-emerging antimicrobial-resistant bacterial pathogens. *Current Opinion in Microbiology* 1(1):125–129.

McGee L, McDougal L, Zhou J, Spratt BG, Tenover FC, George R, Hakenbeck R, Hryniewicz W, Lefevre JC, Tomasz A, Klugman KP. 2001. Nomenclature of major antimicrobial-resistant clones of *Streptococcus pneumoniae* defined by the pneumococcal molecular epidemiology network. *Journal of Clinical Microbiology* 39(7):2565–2571. Available at: http://jcm.asm.org/cgi/content/full/39/7/2565?view=full&pmid=11427569.

Pinho MG, Filipe SR, de Lencastre H, Tomasz A. 2001. Complementation of the essential peptidoglycan transpeptidase function of penicillin-binding protein 2 (PBP2) by the drug resistance protein PBP2A in *Staphylococcus aureus*. *Journal of Bacteriology* 183(22):6525–6531. Available at: http://jb.asm.org/cgi/content/full/183/22/6525?view=full&pmid=11673420.

Somoskovi A, Parsons LM, Salfinger M. 2001. The molecular basis of resistance to isoniazid, rifampin, and pyrazinamide in *Mycobacterium tuberculosis*. *Respiratory Research* 2(3):164–168. Available at: http://respiratory-research.com/content/2/3/164.

World Health Organization. 2000. *Anti-Tuberculosis Drug Resistance in the World. Report No. 2: Prevalence and Trends*. The WHO/IUATLD Global Project on Anti-Tuberculosis Drug-Resistance Surveillance. Available at: http://www.who.int/gtb/publications/dritw/index.htm.

VIRAL RESISTANCE

Blower SM, Porco TC, Darby G. 1998. Predicting and preventing the emergence of antiviral drug resistance in HSV-2. *Nature Medicine* 4(6):673–678.

Gumina G, Song GY, Chu CK. 2001. Advances in antiviral agents for hepatitis B virus. *Antiviral Chemistry and Chemotherapy* 12 Suppl 1:93–117.

Mital D, Pillay D. 2001. The impact of HIV-1 subtype on drug resistance. *Journal of HIV Therapy* 6(3):56–60.

Pineo GF, Hull RD. 2001. Dalteparin sodium. *Expert Opinion on Pharmacotherapy* 2(8):1325–1337.

Richman DD. 2001. HIV chemotherapy. *Nature* 410(6831):995–1001. Available at: http://www.nature.com/cgi-taf/DynaPage.taf?file=/nature/journal/v410/n6831/full/410995a0_fs.html.

Snell NJ. 2001. Ribavirin—current status of a broad spectrum antiviral agent. *Expert Opinion on Pharmacotherapy* 2(8):1317–1324.

PROTOZOAN RESISTANCE

Bryceson A. 2001. A policy for leishmaniasis with respect to the prevention and control of drug resistance. *Tropical Medicine and International Health* 6(11):928–934.

Carlton JM, Fidock DA, Djimde A, Plowe CV, Wellems TE. 2001. Conservation of a novel vacuolar transporter in plasmodium species and its central role in chloroquine resistance of *P. falciparum*. *Current Opinion in Microbiology* 4(4):415–420.

Gillespie SH, Morrissey I, Everett D. 2001. A comparison of the bactericidal activity of quinolone antibiotics in a *Mycobacterium fortuitum* model. *Journal of Medical Microbiology* 50(6):565–570.

Imwong M, Pukrittakayamee S, Looareesuwan S, Pasvol G, Poirreiz J, White NJ, Snounou G. 2001. Association of genetic mutations in *Plasmodium vivax* dhfr with resistance to sulfadoxine-pyrimethamine: geographical and clinical correlates. *Antimicrobial Agents and Chemotherapy* 45(11):3122–3127. Available at: http://aac.asm.org/cgi/content/full/45/11/3122?view=full&pmid=11600366.

Nomura T, Carlton JM, Baird JK, del Portillo HA, Fryauff DJ, Rathore D, Fidock DA, Su X, Collins WE, McCutchan TF, Wootton JC, Wellems TE. 2001. Evidence for different mechanisms of chloroquine resistance in 2 Plasmodium species that cause human malaria. *The Journal of Infectious Diseases* 183(11):1653–1661. Available at: http://www.journals.uchicago.edu/JID/journal/issues/v183n11/001437/001437.html.

Wellems TE, Plowe CV. 2001. Chloroquine-resistant malaria. *The Journal of Infectious Diseases* 184(6):770–776. Available at: http://www.journals.uchicago.edu/JID/journal/issues/v184n6/010488/010488.html.

White N. 1999. Editorial: Antimalarial drug resistance and mortality in falciparum malaria. *Tropical Medicine and International Health* 4(7):469–470.

HELMINTH RESISTANCE

Barnes EH, Dobson RJ, Stein PA, Le Jambre LF, Lenane IJ. 2001. Selection of different genotype larvae and adult worms for anthelmintic resistance by persistent and short-acting avermectin/milbemycins. *International Journal for Parasitology* 31(7):720–727.

Gryseels B, Mbaye A, De Vlas SJ, Stelma FF, Guisse F, Van Lieshout L, Faye D, Diop M, Ly A, Tchuem-Tchuente LA, Engels D, Polman K. 2001. Are poor responses to praziquantel for the treatment of *Schistosoma mansoni* infections in Senegal due to resistance? An overview of the evidence. *Tropical Medicine and International Health* 6(11):864–873.

King CH, Muchiri EM, Ouma JH. 2000. Evidence against rapid emergence of praziquantel resistance in *Schistosoma haematobium*, Kenya. *Emerging Infectious Diseases* 6(6):585–594. Available at: http://www.cdc.gov/ncidod/eid/vol6no6/king.htm.

Sturrock RF. 2001. Schistosomiasis epidemiology and control: how did we get here and where should we go? *Memórias do Instituto Oswaldo Cruz* 96 Suppl:17–27.

Yu DB, Li Y, Sleigh AC, Yu XL, Li YS, Wei WY, Liang YS, McManus DP. 2001. Efficacy of praziquantel against *Schistosoma japonicum*: field evaluation in an area with repeated chemotherapy compared with a newly identified endemic focus in Hunan, China. *Transactions of the Royal Society of Tropical Medicine and Hygiene* 95(5):537–541.

VACCINE-RESISTANT MUTANTS

Barouch DH, Kunstman J, Kuroda MJ, Schmitz JE, Santra S, Peyerl FW, Krivulka GR, Beaudry K, Lifton MA, Gorgone DA, Montefiori DC, Lewis MG, Wolinsky SM, Letvin NL. 2002. Eventual AIDS vaccine failure in a rhesus monkey by viral escape from cytotoxic T lymphocytes. *Nature* 415(6869):335–339. Available at: http://www.nature.com/cgi-taf/DynaPage.taf?file=/nature/journal/v415/n6869/full/415335a_fs.html.

McLean AR. 1995. Vaccination, evolution and changes in the efficacy of vaccines: a theoretical framework. *Proceedings of the Royal Society of London.* Series B. Biological sciences. 261(1362):389–393.

Wilson JN, Nokes DJ, Carman WF. 2000. Predictions of the emergence of vaccine-resistant hepatitis B in The Gambia using a mathematical model. *Epidemiology and Infection* 124(2):295–307.

FACTORS OF EMERGENCE

Bennish ML. 1999. Animals, humans, and antibiotics: implications of the veterinary use of antibiotics on human health. *Advances in Pediatric Infectious Disease* 14:269–290.

Boyce JM. Consequences of inaction: importance of infection control practices. 2001. *Clinical Infectious Diseases* 33 Suppl 3:S133–S137.

Gerberding JL, McGowan JE Jr, Tenover FC. 1999. Emerging nosocomial infections and antimicrobial resistance. *Current Clinical Topics in Infectious Disease* 19:83–98.

Gross R, Morgan AS, Kinky DE, Weiner M, Gibson GA, Fishman NO. 2001. Impact of a hospital-based antimicrobial management program on clinical and economic outcomes. *Clinical Infectious Diseases* 33(3):289–295. Available at: http://www.journals.uchicago.edu/CID/journal/issues/v33n3/001003/001003.html.

Hryniewicz W, Grzesiowski P, Ozorowski T. 2001. Hospital infection control in Poland. *Journal of Hospital Infection* 49(2):94–98.

Nicolle LE. Preventing infections in non-hospital settings: long-term care. 2001. *Emerging Infectious Diseases* 7(2):205–207. Available at: http://www.cdc.gov/ncidod/eid/vol7no2/nicolle.htm.

Nicolle LE, Bentley DW, Garibaldi R, Neuhaus EG, Smith PW. 2000. Antimicrobial use in long-term-care facilities. SHEA Long-Term-Care Committee. *Infection Control and Hospital Epidemiology* 21(8):537–545.

Okeke IN, Lamikanra A, Edelman R. 1999. Socioeconomic and behavioral factors leading to acquired bacterial resistance to antibiotics in developing countries. *Emerging Infectious Diseases* 5(1):18–27. Available at: http://www.cdc.gov/ncidod/eid/vol5no1/okeke.htm.

Pechere JC. 2001. Patients' interviews and misuse of antibiotics. *Clinical Infectious Diseases* 33 Suppl 3:S170–S173.

Roberts R, Cordell R, Scott RD. *Issues Concerning Studies on the Impact of Health Care Associated Infections with Antimicrobial Resistant Pathogens.* Available at: http://www.carp-net.org/Cost/study1/cost_study_1.htm.

Schierholz JM, Beuth J. 2001. Implant infections: a haven for opportunistic bacteria. *Journal of Hospital Infection* 49(2):87–93.

Shryock TR. 1999. Relationship between usage of antibiotics in food-producing animals and the appearance of antibiotic resistant bacteria. *International Journal of Antimicrobial Agents* 12(4):275–278.

Strausbaugh LJ, Crossley KB, Nurse BA, Thrupp LD. 1996. Antimicrobial resistance in long-term-care facilities. *Infection Control and Hospital Epidemiology* 17(2):129–140

Teuber M. 2001.Veterinary use and antibiotic resistance. *Current Opinion in Microbiology*. 4(5):493–499.
Thamlikitkul V, Jintanothaitavorn D, Sathitmethakul R, Vaithayaphichet S, Trakulsomboon S, Danchaivijitr S. 2001. Bacterial infections in hospitalized patients in Thailand in 1997 and 2000. *Journal of the Medical Association of Thailand* 84(5):666–673.
Weinstein RA. 2001. Controlling antimicrobial resistance in hospitals: infection control and use of antibiotics. *Emerging Infectious Diseases* 7(2):188–192. Available at: http://www.cdc.gov/ncidod/eid/vol7no2/weinstein.htm.

VECTOR RESISTANCE

Gratz NG, Jany WC. 1994. What role for insecticides in vector control programs? *American Journal of Tropical Medicine and Hygiene* 50(6 Suppl):11–20.
Gubler DJ. 1998. Resurgent vector-borne diseases as a global health problem. *Emerging Infectious Diseases* 4(3):442–450. Available at: http://www.cdc.gov/ncidod/eid/vol4no3/gubler.htm.
Guillet P, N'Guessan R, Darriet F, Traore-Lamizana M, Chandre F, Carnevale P. 2001. Combined pyrethroid and carbamate 'two-in-one' treated mosquito nets: field efficacy against pyrethroid-resistant *Anopheles gambiae* and *Culex quinquefasciatus*. *Medical and Veterinary Entomology* 15(1):105–112.
Hemingway J, Ranson H. 2000. Insecticide resistance in insect vectors of human disease. *Annual Review of Entomology* 45:371–391.
Pittendrigh BR, Gaffney PJ. 2001. Pesticide resistance: can we make it a renewable resource? *Journal of Theoretical Biology* 211(4):365–375.
Regis L, Silva-Filha MH, Nielsen-LeRoux C, Charles JF. 2001. Bacteriological larvicides of dipteran disease vectors. *Trends in Parasitology* 17(8):377–380.
Roberts DR, Andre RG. Insecticide resistance issues in vector-borne disease control. 1994. *American Journal of Tropical Medicine and Hygiene* 50(6 Suppl):21–34.
Roberts DR, Laughlin LL, Hsheih P, Legters LJ. 1997. DDT, global strategies, and a malaria control crisis in South America. *Emerging Infectious Diseases* 3(3):295–302. Available at: http://www.cdc.gov/ncidod/eid/vol3no3/roberts.htm.

EMERGING TECHNOLOGY AND TOOLS TO COMBAT RESISTANCE

Research and Technology

Bax R, Mullan N, Verhoef J. 2000. The millennium bugs—the need for and development of new antibacterials. *International Journal of Antimicrobial Agents* 16(1):51–59.
Fischetti VA. 2001. Phage antibacterials make a comeback. *Nature Biotechnology* 19(8):734–735. Available at: http://www.nature.com/cgitaf/DynaPage.taf?file=/nbt/journal/v19/n8/full/nbt0801_734.html.
Loeffler JM, Nelson D, Fischetti VA. 2001. Rapid killing of *Streptococcus pneumoniae* with bacteriophage cell wall hydrolase. *Science* 294(5549):2170–2172. Available at: http://www.sciencemag.org/cgi/content/full/294/5549/2170.
Mangel WF, Brown MT, Baniecki ML, Barnard D, McGrath WJ. 2001. Prevention of viral drug resistance by novel combination therapy. *Current Opinion in Investigational Drugs* 2(5):613–616.
Tang C, Holden D. 1999. Pathogen virulence genes—implications for vaccines and drug therapy. *British Medical Bulletin* 55(2):387–400.

Wright GD. 2000. Resisting resistance: new chemical strategies for battling superbugs. *Chemistry and Biology* 7(6):R127–R132.

Tools

Bax R, Bywater R, Cornaglia G, Goossens H, Hunter P, Isham V, Jarlier V, Jones R, Phillips I, Sahm D, Senn S, Struelens M, Taylor D, White A. 2001. Surveillance of antimicrobial resistance—what, how and whither? *Clinical Microbiology and Infection* 7(6):316–325.

Centers for Disease Control and Prevention. 2000. Laboratory capacity to detect antimicrobial resistance, 1998. *Morbidity and Mortality Weekly Report* 48(51-52):1167–1171.

Guan J, Fan C, Liao L. 2000. Protein secretion from drug-resistant bacteria—a suitable target for new antibiotics. *Ying Yong Sheng Tai Xue Bao* 11(6):947–950.

Kristinsson KG. 2001. Mathematical models as tools for evaluating the effectiveness of interventions: a comment on Levin. *Clinical Infectious Diseases* 33 Suppl 3:S174–S179.

Laxminarayan R, Brown GM. 2001. Economics of antibiotic resistance: a theory of optimal use. *Journal of Environmental Economics and Management* 42(2):183–206.

Peck SL. 2001. Antibiotic and insecticide resistance modeling—is it time to start talking? *Trends in Microbiology* 9(6):286–292.

Simpson JA, Watkins ER, Price RN, Aarons L, Kyle DE, White NJ. 2000. Mefloquine pharmacokinetic-pharmacodynamic models: implications for dosing and resistance. *Antimicrobial Agents and Chemotherapy* 44(12):3414–3424. Available at: http://aac.asm.org/cgi/content/full/44/12/3414?view=full&pmid=11083649.

Vacek V. 2001. Antibacterial chemotherapy—are we really at the end of the antibiotic era? *Casopís lékar°u ceskych* 140(19):592–595.

CONTAINMENT STRATEGIES

Antimicrobial Resistance

Amaral L, Viveiros M, Kristiansen JE. 2001. Phenothiazines: potential alternatives for the management of antibiotic resistant infections of tuberculosis and malaria in developing countries. *Tropical Medicine and International Health* 6(12):1016–1022.

Blower SM, Gerberding JL. 1998. Understanding, predicting and controlling the emergence of drug-resistant tuberculosis: a theoretical framework. *Journal of Molecular Medicine* 76(9):624–636.

Carbon C, Bax RP. 1998. Regulating the use of antibiotics in the community. *British Medical Journal* 317(7159):663–665. Available at: http://bmj.com/cgi/content/full/317/7159/663?view=full&pmid=9728001.

Enserink M. 2001. Driving a stake into resurgent TB. *Science* 293(5528):234–235. Available at: http://www.sciencemag.org/cgi/content/full/293/5528/234.

Escalante P, Graviss EA, Griffith DE, Musser JM, Awe RJ. 2001.Treatment of isoniazid-resistant tuberculosis in southeastern Texas. *Chest* 119(6):1730–1736. Available at: http://www.chestjournal.org/cgi/content/full/119/6/1730

Goldmann DA, Weinstein RA, Wenzel RP, Tablan OC, Duma RJ, Gaynes RP, Schlosser J, Martone WJ. 1996. Strategies to prevent and control the emergence and spread of antimicrobial-resistant microorganisms in hospitals. A challenge to hospital leadership. *Journal of the American Medical Association* 275(3):234–240.

Interagency Task Force on Antimicrobial Resistance. 2001. *A Public Health Action Plan to Combat Antimicrobial Resistance (Part 1: Domestic Issues)*. Executive Summary. Available at: http://www.cdc.gov/drugresistance/actionplan/aractionplan.pdf.

Medina-Cuevas F, Navarrete-Navarro S, Avila-Figueroa C, Santos-Preciado JI. 2000. FARMAC: a program designed for monitoring the prescription of antimicrobials in hospitals (abstract only). *Gaceta médica de México* 136(2):107–111.

OIE (Office International des Epizooties). The Use of Antibiotics in Animals—Ensuring the Protection of Public Health. March 24–26, 1999. Summary and Recommendations from the European Scientific Conference. Available at: http://www.antibiotics-conference.net/site/conclusn/summary.htm.

Schentag JJ, Gilliland KK, Paladino JA. 2001. What have we learned from pharmacokinetic and pharmacodynamic theories? *Clinical Infectious Diseases* 32 Suppl 1:S39–S46. Available at: http://www.journals.uchicago.edu/CID/journal/issues/v32nS1/000683/000683.html.

Schrag SJ, Beall B, Dowell SF. 2000. Limiting the spread of resistant pneumococci: biological and epidemiologic evidence for the effectiveness of alternative interventions. *Clinical Microbiology Reviews* 13(4):588–601. Available at: http://cmr.asm.org/cgi/content/full/13/4/588?view=full&pmid=11023959.

Shlaes DM, Gerding DN, John JF Jr, Craig WA, Bornstein DL, Duncan RA, Eckman MR, Farrer WE, Greene WH, Lorian V, Levy S, McGowan JE Jr, Paul SM, Ruskin J, Tenover FC, Watanakunakorn C. 1997. Society for Healthcare Epidemiology of America and Infectious Diseases Society of America Joint Committee on the Prevention of Antimicrobial Resistance: Guidelines for the Prevention of Antimicrobial Resistance in Hospitals. *Infection Control and Hospital Epidemiology* 18(4):275–291.

World Health Organization. 2001. WHO Global Strategy for Containment of Antimicrobial Resistance. Available at: http://www.who.int/emc/amrpdfs/WHO_Global_Strategy_English.pdf.

Insecticide Resistance/Vector Control

Insecticide Resistance Management: A Driving Force for New Insecticide Development. 2001. *Down to Earth* 56(1): 8–9. Available at: http://www.dowagro.com/webapps/lit/litorder.asp?objid=09002f138016e140&filepath=/noreg.

McGaughey WH, Gould F, Gelernter W. 1998. Bt resistance management. *Nature Biotechnology* 16(2):144–146.

Rose RI. 2001. Pesticides and public health: integrated methods of mosquito management. *Emerging Infectious Diseases* 7(1):17–23. Available at: http://www.cdc.gov/ncidod/eid/vol7no1/rose.htm.

Sina BJ, Aultman K. 2001. Resisting resistance. *Trends in Parasitology* 17(7):305–306.

World Health Organization Communicable Disease Control, Prevention and Eradication, WHO Pesticide Evaluation Scheme (WHOPES). 2000. Report of the Second Meeting of the Global Collaboration for Development of Pesticides for Public Health (GCDPP). April 6–7, 2000. Available at: http://www.who.int/ctd/whopes/gcdpp2.pdf.

Appendix D

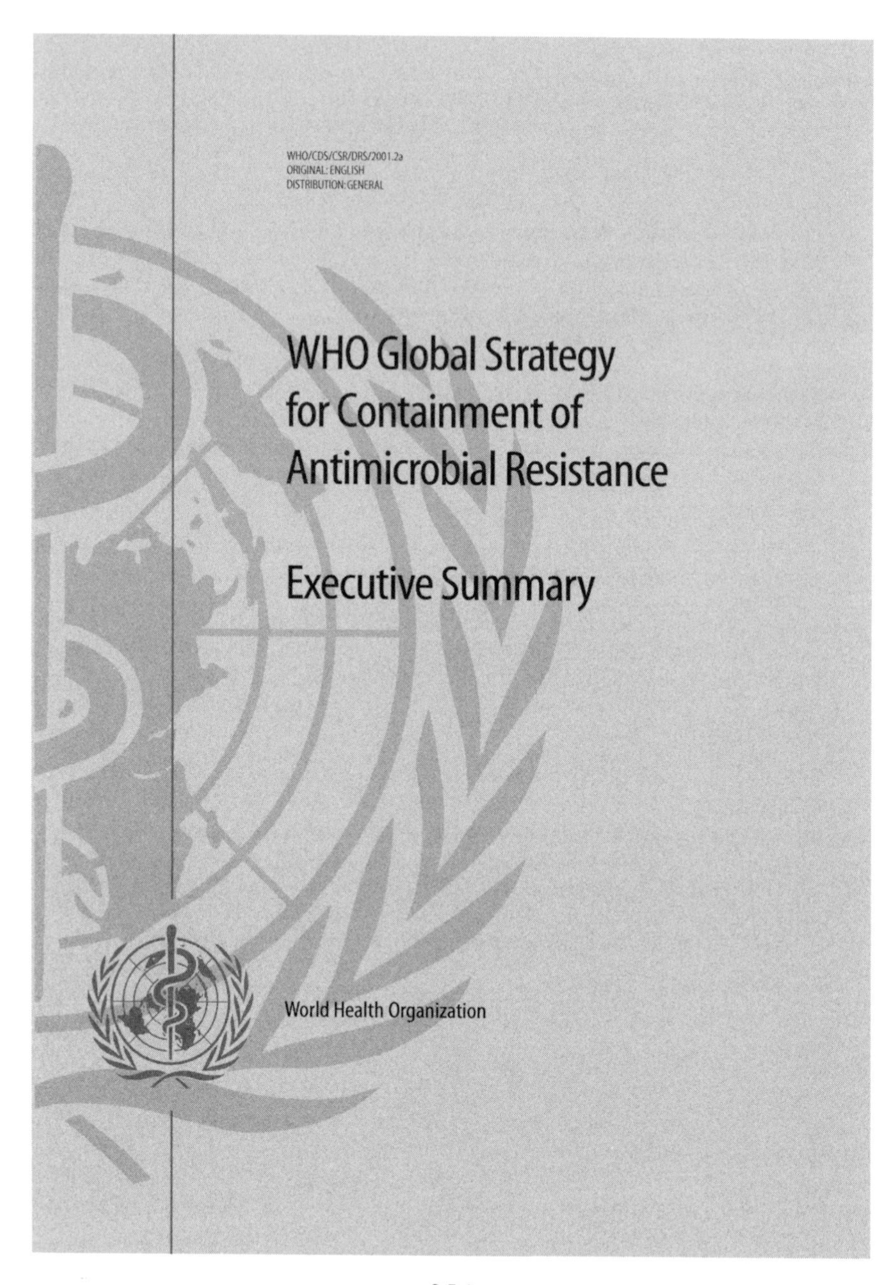
WHO/CDS/CSR/DRS/2001.2a
ORIGINAL: ENGLISH
DISTRIBUTION: GENERAL

WHO Global Strategy for Containment of Antimicrobial Resistance

Executive Summary

World Health Organization

Designed by minimum graphics
Printed in Switzerland

Acknowledgements

The World Health Organization (WHO) wishes to acknowledge with gratitude the significant support from the United States Agency for International Development (USAID) and additional assistance for this work from the United Kingdom Department for International Development and the Ministry of Health, Labour and Welfare, Japan.

This strategy is the product of collaborative efforts across WHO, particularly in the clusters of Communicable Diseases, Health Technology and Pharmaceuticals, and Family and Community Health, with significant input from the staff at WHO Regional Offices and from many partners working with WHO worldwide. In particular, WHO would like to acknowledge the important contributions made to the drafting of the strategy by Professor W Stamm, Professor ML Grayson, Professor L Nicolle and Dr M Powell, and the generosity of their respective institutions—Infectious Diseases Department, Harborview Medical Center, University of Washington, Seattle, USA; Infectious Diseases and Clinical Epidemiology Department, Monash Medical Centre, Monash University, Melbourne, Australia; Department of Internal Medicine, University of Manitoba, Winnipeg, Canada; Medicines Control Agency, London UK—that enabled them to spend time at WHO.

WHO also wishes to thank all those who participated and contributed their expertise in the consultations and those individuals and organizations that provided valuable comments on drafts of this document.

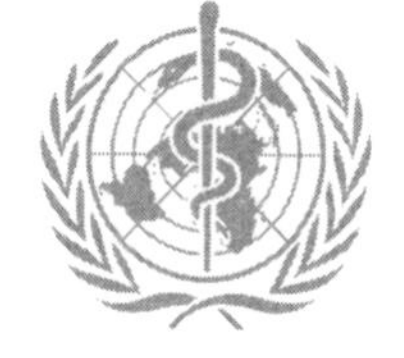

Executive Summary

■ Deaths from acute respiratory infections, diarrhoeal diseases, measles, AIDS, malaria and tuberculosis account for more than 85% of the mortality from infection worldwide. Resistance to first-line drugs in most of the pathogens causing these diseases ranges from zero to almost 100%. In some instances resistance to second- and third-line agents is seriously compromising treatment outcome. Added to this is the significant global burden of resistant hospital-acquired infections, the emerging problems of antiviral resistance and the increasing problems of drug resistance in the neglected parasitic diseases of poor and marginalized populations.

■ Resistance is not a new phenomenon; it was recognized early as a scientific curiosity and then as a threat to effective treatment outcome. However, the development of new families of antimicrobials throughout the 1950s and 1960s and of modifications of these molecules through the 1970s and 1980s allowed us to believe that we could always remain ahead of the pathogens. By the turn of the century this complacency had come to haunt us. The pipeline of new drugs is running dry and the incentives to develop new antimicrobials to address the global problems of drug resistance are weak.

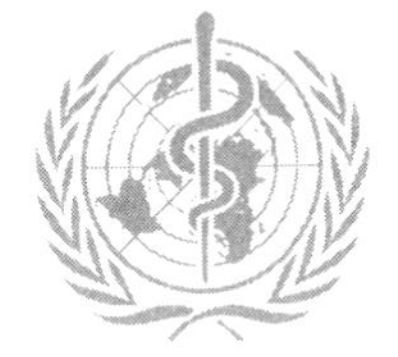

■ Resistance costs money, livelihoods and lives and threatens to undermine the effectiveness of health delivery programmes. It has recently been described as a threat to global stability and national security. A few studies have suggested that resistant clones can be replaced by susceptible ones; in general, however, resistance is slow to reverse or is irreversible.

- Antimicrobial use is the key driver of resistance. Paradoxically this selective pressure comes from a combination of overuse in many parts of the world, particularly for minor infections, misuse due to lack of access to appropriate treatment and underuse due to lack of financial support to complete treatment courses.

- Resistance is only just beginning to be considered as a societal issue and, in economic terms, as a negative externality in the health care context. Individual decisions to use antimicrobials (taken by the consumer alone or by the decision-making combination of health care worker and patient) often ignore the societal perspective and the perspective of the health service.

- The World Health Assembly (WHA) Resolution of 1998[1] urged Member States to develop measures to encourage appropriate and cost-effective use of antimicrobials, to prohibit the dispensing of antimicrobials without the prescription of a qualified health care professional, to improve practices to prevent the spread of infection and thereby the spread of resistant pathogens, to strengthen legislation to prevent the manufacture, sale and distribution of counterfeit antimicrobials and the sale of antimicrobials on the informal market, and to reduce the use of antimicrobials in food-animal production. Countries were also encouraged to develop sustainable systems to detect resistant pathogens, to monitor volumes and patterns of use of antimicrobials and the impact of control measures.

- Since the WHA Resolution, many countries have expressed growing concern about the problem of antimicrobial resistance and some have developed national action plans to address the problem. Despite the mass of literature on antimicrobial resistance, there is depressingly little on the true

[1] World Health Organization. World Health Assembly (fifty-first). ***Emerging and other communicable diseases: antimicrobial resistance.*** WHA51.17, 1998, agenda item 21.3.

costs of resistance and the effectiveness of interventions. Given this lack of data in the face of a growing realization that actions need to be taken now to avert future disaster, the challenge is *what to do* and *how to do it*.

■ The WHO Global Strategy for Containment of Antimicrobial Resistance addresses this challenge. It provides a framework of interventions to slow the emergence and reduce the spread of antimicrobial-resistant microorganisms through:

— reducing the disease burden and the spread of infection

— improving access to appropriate antimicrobials

— improving use of antimicrobials

— strengthening health systems and their surveillance capabilities

— enforcing regulations and legislation

— encouraging the development of appropriate new drugs and vaccines.

■ The strategy highlights aspects of the containment of resistance and the need for further research directed towards filling the existing gaps in knowledge.

■ The strategy is people-centred, with interventions directed towards the groups of people who are involved in the problem and need to be part of the solution, i.e. prescribers and dispensers, veterinarians, consumers, policy-makers in hospitals, public health and agriculture, professional societies and the pharmaceutical industry.

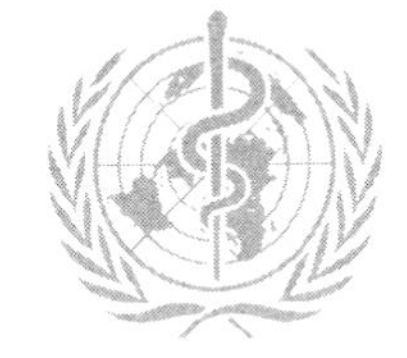

■ The strategy addresses antimicrobial resistance in general rather than through a disease-specific approach, but is particularly focused on resistance to antibacterial drugs.

■ Much of the responsibility for implementation of the strategy will fall on individual countries. Governments have a critical role to play in the provision of public goods such as information, in surveillance, analysis of cost-effectiveness and cross-sectoral coordination.

■ Given the complex nature of antimicrobial resistance, the strategy necessarily contains a large number of recommendations for interventions. Prioritization of the implementation of these interventions needs to be customized to national realities. To assist in this process an implementation approach has been defined together with indicators for monitoring implementation and outcomes.

■ Recognition that the problem of resistance exists and the creation of effective national intersectoral task forces are considered critical to the success of implementation and monitoring of interventions. International interdisciplinary cooperation will also be essential.

■ Improving antimicrobial use must be a key action in efforts to contain resistance. This requires improving access and changing behaviour; such changes take time.

■ Containment will require significant strengthening of the health systems in many countries and the costs of implementation will not be negligible. However, such costs must be weighed against future costs averted by the containment of widespread antimicrobial resistance.

Summary of recommendations for intervention

Patients and the general community and prescribers and dispensers

The emergence of antimicrobial resistance is a complex problem driven by many interconnected factors, in particular the use and misuse of antimicrobials. Antimicrobial use, in turn, is influenced by an interplay of the knowledge, expectations and interactions of prescribers and patients, economic incentives, characteristics of the health system(s) and the regulatory environment. In the light of this complexity, coordinated interventions are needed that simultaneously target the behaviour of providers and patients and change important features of the environments in which they interact. These interventions are most likely to be successful if the following factors are understood within each health setting:

- which infectious diseases and resistance problems are important
- which antimicrobials are used and by whom
- what factors determine patterns of antimicrobial use
- what the relative costs and benefits are from changing use
- what barriers exist to changing use.

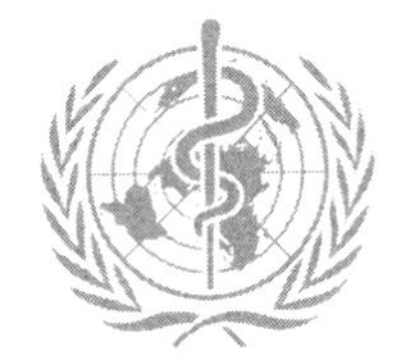

Although the interventions directed towards providers and patients are presented separately (1 and 2) for clarity, they will require implementation in an integrated fashion.

1 PATIENTS AND THE GENERAL COMMUNITY

Education

1.1 Educate patients and the general community on the appropriate use of antimicrobials.

1.2 Educate patients on the importance of measures to prevent infection, such as immunization, vector control, use of bednets, etc.

1.3 Educate patients on simple measures that may reduce transmission of infection in the household and community, such as handwashing, food hygiene, etc.

1.4 Encourage appropriate and informed health care seeking behaviour.

1.5 Educate patients on suitable alternatives to antimicrobials for relief of symptoms and discourage patient self-initiation of treatment, except in specific circumstances.

2 PRESCRIBERS AND DISPENSERS

Education

2.1 Educate all groups of prescribers and dispensers (including drug sellers) on the importance of appropriate antimicrobial use and containment of antimicrobial resistance.

2.2 Educate all groups of prescribers on disease prevention (including immunization) and infection control issues.

2.3 Promote targeted undergraduate and postgraduate educational programmes on the accurate diagnosis and management of common infections for all health care workers, veterinarians, prescribers and dispensers.

2.4 Encourage prescribers and dispensers to educate patients on antimicrobial use and the importance of adherence to prescribed treatments.

2.5 Educate all groups of prescribers and dispensers on factors that may strongly influence their prescribing habits, such as economic incentives, promotional activities and inducements by the pharmaceutical industry.

Management, guidelines and formularies

2.6 Improve antimicrobial use by supervision and support of clinical practices, especially diagnostic and treatment strategies.

2.7 Audit prescribing and dispensing practices and utilize peer group or external standard comparisons to provide feedback and endorsement of appropriate antimicrobial prescribing.

2.8 Encourage development and use of guidelines and treatment algorithms to foster appropriate use of antimicrobials.

2.9 Empower formulary managers to limit antimicrobial use to the prescription of an appropriate range of selected antimicrobials.

Regulation

2.10 Link professional registration requirements for prescribers and dispensers to requirements for training and continuing education.

Hospitals

Although most antimicrobial use occurs in the community, the intensity of use in hospitals is far higher; hospitals are therefore particularly important in the containment of antimicrobial resistance. In hospitals it is crucial to develop integrated approaches to improving the use of antimicrobials, reducing the incidence and spread of hospital-acquired (nosocomial) infections, and linking therapeutic and drug supply decision-making. This will require training of key individuals and the allocation of resources to effective surveillance, infection control and therapeutic support.

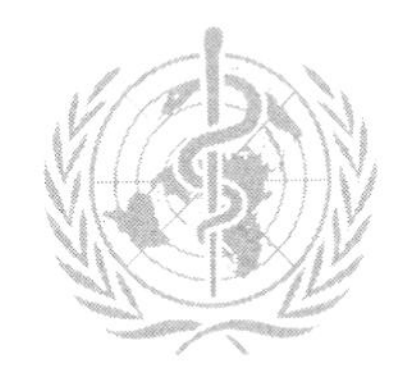

3 HOSPITALS

Management

3.1 Establish infection control programmes, based on current best practice, with the responsibility for effective management of antimicrobial resistance in hospitals and ensure that all hospitals have access to such a programme.

3.2 Establish effective hospital therapeutics committees with the responsibility for overseeing antimicrobial use in hospitals.

3.3 Develop and regularly update guidelines for antimicrobial treatment and prophylaxis, and hospital antimicrobial formularies.

3.4 Monitor antimicrobial usage, including the quantity and patterns of use, and feedback results to prescribers.

Diagnostic laboratories

3.5 Ensure access to microbiology laboratory services that match the level of the hospital, e.g. secondary, tertiary.

3.6 Ensure performance and quality assurance of appropriate diagnostic tests, microbial identification, antimicrobial susceptibility tests of key pathogens, and timely and relevant reporting of results.

3.7 Ensure that laboratory data are recorded, preferably on a database, and are used to produce clinically- and epidemiologically-useful surveillance reports of resistance patterns among common pathogens and infections in a timely manner with feedback to prescribers and to the infection control programme.

Interactions with the pharmaceutical industry

3.8 Control and monitor pharmaceutical company promotional activities within the hospital environment and ensure that such activities have educational benefit.

Use of antimicrobials in food-producing animals

A growing body of evidence establishes a link between the use of antimicrobials in food-producing animals and the emergence of resistance among common pathogens. Such resistance has an impact on animal health and on human health if these pathogens enter the food chain. The factors affecting such antimicrobial use, whether for therapeutic, prophylactic or growth promotion purposes, are complex and the required interventions need coordinated implementation. The underlying principles of appropriate antimicrobial use and containment of resistance are similar to those applicable to humans. The WHO global principles for the containment of antimicrobial resistance in animals intended for food[2] were adopted at a WHO consultation in June 2000 in Geneva. They provide a framework of recommendations to reduce the overuse and misuse of antimicrobials in food animals for the protection of human health. Antimicrobials are widely used in a variety of other settings outside human medicine, e.g. horticulture and aquaculture, but the risks to human health from such uses are less well understood and they have not been included in this document.

4 USE OF ANTIMICROBIALS IN FOOD-PRODUCING ANIMALS

This topic has been the subject of specific consultations which resulted in "WHO global principles for the containment of antimicrobial resistance in animals intended for food"[2]. A complete description of all recommendations is contained in that document and only a summary is reproduced here.

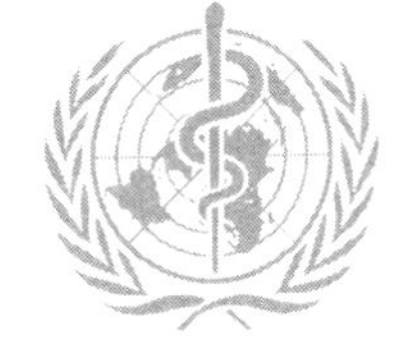

[2] World Health Organization. *WHO global principles for the containment of antimicrobial resistance in animals intended for food.* 2000. www.who.int/emc/diseases/zoo/who_global_principles.html

Summary

4.1 Require obligatory prescriptions for all antimicrobials used for disease control in food animals.

4.2 In the absence of a public health safety evaluation, terminate or rapidly phase out the use of antimicrobials for growth promotion if they are also used for treatment of humans.

4.3 Create national systems to monitor antimicrobial usage in food animals.

4.4 Introduce pre-licensing safety evaluation of antimicrobials with consideration of potential resistance to human drugs.

4.5 Monitor resistance to identify emerging health problems and take timely corrective actions to protect human health.

4.6 Develop guidelines for veterinarians to reduce overuse and misuse of antimicrobials in food animals.

National governments and health systems

Government health policies and the health care systems in which they are implemented play a crucial role in determining the efficacy of interventions to contain antimicrobial resistance. National commitment to understand and address the problem and the designation of authority and responsibility are prerequisites. Effective action requires the introduction and enforcement of appropriate regulations and allocation of appropriate resources for education and surveillance. Constructive interactions with the pharmaceutical industry are critical, both for ensuring appropriate licensure, promotion and marketing of existing antimicrobials and for encouraging the development of new drugs and vaccines. For clarity, interventions relating to these interactions with the industry are shown in separate recommendation groups (6 and 7).

5 NATIONAL GOVERNMENTS AND HEALTH SYSTEMS

Advocacy and intersectoral action

5.1 Make the containment of antimicrobial resistance a national priority.
- Create a national intersectoral task force (membership to include health care professionals, veterinarians, agriculturalists, pharmaceutical manufacturers, government, media representatives, consumers and other interested parties) to raise awareness about antimicrobial resistance, organize data collection and oversee local task forces. For practical purposes such a task force may need to be a government task force which receives input from multiple sectors.
- Allocate resources to promote the implementation of interventions to contain resistance. These interventions should include the appropriate utilization of antimicrobial drugs, the control and prevention of infection, and research activities.
- Develop indicators to monitor and evaluate the impact of the antimicrobial resistance containment strategy.

Regulations

5.2 Establish an effective registration scheme for dispensing outlets.

5.3 Limit the availability of antimicrobials to prescription-only status, except in special circumstances when they may be dispensed on the advice of a trained health care professional.

5.4 Link prescription-only status to regulations regarding the sale, supply, dispensing and allowable promotional activities of antimicrobial agents; institute mechanisms to facilitate compliance by practitioners and systems to monitor compliance.

5.5 Ensure that only antimicrobials meeting international standards of quality, safety and efficacy are granted marketing authorization.

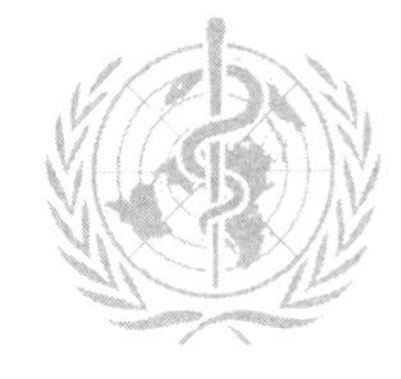

5.6 Introduce legal requirements for manufacturers to collect and report data on antimicrobial distribution (including import/export).

5.7 Create economic incentives for the appropriate use of antimicrobials.

Policies and guidelines

5.8 Establish and maintain updated national Standard Treatment Guidelines (STGs) and encourage their implementation.

5.9 Establish an Essential Drugs List (EDL) consistent with the national STGs and ensure the accessibility and quality of these drugs.

5.10 Enhance immunization coverage and other disease preventive measures, thereby reducing the need for antimicrobials.

Education

5.11 Maximize and maintain the effectiveness of the EDL and STGs by conducting appropriate undergraduate and postgraduate education programmes of health care professionals on the importance of appropriate antimicrobial use and containment of antimicrobial resistance.

5.12 Ensure that prescribers have access to approved prescribing literature on individual drugs.

Surveillance of resistance, antimicrobial usage and disease burden

5.13 Designate or develop reference microbiology laboratory facilities to coordinate effective epidemiologically sound surveillance of antimicrobial resistance among common pathogens in the community, hospitals and other health care facilities. The standard of these laboratory facilities should be at least at the level of recommendation 3.6.

5.14 Adapt and apply WHO model systems for antimicrobial resistance surveillance and ensure data flow to the national intersectoral task force, to authorities responsible for the national STGs and drug policy, and to prescribers.

5.15 Establish systems for monitoring antimicrobial use in hospitals and the community, and link these findings to resistance and disease surveillance data.

5.16 Establish surveillance for key infectious diseases and syndromes according to country priorities, and link this information to other surveillance data.

6 DRUG AND VACCINE DEVELOPMENT

6.1 Encourage cooperation between industry, government bodies and academic institutions in the search for new drugs and vaccines.

6.2 Encourage drug development programmes which seek to optimize treatment regimens with regard to safety, efficacy and the risk of selecting resistant organisms.

6.3 Provide incentives for industry to invest in the research and development of new antimicrobials.

6.4 Consider establishing or utilizing fast-track marketing authorization for safe new agents.

6.5 Consider using an orphan drug scheme where available and applicable.

6.6 Make available time-limited exclusivity for new formulations and/or indications for use of antimicrobials.

6.7 Align intellectual property rights to provide suitable patent protection for new antimicrobial agents and vaccines.

6.8 Seek innovative partnerships with the pharmaceutical industry to improve access to newer essential drugs.

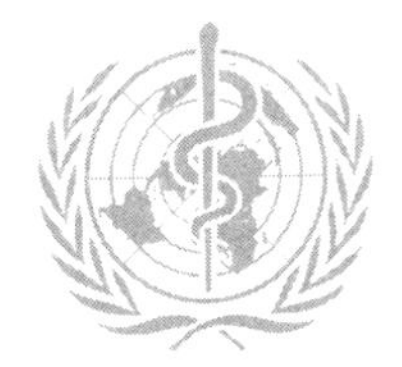

7 PHARMACEUTICAL PROMOTION

7.1 Introduce requirements for pharmaceutical companies to comply with national or international codes of practice on promotional activities.

7.2 Ensure that national or international codes of practice cover direct-to-consumer advertising, including advertising on the Internet.

7.3 Institute systems for monitoring compliance with legislation on promotional activities.

7.4 Identify and eliminate economic incentives that encourage inappropriate antimicrobial use.

7.5 Make prescribers aware that promotion in accordance with the datasheet may not necessarily constitute appropriate antimicrobial use.

8 INTERNATIONAL ASPECTS OF CONTAINING ANTIMICROBIAL RESISTANCE

8.1 Encourage collaboration between governments, non-governmental organizations, professional societies and international agencies to recognize the importance of antimicrobial resistance, to present consistent, simple and accurate messages regarding the importance of antimicrobial use, antimicrobial resistance and its containment, and to implement strategies to contain resistance.

8.2 Consider the information derived from the surveillance of antimicrobial use and antimicrobial resistance, including the containment thereof, as global public goods for health to which all governments should contribute.

8.3 Encourage governments, non-governmental organizations, professional societies and international agencies to support the establishment of networks, with trained staff and adequate infrastructures, which can undertake epidemiologically valid surveillance of antimicrobial resistance and antimicrobial use to provide information for the optimal containment of resistance.

8.4 Support drug donations in line with the UN interagency guidelines*.

8.5 Encourage the establishment of international inspection teams qualified to conduct valid assessments of pharmaceutical manufacturing plants.

8.6 Support an international approach to the control of counterfeit antimicrobials in line with the WHO guidelines**.

8.7 Encourage innovative approaches to incentives for the development of new pharmaceutical products and vaccines for neglected diseases.

8.8 Establish an international database of potential research funding agencies with an interest in antimicrobial resistance.

8.9 Establish new, and reinforce existing, programmes for researchers to improve the design, preparation and conduct of research to contain antimicrobial resistance.

* *Interagency Guidelines. Guidelines for Drug Donations*, revised 1999. Geneva, World Health Organization, 1999. WHO/EDM/PAR/99.4.

***Counterfeit drugs. Guidelines for the development of measures to combat counterfeit drugs.* Geneva, World Health Organization, 1999. WHO/EDM/QSM/99.1.

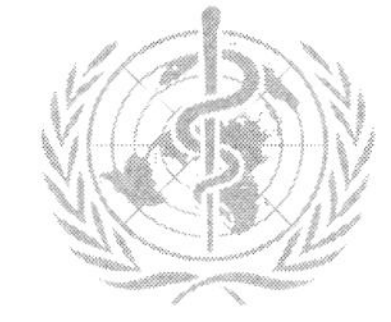

Appendix E
Interventions Against Antimicrobial Resistance: A Review of the Literature and Exploration of Modelling Cost-Effectiveness

A report prepared for the Global Forum for Health Research

Richard D. Smith

Senior Lecturer in Health Economics
Health Economics Group, School of Health Policy and Practice,
University of East Anglia

Joanna Coast

Lecturer in Health Economics, Department of Social Medicine,
University of Bristol

Michael R. Millar

Consultant Microbiologist and Infection Control Doctor,
Barts and The London NHS Trust

Paula Wilton

Research Associate, Health Economics Group
School of Health Policy and Practice, University of East Anglia

Anne-Marie Karcher

Specialist Registrar in Microbiology, Department of Microbiology,
Homerton Hospital

EXECUTIVE SUMMARY

1. Introduction

Antimicrobial resistance (AMR) is one of the biggest challenges to face global public health at the beginning of the third millennium. However, there is little accurate information concerning many aspects of AMR, including, in particular, the cost and/or effectiveness of various strategies which may prevent the emergence of AMR and/or limit the transmission of resistant organisms, or resistance determinants. The Global Forum for Health Research therefore provided funding to:

1. Review current knowledge concerning the cost and/or effectiveness of (medical) interventions aimed at reducing the emergence and transmission of AMR in humans; and
2. Explore the feasibility of, and issues involved in, the development of an economic model to assess the cost-effectiveness of interventions to address AMR in humans.

2. Literature review — Methodology

A systematic literature review was undertaken to describe and critically appraise studies reporting on: (i) the costs and/or effectiveness of strategies to prevent, and control the spread of, AMR; and (ii) the cost impact of resistance. Literature was identified through contact with key international figures and institutions in the field of AMR, and through searching major electronic bibliographic databases. Approximately 155 studies were reviewed, following clearly defined inclusion and exclusion, and quality assessment strategies. Meta-analysis was inappropriate, and thus a qualitative overview provided.

3. Literature review — Results

From this review it would appear that most studies:

1. Are from the developed world (principally the USA);
2. Are mostly hospital/other institution based, with few community level interventions;
3. Are concerned with control of transmission as opposed to prevention of emergence;
4. Cover "micro" interventions, such as hand-washing, and not more "macro" policy interventions, such as legislation, global control of drug availability, tax/subsidy; and

5. Do not measure the cost impact of AMR to the health service, patients or society.

There were few studies examining strategies to reduce AMR in developing countries, although several focusing upon prescribing were reviewed. This may be a reflection of pharmaceuticals being widely available at a community level (with few restrictions governing their availability) and, as a consequence, much inappropriate prescribing. Given the focus on prescribing, it is not surprising that, here, analysis tended to be concentrated at the community level.

Overall, there appears to be no definitive evidence (cost and/or effectiveness) which suggests that one specific control measure (or combination) is particularly more successful than another in containing the spread of AMR. In addition, many interventions that impinge on levels of antimicrobial usage, and thus ultimately levels of resistance, are also not currently being subject to such formal evaluation.

4. Modelling cost-effectiveness —techniques and methods

Modelling is an extrapolation of the main parameters which influence the phenomenon of interest, and then a construction of relationships between these parameters. There are six main forms of modelling in common use which might be applied to AMR:

1. Decision-analytic models
2. Markov-chain models
3. Monte-Carlo simulation
4. Mathematical models
5. Statistical models
6. Macro-economic models

These forms of modelling differ in their theoretical and methodological basis, the purpose for which they are designed, the manner of presentation and the level of data required. The theoretical and methodological features of each of these forms of model are summarised in chapter 4.

5. Modelling cost-effectiveness —factors in model development

In considering the range of possible approaches to modelling for AMR there are several specific factors that are important in determining which is most suitable:

1. Contextual factors, such as socio-economic environment, type of health care system and demographic characteristics of the population;
2. Policy goal of the intervention, such as a focus upon resistance or infection, micro or macro intervention and the prevention of emergence or transmission of AMR;
3. Outcome of interest, referring to a focus upon resistance or health more widely;
4. Temporal factors and the role of changes over time;
5. Extent of endogeneity of parameters within the model (i.e., those explained by the model);
6. Discounting of future costs and benefits; and
7. Handling uncertainty, in both the development of new antimicrobials and the development of resistance.

These will determine the relevant parameters to be collected, and how the relationships between them will be constructed. These factors are outlined in chapter 5.

6. Modelling cost-effectiveness — "minimum" data set

As well as the broader structural issues, outlined in chapter 5, there is a requirement for specification of variables of importance and the collection of data related to them. Although these will vary according to the final model structure, there will likely be a "minimum data set" of variables that would be required whatever the specific model developed. Chapter 6 considers the variables that would likely comprise such a "minimum data set" within categories of:

1. Epidemiological or clinical factors relating to resistance;
2. Cost factors relating to resistance;
3. Pattern of antimicrobial usage;
4. Impact on AMR in humans from non-human consumption of antimicrobials; and
5. Information concerning the costs and effectiveness of the policy evaluated.

7. Discussion and research agenda

In terms of current literature, there is a narrow focus upon the closed hospital system and concentrating upon the effects of policies aimed at reducing *transmission* rather than *emergence* of resistance. However, although it will be easier to identify the impact of strategies aimed at reducing transmission in a closed environment, these are not likely to produce an optimal long-term outcome (i.e., a stable balance of the costs and benefits of antimicrobial use). This is because of the possible irreversibility of AMR and the potentially severe harm which could be imposed as a result. Yet, given the increasing importance of evidence-based medicine, strategies that have been evaluated using experimental methods and well conducted economic evaluations, may be prioritised above these policies, which are much more difficult to evaluate. This is a danger that should be avoided both by awareness among policy makers of the relative challenges associated with evaluating different types of policy, and by awareness among the research community of the importance of evaluating policies which may potentially be more important, even if the rigour with which they can be evaluated is less than for the potentially less important policies.

Overall, there appears to be no definitive evidence (cost and/or effectiveness) which suggests that one specific control measure (or indeed a combination of measures) is particularly successful in containing the spread of AMR. Although it would seem that surveillance is a basic pre-requisite to tackling AMR, in the absence of evidence it is difficult to go further in making recommendations, or in suggesting priorities for research among those interventions assessed here. Readers are referred to the WHO Global Strategy for the Containment of Antimicrobial Resistance as presenting the most current and complete "best advice" on interventions to tackle AMR, how these should be implemented, and research priorities.

In terms of developing a model to assess the cost-effectiveness of strategies to tackle AMR, the appropriate and desirable model will need to satisfy four broad criteria of feasibility, sensitivity, relevance and flexibility. Considering these criteria, and this review of modelling as applied to AMR, two broad options are outlined:

1. A "macro-model" approach which attempts to integrate factors within a broad based model aiming to assess strategies on a more "global" level; and
2. A "suite" of micro sub-models, each "embedded" within a given set of primary parameters, such as country, disease and level of intervention (e.g., hospital or community), which determine which of the "suite" of sub-models is most appropriate for that context.

A definitive recommendation concerning which form of modelling to pursue is not possible at present, as it depends upon both feasibility and relevance to the question and context concerned. However, it is clear that there needs to be further research in to the modelling of AMR. Although such a model will require substantial investment of time and resources, the potential benefits of such a model, if accurately specified and incorporating quality data, could be vast in terms of the potential health benefit to current and future generations.

Appendix F

A Public Health Action Plan to Combat Antimicrobial Resistance

EXECUTIVE SUMMARY

This *Public Health Action Plan to Combat Antimicrobial Resistance (Action Plan)* was developed by an interagency Task Force on Antimicrobial Resistance that was created in 1999. The Task Force is co-chaired by the Centers for Disease Control and Prevention, the Food and Drug Administration, and the National Institutes of Health, and also includes the Agency for Healthcare Research and Quality, the Health Care Financing Administration, the Health Resources and Services Administration, the Department of Agriculture, the Department of Defense, the Department of Veterans Affairs, and the Environmental Protection Agency.

The *Action Plan* reflects a broad-based consensus of federal agencies on actions needed to address antimicrobial[1] resistance (AR). Input from state and local health agencies, universities, professional societies, pharmaceutical companies, health care delivery organizations, agricultural producers, consumer groups, and other members of the public was important in developing the plan. While some actions are already underway, complete implementation of this plan will require close collaboration with all of these

[1]In this document, the term "antimicrobial" is used inclusively to refer to any agent (including an antibiotic) used to kill or inhibit the growth of microorganisms (bacteria, viruses, fungi, or parasites.) This term applies whether the agent is intended for human, veterinary, or agricultural applications.

partners,[2] a major objective of the process. The plan will be implemented incrementally, dependent on the availability of resources.

The *Action Plan* provides a blueprint for specific, coordinated federal actions to address the emerging threat of antimicrobial resistance. This document is Part I of the *Action Plan*, focusing on domestic issues. Since AR transcends national borders and requires a global approach to its prevention and control, Part II of the plan, to be developed subsequently, will identify actions that more specifically address international issues. The *Action Plan*, Part I (Domestic Issues), includes four focus areas: Surveillance, Prevention and Control, Research, and Product Development. A summary of the top priority goals and action items in each focus area follows.

Surveillance

Unless AR problems are detected as they emerge—and actions are taken quickly to contain them—the world may soon be faced with previously treatable diseases that have again become untreatable, as in the pre-antibiotic era. Priority Goals and Action Items in this focus area address ways to:

- Develop and implement a coordinated national plan for AR surveillance;
- Ensure the availability of reliable drug susceptibility data for surveillance;
- Monitor patterns of antimicrobial drug use; and
- Monitor AR in agricultural settings to protect the public's health by ensuring a safe food supply as well as animal and plant health.

A coordinated national surveillance plan for monitoring AR in microorganisms that pose a threat to public health will be developed and implemented. The plan will specify activities to be conducted at national, state, and local levels; define the roles of participants; promote the use of standardized methods; and provide for timely dissemination of data to interested parties, e.g., public health officials, clinicians, and researchers.

[2]Implementation of this *Action Plan* requires working with a wide variety of partners, e.g., state and local health agencies, universities, professional societies, pharmaceutical and biotechnology companies, health care delivery organizations, insurers, agricultural producers, consumer groups, and the public. A wide variety of expertise is needed, e.g., from clinicians, consumers, pharmacists, microbiologists, epidemiologists, behavioral and social scientists, economists, health policy researchers, and others. Partners and expertise needed will vary with different action items.

Needed core capacities at state and local levels will be defined and supported. When possible, the plan will coordinate, integrate, and build on existing disease surveillance infrastructure. All surveillance activities will be conducted with respect for patient and institutional confidentiality.

The availability of reliable drug susceptibility data is essential for AR surveillance. The accuracy of AR detection and reporting will be improved through training and proficiency testing programs for diagnostic laboratories and by promoting and further refining standardized methods for detecting drug resistance in important pathogens, including bacteria, parasites, fungi, and viruses. Public and private sector partners will address barriers to AR testing and reporting, e.g., barriers due to changes in health care delivery.

A plan to monitor patterns of antimicrobial drug use will be developed and implemented as an important component of the national AR surveillance plan. This information is essential to interpret trends and variations in rates of AR, improve our understanding of the relationship between drug use and resistance, identify and anticipate gaps in availability of existing drugs, and identify interventions to prevent and control AR.

Improved surveillance for AR in agricultural settings will allow early detection of resistance trends in pathogens that pose a risk to animal and plant health, as well as in bacteria that enter the food supply. Agricultural surveillance data will also help improve understanding of the relationship between antimicrobial drug and pesticide use and the emergence of drug resistance.

Prevention and Control

The prevention and control of drug-resistant infections requires measures to promote the appropriate use[3] of antimicrobial drugs and prevent the transmission of infections (whether drug-resistant or not). Priority Goals and Action Items in this focus area address ways to:

- Extend the useful life of antimicrobial drugs through appropriate use policies that discourage overuse and misuse;
- Improve diagnostic testing practices;

[3]In this *Action Plan*, appropriate antimicrobial drug use is defined as use that maximizes therapeutic impact while minimizing toxicity and the development of resistance. In practice, this means prescribing antimicrobial therapy when and only when beneficial to a patient; targeting therapy to the desired pathogens; and using the appropriate drug, dose, and duration.

- Prevent infection transmission through improved infection control methods and use of vaccines;
- Prevent and control emerging AR problems in agriculture and human and veterinary medicine; and
- Ensure that comprehensive programs to prevent and control AR involve a wide variety of nonfederal partners and the public so these programs become a part of routine practice nationwide.

Appropriate drug-use policies will be implemented through a public health education campaign on appropriate antimicrobial drug use as a national health priority. Other actions in support of appropriate drug use will include reducing inappropriate prescribing through development of clinical guidelines and computer-assisted decision support, considering regulatory changes, supporting other interventions promoting education and behavior change among clinicians, and informing consumers about the uses and limitations of antimicrobial drugs.

Improved diagnostic practices will be promoted by encouraging the use of rapid diagnostic methods to guide drug prescribing, facilitating direct consultation between clinicians and laboratory personnel with appropriate expertise and authority, and promoting the use of appropriate laboratory testing methods. Guidelines, training, and regulatory and reimbursement policies will be utilized to promote improved diagnostic practices.

Reduced rates of infection transmission will be addressed through public health campaigns that promote vaccination and hygienic practices such as hand washing, safe food handling, and other behaviors associated with prevention of infection transmission. Infection control in health care settings will be enhanced by developing new interventions based on rapid diagnosis, improved understanding of the factors that promote cross-infection, and modified medical devices or procedures that reduce the risk of infection.

The prevention and control of AR in agriculture and veterinary medicine requires 1) improved understanding of the risks and benefits of antimicrobial use and ways to prevent the emergence and spread of resistance; 2) development and implementation of principles for appropriate antimicrobial drug use in the production of food animals and plants; 3) improved animal husbandry and food production practices to reduce the spread of infection; and 4) a regulatory framework to address the need for antimicrobial drug use in agriculture and veterinary medicine while ensuring that such use does not pose a risk to human health.

Comprehensive, multifaceted programs involving a wide variety of nonfederal partners and the public are required to prevent and control AR. The AR Task Force agencies will ensure ongoing input from, review by, and collaboration with nonfederal partners. The appropriate agencies will support demonstration projects that use multiple interventions to prevent and control AR (e.g., through surveillance, appropriate drug use, optimized diagnostic testing, immunization practice, and infection control). The Task Force agencies will encourage the incorporation of effective programs into routine practice by implementing model programs in federal health care systems and promoting the inclusion of AR prevention and control activities as part of quality assurance and accreditation standards for health care delivery nationwide.

Research

Understanding the fundamental processes involved in antimicrobial resistance within microbes and the resulting impact on humans, animals, and the environment forms an important basis for influencing and changing these processes and outcomes. Basic and clinical research provides the fundamental knowledge necessary to develop appropriate responses to antimicrobial resistance emerging and spreading in hospitals, communities, farms, and the food supply. Priority Goals and Action Items in this focus area address ways to:

- Increase understanding of microbial physiology, ecology, genetics, and mechanisms of resistance;
- Augment the existing research infrastructure to support a critical mass of researchers in AR and related fields; and
- Translate research findings into clinically useful products, such as novel approaches to detecting, preventing, and treating antimicrobial-resistant infections.

Needs in the field of AR research will be identified and addressed through a government-wide program review with external input. Additional research is needed, for example, on the epidemiology of resistance genes; on mechanisms of AR emergence, acquisition, spread, and persistence; and on the effects of antibiotics used as agricultural growth promoters on microbes that live in animals, humans, plants, soil, and water. Further study is also required to determine whether variations in drug use regimens may stimulate or reduce AR emergence and spread. Improved understanding of the causes of AR emergence will lead to the development of tools for reducing microbial resistance, as well as for predicting where AR problems are likely to arise.

A comprehensive research infrastructure will help ensure a critical mass of AR researchers who will interact, exchange information, and stimulate new discoveries. This aim will be achieved through the appropriate strategies and scientific conferences that promote research on AR. The AR Task

Force agencies will work with the academic and industrial research communities to attract AR researchers, prioritize needs, identify key opportunities, and optimize the utilization of resources to address AR problems.

The translation of research findings into innovative clinical products to treat, prevent, or diagnose drug-resistant infections is an area in which the federal government can play an important role, focusing on gaps not filled by the pharmaceutical industry or by other nongovernment groups. Special efforts will be placed on the identification, development, and testing of rapid, inexpensive, point-of-care diagnostic methods to facilitate appropriate use of antimicrobials. The AR Task Force agencies will also encourage basic research and clinical testing of diagnostic methods, novel treatment approaches, new vaccines, and other prevention approaches for resistant infections.

Product Development

As antimicrobial drugs lose their effectiveness, new products must be developed to prevent, rapidly diagnose, and treat infections. The Priority Goals and Action Items in this focus area address ways to:

- Ensure that researchers and drug manufacturers are informed of current and projected gaps in the arsenal of antimicrobial drugs, vaccines, and diagnostics and of potential markets for these products (designated here as "AR products");
- Stimulate the development of priority AR products for which market incentives are inadequate, while fostering their appropriate use; and
- Optimize the development and use of veterinary drugs and related agricultural products that reduce the transfer of resistance to pathogens that can infect humans.

Current and projected gaps in the arsenal of AR products and potential markets for these products will be reported to researchers and drug manufacturers through an interagency working group convened to identify and publicize priority public health needs.

The development of urgently needed AR products will be stimulated throughout the process from drug discovery through licensing. The regulatory process for AR products will continue to be streamlined, and incentives that promote the production and appropriate use of priority AR products can be evaluated in pilot programs that monitor costs and assess the return on the public investment.

The production of veterinary AR products that reduce the risk of development and transfer of resistance to drugs used in human clinical medicine will be expedited through a streamlined regulatory and approval process. As with drugs for the treatment of human infections, pilot programs can be initiated to evaluate incentives that encourage the development and appropriate use of priority products that meet critical animal and plant health needs.

Private and public partners will also evaluate ways to improve or reduce the agricultural use of particular antimicrobial drugs, as well as ways to prevent infection, such as the use of veterinary vaccines, changes in animal husbandry, and the use of competitive exclusion products (i.e., treatments that affect the intestinal flora of food animals).

TOP PRIORITY ACTION ITEMS TO COMBAT ANTIMICROBIAL RESISTANCE

(All 13 items have top priority, regardless of their order in the list.)

Surveillance

- With partners, design and implement a national AR surveillance plan that defines national, regional, state, and local surveillance activities and the roles of clinical, reference, public health, and veterinary laboratories. The plan should be consistent with local and national surveillance methodology and infrastructure that currently exist or are being developed. (Action Item #2)
- Develop and implement procedures for monitoring patterns of antimicrobial drug use in human medicine, agriculture, veterinary medicine, and consumer products. (Action Item #5)

Prevention and Control

- Conduct a public health education campaign to promote appropriate antimicrobial use as a national health priority. (Action Item #25)
- In collaboration with many partners, develop and facilitate the implementation of educational and behavioral interventions that will assist clinicians in appropriate antimicrobial prescribing. (Action Item #26)
- Evaluate the effectiveness (including cost-effectiveness) of current and novel infection-control practices for health care and extended care settings and in the community. Promote adherence to practices proven to be effective. (Action Item #39)
- In consultation with stakeholders, refine and implement the proposed FDA framework for approving new antimicrobial drugs for use in

food-animal production and, when appropriate, for re-evaluating currently approved veterinary antimicrobial drugs. (Action Item #58)

- Support demonstration projects to evaluate comprehensive strategies that use multiple interventions to promote appropriate drug use and reduce infection rates, in order to assess how interventions found effective in research studies can be applied routinely and most cost-effectively on a large scale. (Action Item #63)

Research

- Provide the research community genomics and other powerful technologies to identify targets in critical areas for the development of new, rapid diagnostics methodologies, novel therapeutics, and interventions to prevent the emergence and spread of resistant pathogens. (Action Item #70)
- In consultation with academia and the private sector, identify and conduct human clinical studies addressing AR issues of public health significance that are unlikely to be studied in the private sector (e.g., novel therapies, new treatment regimens, and other products and practices). (Action Item #75)
- Identify, develop, test, and evaluate new rapid diagnostic methods for human and veterinary uses with partners, including academia and the private sector. Such methods should be accurate, affordable, and easily implemented in routine clinical settings (e.g., tests for resistance genes, point-of-care diagnostics for patients with respiratory infections and syndromes, and diagnostics for drug resistance in microbial pathogens, including in nonculture specimens). (Action Item #76)
- Encourage basic and clinical research in support of the development and appropriate use of vaccines in human and veterinary medicine in partnership with academia and the private sector. (Action Item #77)

Product Development

- Create an Interagency AR Product Development Working Group to identify and publicize priority public health needs in human and animal medicine for new AR products (e.g., innovative drugs, targeted spectrum antibiotics, point-of-care diagnostics, vaccines and other biologics, anti-infective medical devices, and disinfectants). (Action Item #79)
- Identify ways (e.g., financial and/or other incentives or investments) to promote the development and/or appropriate use of priority AR products, such as novel compounds and approaches, for human and veterinary medicine for which market incentives are inadequate. (Action Item #80)

Appendix G

Forum Member, Speaker, and Staff Biographies

FORUM MEMBERS

ADEL A.F. MAHMOUD, M.D., Ph.D., *(Chair),* is President of Merck Vaccines at Merck & Co., Inc. He formerly served Case Western Reserve University and University Hospitals of Cleveland as Chairman of Medicine and Physician-in-Chief from 1987 to 1998. Prior to that, Dr. Mahmoud held several positions, spanning 25 years, at the same institutions. Dr. Mahmoud and his colleagues conducted pioneering investigations on the biology and function of eosinophils. He prepared the first specific anti-eosinophil serum, which was used to define the role of these cells in host resistance to helminthic infections. Dr. Mahmoud also established clinical and laboratory investigations in several developing countries, including Kenya, Egypt, and The Philippines, to examine the determinants of infection and disease in schistosomiasis and other infectious agents. This work led to the development of innovative strategies to control those infections, which have been adopted by the World Health Organization (WHO) as selective population chemotherapy. In recent years, Dr. Mahmoud turned his attention to developing a comprehensive set of responses to the problems associated with emerging infections in the developing world. He was elected to membership of the American Society for Clinical Investigation in 1978, the Association of American Physicians in 1980, and the Institute of Medicine of the National Academy of Sciences in 1987. He received the Bailey K. Ashford Award of the American Society of Tropical Medicine and Hygiene in 1983, and the Squibb Award of the Infectious Diseases Society of America in 1984. Dr. Mahmoud currently serves as Chair of the Forum on Emerging Infections and is a member of the Board on Global Health, both of the Institute of Medicine. He also chairs the U.S. Delegation to the U.S.-Japan Cooperative Medical Science Program.

STANLEY M. LEMON, M.D., *(Vice-Chair),* is Dean of the School of Medicine at the University of Texas Medical Branch at Galveston. He received his undergraduate degree in biochemical sciences from Princeton University summa cum laude, and his M.D. with honors from the University of Rochester. He completed postgraduate training in internal medicine and infectious diseases at the University of North Carolina at Chapel Hill, and is board-certified in both. From 1977 to 1983, he served with the U.S. Army Medical Research and Development Command, directing the Hepatitis Laboratory at the Walter Reed Army Institute of Research. He joined the faculty of the University of North Carolina School of Medicine in 1983, serving first as Chief of the Division of Infectious Diseases, and then Vice Chair for Research of the Department of Medicine. In 1997, Dr. Lemon moved to the University of Texas Medical Branch as Professor and Chair of the Department of Microbiology & Immunology. He was subsequently appointed Dean *pro tem* of the School of Medicine in 1999, and permanent Dean of Medicine in 2000. Dr. Lemon's research interests relate to the molecular virology and pathogenesis of the positive-stranded RNA viruses responsible for hepatitis C and hepatitis A. He is particularly interested in the molecular mechanisms controlling replication of these RNA genomes and related mechanisms of disease pathogenesis. He has published over 180 papers, and numerous textbook chapters related to hepatitis and other viral infections, and has a longstanding interest in vaccine development. He has served previously as chair of the Anti-Infective Drugs Advisory Committee and the Vaccines and Related Biologics Advisory Committee of the U.S. Food and Drug Administration, and is past chair of the Steering Committee on Hepatitis and Poliomyelitis of WHO's Programme on Vaccine Development. He presently serves as Chairman of the U.S. Hepatitis Panel of the U.S.-Japan Cooperative Medical Sciences Program, and recently chaired an Institute of Medicine study committee related to vaccines for the protection of the military against naturally occurring infectious disease threats.

DAVID ACHESON, M.D., is Chief Medical Officer at the Center for Food Safety and Applied Nutrition, U.S. Food and Drug Administration. He received his medical degree at the University of London. After completing internships in general surgery and medicine, he continued his postdoctoral training in Manchester, England, as a Wellcome Trust Research Fellow. He subsequently was a Wellcome Trust Training Fellow in Infectious Diseases at the New England Medical Center and at the Wellcome Research Unit in Vellore, India. Dr. Acheson was Associate

Professor of Medicine, Division of Geographic Medicine and Infectious Diseases, New England Medical Center until 2001. He then joined the faculties of the Department of Epidemiology and Preventive Medicine and Department of Microbiology and Immunology at the University of Maryland Medical School. Currently at the FDA, his research concentration is on foodborne pathogens and encompasses a mixture of molecular pathogenesis, cell biology, and epidemiology. Specifically, his research focuses on Shiga toxin-producing *E. coli* and understanding toxin interaction with intestinal epithelial cells using tissue culture models. His laboratory has also undertaken a study to examine Shiga toxin-producing *E. coli* in food animals in relation to virulence factors and antimicrobial resistance patterns. More recently, Dr. Acheson initiated a project to understand the molecular pathogenesis of *Campylobacter jejuni.* Other studies have undertaken surveillance of diarrheal disease in the community to determine causes, outcomes, and risk factors of unexplained diarrhea. Dr. Acheson has authored/co-authored over 72 journal articles and 42 book chapters and reviews, and is coauthor of the book *Safe Eating* (Dell Health, 1998). He is reviewer of more than 10 journals and is on the editorial board of *Infection and Immunity* and *Clinical Infectious Diseases*. Dr. Acheson is a Fellow of the Royal College of Physicians, a Fellow of the Infectious Disease Society of America, and holds several patents.

STEVEN J. BRICKNER, Ph.D., is Research Advisor, Antibacterials Chemistry, at Pfizer Global Research and Development. He received his Ph.D. in organic chemistry from Cornell University and was a NIH Postdoctoral Research Fellow at the University of Wisconsin-Madison. Dr. Brickner is a medicinal chemist with nearly 20 years of research experience in the pharmaceutical industry, all focused on the discovery and development of novel antibacterial agents. He is an inventor/co-inventor on 21 U.S. patents, and has published numerous scientific papers, primarily within the area of the oxazolidinones. Prior to joining Pfizer in 1996, he led a team at Pharmacia and Upjohn that discovered and developed linezolid, the first member of a new class of antibiotics to be approved in the last 35 years.

GAIL H. CASSELL, Ph.D., is Vice President, Scientific Affairs, Distinguished Lilly Research Scholar for Infectious Diseases, Eli Lilly & Company. Previously, she was the Charles H. McCauley Professor and (since 1987) Chair, Department of Microbiology, University of Alabama Schools of Medicine and Dentistry at Birmingham, a department which, under her leadership, has ranked first in research funding from the National Institutes of Health since 1989. She is a member of the Director's Advisory Committee of the Centers for Disease Control and Prevention. Dr. Cassell is past president of the American Society for Microbiology (ASM) and is serving her third three-year term as chairman of the Public and Scientific Affairs Board of ASM. She is a former member of the National Institutes of

Health Director's Advisory Committee and a former member of the Advisory Council of the National Institute of Allergy and Infectious Diseases. She has also served as an advisor on infectious diseases and indirect costs of research to the White House Office on Science and Technology and was previously chair of the Board of Scientific Counselors of the National Center for Infectious Diseases, Centers for Disease Control and Prevention. Dr. Cassell served eight years on the Bacteriology-Mycology-II Study Section and served as its chair for three years. She serves on the editorial boards of several prestigious scientific journals and has authored over 275 articles and book chapters. She has been intimately involved in the establishment of science policy and legislation related to biomedical research and public health. Dr. Cassell has received several national and international awards and an honorary degree for her research on infectious diseases.

GORDON DEFRIESE, Ph.D., is Professor of Social Medicine and Professor of Medicine (in the Division of General Medicine and Clinical Epidemiology) at the UNC-CH School of Medicine. In addition, he holds appointments as Professor of Epidemiology and Health Policy and Administration in the UNC-CH School of Public Health and as Professor of Dental Ecology in the UNC-CH School of Dentistry. From 1986–2000, he served as Co-Director of the Robert Wood Johnson Clinical Scholars Program, cosponsored by the UNC-CH School of Medicine and the Cecil G. Sheps Center for Health Services Research. He received his Ph.D. from the University of Kentucky College of Medicine. Some of his research interests are in the areas of health promotion and disease prevention, medical sociology, primary health care, rural health care, cost-benefit analysis, and cost-effectiveness. He is a past president of the Association for Health Services Research and a fellow of the New York Academy of Medicine. He is founder of the Partnership for Prevention, a coalition of private-sector business and industry organizations, voluntary health organizations, and state and federal public health agencies based in Washington, D.C. that have joined together to work toward the elevation of disease prevention among the nation's health policy priorities. He is an at-large member of the National Board of Medical Examiners. Since 1994 he has served as President and CEO of the North Carolina Institute of Medicine. He is Editor-in-Chief and Publisher of the *North Carolina Medical Journal*.

CEDRIC E. DUMONT, M.D., is Medical Director for the Office of Medical Services (MED) at the U.S. Department of State. Dr. Dumont graduated from Columbia University with a B.A. in 1975 and obtained his medical degree from Tufts University School of Medicine in 1980. Dr. Dumont is a board-certified internist with subspecialty training in infectious diseases. He completed his internal medicine residency in 1983 and infectious diseases fellowship in 1988 at Georgetown University Hospital in Washington, D.C. Dr. Dumont has been a medical practitioner for over 22 years, 2 of which included service in the Peace Corps. Since joining the Department of State in 1990, he has had substantial experience overseas in Dakar, Bamako, Kinshasa, and Brazzaville. For the past 6 years, as the Medical Director for the Department of State, Dr. Dumont has promoted the health of all United States government employees serving overseas by encouraging their participation in a comprehensive health maintenance program and by facilitating their access to high-quality medical care. Dr. Dumont is a very strong supporter of the professional development and advancement of MED's highly qualified professional staff. In addition, he has supported and encouraged the use of an electronic medical record, which will be able to monitor the health of all its beneficiaries, not only during a specific assignment but also throughout their career in the Foreign Service. In the aftermath of the bombings in Nairobi and Dar es Salaam, Dr. Dumont has led in the development and implementation of a comprehensive medical response plan to terrorist attacks on USG missions overseas, including events involving chemical and biological weapons. He also has initiated the development and implementation of a Health Promotion and Wellness program designed for all Department employees and family members.

JESSE L. GOODMAN, M.D., M.P.H., was professor of medicine and Chief of Infectious Diseases at the University of Minnesota, and is now serving as Deputy Director for the U.S. Food and Drug Administration's (FDA) Center for Biologics Evaluation and Research, where he is active in a broad range of scientific, public health, and policy issues. After joining the FDA commissioner's office, he has worked closely with several centers and helped coordinate FDA's response to the antimicrobial resistance problem. He was co-chair of a recently formed federal interagency task force which developed the national Public Health Action Plan on antimicrobial resistance. He graduated from Harvard College and attended the Albert Einstein College of Medicine followed by internal medicine, hematology, oncology, and infectious diseases training at the University of Pennsylvania and University of California Los Angeles, where he was also chief medical resident. He received his master's of public health from the University of Minnesota. He has been active in community public health activities, including creating an environmental health partnership in St. Paul, Minnesota. In recent years, his laboratory's research has focused on the molecular pathogenesis of tickborne diseases. His laboratory isolated the etiological intracellular agent of the emerging tickborne infection, human granulocytic ehrlichiosis, and identified its leukocyte receptor. He has also been an active clinician and teacher and has directed or participated in major multi-center clinical studies. He is a Fellow of the Infectious Diseases Society of America and, among several honors, has been elected to the American Society for Clinical Investigation.

RENU GUPTA, M.D., is Vice President and Head, U.S. Clinical Research and Development at Novartis Pharmaceuticals. Previously, she was Vice President, Medical, Safety, and Therapeutics at Covance. Dr. Gupta is a board-certified pediatrician, with subspecialty training in Infectious Diseases from Children's Hospital of Philadelphia and the University of Pennsylvania. She was also Postdoctoral Research Fellow in Microbiology at the University of Pennsylvania and the Wistar Institute of Anatomy and Biology, where she conducted research on the pathogenesis of infectious diseases. Dr. Gupta received her M.B., Ch.B with distinction from the University of Zambia, where she examined the problem of poor compliance in the treatment of tuberculosis in rural and urban Africa. She is currently active in a number of professional societies, including the Infectious Diseases Society of America and the American Society of Microbiology. She is a frequent presenter at the Interscience Conference on Antimicrobial Agents and Chemotherapy and other major congresses, and has been published in leading infectious diseases periodicals. From 1989 to mid-1998, Dr. Gupta was with Bristol-Myers Squibb Company, where she directed clinical research as well as strategic planning for the Infectious Diseases and Immunology Divisions. For the past several years, her work has focused on a better understanding of the problem of emerging infections. This has led to her pioneering efforts in establishing the Global Antimicrobial Surveillance Program, SENTRY, a private-academic-public sector partnership. Dr. Gupta chaired the steering committee for the SENTRY Antimicrobial Surveillance Program. She remains active in women's and children's health issues, and is currently furthering education and outreach initiatives. More recently, Dr. Gupta has been instrumental in the formation of the Harvard-Pharma Management Board, of which she is a member, to further the educational goals of the Scholars in Clinical Science Program at the Harvard Medical School.

MARGARET A. HAMBURG, M.D., is Vice President for Biological Programs at Nuclear Threat Initiative (NTI), a charitable organization working to reduce the global threat from nuclear, biological, and chemical weapons. Dr. Hamburg is in charge of the biological program area. Before taking on her current position, Dr. Hamburg was the Assistant Secretary for Planning and Evaluation, U.S. Department of Health and Human Services, serving as a principal policy advisor to the Secretary of Health and Human Services with responsibilities including policy formulation and analysis, the development and review of regulations and/or legislation, budget analysis, strategic planning, and the conduct and coordination of policy research and program evaluation. Prior to this, she served for almost six years as the Commissioner of Health for the City of New York. As chief health officer in the nation's largest city, Dr. Hamburg's many accomplishments included the design and implementation of an internationally recognized tuberculosis control program that produced dramatic declines in tuberculosis cases; the development of initiatives that raised childhood immunization rates to record levels; and the creation of the first public health bioterrorism preparedness program in the nation. She completed her internship and residency in Internal Medicine at the New York Hospital/Cornell University Medical Center and is certified by the American Board of Internal Medicine. Dr. Hamburg is a graduate of Harvard College and Harvard Medical School. She currently serves on the Harvard University Board of Overseers. She has been elected to membership in the Institute of Medicine, the New York Academy of Medicine, and the Council on Foreign Relations, and is a Fellow of the American Association for the Advancement of Science and the American College of Physicians.

CAROLE A. HEILMAN, Ph.D., is Director of the Division of Microbiology and Infectious Diseases (DMID) of the National Institute of Allergy and Infectious Diseases (NIAID). Dr. Heilman received her bachelor's degree in biology from Boston University in 1972, and earned her master's degree and doctorate in microbiology from Rutgers University in 1976 and 1979, respectively. Dr. Heilman began her career at the National Institutes of Health as a postdoctoral research associate with the National Cancer Institute where she carried out research on the regulation of gene expression during cancer development. In 1986, she came to NIAID as the influenza and viral respiratory diseases program officer in DMID and, in 1988, she was appointed chief of the respiratory diseases branch where she coordinated the development of acellular pertussis vaccines. She joined the Division of AIDS as deputy director in 1997 and was responsible for developing the Innovation Grant Program for Approaches in HIV Vaccine Research. She is the recipient of several notable awards for outstanding achievement. Throughout her extramural career, Dr. Heilman has contributed articles on vaccine design and development to many scientific journals and has served as a consultant to the World Bank and WHO in this area. She is also a member of several professional societies, including the Infectious Diseases Society of America, the American Society for Microbiology, and the American Society of Virology.

DAVID L. HEYMANN, M.D., is currently the Executive Director of the World Health Organization (WHO) Communicable Diseases Cluster. From October 1995 to July 1998 he was Director of the WHO Programme on Emerging and Other Communicable Diseases Surveillance and Control. Prior to becoming director of this program, he was the chief of research activities in the Global Programme on AIDS. From 1976 to 1989, prior to joining WHO, Dr Heymann spent 13 years working as a medical epidemiologist in sub-Saharan Africa (Cameroon, Ivory Coast, the former Zaire, and Malawi) on assignment from the Centers for Disease Control and Prevention (CDC) in CDC-supported activities aimed at strengthening capacity in surveillance of infectious diseases and their control, with special emphasis on the childhood immunizable diseases, African hemorrhagic fevers, pox viruses, and malaria. While based in Africa, Dr. Heymann participated in the investigation of the first outbreak of Ebola in Yambuku (former Zaire) in 1976, then again investigated the second outbreak of Ebola in 1977 in Tandala, and in 1995 directed the international response to the Ebola outbreak in Kikwit. Prior to 1976, Dr. Heymann spent two years in India as a medical officer in the WHO Smallpox Eradication Programme. Dr. Heymann holds a B.A. from the Pennsylvania State University, an M.D. from Wake Forest University, and a Diploma in Tropical Medicine and Hygiene from the London School of Hygiene and Tropical Medicine, and completed practical epidemiology training in the Epidemic Intelligence Service (EIS) training program of the CDC. He has published 131 scientific articles on infectious diseases in peer-reviewed medical and scientific journals.

JAMES M. HUGHES, M.D., received his B.A. in 1966 and M.D. in 1971 from Stanford University. He completed a residency in internal medicine at the University of Washington and a fellowship in infectious diseases at the University of Virginia. He is board-certified in internal medicine, infectious diseases, and preventive medicine. He first joined CDC as an Epidemic Intelligence Service officer in 1973. During his CDC career, he has worked primarily in the areas of foodborne disease and infection control in health care settings. He became Director of the National Center for Infectious Diseases in 1992. The center is currently working to address domestic and global challenges posed by emerging infectious diseases and the threat of bioterrorism. He is a member of the Institute of Medicine and a fellow of the American College of Physicians, the Infectious Diseases Society of America, and the American Association for the Advancement of Science. He is an Assistant Surgeon General in the Public Health Service.

SAMUEL L. KATZ, M.D., is Wilburt C. Davison Professor and chairman emeritus of pediatrics at Duke University Medical Center. He has concentrated his research on infectious diseases, focusing primarily on vaccine research, development, and policy. Dr. Katz has served on a number of scientific advisory committees and is the recipient of many prestigious awards and honorary fellowships in international organizations. He attained his M.D. from Harvard Medical School and completed his residency training at Boston hospitals. He became a staff member at Children's Hospital, working with Nobel laureate John Enders, during which time they developed the attenuated measles virus vaccine now used throughout the world. He has chaired the Committee on Infectious Diseases of the American Academy of Pediatrics (the Redbook Committee), the Advisory Committee on Immunization Practices (ACIP) of the Centers for Disease Control and Prevention, the Vaccine Priorities Study of the Institute of

Medicine (IOM), and several WHO and Children's Vaccine Initiative panels on vaccines. He is a member of many scientific advisory committees including those of the NIH, IOM, and WHO. Dr. Katz's published studies include abundant original scientific articles, chapters in textbooks, and many abstracts, editorials, and reviews. He is the coeditor of a textbook on pediatric infectious diseases and has given many named lectures in the United States and abroad. Currently he co-chairs the Indo-U.S. Vaccine Action Program as well as the National Network for Immunization Information (NNii).

COLONEL PATRICK KELLEY, M.D., M.P.H., Dr.P.H., is Director of the Department of Defense Global Emerging Infections System and the Director of the Division of Preventive Medicine at the Walter Reed Army Institute of Research (WRAIR), Silver Spring, Maryland. He obtained his M.D. from the University of Virginia and a Dr.P.H. in infectious disease epidemiology from the Johns Hopkins Bloomberg School of Public Health. He is board-certified in general preventive medicine and a fellow of the American College of Preventive Medicine. For many years he directed the Army General Preventive Medicine Residency at WRAIR. Colonel Kelley has extensive experience leading military infectious disease studies and in managing domestic and international public health surveillance efforts. He has spoken before professional audiences in over 15 countries and has authored or co-authored over 50 scientific papers and book chapters on a variety of infectious disease and preventive medicine topics. He serves as the specialty editor for a textbook entitled, *Military Preventive Medicine: Mobilization and Deployment.*

MARCELLE LAYTON, M.D., is the Assistant Commissioner for the Bureau of Communicable Diseases at the New York City Department of Health. This bureau is responsible for the surveillance and control of 62 infectious diseases and conditions reportable under the New York City Health Code. Current areas of concern include antibiotic resistance; foodborne, waterborne, and tickborne diseases; hepatitis C; and biological disaster planning for the potential threats of bioterrorism and pandemic influenza. Dr. Layton received her medical degree from Duke University. She completed an internal medicine residency at the University Health Science Center in Syracuse, New York, and an infectious disease fellowship at Yale University. In addition, Dr. Layton spent two years with the Centers for Disease Control and Prevention as a fellow in the Epidemic Intelligence Service, where she was assigned to the New York City Department of Health. In the past, she has volunteered or worked with the Indian Health Service, the Alaskan Native Health Service, and clinics in northwestern Thailand and central Nepal.

JOSHUA LEDERBERG, Ph.D., is Professor emeritus of Molecular Genetics and Informatics and Sackler Foundation Scholar at The Rockefeller

University, New York, New York. His lifelong research, for which he received the Nobel Prize in 1958, has been in genetic structure and function in microorganisms. He has a keen interest in international health and was co-chair of a previous Institute of Medicine Committee on Emerging Microbial Threats to Health (1990–1992) and currently is co-chair of the Committee on Emerging Microbial Threats to Health in the 21st Century. He has been a member of the National Academy of Sciences since 1957 and is a charter member of the Institute of Medicine.

CARLOS LOPEZ, Ph.D., is Research Fellow, Research Acquisitions, Eli Lilly Research Laboratories. He received his Ph.D. from the University of Minnesota in 1970. Dr. Lopez was awarded the NTRDA postdoctoral fellowship. After his fellowship he was appointed assistant professor of pathology at the University of Minnesota, where he did his research on cytomegalovirus infections in renal transplant recipients and the consequences of those infections. He was next appointed assistant member and head of the Laboratory of Herpesvirus Infections at the Sloan Kettering Institute for Cancer Research, where his research focused on herpes virus infections and the resistance mechanisms involved. Dr. Lopez's laboratory contributed to the immunological analysis of the earliest AIDS patients at the beginning of the AIDS epidemic in New York. He is co-author of one of the seminal publications on this disease, as well as many scientific papers, and co-editor of six books. Dr. Lopez has been a consultant to numerous agencies and organizations including the National Institutes of Health, the Department of Veterans Affairs, and the American Cancer Society.

LYNN MARKS, M.D., is board-certified in internal medicine and infectious diseases. He was on faculty at the University of South Alabama College of Medicine in the Infectious Diseases department focusing on patient care, teaching, and research. His academic research interest was on the molecular genetics of bacterial pathogenicity. He subsequently joined SmithKline Beecham's (now GlaxoSmithKline) anti-infectives clinical group and later progressed to global head of the Consumer Healthcare division Medical and Regulatory group. He then returned to pharmaceutical research and development as global head of the Infectious Diseases Therapeutic Area Strategy Team for GlaxoSmithKline.

STEPHEN S. MORSE, Ph.D., is Director of the Center for Public Health Preparedness at the Mailman School of Public Health of Columbia University, and a faculty member in the Epidemiology Department. Dr. Morse recently returned to Columbia from four years in government service as Program Manager at the Defense Advanced Research Projects Agency (DARPA), where he co-directed the Pathogen Countermeasures program and subsequently directed the Advanced Diagnostics program. Before coming to Columbia, he was Assistant Professor (Virology) at The Rockefeller University in New York, where he remains an adjunct faculty member. Dr. Morse is the editor of two books, *Emerging Viruses* (Oxford University Press, 1993; paperback, 1996) (selected by *American Scientist* for its list of "100 Top Science Books of the 20th Century"), and *The Evolutionary Biology of Viruses* (Raven Press, 1994). He currently serves as a Section Editor of the CDC journal *Emerging Infectious Diseases* and was formerly an Editor-in-Chief of the Pasteur Institute's journal *Research in Virology*. Dr. Morse was Chair and principal organizer of the 1989 NIAID/NIH Conference on Emerging Viruses (for which he originated the term and concept of emerging viruses/infections); served as a member of the Institute of Medicine-National Academy of Sciences' Committee on Emerging Microbial Threats to Health (and chaired its Task Force on Viruses), and was a contributor to its report, *Emerging Infections* (1992); was a member of the IOM's Committee on Xenograft Transplantation; currently serves on the Steering Committee of the Institute of Medicine's Forum on Emerging Infections, and has served as an adviser to WHO, PAHO (Pan-American Health Organization), FDA, the Defense Threat Reduction Agency (DTRA), and other agencies. He is a Fellow of the New York Academy of Sciences and a past Chair of its Microbiology Section. He was the founding Chair of ProMED (the nonprofit international Program to Monitor Emerging Diseases) and was one of the originators of ProMED-mail, an international network inaugurated by ProMED in 1994 for outbreak reporting and disease monitoring using the Internet. Dr. Morse received his Ph.D. from the University of Wisconsin-Madison.

MICHAEL T. OSTERHOLM, Ph.D., M.P.H., is Director of the Center for Infectious Disease Research and Policy at the University of Minnesota where he is also Professor at the School of Public Health. Previously, Dr. Osterholm was the state epidemiologist and Chief of the Acute Disease Epidemiology Section for the Minnesota Department of Health. He has received numerous research awards from the National Institute of Allergy and Infectious Diseases and the Centers for Disease Control and Prevention (CDC). He served as principal investigator for the CDC-sponsored Emerging Infections Program in Minnesota. He has published more than 240 articles and abstracts on various emerging infectious disease problems and is the author of the best selling book, *Living Terrors: What America Needs to Know to Survive the Coming Bioterrorist Catastrophe*. He is past president of the Council of State and Territorial Epidemiologists. He currently serves on the National Academy of Sciences, Institute of Medicine (IOM) Forum on Emerging Infections. He has also served on the IOM Committee, Food Safety, Production to Consumption and the IOM Committee on the Department of Defense Persian Gulf Syndrome Comprehensive Clinical Evaluation Program, and as a reviewer for the IOM report on chemical and biological terrorism.

GARY A. ROSELLE, M.D., received his M.D. from Ohio State

University School of Medicine in 1973. He served his residency at Northwestern University School of Medicine and his Infectious Diseases fellowship at the University of Cincinnati School of Medicine. Dr. Roselle is the Program Director for Infectious Diseases for the VA Central Office in Washington, D.C., as well as the Chief of the Medical Service at the Cincinnati VA Medical Center. He is a professor of medicine in the Department of Internal Medicine, Division of Infectious Diseases at the University of Cincinnati College of Medicine. Dr. Roselle serves on several national advisory committees. In addition, he is currently heading the Emerging Pathogens Initiative for the Department of Veterans Affairs. Dr. Roselle has received commendations from the Cincinnati Medical Center Director, the Under Secretary for Health for the Department of Veterans Affairs, and the Secretary of Veterans Affairs for his work in the infectious diseases program for the Department of Veterans Affairs. He has been an invited speaker at several national and international meetings, and has published over 80 papers and several book chapters.

DAVID M. SHLAES, M.D., Ph.D., is Executive Vice President for Research and Development at Idenix Pharmaceuticals. Previously, he spent six years as Vice President and Therapeutic Area Co-Leader for Infectious Diseases at Wyeth Research. Before joining Wyeth, Dr. Shlaes was professor of medicine at the Case Western Reserve University School of Medicine and chief of the Infectious Diseases Section and the Clinical Microbiology Unit at the Veterans Affairs Medical Center in Cleveland, Ohio. His major research interest has been the mechanisms and epidemiology of antimicrobial resistance in bacteria, in which area he has published widely. He has recently become more involved in the area of public policy as it relates to the discovery and development of antibiotics. He has served on the Institute of Medicine's Forum on Emerging Infections since 1996.

JANET SHOEMAKER is director of the American Society for Microbiology's Public Affairs Office, a position she has held since 1989. She is responsible for managing the legislative and regulatory affairs of this 42,000-member organization, the largest single biological science society in the world. She has served as principal investigator for a project funded by the National Science Foundation (NSF) to collect and disseminate data on the job market for recent doctorates in microbiology and has played a key role in American Society for Microbiology (ASM) projects, including the production of the ASM *Employment Outlook in the Microbiological Sciences* and *The Impact of Managed Care and Health System Change on Clinical Microbiology*. Previously, she held positions as Assistant Director of Public Affairs for ASM, as ASM coordinator of the U.S./U.S.S.R. Exchange Program in Microbiology, a program sponsored and coordinated by the National Science Foundation and the U.S. Department of State, and as a freelance editor and writer. She received her baccalaureate, cum laude, from the University of Massachusetts, and is a graduate of the George Washington University programs in public policy and in editing and publications. She has served as commissioner to the Commission on Professionals in Science and Technology, and as the ASM representative to the ad hoc Group for Medical Research Funding, and is a member of Women in Government Relations, the American Society of Association Executives, and the American Association for the Advancement of Science. She has co-authored published articles on research funding, biotechnology, biological weapons control, and public policy issues related to microbiology.

P. FREDERICK SPARLING, M.D., is J. Herbert Bate Professor emeritus of Medicine, Microbiology and Immunology at the University of North Carolina (UNC) at Chapel Hill, and is Director of the North Carolina Sexually Transmitted Infections Research Center. Previously, he served as chair of the Department of Medicine and chair of the Department of Microbiology and Immunology at UNC. He was president of the Infectious Disease Society of America in 1996–1997. He was also a member of the Institute of Medicine's Committee on Microbial Threats to Health (1991–1992). Dr. Sparling's laboratory research is in the molecular biology of bacterial outer membrane proteins involved in pathogenesis, with a major emphasis on gonococci and meningococci. His current studies focus on the biochemistry and genetics of iron-scavenging mechanisms used by gonococci and meningococci and the structure and function of the gonococcal porin proteins. He is pursuing the goal of a vaccine for gonorrhea.

MICHAEL ZEILINGER, D.P.M., M.P.H., is Infectious Disease Team Leader at the Office of Health and Nutrition, Environmental Health Division at the U.S. Agency for International Development. Dr. Zeilinger serves as the senior advisor and manager of the infectious disease strategic objective team which encompasses four sub-teams: malaria, tuberculosis, antimicrobial resistance, and surveillance. He is also the Cognizant Technical Officer for USAID's umbrella Inter-Agency Agreement with the Centers for Disease Control and Prevention. Prior to his work at USAID/W, Dr. Zeilinger was the Program Director for Project HOPE in the Central Asian republics, which included public and private sector-funded TB control projects in Kazakhstan, Uzbekistan, Kyrgyzstan, and Turkmenistan. His work in Central Asia also included humanitarian assistance and child survival programs. Prior to that, he worked with Birch and Davis on the Department of Defense's Military Health Service System, and the Public Health Foundation on a U.S. Department of Health and Human Services-funded Empowerment Zones/Enterprise Communities Health Benchmarks Demonstration Project. Dr. Zeilinger is a Doctor of Podiatric Medicine and managed several community health programs during his surgical residency. He also has a master's degree in public health (International Health

Promotion) from The George Washington University and is currently an Adjunct Professor at their School of Public Health.

SPEAKERS

DAVID M. BELL, M.D., is Assistant to the Director for Antimicrobial Resistance, National Center for Infectious Diseases, Centers for Disease Control and Prevention (CDC), Atlanta. In this capacity, he coordinates CDC's efforts to address antimicrobial resistance. He is also co-chair of the U.S. Federal Interagency Task Force on Antimicrobial Resistance and clinical assistant professor of pediatric infectious diseases at Emory University School of Medicine, Atlanta. From 1987 to 1997, Dr. Bell directed CDC's efforts to assess and reduce the risk of HIV transmission to workers and patients in healthcare settings. Previously, he was Director of the Diagnostic Virology Laboratory at the University of Tennessee, Memphis, and practiced general pediatrics. He is co-author of 90 scientific publications and book chapters dealing with the public health, clinical, and laboratory aspects of infectious diseases. In 2000, he chaired the WHO Consultation to develop Global Principles for the Containment of Antimicrobial Resistance due to Antimicrobial Use in Animals Intended for Food. Dr. Bell graduated from Princeton University (A.B., 1973) and Harvard Medical School (M.D., 1977). His training included residency at Boston Children's Hospital, the Epidemic Intelligence Service Program at CDC, and fellowship in pediatric infectious diseases at the University of Rochester.

WILLIAM G. BROGDON, Ph.D., has been Chief of the Vector Biology and Toxicology Section, Entomology Branch, Division of Parasitic Diseases, National Center for Infectious Diseases, Centers for Disease Control and Prevention, since 1996. With over 24 years as a research entomologist with the CDC, Dr. Brogdon has developed an applied research program on insecticide resistance in arthropod vectors of disease. Studies have been conducted both in the United States and in 20 countries on insecticide resistance in Aedes, Culex, and Anopheles mosquito vectors. Dr. Brogdon has developed novel biological, biochemical, and molecular approaches to detecting insecticide resistance and its mechanisms in individual insects. With support from the Emerging Infectious Diseases program, he has operated a Resistance Surveillance Laboratory since 1995 and a WHO Collaborating Center on Insecticide Resistance. Dr. Brogdon has served as a member of the WHO Expert Committee on Vector Control.

THOMAS B. ELLIOTT, Ph.D., is a research microbiologist at The Armed Forces Radiobiology Research Institute, Bethesda, Maryland, where he has studied susceptibility to infectious agents and therapy for bacterial infections in irradiated animal models and the inactivation of bacteria and viruses by ionizing radiation. His work contributed to the recommended therapy for sepsis in victims of radiation accidents, development of combined therapy with non-specific biological response modifiers together with antimicrobial agents, and the discovery that pulmonary infections of *Bacillus anthracis* induce a unique polymicrobial sepsis following sub-lethal doses of gamma radiation. Dr. Elliott directs research projects for students in the Master of Public Health and the Laboratory Animal Medicine Residency programs in the Department of Preventive Medicine and Biometrics, Uniformed Services University of the Health Sciences. Previously, Dr. Elliott was a clinical chemist, performed industrial microbiological studies, and taught microbiology and immunology at The George Washington University and the Foundation for Advancement of Education in the Sciences, National Institutes of Health. He is currently serving on two advisory committees, which are coordinated by the Office of Science and Technology Policy, Executive Office of the President, on inactivation of microorganisms and the Interagency Working Committee on Test Methods and Surrogates for Anthrax, Environmental Protection Agency. He has participated on advisory committees, the Human Response Dose Committee, Defense Threat Reduction Agency; and U.S. Army Specific Military Requirements, U.S. Army Nuclear and Chemical Agency. Dr. Elliott is a member of the American Society for Microbiology and the Society of the Sigma Xi.

VINCENT A. FISCHETTI, Ph.D., has been a professor and chairman of the Laboratory of Bacterial Pathogenesis and Immunology at the Rockefeller University, New York, New York, since 1990. He is a fellow of the American Academy of Microbiology and the recipient of two NIH MERIT awards. He has been editor-in-chief of the scientific journal *Infection and Immunity* for 10 years, and serves as advisory editor for the *Journal of Experimental Medicine* and *Trends in Microbiology*. Dr. Fischetti serves on the scientific advisory board and as trustee of the Trudeau Institute. He has published approximately 130 primary research articles and 77 textbook chapters as well as being an inventor on over 37 issued patents. Dr. Fischetti received a Ph.D. in microbiology from New York University. His research career has been directed toward the understanding of infection by gram-positive bacteria. He has focused his attention on group A streptococcus and has developed new strategies to control infection by these bacteria. He currently has a vaccine in clinical trial to control strep infections and a novel target for antibiotic development being tested by a major pharmaceutical company. In recent years he has directed his attention to the use of bacteriophage lytic enzymes to control colonizing pathogenic bacteria, particularly those that are resistant to current antibiotics.

JULIE L. GERBERDING, M.D., M.P.H., is Director of the Centers for Disease Control and Prevention (CDC), an associate clinical professor of medicine (infectious diseases) at Emory University, and an associate professor of medicine (infectious diseases) and epidemiology and biostatistics at the University of California, San Francisco (UCSF). She earned her B.A. degree magna cum laude in chemistry and biology and M.D. degree at Case Western Reserve University and then completed her internship and residency in internal medicine at UCSF, where she also served as chief medical resident before completing her fellowship in clinical pharmacology and infectious diseases at UCSF. She earned her M.P.H. at the University of California, Berkeley in 1990. Dr. Gerberding is a member of Phi Beta Kappa, Alpha Omega Alpha, the American Society for Clinical Investigation (ASCI), and the American College of Physicians, and is a fellow in the Infectious Diseases Society of America (IDSA). She has served as chair and co-chair of the IDSA's Committee on Professional Development and Diversity and co-chair of the Annual Program Committee, and was elected to serve as a member of the nominations committee. Dr. Gerberding is also a member of the Society for Healthcare Epidemiology of America and has served as a member of the AIDS/Tuberculosis Committee and as Academic Counselor on the SHEA Board, and will be president of SHEA in 2003. In the past, she served as a member of NCID/CDC Board of Scientific Counselors, the CDC HIV Advisory Committee, and the Scientific Program Committee, National Conference on Human Retroviruses. She has also been a consultant to NIH, AMA, CDC, OSHA, the National AIDS Commission, Office of Technology Assessment, and WHO. Her editorial activities have included appointments to the Editorial Board, *Annals of Internal Medicine*; Associate Editor, *American Journal of Medicine*, and service as a peer reviewer for numerous journals. She has authored/co-authored more than 120 publications. Her scientific interests encompass infection prevention/health care quality promotion among patients and their health care providers and emerging infectious diseases threats.

MARK J. GOLDBERGER, M.D., M.P.H., received his medical degree from the Columbia University College of Physicians and Surgeons. He did his postgraduate training at the Presbyterian Hospital in New York City and with the Centers for Disease Control and Prevention and is board-certified in internal medicine and infectious diseases and a fellow of the Infectious Diseases Society of America. Dr. Goldberger was on the faculty of Columbia University for nine years and has been with the Food and Drug Administration since 1989. He is currently the director of the Office of Drug Evaluation IV within the Center for Drugs at FDA. This office is responsible for the regulation of all anti-infective drugs as well as drugs for solid organ transplantation. He also serves as the lead in coordinating drug shortage activities within the Center.

TERRY GREEN is a Senior Program Associate with Management Sciences for Health where he is the team leader for the RPM Plus Infectious

Disease/Antimicrobial Resistance activity. He is responsible for the implementation of global and national antimicrobial resistance containment strategies, including infection control activities. This work also includes the development and implementation of training materials for international drug and therapeutics committee training courses. He has facilitated courses in Thailand, The Philippines, Indonesia, Kenya, and Nepal. Green is a pharmacist with 22 years of experience with the U.S. Public Health Service and 4 years experience in international health. Experience includes serving on drug and therapeutics committees, development and implementation of pharmacy quality assurance programs, providing drug information services, and development of pharmacy-based primary care programs. International experience prior to working with Management Sciences for Health includes pharmacy assessments in Montenegro, Nicaragua, Micronesia, the Virgin Islands, and three years of pharmacy development work in the Republic of Palau.

JANET HEMINGWAY, Ph.D., is the current Director of the Liverpool School of Tropical Medicine. She received her B.Sc. in Genetics from Sheffield University and her Ph.D. in Tropical Medicine from the London School of Hygiene and Tropical Medicine. She then proceeded to a lecturership in Toxicology at the University of California, Riverside, followed by a Royal Society Research Fellowship at the London School of Hygiene and Tropical Medicine. Prior to her current post, she was Professor of Insect Molecular Biology and Director of Biosciences research at Cardiff University. Her major research interests are the development and spread of insecticide resistance in insect vectors of disease. Dr. Hemingway currently has a research group of 33 scientists at post-doctoral and post-graduate levels looking at numerous aspects of resistance from the molecular biology of resistance gene amplification and control of resistance gene expression, through positional cloning for resistance gene identification, to field-based resistance management programs in Africa and Latin America. The group is also looking at the interaction of insecticide resistance and vectorial capacity in filarial and malarial systems using genomic approaches.

WILLIAM JACK, D.Phil., is an Assistant Professor in the Economics Department at Georgetown University. He has held positions at the Australian National University and the University of Sydney, and has worked as a staff member of the International Monetary Fund and the Joint Committee on Taxation of the U.S. Congress. He has undertaken studies on health reform in Latin America and Eastern Europe for the World Bank. In addition to publications in academic journals on health care, health insurance, and public economics, he has written *Principles of Health Economics for Developing Countries*, a text published through the World Bank for health policy makers, students, and researchers.

CHARLES H. KING, M.D., M.S., is an associate professor of Medicine,

International Health, and Epidemiology and Biostatistics at Case Western Reserve University in Cleveland, Ohio. He is a specialist in the areas of Infectious Diseases and Travel Medicine at University Hospitals of Cleveland, and is a full-time faculty member at CWRU School of Medicine. He received his B.S. from the Massachusetts Institute of Technology, his M.D. from the State University of New York Downstate Medical Center, and his M.S. in Statistics from the University of Michigan School of Public Health. His current research focuses on the modeling of transmission of infectious diseases and the prevention of disease due to helminthic infections. He is director of two NIH-funded research projects based in Coast Province, Kenya, which focus, respectively, on the ecology of *Schistosoma haematobium* transmission and on drug-based control of human urinary schistosomiasis.

RAMANAN LAXMINARAYAN, Ph.D., M.P.H., is a fellow in the Energy and Natural Resources Division at Resources for the Future (RFF). Laxminarayan received his undergraduate degree in engineering from the Birla Institute of Technology and Science in Pilani, India, and both his master's degree in public health and doctorate in economics from the University of Washington in Seattle. His research deals with the integration of epidemiological models of infectious disease transmission and acquisition of bacterial and parasite resistance into the economic analysis of public health problems. His research on "resistance economics" is focused on improving the analytical framework to study problems such as bacterial resistance to antibiotics and pest resistance to genetically modified crops. He has worked with WHO on evaluating malaria treatment policy in Africa, has organized two conferences on the Economics of Resistance, and is editor of a forthcoming book, *Battling Resistance to Antibiotics and Pesticides: An Economic Approach.*

STUART B. LEVY, M.D., is Professor of Medicine and of Molecular Biology and Microbiology and the Director of the Center for Adaptation Genetics and Drug Resistance at Tufts University School of Medicine, and Staff Physician at the New England Medical Center. He also serves as President of the Alliance for the Prudent Use of Antibiotics, an international organization with members in over 100 countries. He is a past president of the 42,000 member American Society for Microbiology. He is co-founder and Chief Scientific Officer of Paratek Pharmaceuticals, Inc. Dr. Levy has published over 250 papers on antibiotic use and resistance, and has edited four books and two special journal editions devoted to the subject. The new edition of his book, *The Antibiotic Paradox: How Misuse of Antibiotics Destroys Their Curative Powers,* was released in January 2002 by Perseus Books. Dr. Levy is a Fellow of the American College of Physicians, Infectious Disease Society of America, and the American Academy of Microbiology. He has organized and chaired four international meetings on drug resistance and was Chairperson of the NIH Fogarty Center three-year international study of antibiotic use and resistance worldwide. He was awarded the 1995 Hoechst-Roussel Award for esteemed research in antimicrobial chemotherapy by the American Society for Microbiology. He was awarded an honorary degree in biology from Wesleyan University in 1998 and one from Des Moines University in 2001. Dr. Levy has been featured and quoted for his work on antibiotic use and resistance in major national and international newspapers and magazines including *Time*, *Newsweek*, *U.S. News and World Report*, *The New Yorker*, *The New York Times*, *The Washington Post*, and *USA Today*. He has appeared on Good Morning America, Nova, The Today Show, Fox TV Front Page, ABC Prime Time, CBS 48 Hours, the Jim Lehrer News Hour, CNN, and all major U.S. television network news shows.

MURRAY M. LUMPKIN, M.D., M.Sc., is presently the Acting Deputy Commissioner of the Food and Drug Administration. He is also the FDA's Senior Associate Commissioner for International Activities and Strategic Initiatives and the Senior Medical Officer in the Office of the Commissioner. In addition to overseeing all FDA international initiatives, he is responsible for leading the FDA response to several national public health issues that cut across several of the programmatic centers at FDA, including the agency's response to the threat of bovine spongiform encephalopathy (BSE) and antimicrobial resistance. Dr. Lumpkin received his B.A. in German from Davidson College and his medical degree from Wake Forest University. He completed a residency in pediatrics at the Mayo Clinic followed by a fellowship in pediatric infectious diseases. He attended the London School of Hygiene and Tropical Medicine as a Fulbright Fellow and received an M.Sc. in Medical Parasitology from the University of London. His professional certifications include pediatrics and tropical medicine. In 1989 he joined the FDA as Director of the Division of Anti-Infective Drug Products, Center for Drug Evaluation and Research (CDER), which is charged with the primary oversight and approval responsibilities for drugs classified as antimicrobials as well as dermatological and ophthalmological drug products. He then served as Deputy Center Director for CDER. He has represented the FDA in numerous bilateral initiatives with various governments, including those of Canada, Great Britain, Singapore, Germany, France, Taiwan, and Australia, along with the European Commission. His prior professional experience includes working as a clinical worker in a refugee camp in Bangladesh; head of pediatric infectious diseases at East Tennessee Children's Hospital in Knoxville; and Medical Director at Abbott Laboratories where he was in a senior leadership position on the multidisciplinary, global team responsible for the worldwide development of a new antimicrobial (clarithromycin).

SHAHRIAR MOBASHERY, Ph.D., is a Professor in the Departments of Chemistry, Pharmacology and Biochemistry and Molecular Biology at Wayne State University. He received his undergraduate and graduate degrees from the University of Southern California and the University of Chicago, respectively. After a two-year postdoctoral research program at the Rockefeller University, he joined the faculty at Wayne State University. He leads a multidisciplinary research group that integrates research in organic chemistry, biochemistry, molecular biology, structural biology, and computational sciences. The research interests of the group are diverse, spanning investigations of the mechanisms of drug resistance to antibiotics, development of novel classes of antibiotics, studies of the structural aspects of the bacterial envelope, and cancer metastasis. He has served on numerous advisory committees for the government and the private sector. He is currently on the editorial boards of a number of scientific journals, serves on the Scientific Advisory Board of Newbiotics, Inc., and is a member of the NIH Bioorganic and Natural Products study section. Dr. Mobashery assumes the position of the Navari Professor of Chemistry and Biochemistry at the University of Notre Dame in 2003.

LINDSAY E. NICOLLE, M.D., F.R.C.P.C., is Professor of Internal Medicine and Medical Microbiology at the University of Manitoba and Consultant in Infectious Diseases at the Health Sciences Centre and St. Boniface Hospital in Winnipeg, Manitoba, Canada. She is also currently Acting Director, Infection Control at St. Boniface Hospital. She has recently completed a sabbatical at WHO where she participated in development of the Global Strategy for Antimicrobial Resistance. Dr. Nicolle is currently Chairperson of the Infection Control Guidelines Committee of the Laboratory Centre for Disease Control in Canada. She was Chairperson of the Long Term Care Committee of the Society for Health Care Epidemiology of America from 1994 to 2002, and was previously secretary of this organization. She has also served as President of the Canadian Infectious Diseases Society, member of the Board of the Community and Hospital Infection Control Association, and of the Canadian Society for Clinical Investigation, and is previous co-chair and founder of the Canadian Nosocomial Infection Surveillance Program. Other activities include membership on the Health Canada Expert Committee on Blood Regulation, Pandemic Influenza Planning Committee, and Minister's Advisory Committee for Chemical, Biological, and Radioactive Safety. Dr. Nicolle's research interests have been in hospital-acquired infections, infections in the elderly, and urinary tract infections. She is the Editor-in-Chief of the *Canadian Journal of Infectious Diseases*, and a member of the Editorial Board of *Infection Control and Hospital Epidemiology*. She has authored/ co-authored over 300 publications and book chapters, and contributed to the development of many position papers and consensus documents on infection control and infectious diseases.

IRUKA OKEKE, Ph.D., is Assistant Professor of Microbiology at the Department of Biology, Haverford College, Pennsylvania. She undertook undergraduate and graduate training in pharmacy and microbiology at Obafemi Awolowo University, Ile-Ife, Nigeria, where she studied the antibiotic resistance and virulence of fecal *Escherichia coli*. Since then, she has continued to research the antibiotic resistance and pathogenesis of *E. coli*, first as post-doctoral fellow at Uppsala Universitet, Sweden, and the University of Maryland, and more recently as Career Development Lecturer in microbiology at the University of Bradford, U.K. Her current research focuses on the molecular epidemiology, pathogenesis, and antibiotic resistance of enterovirulent *E. coli*.

STEPHEN R. PALUMBI, Ph.D., received his Ph.D. from the University of Washington in 1984. His research group engages in the study of rapid evolutionary change, including the genetics, evolution, conservation, population biology, and systematics of a diverse array of marine organisms. Professor Palumbi has published on the genetics and evolution of a wide variety of organisms including sea urchins, whales, cone snails, corals, sharks, spiders, shrimps, bryozoans, and butterflyfishes. Palumbi's latest book, *The Evolution Explosion: How Humans Cause Rapid Evolutionary Change* (W.W. Norton), shows how rapid evolution is central to emerging problems in modern society, and has been cited for its easy readability by non-scientists. A primary research focus of his is the use of molecular genetic techniques in conservation, including for the identification of whale and dolphin products available in commercial markets. Current conservation work centers on the genetics of marine reserves designed for conservation and fisheries enhancement, with projects in The Philipppines, the Bahamas, and off the west coast of the United States. In addition, basic work on the molecular evolution of reproductive isolation and its influence on patterns of speciation uses marine model systems such as sea urchins. This work is expanding our view of the evolution of gamete morphology and the genes involved. In fall 2002, Steve appeared on the TV series, "The Future Is Wild," a computer-animated exploration of the possible courses of evolution in the next few hundred million years.

STEVEN L. PECK, Ph.D., earned his master's degree at the University of North Carolina at Chapel Hill in Biostatistics. He completed his Ph.D. work in Biomathematics, on the spread of resistance in spatially structured systems, at the North Carolina State University. This work was used by the EPA to set refuge sizes for delaying resistance development in transgenic crops. Currently he is assistant professor in the Zoology Department of Brigham Young University where he continues to work on modeling the spatial aspects in the spread of resistance and on rates of evolution in spatially subdivided populations.

DONALD R. ROBERTS, Ph.D., is a Professor of Tropical Public Health in the Division of Tropical Public Health at the Uniformed Services University of the Health Sciences (USUHS) in Bethesda, Maryland. He is also the Director of the Center for Applications of Remote Sensing and geographical information systems in Public Health. The center has a multidisciplinary staff of researchers who are involved in field research in Peru, Belize, and Thailand. Dr. Roberts has 94 peer-reviewed publications, with several others in press, under review, or in preparation. His special area of interest is malaria control, especially the control of malaria by spraying insecticide residues on house walls. He has published several original papers on behavioral responses of malaria vectors to insecticide residues and the re-emergence of malaria when house spray programs are abandoned. Additionally, he is interested in applications of GIS and remote sensing technologies for research and control of arthropod-borne diseases. Although he has conducted research in Asia, his primary area of interest is malaria control in Central and South America.

ANTHONY SAVELLI is a Principal Program Associate with the Management Sciences for Health (MSH) Center for Pharmaceutical Management (CPM). He is currently Director of the USAID-funded Rational Pharmaceutical Management Plus (RPM Plus) Program. This five-year program includes global, regional, and country-level initiatives working in the areas of general pharmaceutical system strengthening, as well as child survival, maternal health, HIV/AIDS, malaria, TB, and antimicrobial resistance. Since October 2000, RPM Plus has worked in Haiti, the Dominican Republic, Honduras, Peru, Nepal, Bangladesh, Vietnam, Zambia, Kenya, Senegal, Uganda, South Africa, Albania, Moldova, Romania, Tajikistan, Uzbekistan, and Turkmenistan. Prior to his work with RPM Plus, Savelli was director of the predecessor Rational Pharmaceutical Management Project, and the Rational Pharmaceutical Management/Russia Project. He has held long-term pharmacy advisor positions in The Commonwealth of Dominica, Swaziland, and Russia. Savelli is a pharmacist and has a master's degree in Public and International Affairs.

JEROME J. SCHENTAG, Pharm.D., earned his bachelor's degree in Pharmacy from the University of Nebraska in Omaha, and his Doctor of Pharmacy degree from the Philadelphia College of Pharmacy in Philadelphia, Pennsylvania. He completed a postdoctoral fellowship in Clinical Pharmacokinetics at the State University of New York (SUNY) in Buffalo, then joined the department faculty. Presently, Dr. Schentag is Professor of Pharmaceutics and Pharmacy, University at Buffalo School of Pharmacy. Dr. Schentag also holds the title of Fellow, Center for

Entrepreneurial Leadership, SUNY at Buffalo School of Management. He is a member of numerous professional societies and holds several professional distinctions, including the status of Fellow in the American College of Clinical Pharmacy. Dr. Schentag has authored or co-authored more than 260 publications and serves or has served on the editorial boards of the journals *Pharmacotherapy, Annals of Pharmacotherapy, Antimicrobial Agents and Chemotherapy, Pharmaceutical Research*, and *Clinical Pharmacology and Therapeutics*. His research interests include the effects of diseases on the pharmacokinetics and pharmacodynamics of antibiotics, oncolytics, and cardiovascular medications, and the relationships between pharmacokinetics and toxicity of medications used in critically ill patients.

THOMAS R. SHRYOCK, Ph.D., is a Senior Technical Microbiology Advisor for Elanco Animal Health, a division of Eli Lilly & Co., where his responsibilities include interacting with regulatory authorities, animal production companies, and industry trade organizations on issues surrounding the use of antibiotics in food animals as they pertain to antibiotic resistance. Dr. Shryock was initially involved with the in vitro and in vivo efficacy evaluation of new antibacterial products in Elanco Discovery. In addition, Dr. Shryock is the Chairholder of the NCCLS Veterinary Antimicrobial Susceptibility Testing subcommittee and a Member of the NCCLS Area Committee on Microbiology. He is also currently Division Advisor of Division Z, Animal Health Microbiology, which he co-founded and previously served as Acting Chair and Chair. Dr. Shryock was previously employed as an Assistant Professor of Life Sciences at the Indiana State University, participating in the Medical Technology Program. Prior to that position, he was a Research Microbiologist with Pfizer Animal Health for four years. Dr. Shryock received his B.S. in Biology from the University of Toledo and his doctorate in Medical Microbiology and Immunology from Ohio State University. He subsequently completed two post-doctoral fellowships conducting research in the area of cystic fibrosis pulmonary infection and immune response. Dr. Shryock has authored and/or co-authored over 40 research papers on infectious disease topics. He has been an editor for *Antimicrobial Agents and Chemotherapy* for nine years and has given presentations in numerous meetings around the world on the topic of antibiotic use in food animals.

RICHARD D. SMITH, M.Sc., graduated in economics and completed postgraduate studies in Health Economics at the University of York in 1991. He has since held positions in Sydney, Cambridge, Bristol, and Melbourne, joining the University of East Anglia as Senior Lecturer in Health Economics in June 1999. He is also an Honorary Associate Professor at the University of Hong Kong. Smith's research interests and experience range extensively across many facets of health economics and he has over 70 published works, including over 20 journal papers and chapters concerning the economics of antimicrobial resistance. His research has focused mainly on: (i) the valuation of benefits resulting from health care interventions, in particular the theory and method of willingness-to-pay, and the interface of cost-benefit analysis with cost-utility analysis; (ii) the economics of antimicrobial resistance; and (iii) primary care reform. More recently, he has become involved in the application of public goods theory in health, with a forthcoming book on this topic (*Global Public Goods for Health: A Health Economic and Public Health Perspective*) published by Oxford University Press. In recent years Smith has worked extensively with WHO, both in the development of the *WHO Global Strategy for the Containment of Resistance* and, more recently, in aspects of globalization and health. Smith has also taught widely to economic and medical undergraduates and postgraduates as well as a variety of health service professionals in the U.K., Australia, Hong Kong, and The Philippines. He is currently Director of Postgraduate Programmes within the School of Medicine, Health Policy and Practice at the University of East Anglia.

ALEXANDER TOMASZ, Ph.D., has a Ph.D. in Biochemistry from Columbia University, New York. He is currently Professor and Head of the Laboratory of Microbiology at The Rockefeller University. Dr. Tomasz's contributions include studies on molecular steps in DNA uptake during genetic transformation of pneumococci; the isolation of the first bacterial quorum-sensing agent, the polypeptide hormone (also called "activator") responsible for the triggering of the physiological state of competence for genetic transformation; the discovery of antibiotic tolerance in bacteria and elucidation of the mechanism of penicillin resistance through alteration of penicillin-binding proteins in pneumococci; the discovery of penicillin-binding protein 2A, the gene product of *mecA*, which is the central genetic determinant of methicillin resistance in staphylococci; the first high-resolution biochemical analysis of gram-positive bacterial cell walls (pneumococcus, staphylococcus) including identification of the unique phosphocholine-containing teichoic acid of pneumococci; and the first demonstration of inflammatory activity and cytokine-inducing activity of bacterial cell wall components. Most recent contributions include mechanism of staphylococcal glycopeptide resistance; identification of multi-drug-resistant epidemic clones of pneumococci, staphylococci; and organization of a New York-based (Bacterial Antibiotic Resistance, BAR) initiative and an international surveillance network (CEM/NET) for the tracking of antibiotic-resistant bacterial pathogens. Dr. Tomasz has received the prestigious Hoechst-Roussel Award and the Selman A. Waksman Award of the American Society for Microbiology, in recognition of contributions to the field of antibiotic resistance in bacteria, and received an Endowed Chair in Infectious Diseases in 1998 at The Rockefeller University. He is a member of several task forces evaluating the impacts of antibiotic-resistant bacteria (Congress of the United States, Office of Technology Assessment; the American Society for Microbiology; Advisory Board of the WHO), and the author of over 300 publications. He is on the editorial board of several journals, and is Editor-in-Chief of the journal *Microbial Drug Resistance*.

MARY E. TORRENCE, D.V.M., Ph.D., is the National Program Leader for Food Safety at USDA's Cooperative State Research Education and Extension Service. As a National Program Leader, Dr. Torrence provides leadership and direction to universities, particularly land grant universities, in food safety research. Dr. Torrence is also the program director for the National Research Initiative's grant program entitled Epidemiologic Approaches for Food Safety. Before taking this position, Dr. Torrence was the branch chief of the Epidemiology Branch in the Office of Surveillance and Biometrics in the Center for Devices and Radiological Health, FDA. She has also worked at the Center for Veterinary Medicine, FDA, and at Purdue University. In her current position, she is responsible for providing leadership on a national level to land grant universities. She is a member of numerous federal food safety committees, including the Risk Assessment Consortium and the National Food Safety System. She received her D.V.M. from Ohio State University and her Ph.D. in epidemiology and public health from Virginia Tech. She is a Diplomate in the American College of Veterinary Preventive Medicine. She was co-organizer of a Workshop on Epidemiologic Methods and Approaches for Food Safety and, recently, a co-chair for a research colloquium for the American Academy of Micro-biology on the "Impact of Antimicrobial Resistance on Agriculture: A Critical Scientific Assessment." She is author of the book (Mosby, Inc.) entitled *Understanding Epidemiology*. She is co-editor of *Microbial Food Safety in Animal Agriculture: Current Topics*, which is due to be published by Iowa State Press in March, 2003.

ROBERT G. WEBSTER, Ph.D., is Professor of Virology in the department of Infectious Diseases at St. Jude Children's Research Hospital. A native of New Zealand, Dr. Webster received his B.Sc. and M.Sc. in Microbiology from the Otago University in New Zealand. In 1962, he earned his Ph.D. from the Australian National University and went on to spend the next two years as a Fulbright Scholar working on influenza with Dr. Tommy Francis in the Department of Epidemiology, School of Public Health, at the University of Michigan, Ann Arbor. Since 1968, Dr. Webster has been at St. Jude Children's Research Hospital, Memphis, Tennessee, and in 1988, he was appointed to the Rose Marie Thomas Chair in Virology. In 1989, Dr. Webster was admitted to the highly prestigious Royal Society of London in recognition for his contribution to influenza virus research. In 1998, he was selected for membership to the National Academy of Sciences. In addition to his position at St. Jude, Dr. Webster is Director of the U.S. Collaborating Center of the WHO dealing with the ecology of animal influenza viruses. Dr. Webster's interests include the structure and function of influenza virus proteins and the development of new vaccines and antivirals, and the importance of influenza viruses in wild birds as a major reservoir of influenza viruses and their role in the evolution of new pandemic strains for humans and lower animals. His curriculum vitae contains over 400 original articles and reviews on influenza viruses. He has mentored many individuals who have been successful in contributing to our knowledge of influenza as an emerging pathogen.

THOMAS E. WELLEMS, M.D., Ph.D., is Chief of the Laboratory for Malaria and Vector Research at the National Institute of Allergy and Infectious Diseases, Bethesda, Maryland. The laboratory supports multidisciplinary research programs on malaria parasites, their transmission by mosquitoes, and their pathology in humans. Dr. Wellems began his work in malaria in 1984 after completing his medical residency at the Hospital of the University of Pennsylvania. His discoveries have been honored by the Director's Award of the National Institutes of Health, the Bailey K. Ashford Medal of the American Society of Tropical Medicine and Hygiene, the Smadel Medal of the Infectious Diseases Society of America, and the Lincei Golgi Medal of the Accademia Nazionale dei Lincei in Rome. Dr. Wellems' specific interests focus on drug resistance, immune evasion, and the virulence of *Plasmodium falciparum*, the parasite that causes the most deadly form of human malaria. Two key findings from his laboratory research have been the *P. falciparum* transporter for chloroquine resistance and the gene family responsible for antigenic variation of parasitized red blood cells. In field investigations, his efforts have led to new diagnostic assays for drug-resistant malaria strains and new information on hemoglobin mutations that confer protection against the severe complications of malaria.

FORUM STAFF

STACEY L. KNOBLER is Director of the Forum on Emerging Infections at the Institute of Medicine (IOM). She previously served as the co-director of the IOM Board on Global Health's study, *Neurological, Psychiatric, and Developmental Disorders in Developing Countries,* and research associate for the *Assessment of Future Scientific Needs for Live Variola Virus.* Ms. Knobler is actively involved in program research and development for the Board on Global Health. Previously, she has held positions as a Research Associate at the Brookings Institution, Foreign Policy Studies Program and as an Arms Control and Democratization Consultant for the Organization for Security and Cooperation in Europe in Vienna and Bosnia-Herzegovina. Ms. Knobler has also worked as a research and negotiations analyst in Israel and Palestine. She is currently a member of the CBACI Senior Working Group for Health, Security, and U.S. Global

Leadership. Ms. Knobler has conducted research and co-authored published articles on biological and nuclear weapons control, foreign aid, health in developing countries, poverty and public assistance, and the Arab-Israeli peace process.

MARJAN NAJAFI, M.P.H., is a research associate for the Forum on Emerging Infections in the Board on Global Health. She has also worked with the IOM committee that produced *Veterans and Agent Orange: Update 2000*. She received her undergraduate degrees in chemical engineering and applied mathematics from the University of Rhode Island. Ms. Najafi served as a public health engineer with the Maryland Department of Environment and, later, the Research Triangle Institute. After obtaining a master's of public health from the Bloomberg School of Public Health at Johns Hopkins University, she managed a lead poisoning prevention program in Micronesia with a grant from the U.S. Department of Health and Human Services. Prior to joining IOM, she worked on a study researching the effects of cellular phone radiation on human health.

LAURIE A. SPINELLI is a project assistant for the Forum on Emerging Infections in the Board on Global Health. Ms. Spinelli joined the IOM in July 2000, and has worked with the IOM committee that generated the *Neurological, Psychiatric, and Developmental Disorders: Meeting the Challenge in the Developing World* report. Currently, she is working on two forthcoming reports: *Reducing the Impact of Birth Defects in Developing Countries* and *Improving Birth Outcomes in Developing Countries*. Prior to joining IOM, she graduated from Syracuse University with a bachelor of arts degree in speech communications. Ms. Spinelli also teaches an interpersonal communication course at the College of Southern Maryland.

EXCEL GUIDE

TO ACCOMPANY

UNDERSTANDABLE STATISTICS

SEVENTH EDITION

BRASE/BRASE

Charles Henry Brase
Regis University

Corrinne Pellillo Brase
Arapahoe Community College

Laurel Tech Integrated Publishing Services

HOUGHTON MIFFLIN COMPANY BOSTON NEW YORK

Sponsoring Editor: Lauren Schultz
Assitant Editor: Marika Hoe
Senior Manufacturing Coordinator: Priscilla Bailey
Marketing Manager: Ben Rivera

Printed in the U.S.A.

ISBN: 0-618-20556-X

4 5 6 7 8 9 - MA - 07 06 05 04

Preface

The use of computing technology can greatly enhance a student's learning experience in statistics. This *Excel Guide* provides basic instruction, examples, and lab activities for

Microsoft® Excel 97
with Analysis ToolPak
for Windows®

The commands and menu selections for Excel 2002 are essentially the same as those shown in this manual.

The Analysis ToolPak is part of Excel and can be installed from the same source as the basic Excel program (normally, a CD-ROM) as an option on the installer program's list of Add-Ins. Details for getting started with the Analysis ToolPak are in Chapter 1 of this guide. No additional software is required to use the Excel functions described.

The lab activities that follow accompany the text *Understandable Statistics,* 7th edition by Brase and Brase. On the following page is a table to coordinate this guide with *Understanding Basic Statistics,* 2nd edition by Brase and Brase. Both texts are published by Houghton Mifflin.

In addition, over one hundred data files from referenced sources are described in the Appendix. These data files are available on the HM-StatPass CD-ROM that is packaged with the student textbook and can be viewed on-line at the Brase/Brase Statistics site. You can access this site from the Houghton Mifflin Web site at

http://math.college.hmco.com/students

Excel is an all-purpose spreadsheet software package. This guide shows how to use Excel's built-in statistical functions and how to produce some useful graphs. Excel is not designed to be a complete statistical software package. In many cases, macros can be created to produce special graphs, such as box-and-whisker plots. However, this guide only shows how to use the existing, built-in features. In most cases, the operations omitted from Excel are easily carried out on an ordinary calculator.

Correlation Guide for *Understanding Basic Statistics*

In *Understanding Basic Statistics,* 2nd edition, the arrangement of topics is slightly different than in *Understandable Statistics,* 7th edition. The chart below shows how to use this *Excel Guide* with *Understanding Basic Statistics.*

***Understanding Basic Statistics,* 2nd ed.**	**Corresponding *Excel Guide* Material**
1 Organizing Data	**1** Getting Started and **2** Organizing Data (excluding Ogives)
2 Averages and Variation	**3** Averages and Variation
3 Regression and Correlation	**10** Regression and Correlation • Linear Regression: Two Variables (excluding Standard Error)
4 Elementary Probability Theory	**4** Elementary Probability Theory
5 Introduction to Probability Distributions and the Binomial Probability Distribution	**5** The Binomial Probability Distribution and Related Topics
6 Normal Distributions	**6** Normal Distributions
7 Introduction to Sampling Distributions	**7** Introduction to Sampling Distributions
8 Estimation	**8** Estimation
9 Hypothesis Testing Involving One Population	**9** Hypothesis Testing • Testing a Single Population Mean
10 Inferences About Differences	**9** Hypothesis Testing • Tests Involving Paired Differences • Tests of Difference of Means
11 Additional Topics Using Inference • Part I: Hypothesis Tests Using the Chi-Square Distribution	**11** Chi-Square and *F* Distributions • Chi-Square Tests of Independence
11 Additional Topics Using Inference • Part II: Inferences Related to Linear Regression	**10** Regression and Correlation • Linear Regression: Two Variables (Standard Error)

Contents

CHAPTER 1 GETTING STARTED

GETTING STARTED WITH EXCEL

Microsoft® Excel is an all-purpose spreadsheet application with many functions. We will be using Excel 97. This guide is not a general Excel manual, but it will show you how to use many of Excel's built-in statistical functions. You may need to install the Analysis ToolPak from the original Excel software if your computer does not have it. To determine if your installation of Excel includes the Analysis ToolPak, open Excel, click on **Tools** in the main menu, and then see if the ToolPak is listed in the **Add-Ins** dialog box. If it is, place a check by Analysis ToolPak. If you do not see a listing for Analysis ToolPak, then you will need to install it from the original Excel installation source.

If you are familiar with Windows-based programs, you will find that many of the editing, formatting, and file handling procedures of Excel are similar to those you have used before. You use the mouse to select, drag, click and double-click as you would in any other Windows program.

If you have any questions about Excel not answered in this guide, consult the Excel manual or select **Help** on the menu bar.

The Excel Window

When you have opened Excel, you should see a window like this:

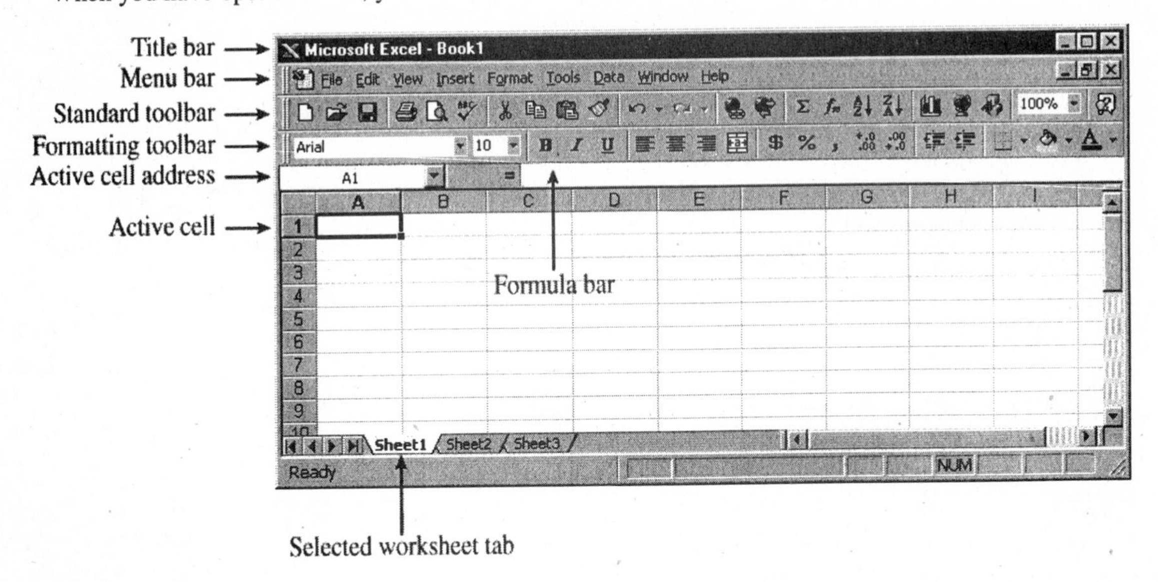

The Excel Workbook

An Excel file is called a Workbook. Notice that in the display shown above, the title bar shows Microsoft Excel - Book1. This means that we are working in Book 1.

Each workbook consists of one or more worksheets. In the worksheet above, the tabs near the bottom of the screen show that we are working with Sheet 1. To change worksheets, click on the appropriate tab. Alternatively, you can right-click the arrows just to the left of the worksheet tabs to get a list of all the worksheets in the projects, and then select a worksheet.

The Cells in the Worksheet

When you look at a worksheet, you should notice horizontal and vertical grid lines. If they are missing, you will need to activate that feature. To do so,

1. Select **Tools** from the menu, and then select **Options** from the drop-down menu.
2. Click on the tab showing **View.** Be sure that the **Gridlines** option is checked.

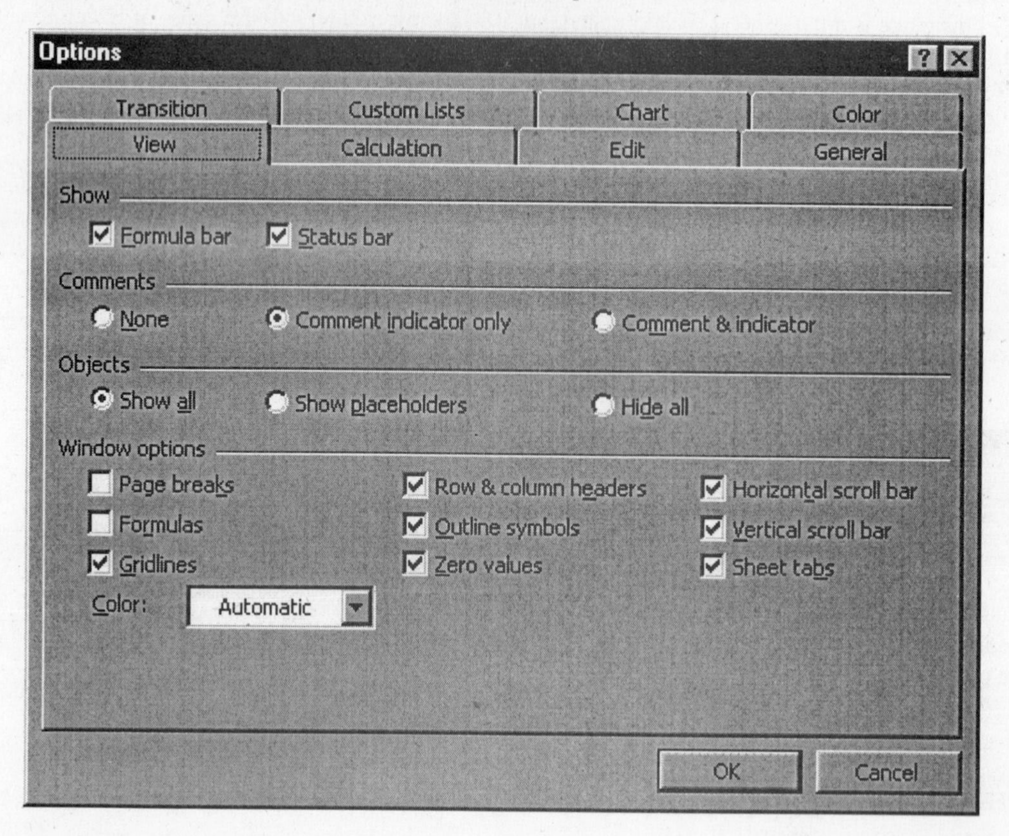

It is convenient to have checks by all the options shown above.

Cell Addresses

The cells are formed by intersecting rows and columns. A cell's address consists of a column letter followed by a row number. For example, the address B3 designates the cell that lies in Column B, Row 3. When Cell B3 is highlighted, it is the active cell. This means we can enter text or numbers into Cell B3.

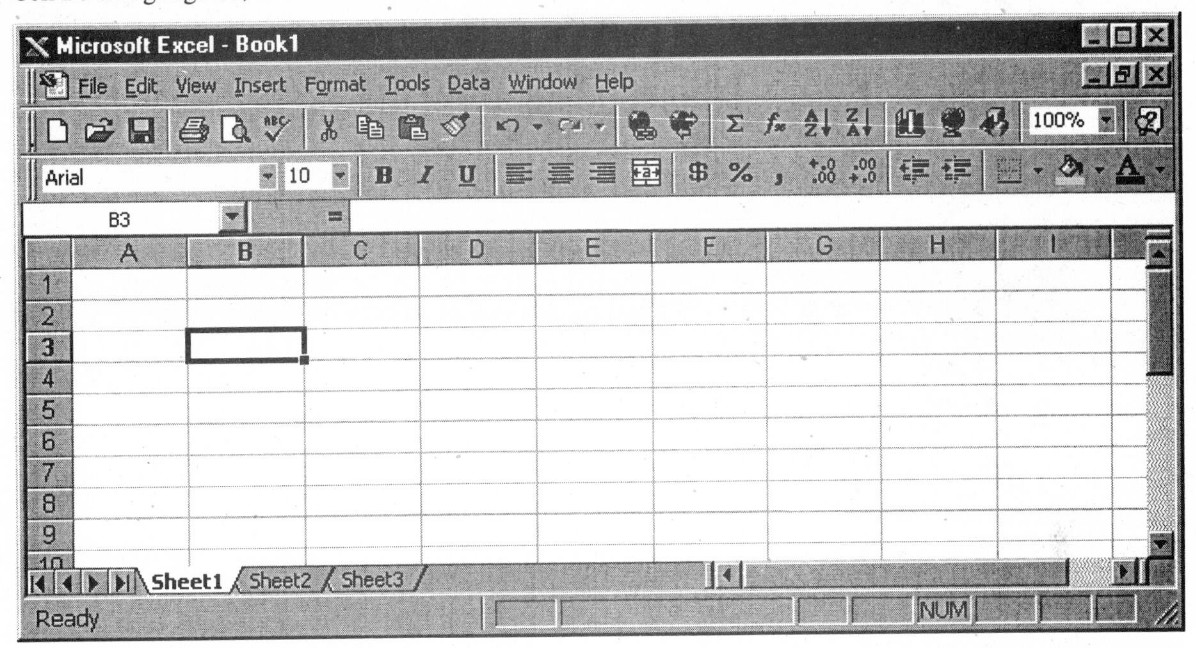

Selecting Cells

To select a cell, position the cursor in the cell and click the left mouse button.

Sometimes you will want to select several cells at once, in order to format them (as described next). To select a rectangular block of cells, position the cursor in a corner cell of the block, hold down the left mouse button, drag the cursor to the cell in the block's opposite corner, and release the button. The selected cells will be highlighted, as shown below.

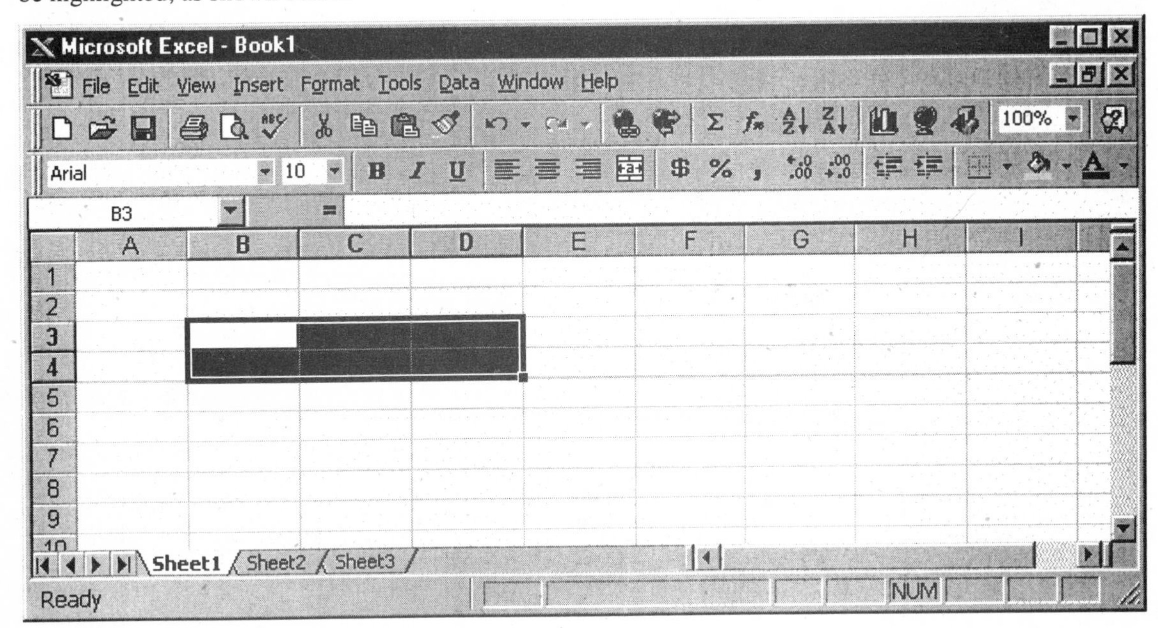

To select an entire column, click on the letter above it; to select an entire row, click on the number to its left. To select every cell in the worksheet, click on the gray blank rectangle in the upper left corner of the worksheet (above row header 1 and left of column header A).

You can also select a block of cells by typing the two corner cells into the active cell address window. The block highlighted on the preceding page would be selected by typing B3:E4 and pressing Enter.

Formatting Cell Contents

In Excel, you may place text or numbers in a cell. As in other Windows applications, you can format the text or numbers by using the formatting toolbar buttons for bold (**B**), italics (***I***), underline (**U**), etc. Other options include left, right, and centered alignment within a cell.

Numbers can be formatted to represent dollar amounts ($) or percents (%) and can be shown with commas in large numbers (**,**). The number of decimal places to which numbers are carried is also adjustable. All these options appear on the formatting menu bar. Other options are accessible through **Cells** under the menu command **Format.**

Changing Cell Width

To change the column widths and row heights for selected cells, use **Column** and **Row** under the **Format** menu option.

Column widths and row heights can also be adjusted by placing the cursor between two columns letters or row numbers. When the cursor changes appearance, hold down the left mouse button, move the column or row boundary, and release.

All these instructions may seem a little mysterious. Once you try them, however, you will find that they are fairly easy to remember.

ENTERING DATA

In Excel we enter data and labels in the cells. It is common to select a column for the data and place a label as the first entry in the column.

Let's enter some data on television advertising. For each of twenty hours of prime-time viewing, both the number of ads and the time devoted to ads were recorded. We will enter the data in two columns, as shown:

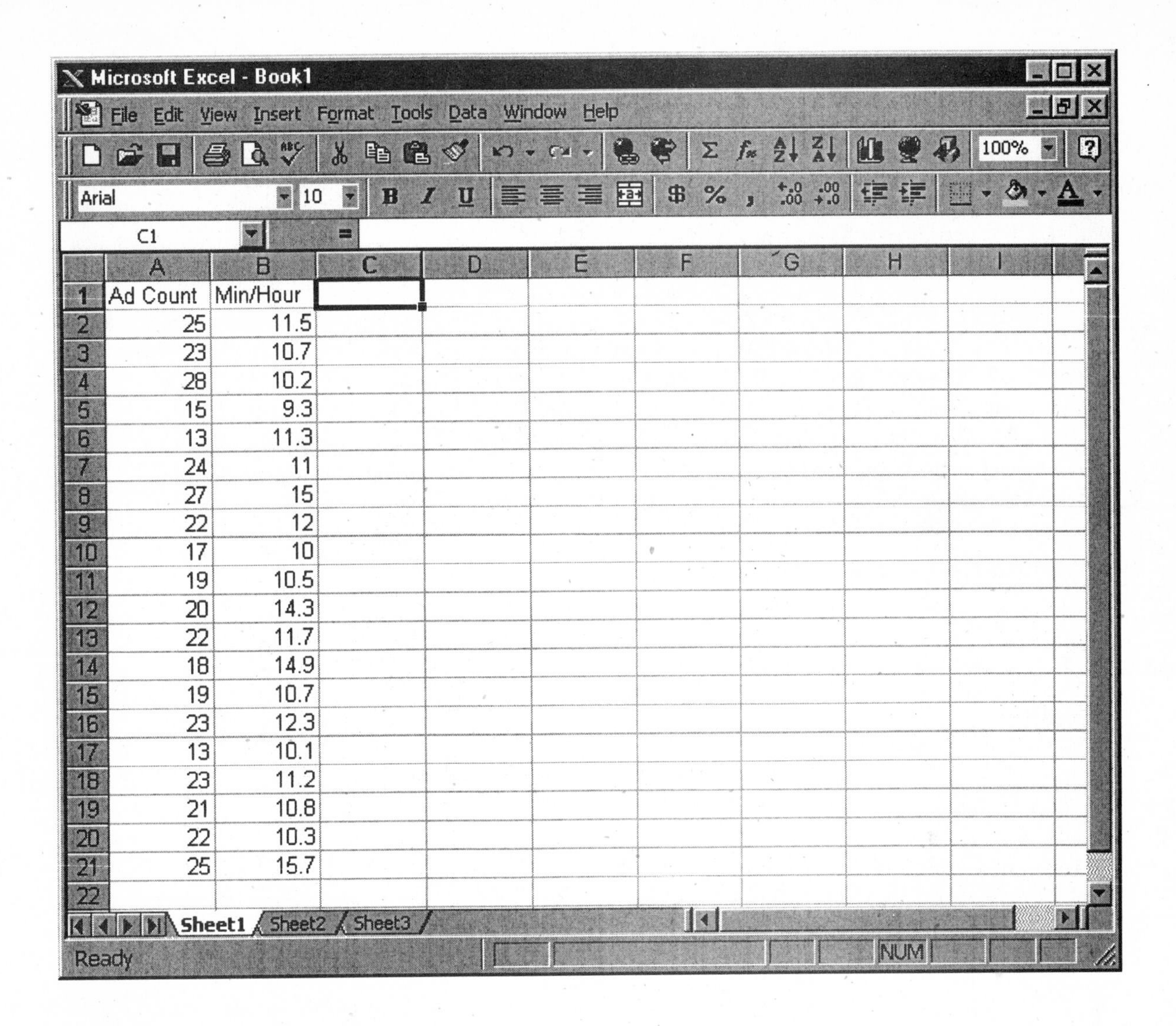

Ad Count	Min/Hour
25	11.5
23	10.7
28	10.2
15	9.3
13	11.3
24	11
27	15
22	12
17	10
19	10.5
20	14.3
22	11.7
18	14.9
19	10.7
23	12.3
13	10.1
23	11.2
21	10.8
22	10.3
25	15.7

Entering and Correcting Data

To select a cell for content entry, move the mouse pointer to the cell and click. Then type the label or data and press Enter. Excel automatically moves to select the next cell in the same column. If you want to enter information in a different cell, just click on it.

Errors are easily fixed. If you notice a mistake before you press Enter, simply back-arrow to the mistake and correct it. If you notice the error after you have pressed Enter, select the affected cell and then click on the formula bar to add a typing cursor to the cell contents displayed. Use standard keyboard editing techniques to make corrections, then press Enter.

If you want to erase the contents of a cell or range of cells but keep the formatting, select the cells and use **➤ Edit ➤ Clear ➤ Contents** from the main menu (or just press Delete). Other options under **Edit ➤ Clear** have slightly different effects. The **➤ Clear ➤ Format** option keeps the content but clears the format. The **➤ Clear ➤ All** option clears both content and format. **➤ Clear ➤ Format** is especially useful for changing percent data back into decimal format.

Arithmetic Options on the Standard Toolbar

Summing Data in a Column

On the standard toolbar, the Σ button automatically sums the values in the selected cells. When we sum the contents of an entire column, Excel places the sum under the selected cells. It is a good idea to type the label *total* next to the cell where the total appears. Below, we selected Column A, pressed the Σ button, and then typed the word *total* in the corresponding row of Column C. We see that the total of Column A is 419.

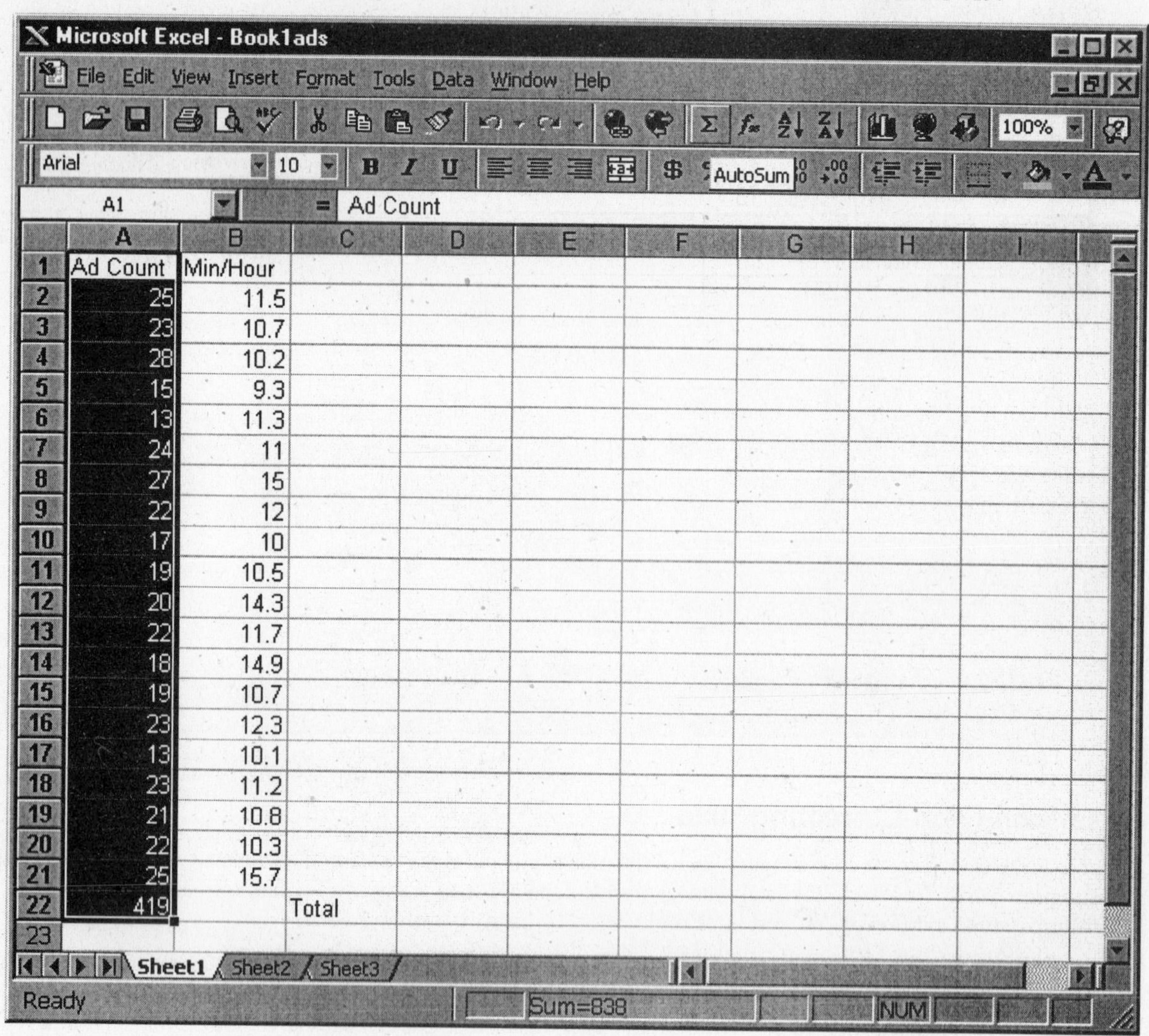

	A	B	C
1	Ad Count	Min/Hour	
2	25	11.5	
3	23	10.7	
4	28	10.2	
5	15	9.3	
6	13	11.3	
7	24	11	
8	27	15	
9	22	12	
10	17	10	
11	19	10.5	
12	20	14.3	
13	22	11.7	
14	18	14.9	
15	19	10.7	
16	23	12.3	
17	13	10.1	
18	23	11.2	
19	21	10.8	
20	22	10.3	
21	25	15.7	
22	419		Total
23			

Sorting Data

The two buttons and sort the data in ascending and descending order, respectively. To sort just one column, highlight that column and press one of the buttons. To sort two or more columns by ascending or descending order of the data in the first column, highlight all the columns and click the appropriate button. In general, we will simply sort one column of data at a time, as shown.

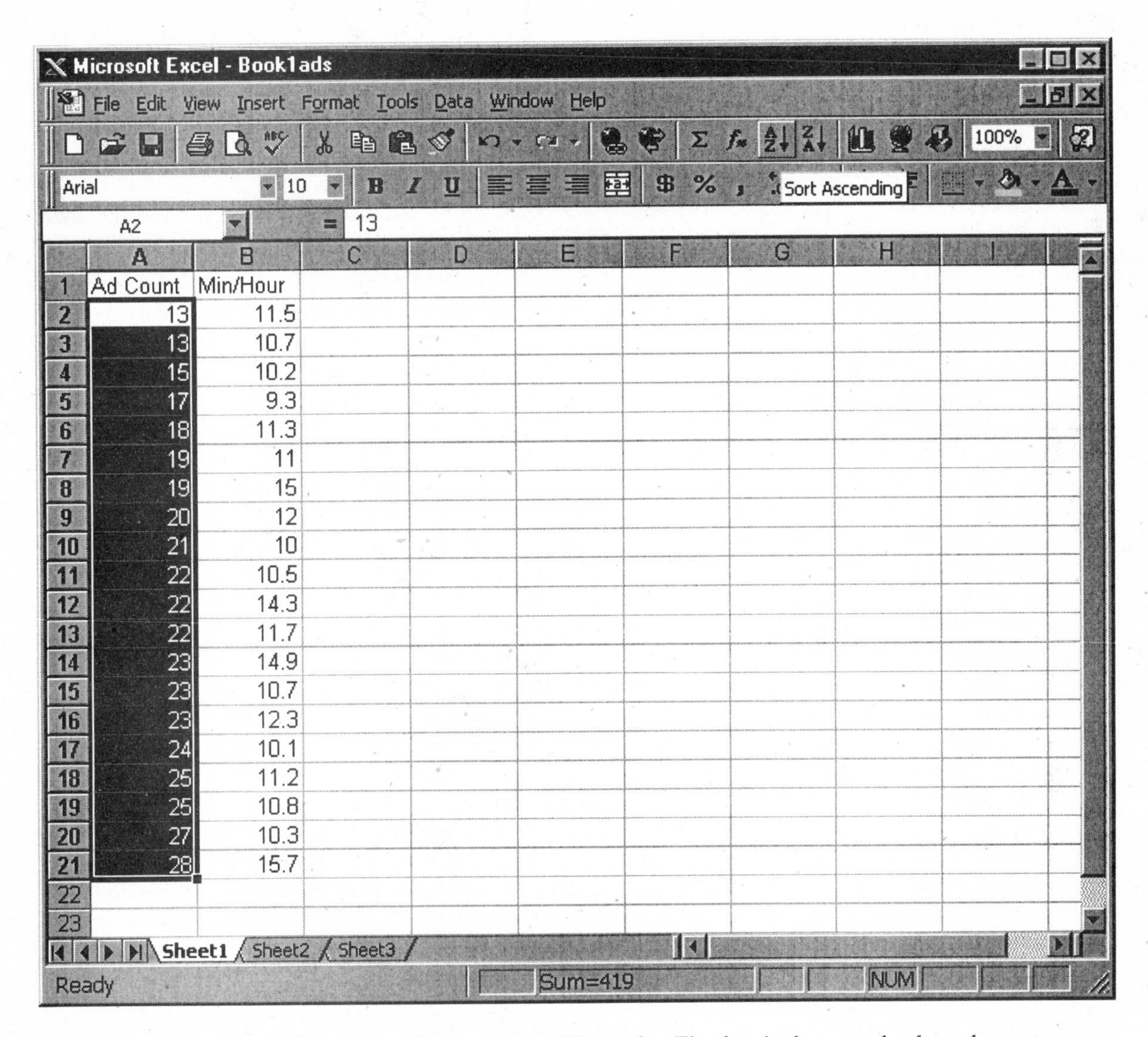

	A	B	C	D	E	F	G	H	I
1	Ad Count	Min/Hour							
2	13	11.5							
3	13	10.7							
4	15	10.2							
5	17	9.3							
6	18	11.3							
7	19	11							
8	19	15							
9	20	12							
10	21	10							
11	22	10.5							
12	22	14.3							
13	22	11.7							
14	23	14.9							
15	23	10.7							
16	23	12.3							
17	24	10.1							
18	25	11.2							
19	25	10.8							
20	27	10.3							
21	28	15.7							
22									
23									

Notice that the data in the first column is now in ascending order. The data in the second column has not moved.

If you decide that it was a mistake to sort the data this way, and you have not made any other changes since you did the sort, you can use ➤ **Edit** ➤ **Undo** from the main menu. The data will appear in their original order.

Copying Cells

To copy one cell or a block of cells to another location on the worksheet,

(a) Select the cells you wish to copy

(b) From the main menu, select ➤ **Edit** ➤ **Copy.** (The shortcut for this process is **Ctrl-C.**) Notice that the range of cells being copied now has a blinking border around it.

(c) Select the upper-left cell of the block that will receive the copy.

(d) Press Enter. When you press Enter, the copy process is complete and the blinking border around the original cells disappears.
Note: Even if you use ➤ **Edit** ➤ **Paste** or the shortcut Ctrl-V to paste, you must still press Enter to remove the blinking border around the original cells.

To copy one cell or a range of cells to another worksheet or workbook, follow steps (a) and (b) above. For step (c), be sure you are in the destination worksheet or workbook and that the worksheet or workbook is activated. Then proceed with step (d).

USING FORMULAS

A formula is an expression that generates a numerical value in a cell, usually based on values in other cells. Formulas usually involve standard arithmetic operations. Excel uses + for addition, - (hyphen) for subtraction, * for multiplication, / for division, and ^ (carat) for exponentiation (raising to a power).

For instance, if we want to divide the contents of Cell A2 by the contents of Cell B2 and place the results in Cell C2, we do the following:

(a) Make Cell C2 the active cell.

(b) Click in the formula bar and type =A2/B2.

(c) Press Enter

The value in Cell C2 will be the quotient of the values in Cells A2 and B2.

If, for a whole series of rows, we wanted to divide the entry in Column A by the entry in Column B and put the results in Column C, we could repeat the above process over and over. However, the typing would be tedious. We can accomplish the same thing more easily by copying and pasting:

(a) Enter =A2/B2 in Cell C2 as described above

(b) Move the cursor to the lower right corner of Cell C2. The cursor should change shape to small black cross (+). Now hold down the left mouse button and drag the + down until all the cells in Column C in which you want the calculation done are highlighted.

(c) Release the mouse button and press Enter. The cell entries in Column C should equal the quotients of the same-row entries in Columns A and B.

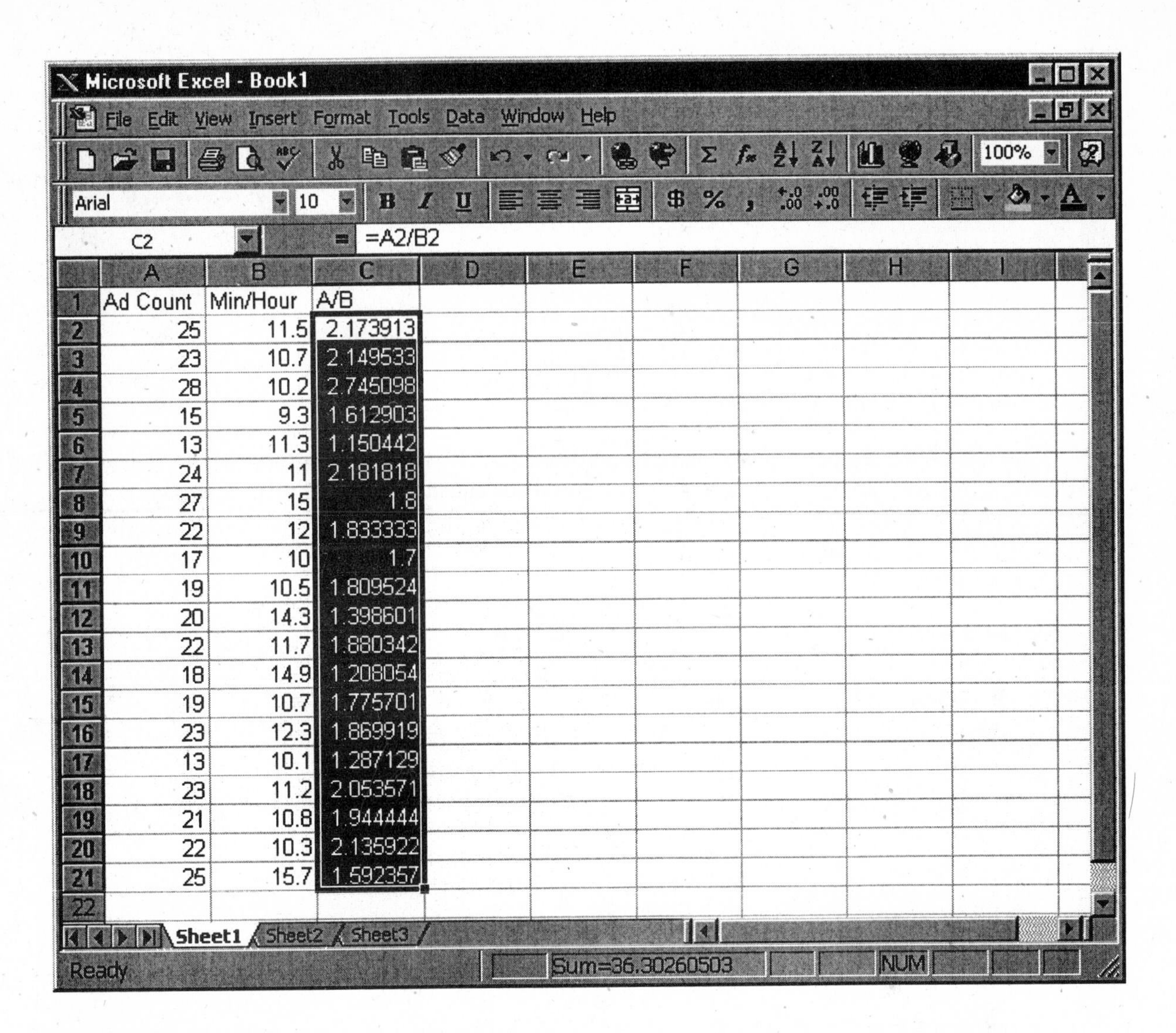

	A	B	C
1	Ad Count	Min/Hour	A/B
2	25	11.5	2.173913
3	23	10.7	2.149533
4	28	10.2	2.745098
5	15	9.3	1.612903
6	13	11.3	1.150442
7	24	11	2.181818
8	27	15	1.8
9	22	12	1.833333
10	17	10	1.7
11	19	10.5	1.809524
12	20	14.3	1.398601
13	22	11.7	1.880342
14	18	14.9	1.208054
15	19	10.7	1.775701
16	23	12.3	1.869919
17	13	10.1	1.287129
18	23	11.2	2.053571
19	21	10.8	1.944444
20	22	10.3	2.135922
21	25	15.7	1.592357
22			

Now, if you click on one of the lower cells in Column C, you will notice that the row number in the cell addresses is not 2 but rather the number of the new cell's row. In general, when a formula is copied from one cell to another, the cell addresses in the formula are automatically adjusted. If the formula =D3+C7 is copied to a new cell three columns right and two rows up from the old one, the pasted formula comes out as =G1+F5. (Three columns right from D is G, two rows up from 3 is 1, and so on.)

Sometimes you will want to prevent the automatic address adjustment. To do this put a dollar sign before any row or column number you want to keep from changing. When the formula =D$3+$C7 is copied to a new cell three columns right and two rows up from the old one, the pasted formula comes out as =G$3+$C5. We will call an address with two $ signs in an *absolute* address, because it always refers to the same cell, no matter where the formula is copy/pasted to. A cell with only on $ sign in it, or none at all, we will call a *relative* address, because the cell referred to can change as the formula is pasted from one location to another.

SAVING WORKBOOKS

After you have entered data into an Excel spreadsheet, it is a good idea to save it. On the main menu, click ➤ **File** ➤ **Save As.** A dialog box will appear, similar to the one at the top of the next page.

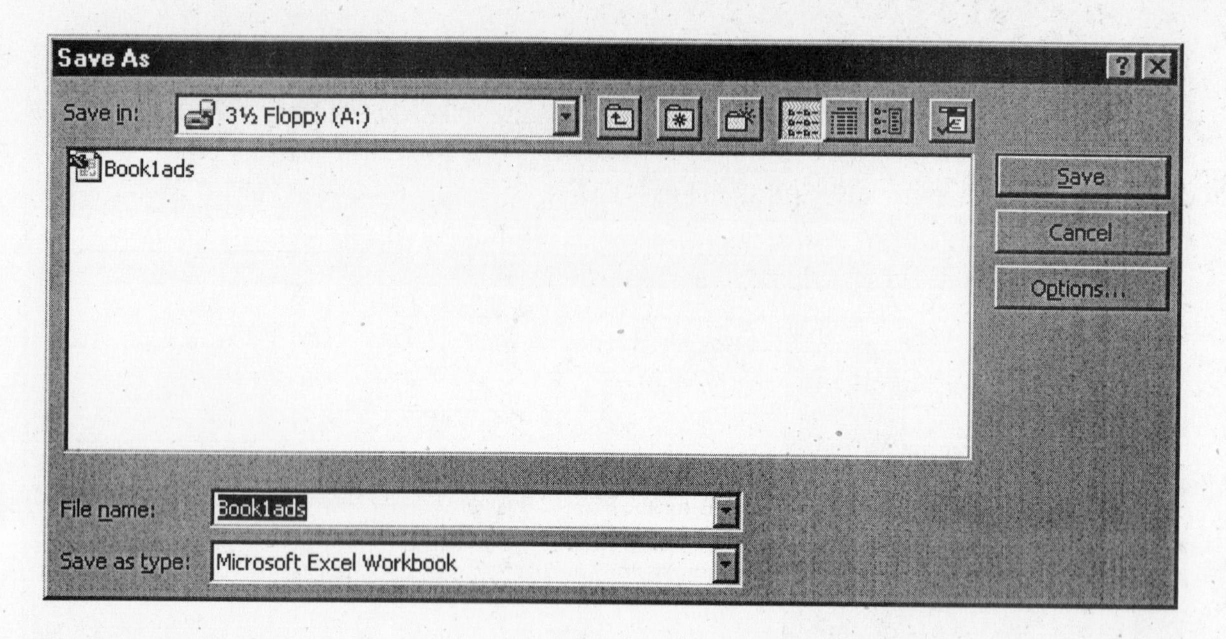

If you are in a college computer lab, you might save your files to a floppy disk. We named the workbook on TV ads Book1ads.

It is a good idea to save your workbook periodically as you are working on it. After you have saved the workbook for the first time, you can save updates during your working session by using the save button on the standard toolbar. This is the third button from the left; it looks like a diskette.

To retrieve an Excel Workbook, go to the main menu and click ➤ **File** ➤ **Open.** Select the drive containing your workbook and then the desired workbook file.

Printing Your Worksheets

Clicking the printer button on the standard toolbar (the icon that looks like a little printer) will open a printer dialog box.

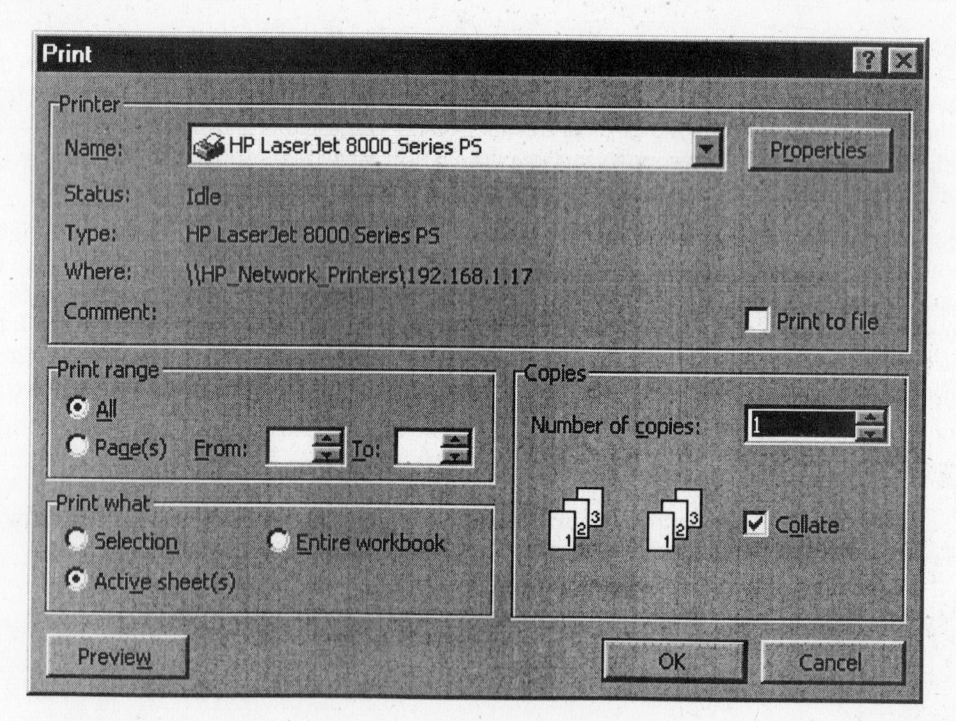

If you select a range of cells on the worksheet before you print, you may print the selected material. Notice that you can tell the printer what to print by clicking next to Selection, Active sheet(s) or Entire Workbook. Clicking the Preview button lets you see what you will print before the page is printed.

LAB ACTIVITIES FOR GETTING STARTED

1. Go to your computer lab (or use your own computer) and open Excel. Check to see if you have the Analysis ToolPak add-in. If so, be sure it is activated.
2. If you have not already done so, enter the TV Ad Count and Min/Hour data into the workbook. Use Column A for the Ad Count and Column B for the Min/Hour data.
3. Save the workbook as Book1ads.
4. Select the cells containing the labels and data and print.
5. (a) In Column C, place the quotients A/B for the Rows 2 through 21. Use the formula bar in Cell C2, and drag with the little + symbol to complete the quotients for all rows. Note that if the calculation mode (see Chapter 2) has been set to Manual, you may need to use the key combination **Shift-F9** after the cells are highlighted.
   (b) Use the sum button Σ on the toolbar to total up the Ad Count column and to total up the Min/Hour column. Place a label in Column D adjacent to the totals.
   (c) Select the data in Columns A, B, C, and D and print it.
6. In this problem we will copy a column of data and sort the copy.
   (a) Select Column A (Ad Count) and copy it to Column D.
   (b) Select Column D and sort it in ascending order (use only the original data, not the sum).
   (c) Select both Column A (Ad Count) and Column B (Min/Hour). Sort these columns by Column A in descending order. Are the data entries of 13 in Column A still next to the data entries 11.3 and 10.1 in Column B? Are the data in Column B sorted?

RANDOM SAMPLES (SECTION 1.2 OF *UNDERSTANDABLE STATISTICS*)

Excel has several random number generators. The one we will find most convenient is the function **RANDBETWEEN(bottom,top).** This function generates a random integer between (inclusively) whatever integer is put in for "bottom" and whatever integer is put in for "top."

To use RANDBETWEEN, select a cell in the active worksheet. Click in the formula bar, type =, and on the standard toolbar click the Paste Function button (called the Insert Function in Excel 2002).

Pressing this button calls up a two-column menu, similar to the one at the top of the next page. Select All in the Function category, and then scroll down on the Function name side until you reach RANDBETWEEN. Note that this command is present only if you have the Analysis ToolPak checked under ➤ **Tools** ➤ **Add-Ins.**

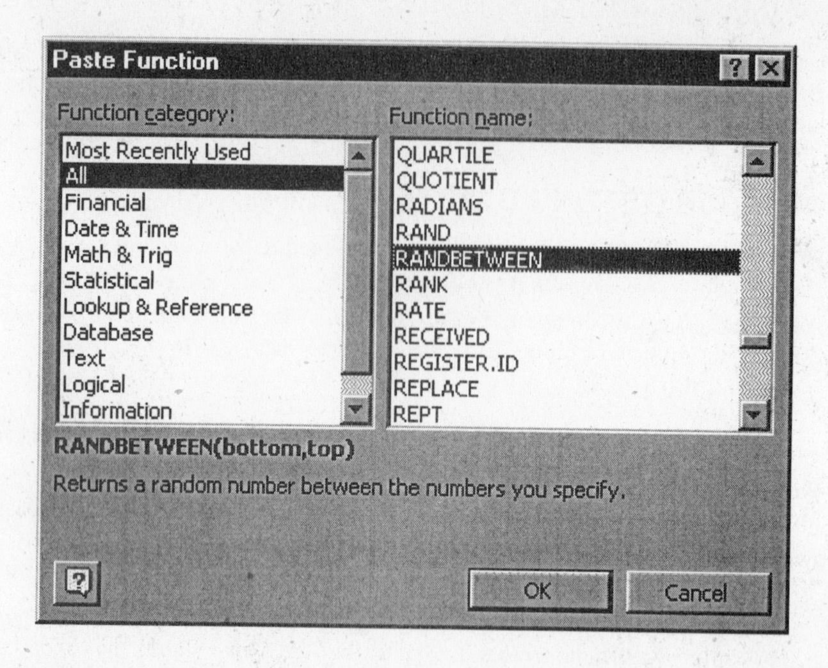

Select RANDBETWEEN and then fill in the bottom and top numbers. Alternatively, you may simply type =RANDBETWEEN(bottom,top) in the formula bar, with numbers in place of bottom and top.

The random number generators of Excel have the characteristic that whenever a command is entered anywhere in the active workbook, the random numbers change because they are recalculated. To prevent this from happening, change the recalculate mode from automatic to manual. Select ➤ **Tools** ➤ **Options,** and then click on the tab labeled Calculation. Select Manual calculation, then press Enter.

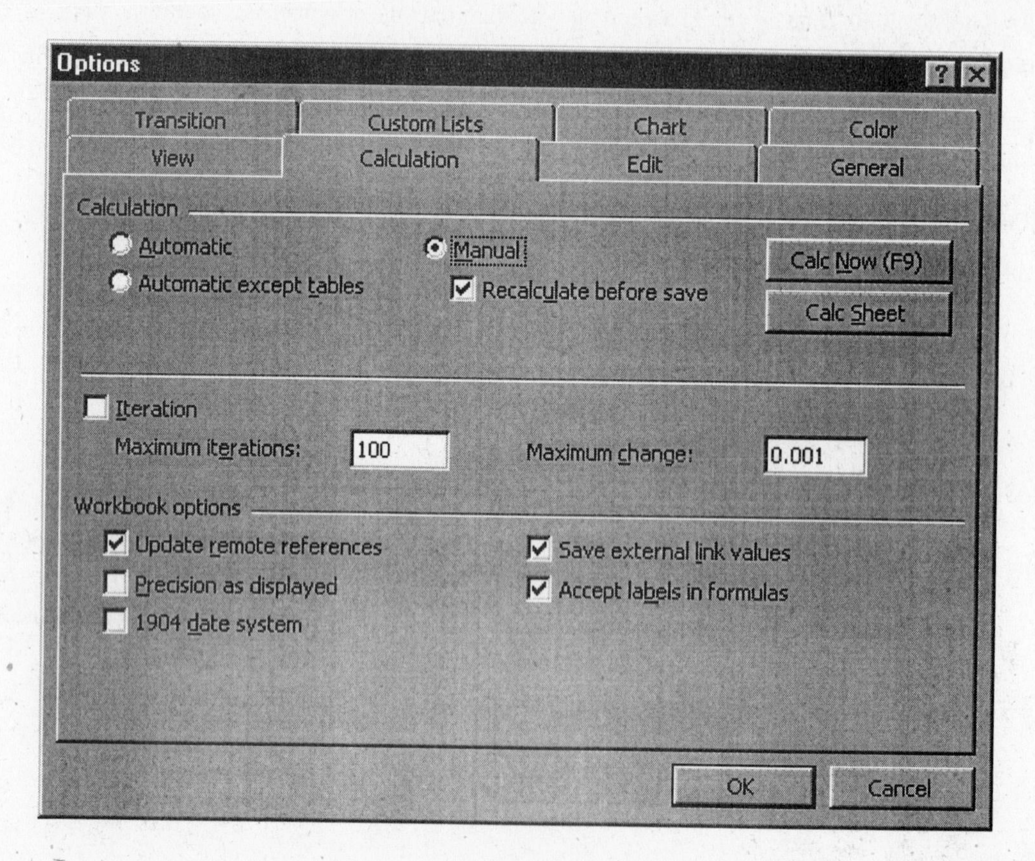

With automatic recalculation disabled, you can still recalculate by pressing the **Shift-F9** key combination. Let us see this in an example, where we select a list of random numbers in a designated range and sort the list in ascending order.

Example

There are 175 students enrolled in a large section of introductory statistics. Draw a random sample of fifteen of the students.

We assign each of the students a distinct number between 1 and 175. To find the numbers of the fifteen students to be included in the sample, we do the following steps.

(a) Change the Calculation mode to Manual.

(b) Type the label Sample in Cell A1.

(c) Select Cell A2.

(d) Type =RANDBETWEEN(1,175) in the formula bar and press Enter.

(e) Position the mouse pointer in the lower right corner of Cell A2 until it becomes a + sign, and click-drag downward until you reach Cell A16. Release. Then press **Shift-F9.**

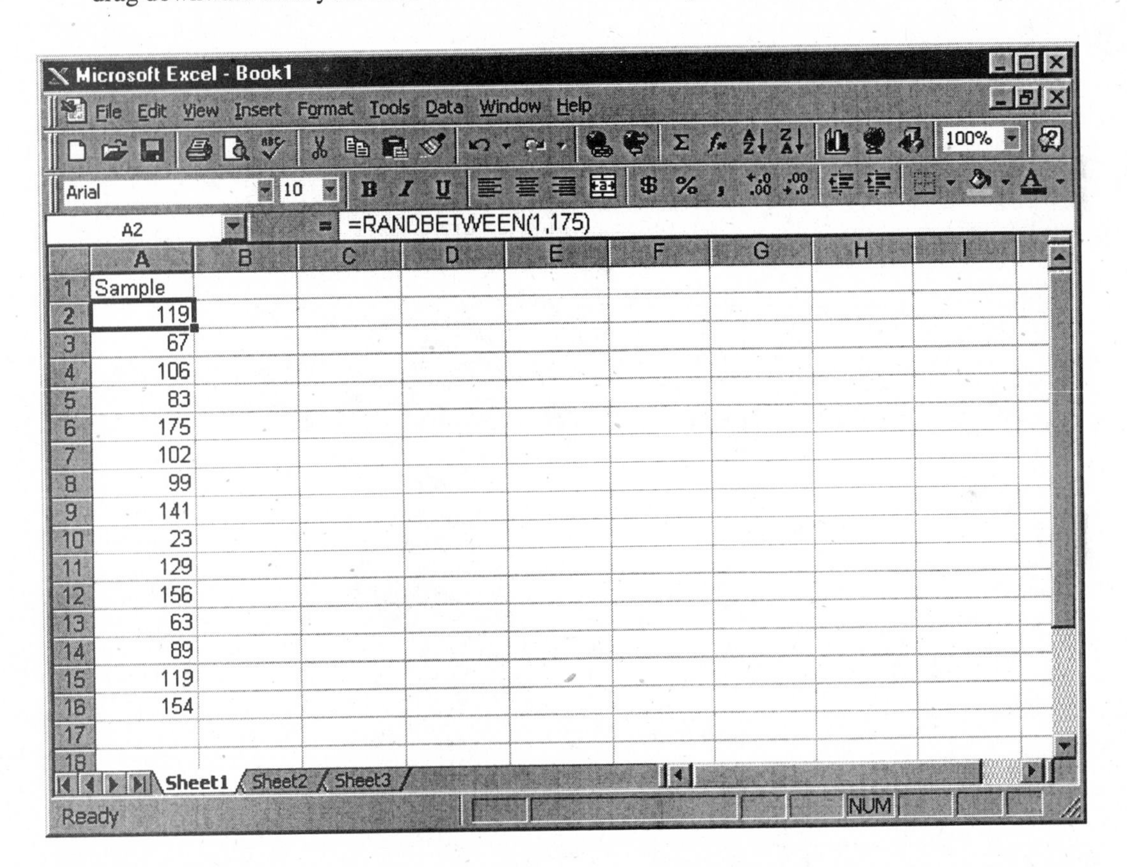

(f) Use one of the Sort buttons to sort the data, so you can easily check for repetitions. If there are repetitions, press **Shift-F9** again and re-sort. Below, with the data sorted, we can verify that there are no repetitions.

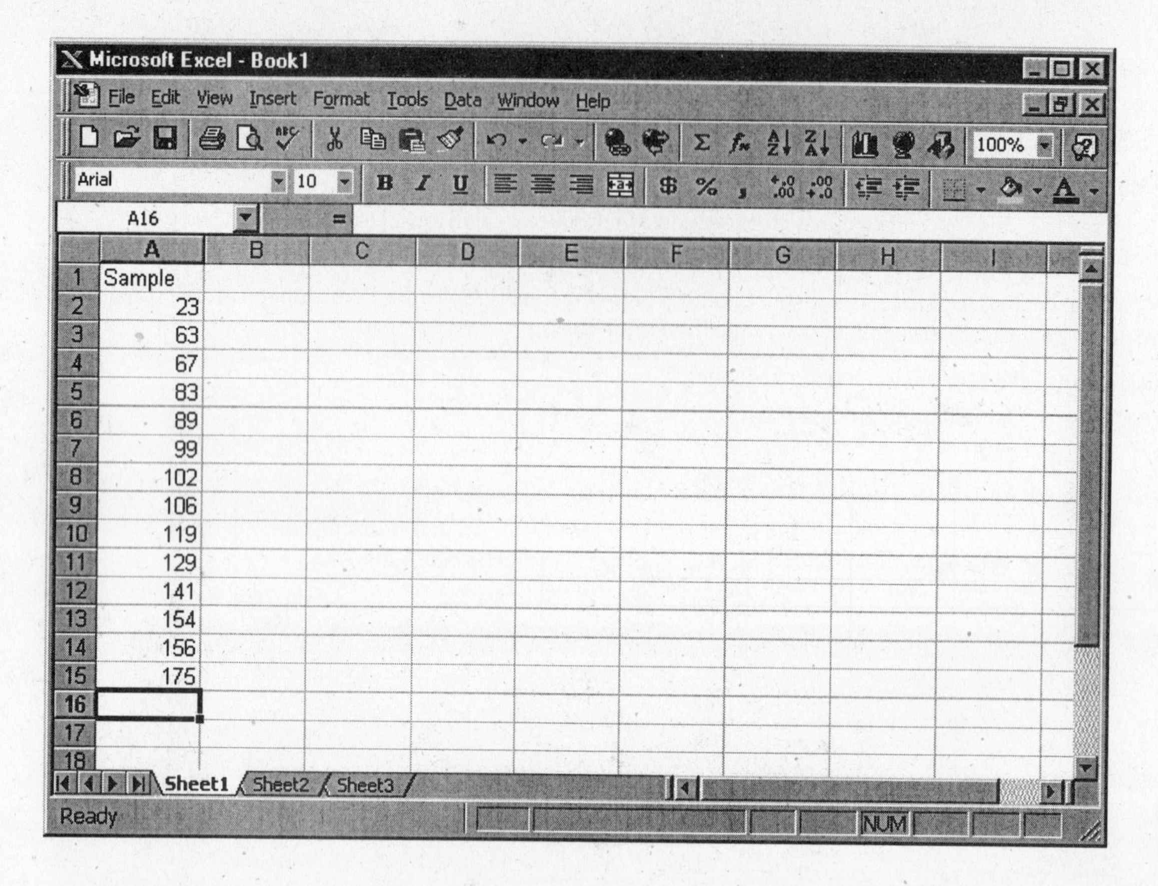

Sometimes we will want to sample from data already in our worksheet. In such case, we can use the **Sampling** dialog box. To reach the **Sampling** dialog box, use the man menu toolbar and select Sampling under **➤ Tools ➤ Data Analysis.**

Example

Enter the even numbers from 0 through 200 in Column A. Then take a sample of size ten, without replacement, from the population of even numbers 0 through 200, and place the results in Column B.

First we need to enter the even numbers 0 through 200 in Column A. Let's type the label Even # in Cell A1. The easiest way to generate the even numbers from 0 through 200 is to use the **Fill** menu selection. To do this, we

(a) Place the value 0 into Cell A2, and finish with Cell A2 highlighted.

(b) From the main menu, select **➤ Edit ➤ Fill ➤ Series.** In the dialog box select Series in Columns, Type Linear. Enter 2 as the Step value and 200 as the Stop value. Press OK.

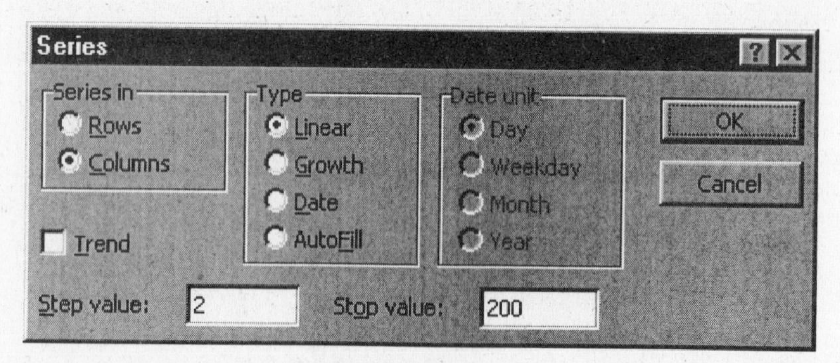

Now Column A should contain the even numbers from 0 to 200.

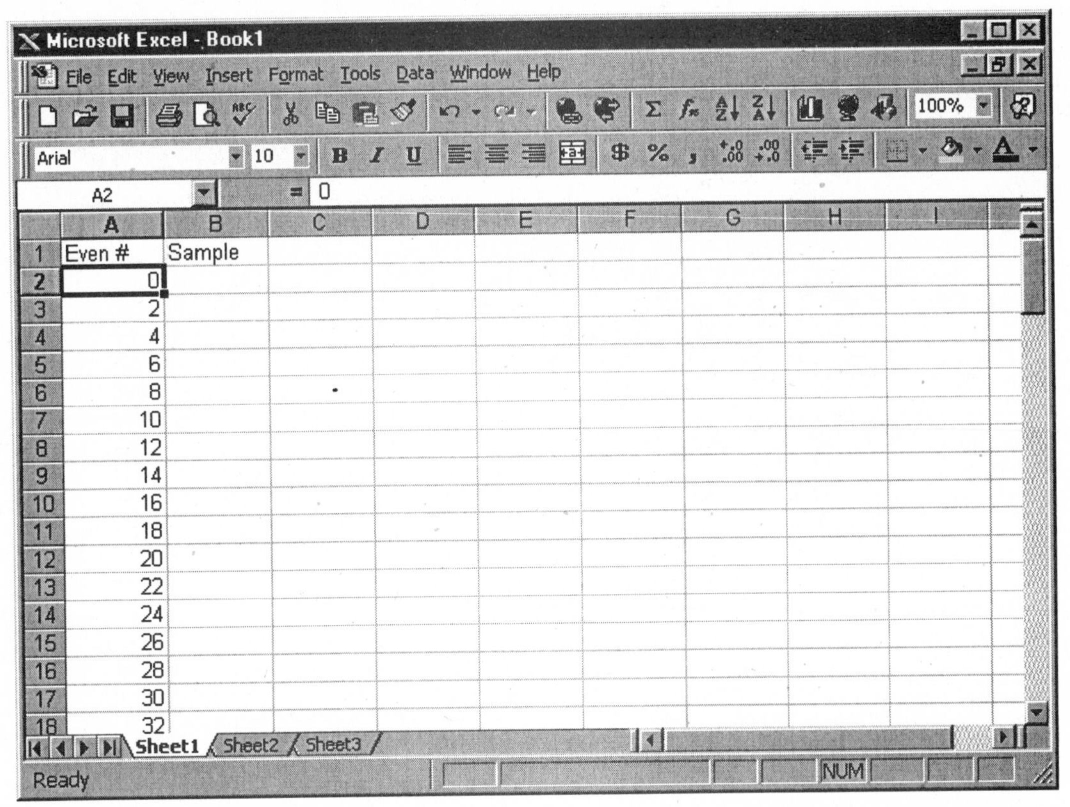

Now we will use the Sampling dialog box to select a sample of size ten from Column A, and we will place the sample in Column B. Notice that we labeled Column B as Sample. To draw the sample,

(a) From the main menu select **➤Tools➤Data Analysis➤Sampling.**

(b) In the dialog box, designate the data range from which we are sampling A1:A102. Also specify that the range contains a label. Select Random and enter 10 as the Number of Samples. Finally select the output range and type the destination B2:B11. Note that B1 already contains the label. Press Enter.

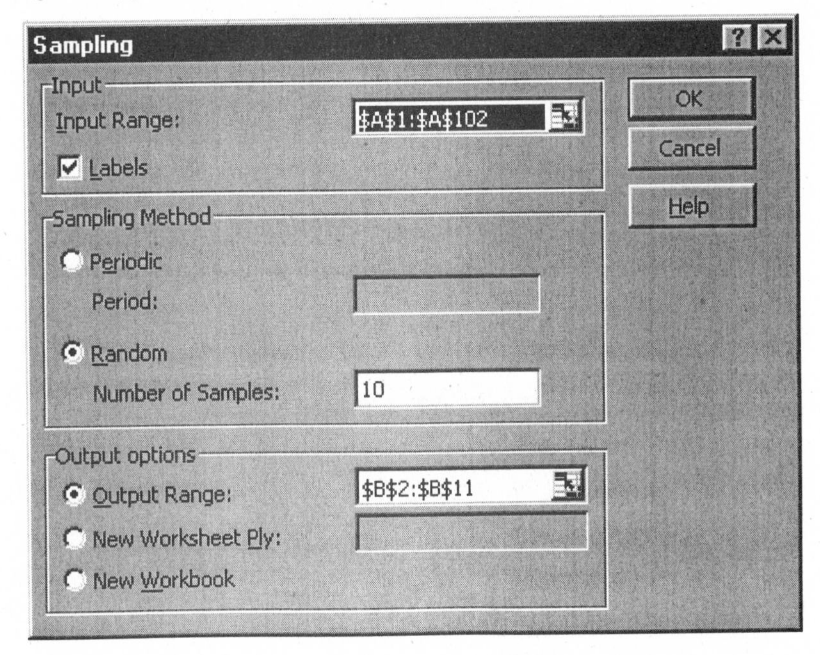

The worksheet now shows the random sample in Column B.

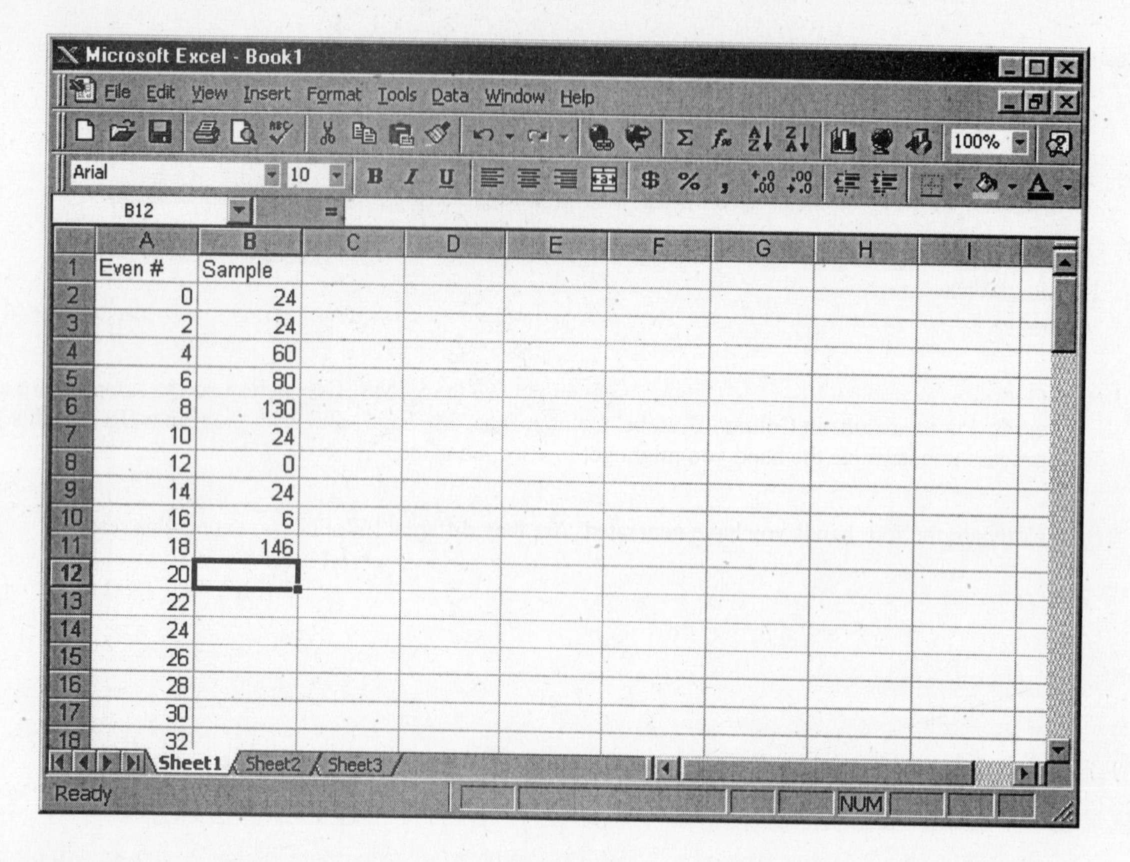

Note: After you finish the random number examples and the lab activities, you may want to set the calculation mode back to Automatic, especially if you are using a school computer.

LAB ACTIVITIES FOR RANDOM SAMPLES

1. Out of a population of 8173 eligible county residents, select a random sample of fifty for prospective jury duty. (Should you sample with or without replacement?) Use the RANDBETWEEN command with bottom value 1 and top value 8173. Then sort the data to check for repetitions. Note: Be sure that Calculation mode is set to manual and use the **Shift-F9** key combination to generate the sample in Rows 2 through 51 of Column A.

2. Retrieve the Excel worksheet Svls02.xls from the data CD-ROM. This file contains weights of a random sample of linebackers on professional football teams. The data is in column form. Use the SAMPLING dialog box to take a random sample of ten of these weights. Print the ten weights included in the sample.

Simulating experiments in which outcomes are equally likely is another important use of random numbers.

3. We can simulate dealing bridge hands by numbering the cards in a bridge deck from 1 to 52. Then we draw a random sample of thirteen numbers without replacement from the population of 52 numbers. A bridge deck has four suits: hearts, diamonds, clubs, and spades. Each suit contains thirteen cards; those numbered 2 through 10, a jack, a queen, a king, and an ace. Decide how to assign the numbers 1 through 52 to the cards in the deck.

(a) Use RANDBETWEEN to generate the numbers of the thirteen cards in one hand. Translate the numbers to specific cards and tell what cards are in the hand. For a second game, the cards would be collected and reshuffled. Use the computer to determine the hand you might get in a second game.

(b) Generate the numbers 1–52 in Column A, and then use the SAMPLING dialog box to sample thirteen cards. Put the results in Column B, Label Column B as "My hand" and print the results. Repeat this process to determine the hand you might get in a second game.

(c) Compare the four hands you have generated. Are they different? Would you expect this result?

4. We can also simulate the experiment of tossing a fair coin. The possible outcomes resulting from tossing a coin are heads or tails. Assign the outcome heads the number 2 and the outcome tails the number 1. Use RANDBETWEEN(1,2) to simulate the act of tossing a coin ten times. Simulate the experiment another time. Do you get the same sequence of outcomes? Do you expect to? Why or why not.

CHAPTER 2 ORGANIZING DATA

BAR GRAPHS, CIRCLE GRAPHS, AND TIME PLOTS (SECTION 2.1 OF *UNDERSTANDABLE STATISTICS*)

Excel has a Chart Wizard that produces a wide variety of charts. To access the Chart Wizard, use the Standard toolbar and select the button with a picture of a chart on it:

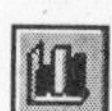

When you press the Chart Wizard button, a dialog box like the following is displayed.

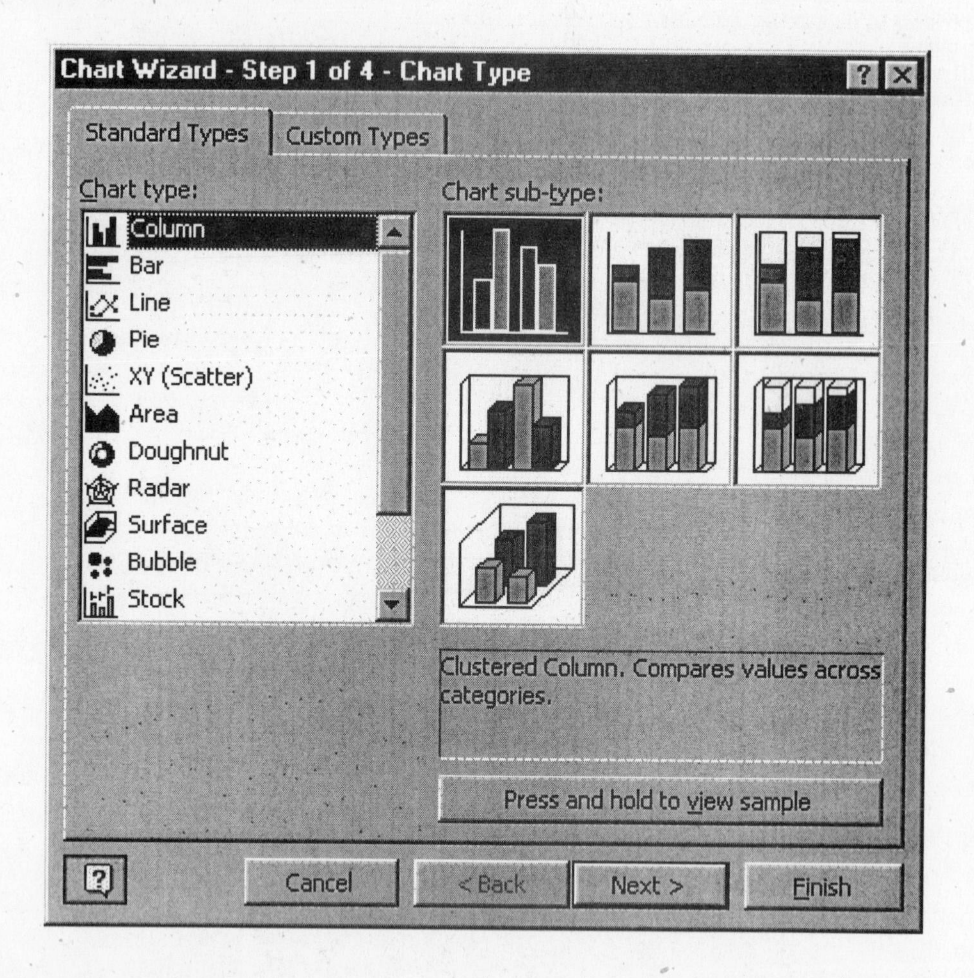

As you can see, you choose from a variety of chart types and select the chart subtype you want.

Bar Graphs

You have the option of making a vertical bar graph (called a column graph in Excel) or a horizontal bar graph (called a bar graph in Excel).

Before making a chart, you must enter the necessary data in a worksheet, in rows or columns with appropriate row and column headers.

Example

If you are out hiking, and the air temperature is 50°F with no wind, a light jacket will keep you comfortable. However, if a wind comes up, you will feel cold, even though the temperature has not changed. This is called wind chill. In the following spreadsheet, wind speeds and equivalent temperatures as a result of wind chill are given for a calm-air temperature of 50°F.

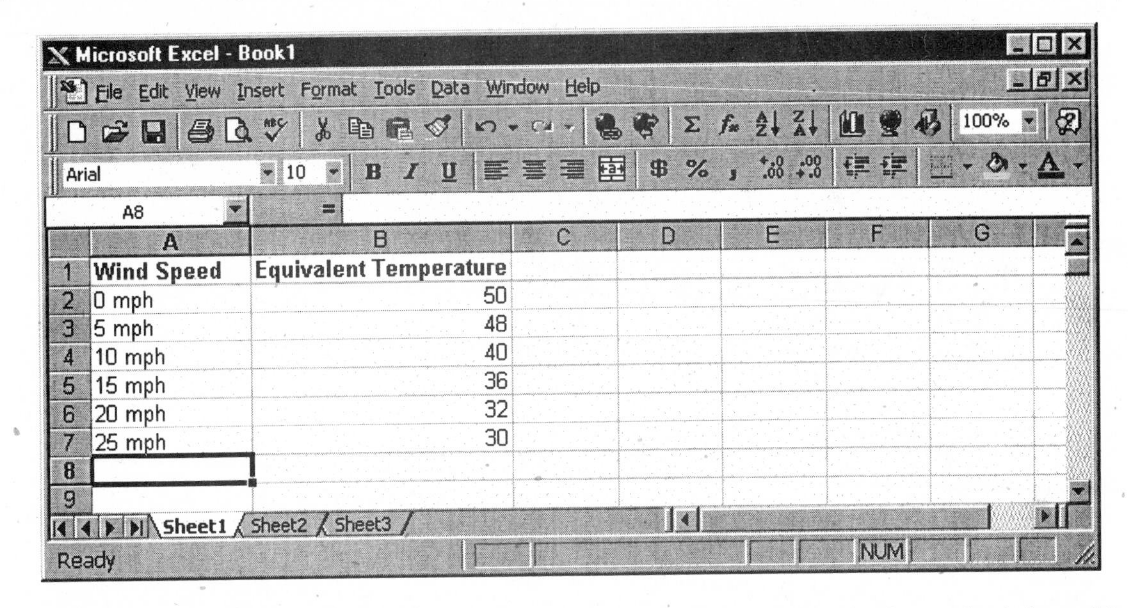

Wind Speed	Equivalent Temperature
0 mph	50
5 mph	48
10 mph	40
15 mph	36
20 mph	32
25 mph	30

Notice that the Columns A and B are widened, and the labels are typed in bold. Also, each wind speed is followed by a label. This will cause Excel to treat the wind speeds as row headers, rather than as numerical values. Now, after making sure that a cell in or touching the data blocks is selected, call up the Chart Wizard, choose the first option, and view a sample chart. The row headers, i.e., the wind speeds, give us the labels on the horizontal axis, while the values in Column B, the equivalent temperatures, appear as bar heights.

In the second step of the Chart Wizard you see this dialog box:

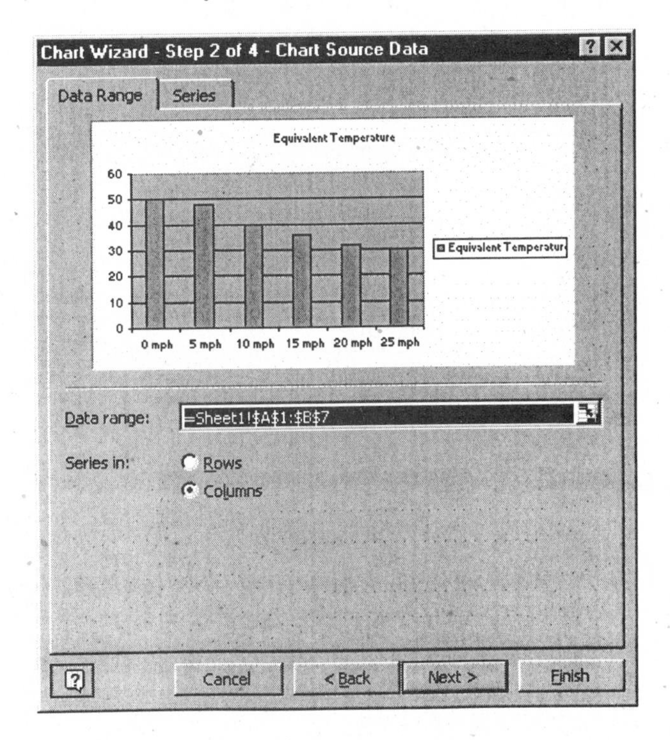

Since the data values are in a column (Column B), we select Series in Columns. Check that the data range is correct. If you click on the Series tab, you can set other parameters. See what happens when you select Series in Rows instead of Series in Columns under the Data Range tab. Click Next. Then click Back and reselect Series in Columns. Again, click Next.

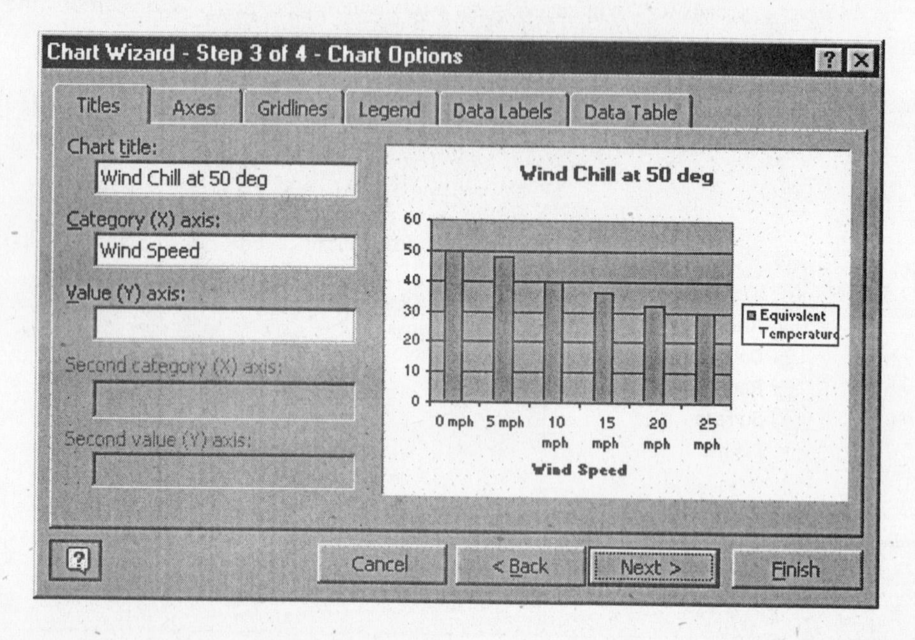

Notice again that there are several tabs. Click on the various tabs to see a variety of options for labeling the axes, setting grids, labeling the heights of the bars, etc. Try different buttons and options. If you do not like the results, deselect the options and return to the Titles tab. Notice that we typed in a title for the graph and also a label for the horizontal axis. Click Next.

The last dialog box asks where we want the graph to appear. If we select "As new sheet," we will get the chart on a worksheet all by itself. Selecting "As object in" places the chart on the designated sheet. It will appear with your data. The chart will have handles on it. When you click inside the chart and hold down the buttons, you can drag the chart to a new location on the worksheet. You can also use the handles to resize the graph. Click outside the chart to remove the chart handles.

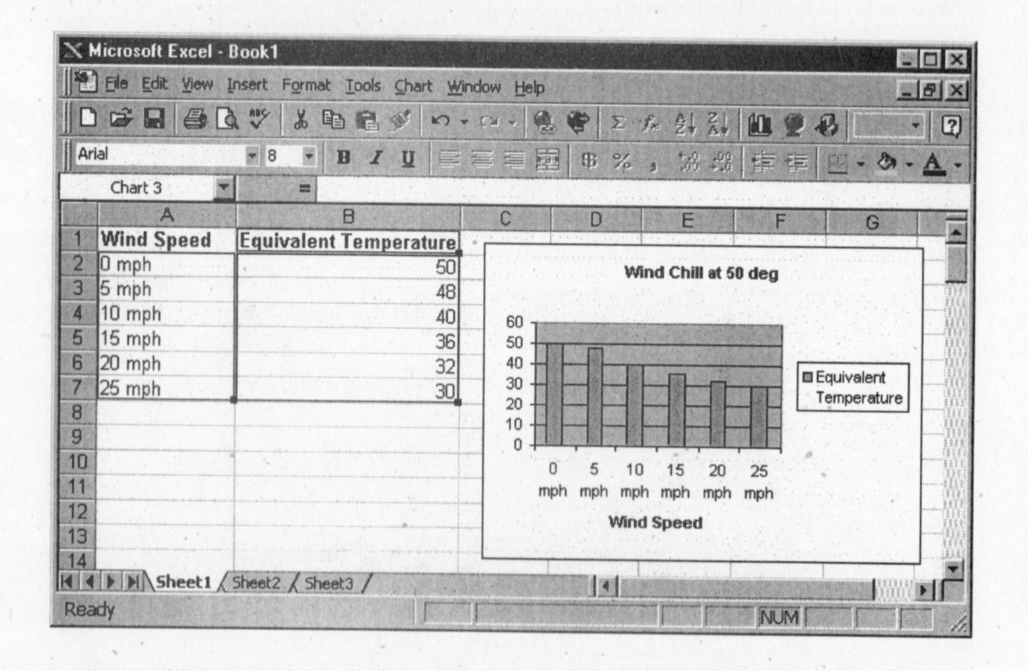

Circle Graphs

Another option available from the Chart Wizard is Pie Chart format.

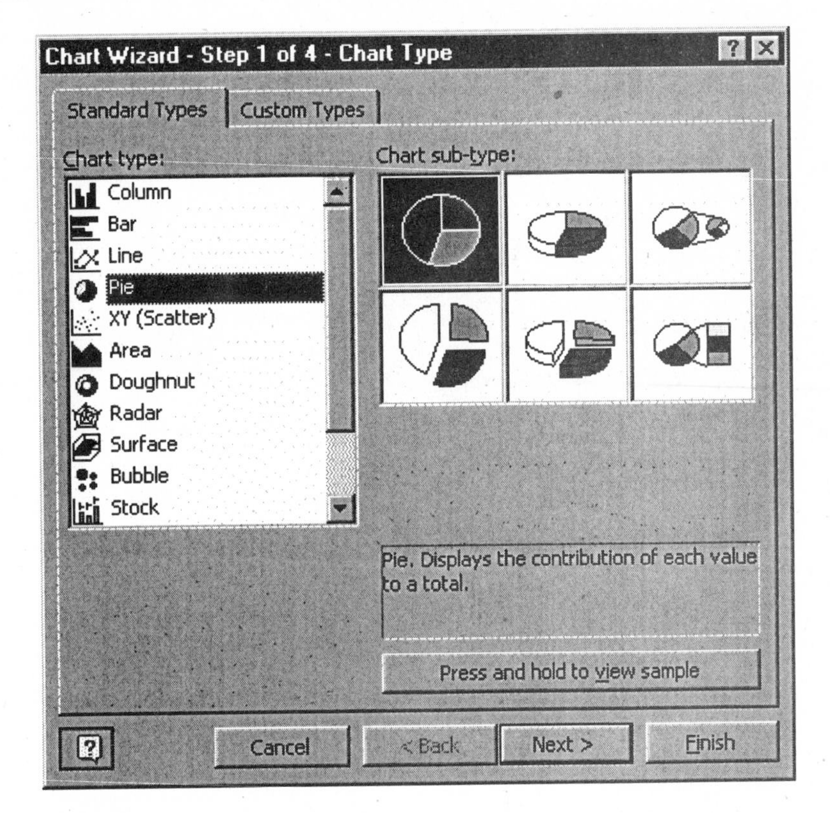

Again, enter the data in the worksheet first.

Example

Where do we hide the mess when company comes? According to *USA Today,* a survey showed that 68% of the respondents hide the mess in the closet, 23% put things under the bed, 6% put things in the bathtub, and 3% put things in the freezer. Make a circle graph for these data. We will put labels in Column A and the percents in Column B.

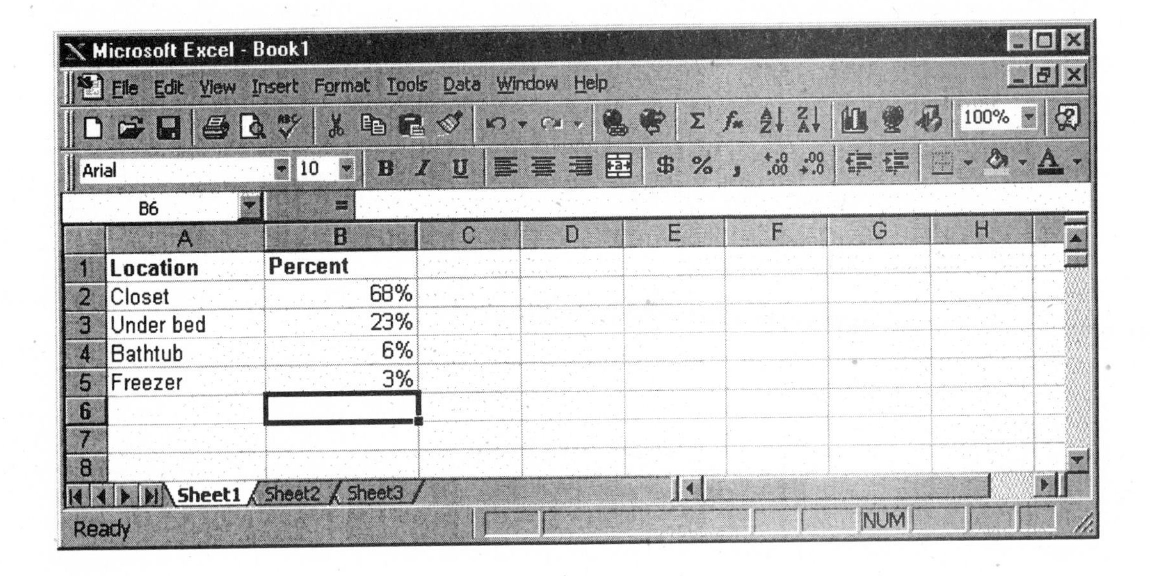

	A	B
1	Location	Percent
2	Closet	68%
3	Under bed	23%
4	Bathtub	6%
5	Freezer	3%

Select the basic pie chart on the Chart Wizard. In the Data Range dialog box, select Series in Columns, then click Next.

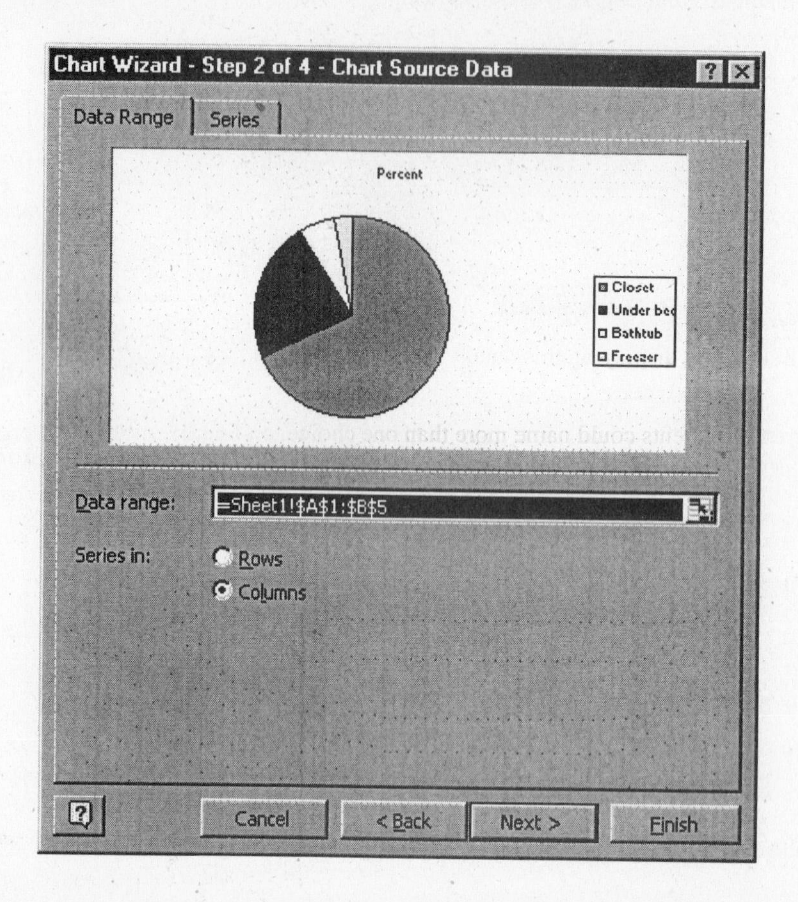

For the title, type "Where We Hide the Mess." Click Next. Select "As object in" and then Finish.

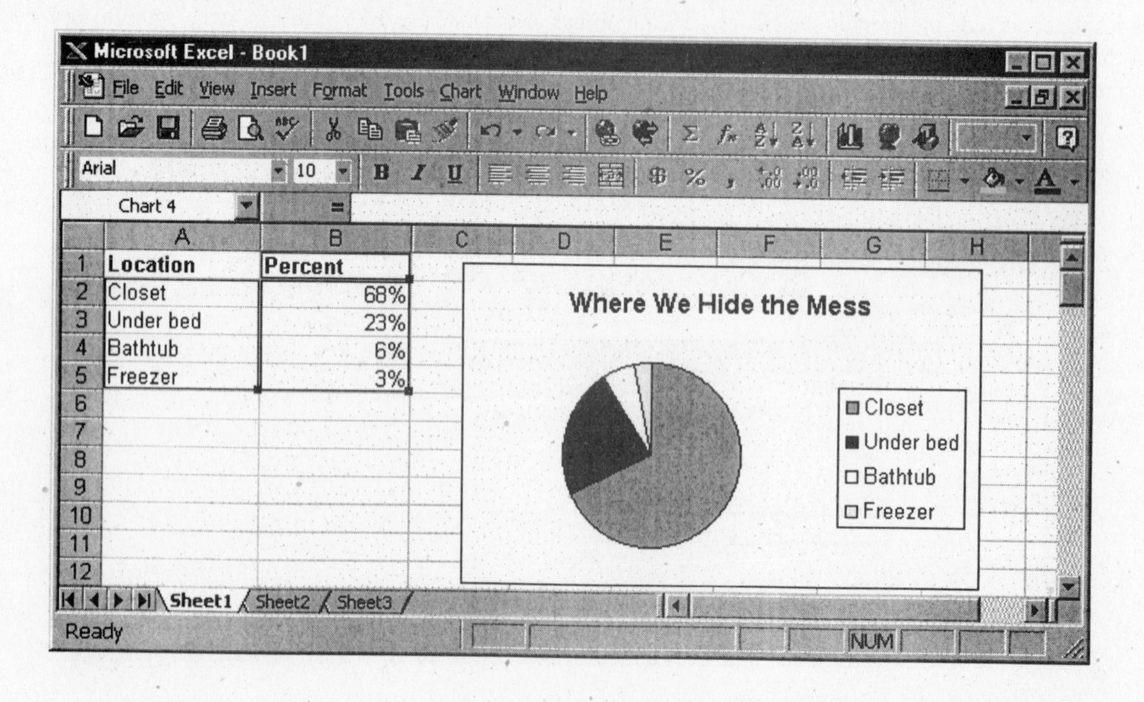

Time Plots

You can make time charts by selecting Line Charts in the Chart Wizard. In step three, select the Axes tab and then choose Time-scale.

LAB ACTIVITIES FOR BAR GRAPHS, CIRCLE GRAPHS, AND TIME PLOTS

1. According to a survey of chief information officers at large companies, the technology skills most in demand are: Networking 33%; Internet/intranet development, 21%; Applications development 18%; Help desk/user support, 8%; Operations, 6%; Project management, 6%, Systems analysis, 5%; Other 3%.

(a) Make a bar graph displaying this data.

(b) Make a circle graph displaying this data.

2. In survey where respondents could name more than one choice, on-line Internet users were asked where they obtained news about current events. The results are: Search engine/directory sites, 49%; Cable news site, 41%; On-line service; 40%; Broadcast news site, 40%; Local newspapers, 30%; National newspaper site; 24%; Other, 13%; National newsweekly site 12%; Haven't accessed news on-line, 11%.

(a) Make a horizontal bar graph displaying this information.

(b) Is this information appropriate for a circle graph display? Why or why not?

3. What percentage of its income does the average household spend on food, and how may workdays are devoted to earning the money spent on food in an average household? The American Farm Bureau Federation gave the following information, by year: In 1930, 25% of a household's budget went to food, and it took 91 workdays to earn the money. In 1960, 17% of the budget was for food, and the money took 64 workdays to earn. In 1990, food was 12% of the budget, earned in 43 workdays. For the year 2000, it was projected that the food budget would 11% of total income and that it would take 40 workdays to earn the money.

(a) Enter these data in an Excel worksheet so you can create graphs.

(b) Make bar charts for both the percent of budget for food, by year, and for the workdays required.

(c) Use the Chart Wizard to make a "double" bar graph that shows side-by-side bars, by year, for the percent of budget and for the number of days of work. (You may need to change the format of the first column of numbers to something other than percent.)

(d) Are these data suitable for a time plot? If so, use the Line graph option in the Chart Wizard to create a time plot that shows both the percent of budget and number of work days consumed on household food.

FREQUENCY DISTRIBUTIONS AND HISTOGRAMS (SECTION 2.2 OF *UNDERSTANDABLE STATISTICS*)

Excel's Histogram dialog box is found under **➤Tools➤Data Analysis➤Histogram.**

Example

Let's make a histogram with four classes, using the data we stored in the workbook Book1ads (created in Chapter 1). Use **➤File➤Open** to locate the workbook, and click on it.

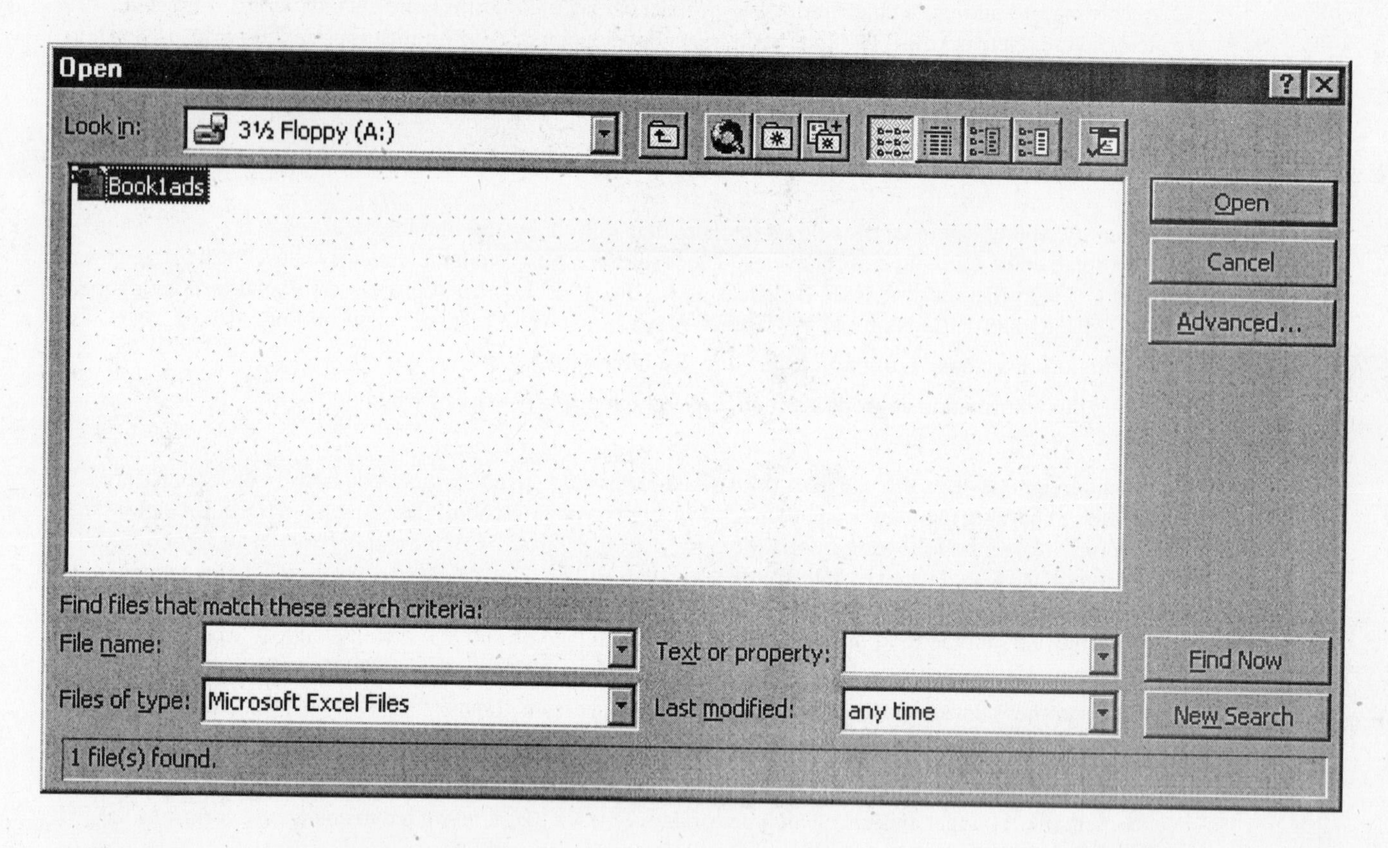

The number of ads per hour of TV is in Column A; we will represent these values in the histogram. We also need to specify class boundaries, and for this we will use Column C. Using methods shown in the text *Understandable Statistics*, we see that the upper class boundaries for four classes are 16.5, 20.5, 24.5, and 28.5.

Label Column C as Ad Count, and below the label enter these values, smallest to largest. The horizontal axis of the histogram will carry the label Ad Count. Note: Excel follows the convention that a data value is counted in a class if the value is less than or equal to the upper boundary (upper bin value) of the class.

Now select **➤Tools➤Data Analysis➤Histogram.** Check the Labels option, and select New workbook for the output option. Finally, check Chart output for the histogram, and check Cumulative percentage to produce an ogive. Note that you can select both options, or just one of the options. Your dialog box should look similar to the one at the top of the next page.

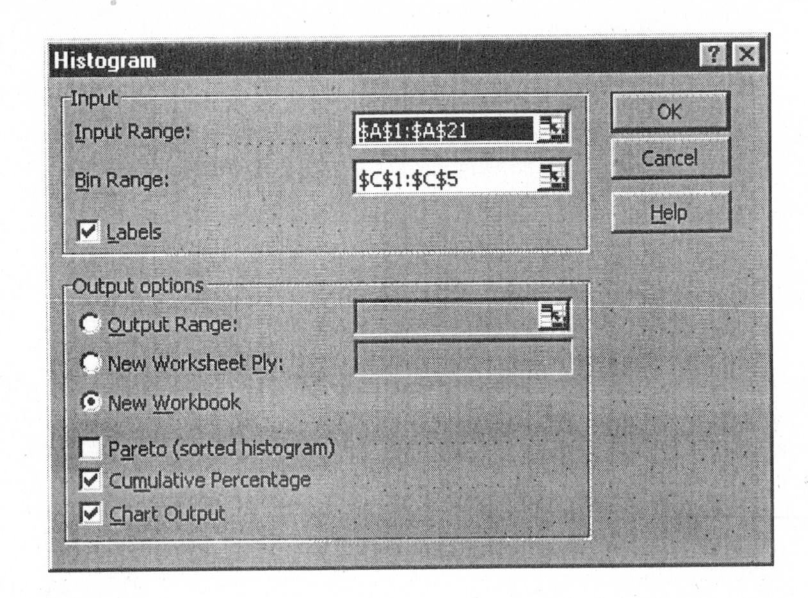

In the resulting worksheet, we moved and resized the chart window. Notice that the class boundaries are not shown directly under the tick marks. The first bar represents all the values less than or equal to 16.5, the second bar is for values greater than 16.5 and less than or equal to 20.5, and so on. There are no values above 28.5.

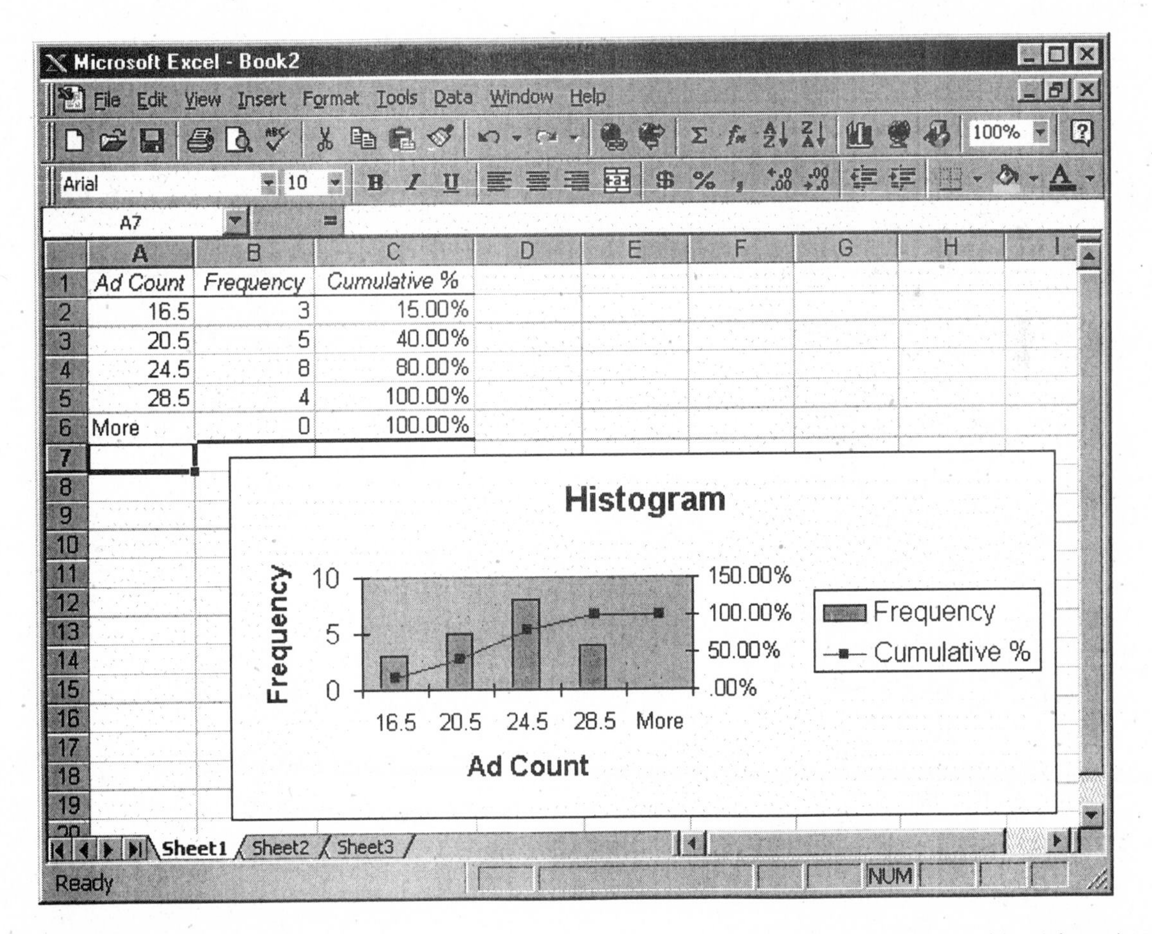

If you do not specify the cells containing the bin range, Excel automatically creates enough bins (classes) to show the data distribution.

Adjusting the Histogram

Excel automatically supplies the "more" category (which will be empty if you specify upper class boundaries). To remove the "more" category, select the row of the frequency table that contains "more". Then, on the main menu bar select **➤Edit➤Delete➤Shift cells up.**

To make the bars touch, *right-click* on one of the bars of the histogram. Then click **Format Data Series** and click the Options tab. Set Gap width to 0. Then press Enter.

The results should be similar to this:

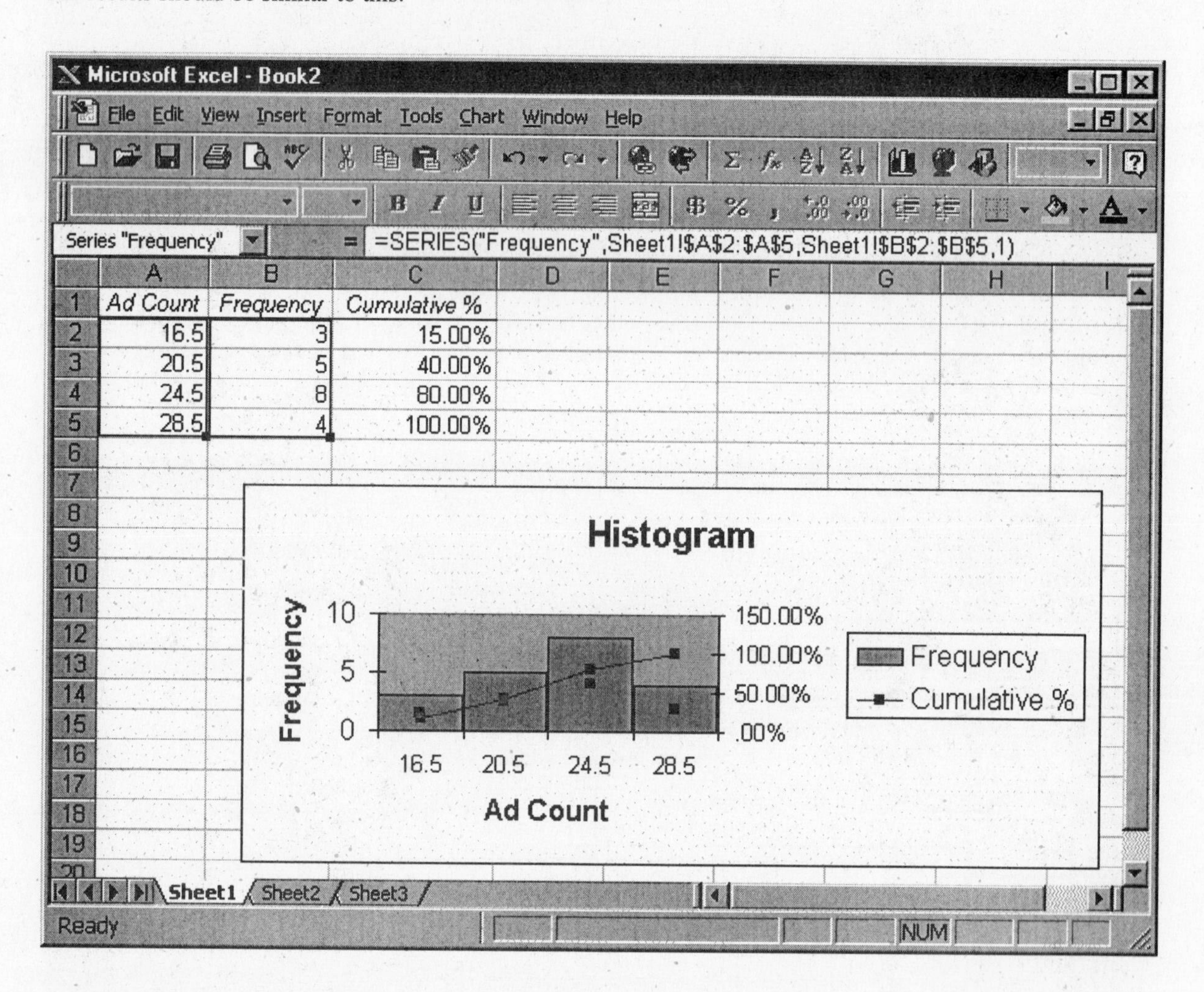

LAB ACTIVITIES FOR FREQUENCY DISTRIBUTIONS AND HISTOGRAMS

1. The Book1ads workbook contains a second column of data, with the minutes of ads per hour of prime time TV. Retrieve the workbook again and use column B to
   - **(a)** Make a histogram letting Excel determine the number of classes (bins).
   - **(b)** Use the Sort button on the standard toolbar, then find the highest and lowest data values. Use the techniques of the text to find the upper class boundaries for five classes. Make a column in your worksheet that contains these boundaries, and label the column Min/Hr. In the Histogram dialog box, use the column containing these upper boundaries as the bin range. Generate a histogram.

2. As a project for her finance class, Linda gathered data about the number of cash requests made at an automatic teller machine located in the student center between the hours of 6 P.M. and 11 P.M. She made a count every day for four weeks. The results follow.

25	17	33	47	22	32	18	21	12	26	43	25
19	27	26	29	39	12	19	27	10	15	21	20
32	24	17	181								

(a) Enter the data.

(b) Repeat part (b) of Problem 1.

3. Choose one of the following workbooks from the Excel data disk.

DISNEY STOCK VOLUME: **Svls01.xls**
WEIGHTS OF PRO FOOTBALL PLAYERS: **Svls02.xls**
HEIGHTS OF PRO BASKETBALL PLAYERS: **Svls03.xls**
MILES PER GALLON GASOLINE CONSUMPTION: **Svls04.xls**
FASTING GLUCOSE BLOOD TESTS: **Svls05.xls**
NUMBER OF CHILDREN IN RURAL CANADIAN FAMILIES: **Svls06.xls**

(a) Make a histogram letting Excel scale it

(b) Make a histogram using five classes. Use the method of part (b) of Problem 1.

4. Histograms are not effective displays for some data. Consider the data

1	2	3	6	7	9	8	4	12	10
1	9	1	12	12	11	13	4	6	206

Enter the data and make a histogram letting Excel do the scaling. Now drop the high value, 206, from the data set. Do you get more refined information from the histogram by eliminating the high and unusual data value?

CHAPTER 3 AVERAGES AND VARIATION

CENTRAL TENDENCY AND VARIATION OF UNGROUPED DATA (SECTIONS 3.1 AND 3.2 OF *UNDERSTANDABLE STATISTICS*)

Sections 3.1 and 3.2 of *Understandable Statistics* describe some of the measures used to summarize the character of a data set. Excel supports these descriptive measures.

On the standard toolbar, click the Paste Function button.

In the dialog box that appears, select Statistical in the left column, and in the right column select the measure of interest. To find the arithmetic mean of a set of numbers, for instance, we use the function AVERAGE.

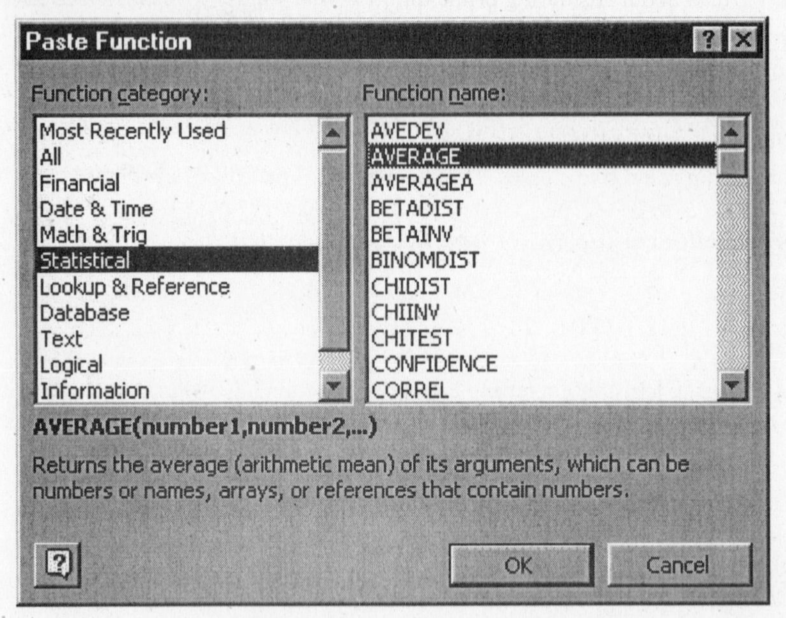

Notice that the bottom of the dialog box contains a brief explanation of how the selected function works.

Of the descriptive measures discussed in Sections 3.1 and 3.2 of the text, Excel supports the following:

AVERAGE(data range)

returns the arithmic mean $\overline{x}$ or μ of the data values in the designated cells.

COUNT(data range)

returns the number of data values in the designated cells.

MEDIAN(data range)

returns the median of the data values in the designated cells.

MODE(data range)

returns the mode of the data values in the designated cells.

STDEV(data range)

returns the sample standard deviation of the data values in the designated cells.

STDEVP(data range)

returns the population standard deviation of the data values in the designated cells.

TRIMMEAN(data range, percent as a decimal)

returns a trimmed mean based on the *total* percentage of data removed from both the bottom and top of the ordered data values. If you want a 5% trimmed mean, implying that 5% of the bottom data and 5% of the top data will be removed, then enter 0.10 for the percent in Excel.

Formatting the Worksheet to Display the Summary Statistics

It is a good idea to create a column in which you type the name of each descriptive measure you use, next to the column where the corresponding computations are performed.

Example

Let's again use the data about ads during prime time TV. We will retrieve Book1ads and find summary statistics for Column B, the time taken up with ads. And we will use Column C as our column of names for the descriptive statistics measures. Notice that we widened the column to accommodate the names. We label Column C to remind us that the summary statistics apply to the number of minutes per hour that ads consume.

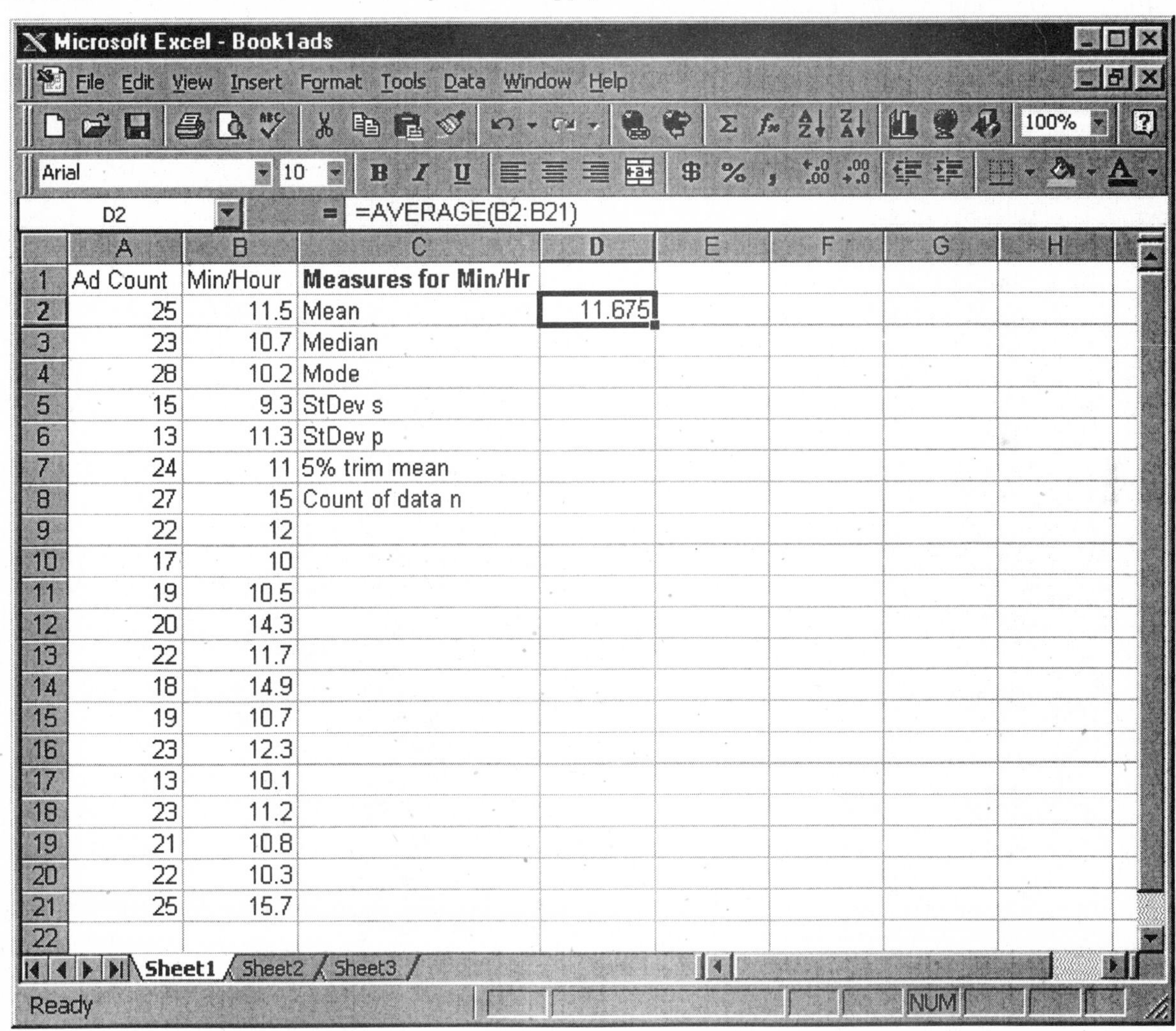

	A	B	C	D
1	Ad Count	Min/Hour	**Measures for Min/Hr**	
2	25	11.5	Mean	11.675
3	23	10.7	Median	
4	28	10.2	Mode	
5	15	9.3	StDev s	
6	13	11.3	StDev p	
7	24	11	5% trim mean	
8	27	15	Count of data n	
9	22	12		
10	17	10		
11	19	10.5		
12	20	14.3		
13	22	11.7		
14	18	14.9		
15	19	10.7		
16	23	12.3		
17	13	10.1		
18	23	11.2		
19	21	10.8		
20	22	10.3		
21	25	15.7		
22				

Notice that Cell D2 is highlighted, and the formula bar shows the command = AVERAGE(B2:B21). The value in Cell D2 is the mean of the data in the Cells B2 through B21.

To compute the other measures, we enter the appropriate formulas in Column D and identify the measures used in Column C, as shown. Notice that you can type the commands directly in the formula bar (don't forget to put = before the command), or you can use the Paste Function button and retrieve the function from the category Statistical.

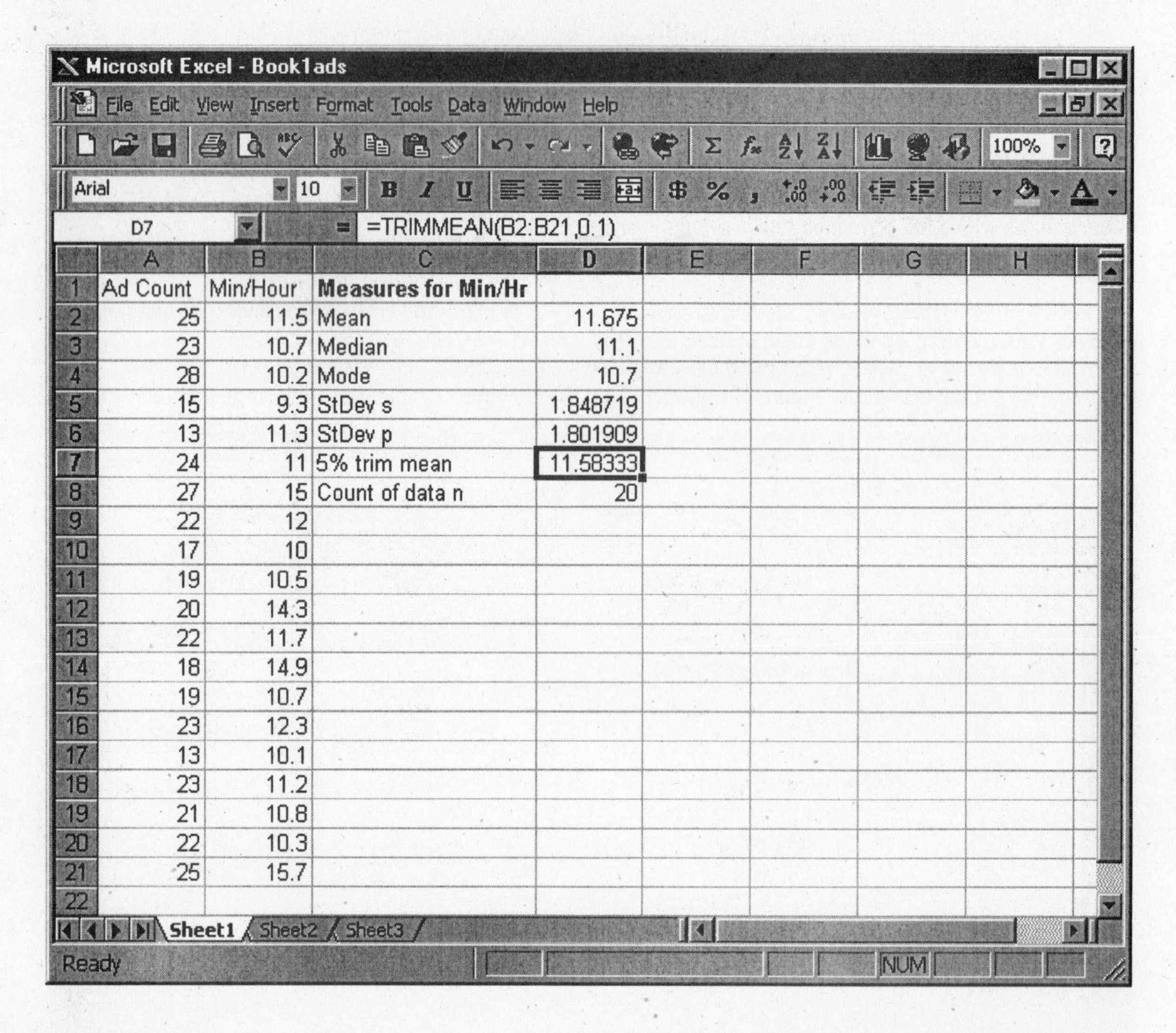

Microsoft Excel - Book1ads

D7 = =TRIMMEAN(B2:B21,0.1)

	A	B	C	D
1	Ad Count	Min/Hour	**Measures for Min/Hr**	
2	25	11.5	Mean	11.675
3	23	10.7	Median	11.1
4	28	10.2	Mode	10.7
5	15	9.3	StDev s	1.848719
6	13	11.3	StDev p	1.801909
7	24	11	5% trim mean	11.58333
8	27	15	Count of data n	20
9	22	12		
10	17	10		
11	19	10.5		
12	20	14.3		
13	22	11.7		
14	18	14.9		
15	19	10.7		
16	23	12.3		
17	13	10.1		
18	23	11.2		
19	21	10.8		
20	22	10.3		
21	25	15.7		
22				

Sheet1 / Sheet2 / Sheet3

Ready NUM

Don't forget that you can control the number of digits displayed after the decimal by using the buttons on the standard toolbar to increase or decrease the number of decimal places.

Another way to obtain a table of some descriptive statistics is to use the menu choices **➤Tools➤Data Analysis➤Descriptive Statistics**. A dialog box appears. If you check Summary statistics, an output table containing the mean, median, mode, and other measures appears.

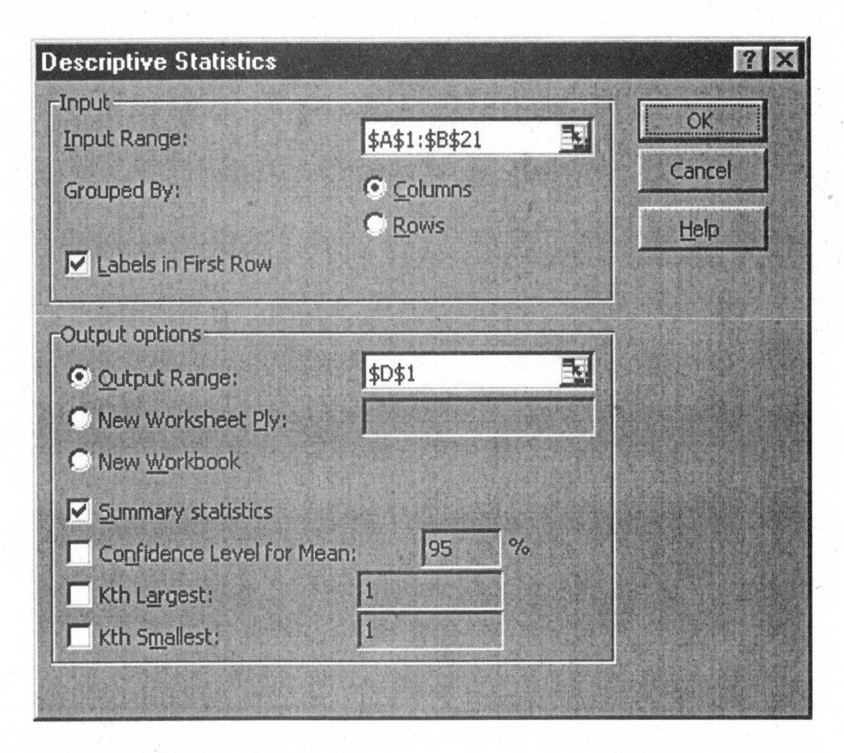

For the Ad count and Min/Hr data the results are.

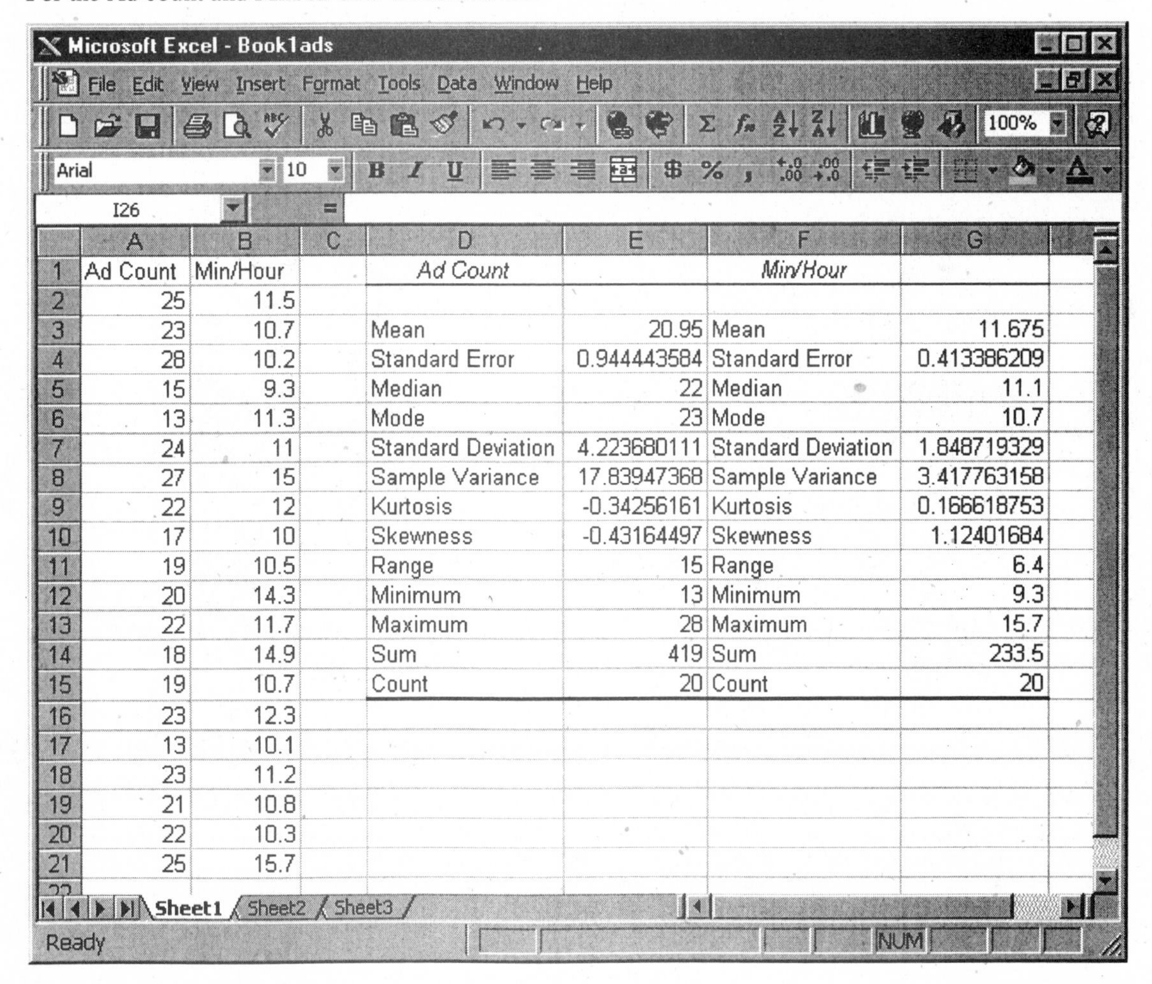

	A	B	C	D	E	F	G
1	Ad Count	Min/Hour		*Ad Count*		*Min/Hour*	
2	25	11.5					
3	23	10.7		Mean	20.95	Mean	11.675
4	28	10.2		Standard Error	0.944443584	Standard Error	0.413386209
5	15	9.3		Median	22	Median	11.1
6	13	11.3		Mode	23	Mode	10.7
7	24	11		Standard Deviation	4.223680111	Standard Deviation	1.848719329
8	27	15		Sample Variance	17.83947368	Sample Variance	3.417763158
9	22	12		Kurtosis	-0.34256161	Kurtosis	0.166618753
10	17	10		Skewness	-0.43164497	Skewness	1.12401684
11	19	10.5		Range	15	Range	6.4
12	20	14.3		Minimum	13	Minimum	9.3
13	22	11.7		Maximum	28	Maximum	15.7
14	18	14.9		Sum	419	Sum	233.5
15	19	10.7		Count	20	Count	20
16	23	12.3					
17	13	10.1					
18	23	11.2					
19	21	10.8					
20	22	10.3					
21	25	15.7					

LAB ACTIVITIES FOR CENTRAL TENDENCY AND VARIATION OF UNGROUPED DATA

1. A random sample of twenty people were asked to dial thirty telephone numbers each. The incidence of numbers misdialed by these people follow:

   3 2 0 0 1 5 7 8 2 6
   0 1 2 7 2 5 1 4 5 3

   Enter the data and use the appropriate commands to find the mean, median, mode, sample standard deviation, population standard deviation, 10% trimmed mean, and data count.

2. Consider the test scores of thirty students in a political science class.

   85 73 43 86 73 59 73 84 100 62
   75 87 70 84 97 62 76 89 90 83
   70 65 77 90 94 80 68 91 67 79

   (a) Use the appropriate commands to find the mean, median, mode, sample standard deviation, 10% trimmed mean, and data count.

   (b) Suppose that Greg, a student in a political science course, missed a several classes because of illness. Suppose he took the final exam anyway and made a score of 30 instead of 85 as listed in the data set. Change the 85 (first entry in the data set) to 30 and use the appropriate commands to find the new mean, median, mode, sample standard deviation, 10% trimmed mean, and data count. Compare the new mean, median and standard deviation with the ones in part (a). Which average was most affected: median or mean? What about the standard deviation?

3. Consider the ten data values

4	7	3	15	9	12	10	2	9	10

   (a) Use the appropriate commands to find the sample standard deviation and the population standard deviation. Compare the two values.

   (b) Now consider these fifty data values in the same general range:

7	9	10	6	11	15	17	9	8	2
2	8	11	15	14	12	13	7	6	9
3	9	8	17	8	12	14	4	3	9
2	15	7	8	7	13	15	2	5	6
2	14	9	7	3	15	12	10	9	10

   Again use the appropriate commands to find the sample standard deviation and the population standard deviation. Compare the two values.

   (c) Compare the results of parts (a) and (b). As the sample size increases, does it appear that the difference between the population and sample standard deviations decreases? Why would you expect this result from the formulas?

4. In this problem we will explode the effects of changing data values by multiplying each data value by a constant, or by adding the same constant to each data value.

   (a) Clear your workbook or begin a new one. Then enter the following data into Column A, with the column label "Original" in Cell A1.

   1 8 3 5 7 2 10 9 4 6 3

(b) Now label Column B as A * 10. Select Cell B2. In the formula bar, type

=A2*10

and press Enter. Select Cell B2 again and move the cursor to the lower right corner of Cell B2. A small black + should appear. Click-drag the + down the column so that Column B contains all the data of Column A, but with each value in Column A multiplied by 10.

(c) Now suppose we add 30 to each data value in Column A and put the new data in Column C.

First label Column E as A + 30. Then select Cell C2. In the formula bar type

=A2+30

and press Enter. Then select Cell C2 again and position the cursor in the lower right corner. The cursor should change shape to a small black +. Click-drag down Column C to generate all the entries of Column A increased by 30.

(d) Predict how you think the mean and the standard deviation of Columns B and C will be similar to or different from those values for column A. Use the **➤Tools➤Data Analysis➤Descriptive Statistics** dialogue box to find the mean and standard deviation for all three columns. Note: use all three columns as input columns in the dialogue box. Compare the actual results to your predictions. What do you predict will happen to these descriptive statistics values if you multiply each data value of Column A by 50? If you add 50 to each data value in Column A?

BOX-AND-WHISKER PLOTS (SECTION 3.4 OF *UNDERSTANDABLE STATISTICS*)

Excel does not have any commands or dialogue boxes that produce box-and-whisker plots directly. Macros can be written to accomplish the task. However, Excel does have commands to produce the five-number summary, and you can then draw a box-and-whisker plot by hand.

The commands for the five-number summary can be found in the dialogue box obtained by pressing the Paste Function (or function wizard) key on the standard tool bar.

MIN(data range) which returns the minimum data value from the designated cells.

QUARTILE(data range, 1) which returns the first quartile for the data in the designated cells.

MEDIAN(data range) which returns the median of the data in the designated cells.

QUARTILE(data range, 3) which returns the third quartile for the data in the designated cells.

MAX(data range) which returns the maximum data value from the designated cells.

Example

Generate the five-number summary for the number of minutes of ads per hour on commercial TV, using the data in Book1ads.

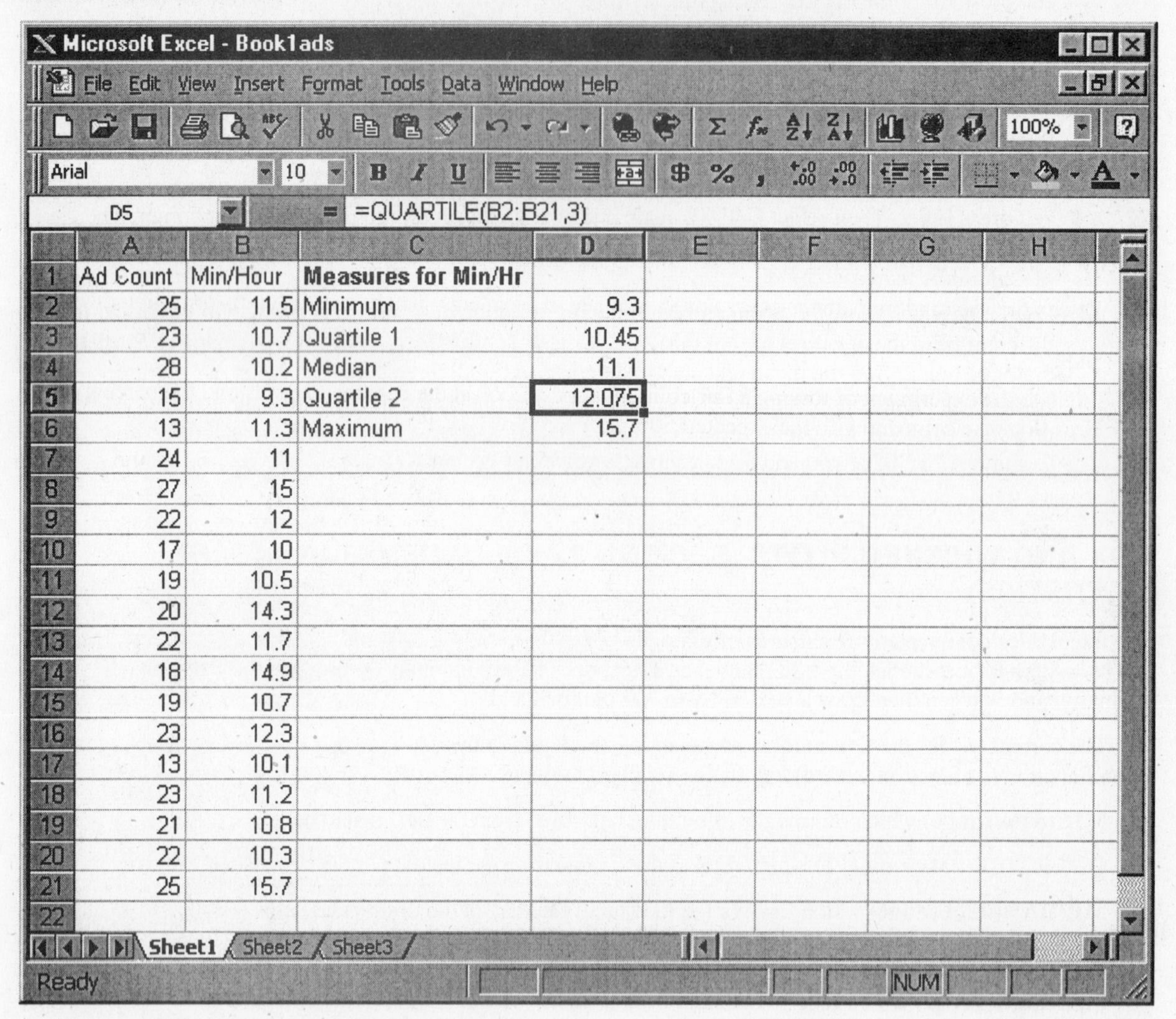

	A	B	C	D
1	Ad Count	Min/Hour	**Measures for Min/Hr**	
2	25	11.5	Minimum	9.3
3	23	10.7	Quartile 1	10.45
4	28	10.2	Median	11.1
5	15	9.3	Quartile 2	12.075
6	13	11.3	Maximum	15.7
7	24	11		
8	27	15		
9	22	12		
10	17	10		
11	19	10.5		
12	20	14.3		
13	22	11.7		
14	18	14.9		
15	19	10.7		
16	23	12.3		
17	13	10.1		
18	23	11.2		
19	21	10.8		
20	22	10.3		
21	25	15.7		
22				

In computing quartiles, Excel uses a slightly different process from the one adopted in *Understandable Statistics.* However, the results will generally be nearly the same.

CHAPTER 4 ELEMENTARY PROBABILITY THEORY

SIMULATIONS

Excel has several random number generators. Recall from Chapter 1 that RANDBETWEEN(Bottom,Top) puts out a random integer between (and including) the bottom and top numbers. Again, the Analysis ToolPak needs to be included as an Add-In to make RANDBETWEEN available. To find the RANDBETWEEN function, click the Paste Function or Function Wizard button on the standard tool bar. Then select All in the left column and scroll down in the right column until you find RANDBETWEEN. You can also type the command directly in the formula bar, but again, remember to type = first.

We can use the random number generator to simulate experiments such as tossing coins or rolling dice.

Example

Simulate the experiment of tossing a fair coin 200 times. Look at the percent of heads and the percent of tails. How do these compare with the expected 50% for each?

Assign the outcome heads to digit 1 and tails to digit 2. We will draw a random sample of size 200 from the distributions of integers from a minimum of 1 to a maximum of 2. When using a random number generator, you are best off setting recalculation to manual. To do this, go to **➤Tools➤Options** and, under Calculation, choose the option Manual Calculation.

Now put the label Coin Toss in Cell A1, and enter = RANDBETWEEN(1,2) in Cell A2. Then press Enter. Reselect Cell A2, move the cursor to the lower right corner until the + symbol appears, and drag down through Cell A201. Since calculation is set to manual, press **Shift-F9** to apply the random integer generation command to each of the selected cells. Column A should now have 200 entries.

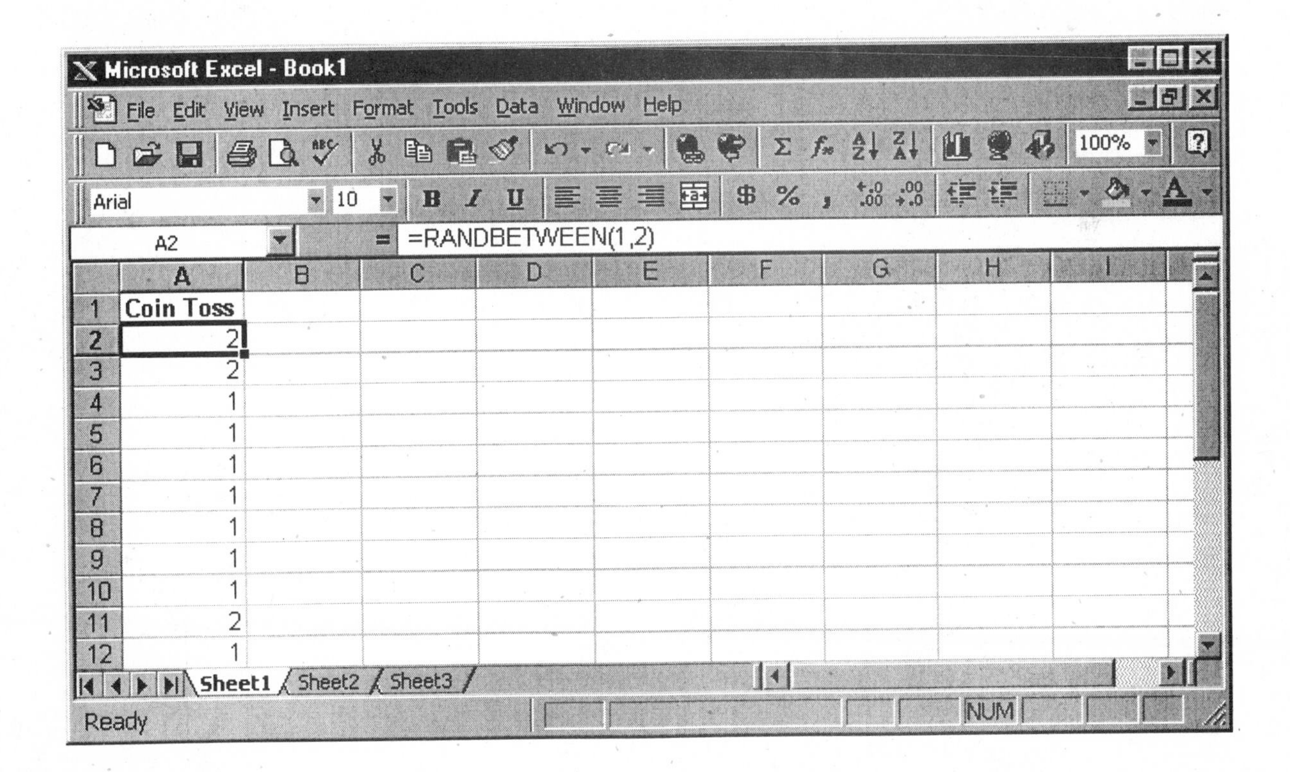

Count the number of heads and the number of tails

Next we want to count the number of 1's and 2's in column A. We will set up a table in Columns C and D to display the counts. Label Cell C1 as Outcome. Type Heads in Cell C2 and Tails in Cell C3. Then Label Cell D1 as Frequency.

We will use the COUNTIF command to count the 1's and 2's. The syntax for the COUNTIF command is

COUNTIF(data range,condition)

Recall that we assigned the number 1 to the outcome heads and the number 2 to the outcome tails. Select Cell D2, and enter

= COUNTIF(A1:A201,1)

This will return the number of 1's, or heads, in the designated cell range. Next select Cell D3, and enter = COUNTIF(A1:A200,2). This will return the number of 2's, or tails, in the same designated cell range.

Compute the relative frequency of each outcome

Let's use column E to display the probability of each outcome. Label Cell E1 as Rel Freq. Select Cell E2. In the formula bar, type

=D2/200

and press Enter. Then select Cell E3 and enter =D3/200. The display should be similar to the one shown.

Notice that the percentages of heads and of tails are each close to 50%. This is what the Law of Large Numbers predict. Of course, each time you repeat the simulation, you will in general get slightly different results.

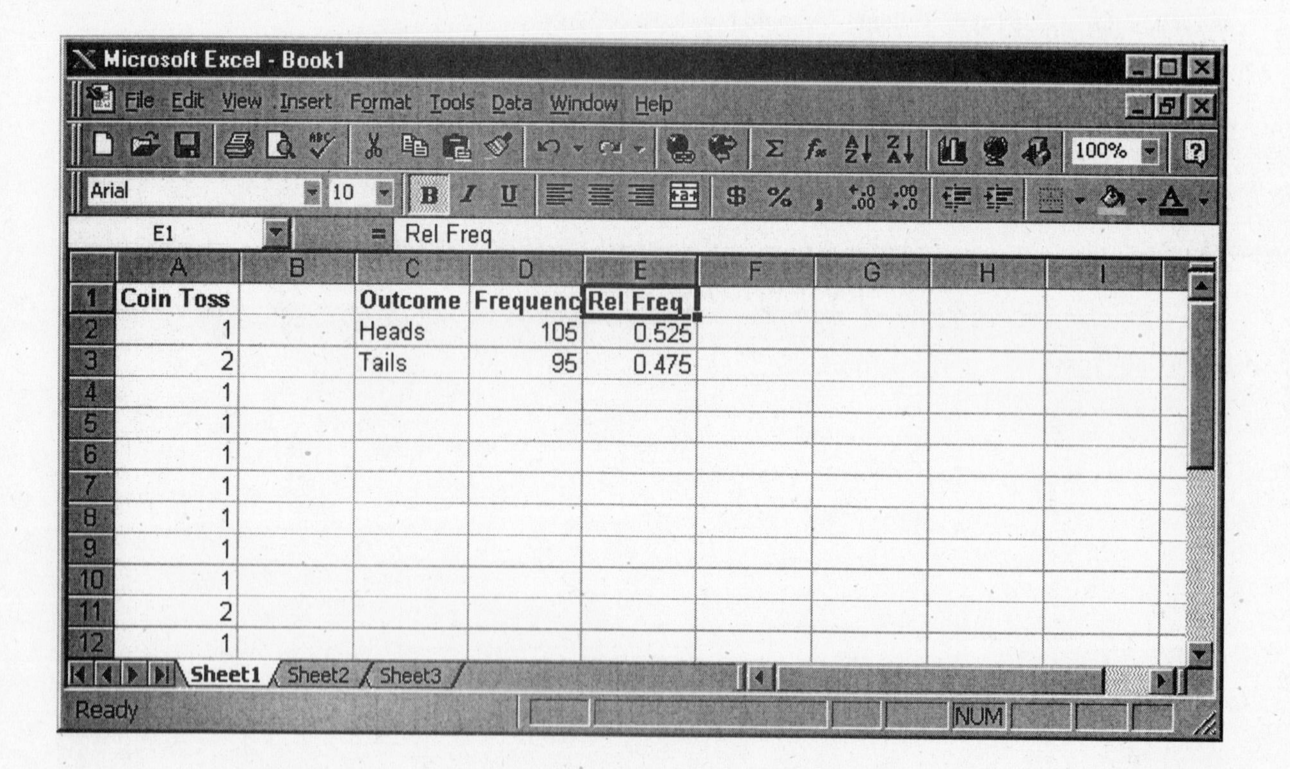

COUNTING

Excel has formulas for permutations and combinations of n objects taken r at a time.

Permut(n,r)

Returns the number of permutations of n objects taken r at a time.

Combin(n,r)

Returns the number of combinations of n objects taken r at a time.

Use the Paste Function to access dialogue boxes for these functions.

LAB ACTIVITIES FOR SIMULATIONS

1. Use the RANDBETWEEN command to simulate 50 tosses of a fair coin. Make a table showing the frequency of the outcomes and the relative frequency. Compare the results with the theoretical expected percents (50% heads, 50% tails). Repeat the process for 500 trials. Are these outcomes closer to the results predicted by theory?
2. Use RANDBETWEEN to simulate 50 rolls of a fair die. Use the number 1 for the bottom value and 6 for the top. Make a table showing the frequency of each outcome and the relative frequency. Compare the results with the theoretical expected percents (16.7% for each outcome). Repeat the process for 500 tosses. Are these outcomes closer to the results predicted by theory?

CHAPTER 5
THE BINOMIAL DISTRIBUTION AND RELATED TOPICS

THE BINOMIAL PROBABILITY DISTRIBUTION

The binomial probability distribution is discussed in Chapter 5 of *Understandable Statistics.* It is a discrete probability distribution controlled by the number of trials, *n,* and the probability of success on a single trial, *p.*

The Excel function that generates binomial probabilities is

BINOMDIST(r,n,p,cumulative)

where *r* represents the number of successes. Using TRUE for cumulative returns the cumulative probability of obtaining no more than *r* successes in *n* trials, and using FALSE returns the probability of obtaining exactly *r* successes in *n* trials.

You can type the command directly in the formula bar (don't forget the preceding equal sign), or you can call up the dialog box by pressing the Paste Function (Function Wizard) button on the standard menu bar, then selecting Statistical in the left column and BINOMDIST in the right column.

To compute the probability of exactly three successes out of four trials where the probability of success on a single trial is 0.50, we would enter the following information into the dialog box. When we press Enter, the formula result 0.25 will appear in the active cell.

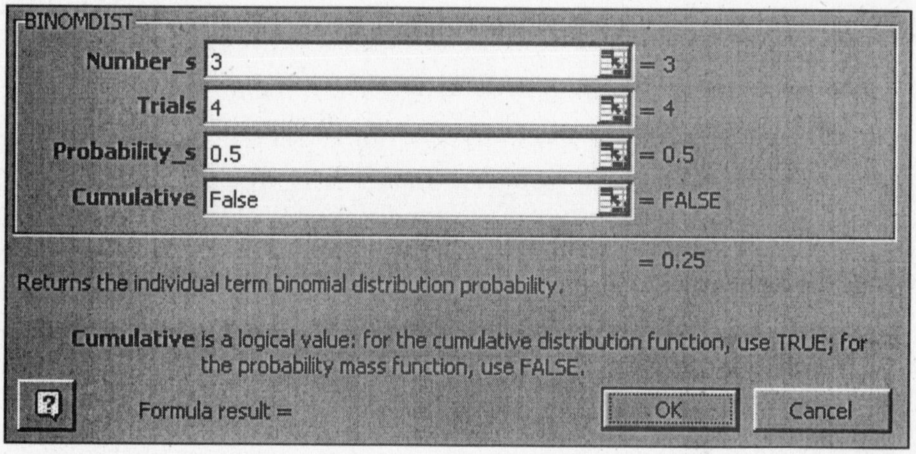

BINOMDIST

Number_s 3 = 3

Trials 4 = 4

Probability_s 0.5 = 0.5

Cumulative False = FALSE

= 0.25

Returns the individual term binomial distribution probability.

Cumulative is a logical value: for the cumulative distribution function, use TRUE; for the probability mass function, use FALSE.

Formula result =

OK Cancel

Example

A surgeon regularly performs a certain difficult operation. The probability of success for any one such operation is $p = 0.73$. Ten similar operations are scheduled. Find the probability of success for 0 through 10 successes out of these operations.

First let's put information regarding the number of trials and probability of success on a single trial into the worksheet. We type n = 10 in Cell A1 and p = 0.73 in Cell B1.

Next, we will put the possible values for the number of successes, *r,* in Cells A3 through A13 with the label **r** in Cell A2. We can also duplicate A2 through A13 in D2 through D13 for easier reading of the finished table. Now place the label **P(r)** in Cell B2 and the label **P(X ≤ r)** in Cell C2. We will have Excel generate the probabilities of the individual number of successes **r** in Cells B3 through B13 and the corresponding cumulative probabilities in Cells C3 through C13.

Generate *P*(*r*) values and adjust format

Select Cell B3 as the active cell. In the formula bar enter

=BINOMDIST(A3,10,0.73,false)

and press Enter. Then select Cell B3 again, and move the cursor to the lower right corner of the cell. When the small black + appears, drag through Cell B13. This process generates the probabilities for each value of **r** in Cells A3 through A13.

The probabilities are expressed in scientific notation, where the value after the E indicates that we are to multiply the decimal value by the given power of 10. To reformat the probabilities, select them all and press the comma button on the formatting tool bar. Then press the button to move the decimal point until you see four digits after it.

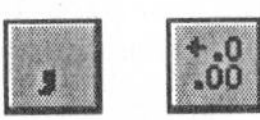

Generate Cumulative Probabilities $P(X \leq r)$ and adjust format

Select Cell C3 as the active cell. In the formula bar enter

=BINOMDIST(A3,10,0.73,true)

and press Enter. Then select Cell C3 again, move the cursor to the lower right corner of the cell, and drag down through Cell C13. This generates the cumulative probabilities for each value of **r** in Cells A3 through A13. Again, reformat the probabilities to show four decimal places.

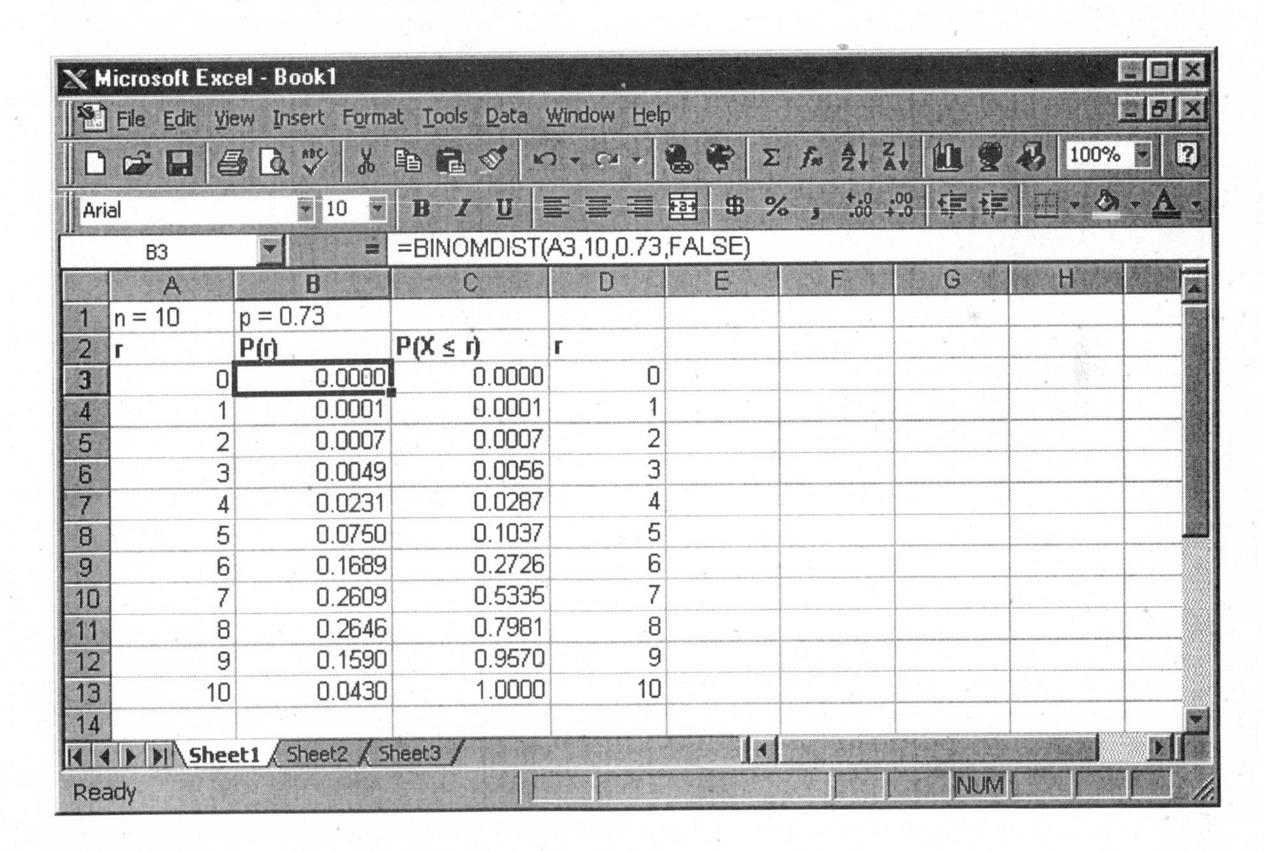
Microsoft Excel - Book1

B3 = =BINOMDIST(A3,10,0.73,FALSE)

	A	B	C	D
1	n = 10	p = 0.73		
2	r	P(r)	P(X ≤ r)	r
3	0	0.0000	0.0000	0
4	1	0.0001	0.0001	1
5	2	0.0007	0.0007	2
6	3	0.0049	0.0056	3
7	4	0.0231	0.0287	4
8	5	0.0750	0.1037	5
9	6	0.1689	0.2726	6
10	7	0.2609	0.5335	7
11	8	0.2646	0.7981	8
12	9	0.1590	0.9570	9
13	10	0.0430	1.0000	10
14				

Next, let's use the Chart Wizard to create a bar graph showing the probability distribution.

Press the Chart Wizard button on the standard tool bar. Select Column and the first sub-type. Press Enter.

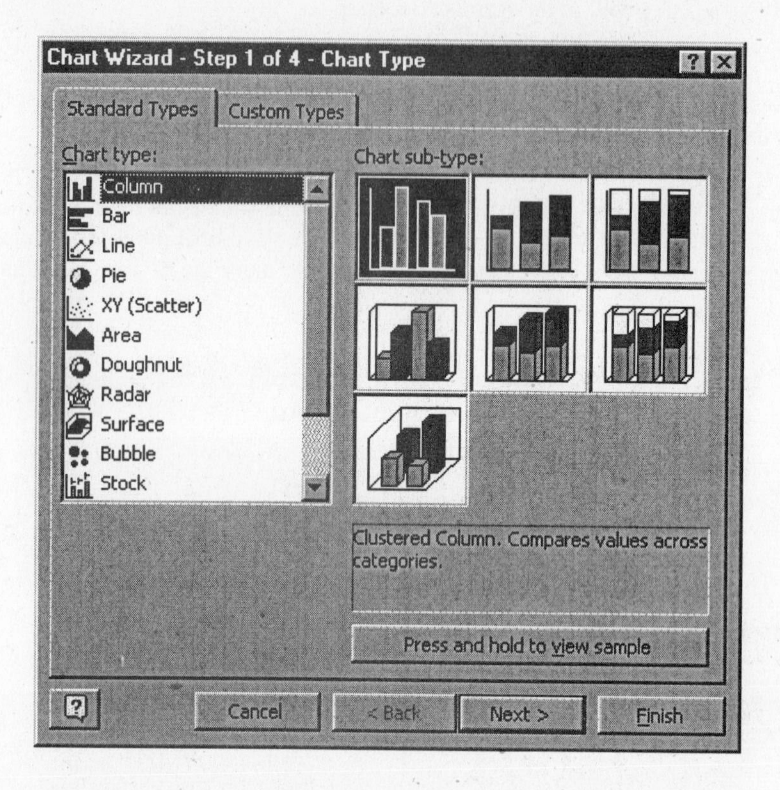

For the data range, activate Cells B2 through B13 and press Enter.

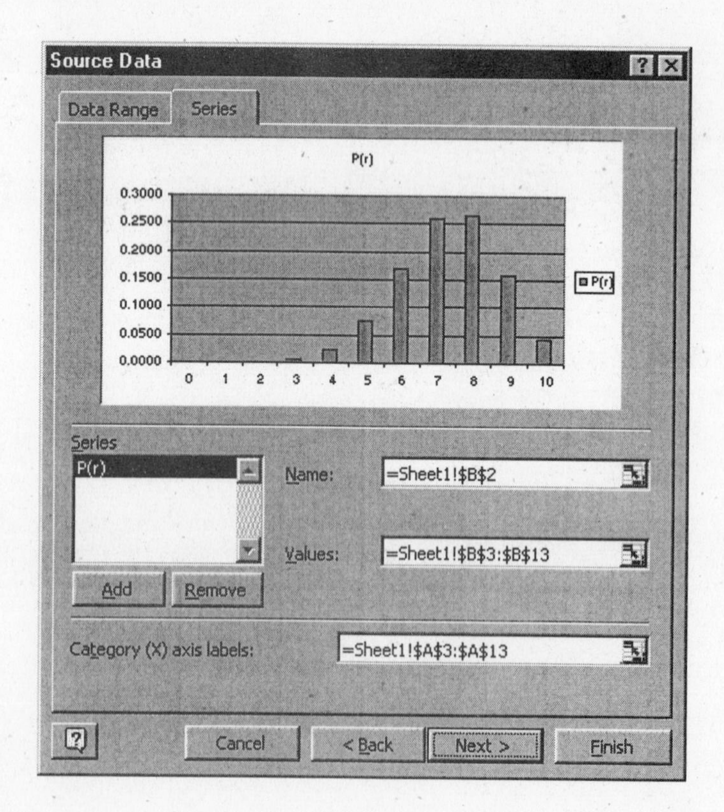

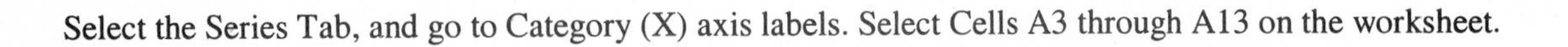

Select the Series Tab, and go to Category (X) axis labels. Select Cells A3 through A13 on the worksheet.

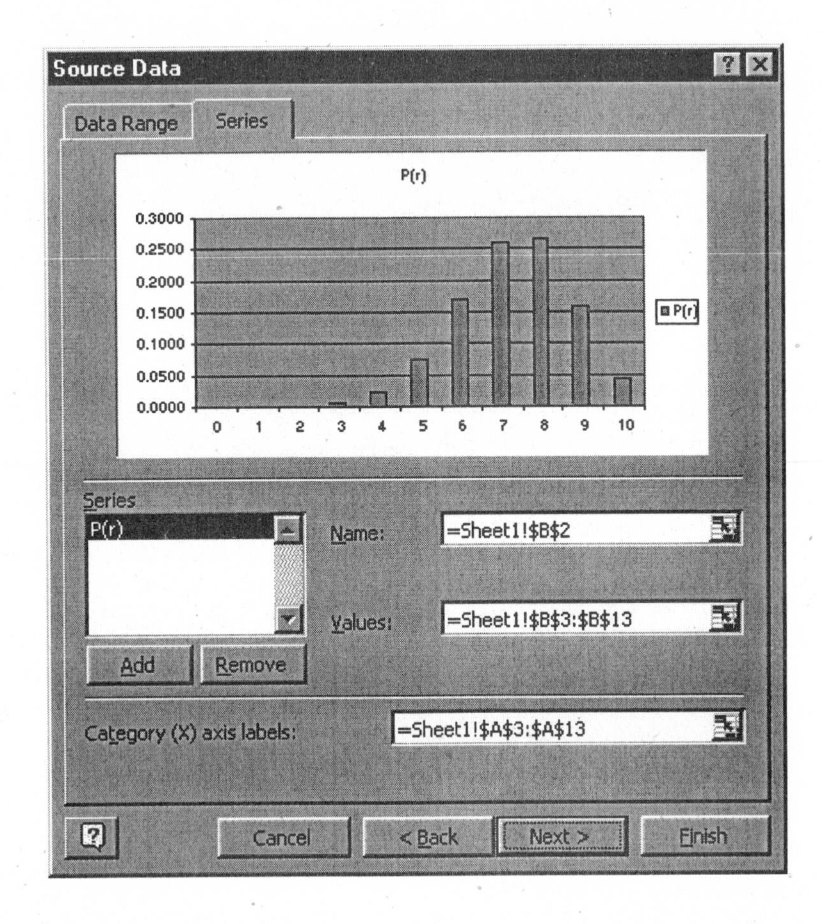

Press Enter or click Next. In the dialog box, fill in the Titles options as shown below and press Finish. The graph will appear on your worksheet.

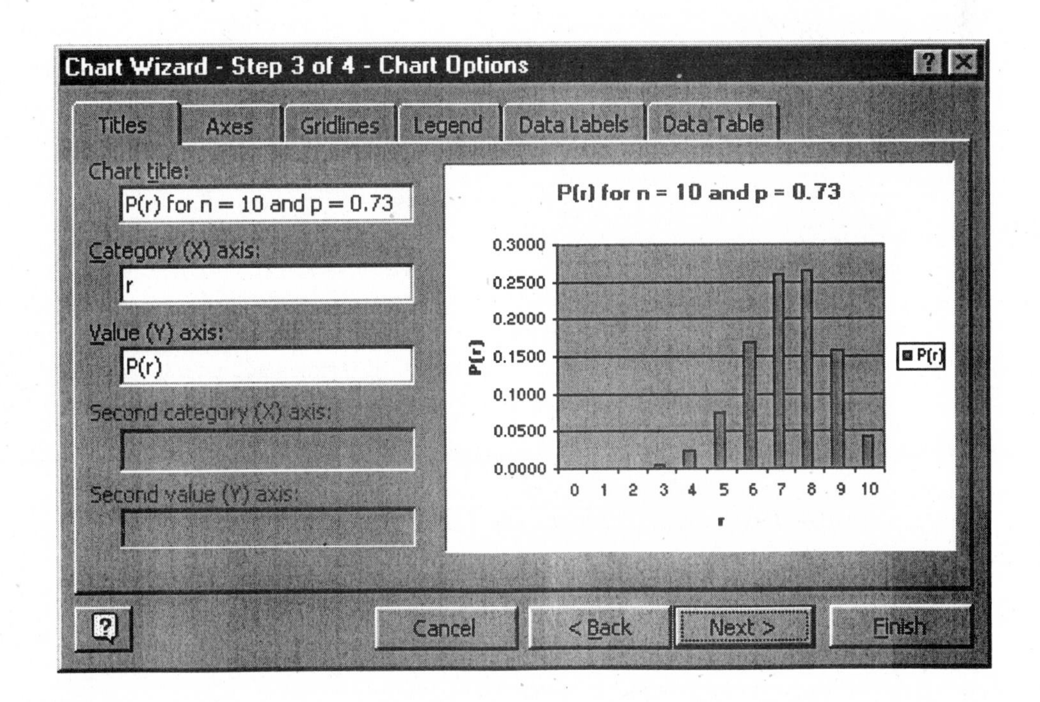

Move the graph so it doesn't block the data columns, and size it as you wish.

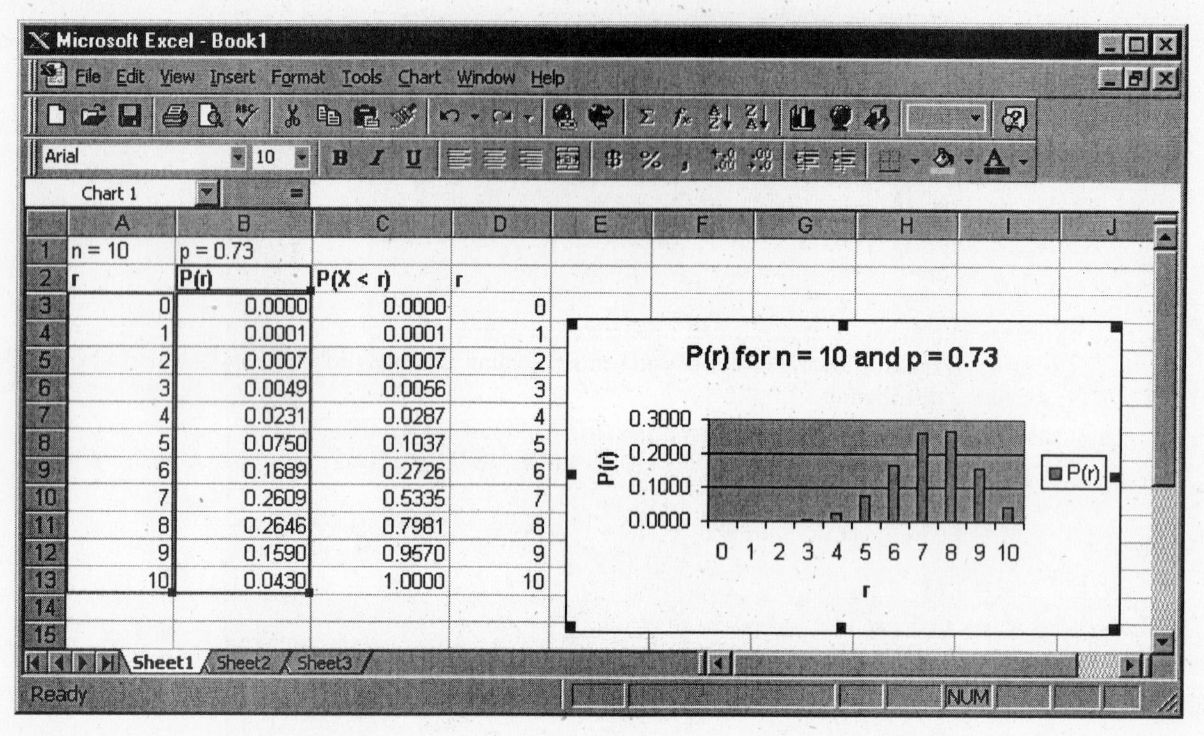

	A	B	C	D
1	n = 10	p = 0.73		
2	r	P(r)	P(X < r)	r
3	0	0.0000	0.0000	0
4	1	0.0001	0.0001	1
5	2	0.0007	0.0007	2
6	3	0.0049	0.0056	3
7	4	0.0231	0.0287	4
8	5	0.0750	0.1037	5
9	6	0.1689	0.2726	6
10	7	0.2609	0.5335	7
11	8	0.2646	0.7981	8
12	9	0.1590	0.9570	9
13	10	0.0430	1.0000	10

LAB ACTIVITIES FOR BINOMIAL PROBABILITY DISTRIBUTIONS

1. You toss a coin n times. Call heads success. If the coin is fair, the probability of success p is 0.5. Use BINOMDIST command with False for cumulative to find each of the following probabilities.
   (a) Find the probability of getting exactly five heads out of eight tosses.
   (b) Find the probability of getting exactly twenty heads out of 100 tosses.
   (c) Find the probability of getting exactly forty heads out of 100 tosses.

2. You toss a coin n times. Call heads success. If the coin is fair, the probability of success p is 0.5. Use BINOMDIST command with True for cumulative to find each of the following probabilities
   (a) Find the probability of getting at least five heads out of eight tosses.
   (b) Find the probability of getting at least twenty heads out of 100 tosses.
   (c) Find the probability of getting at least forty heads out of 100 tosses.
   Hint: Keep in mind how BINOMDIST works. Which should be larger, the value in (b) or the value in (c)?

3. A bank examiner's record shows that the probability of an error in a statement for a checking account at Trust Us Bank is 0.03. The bank statements are sent monthly. What is the probability that exactly two of the next twelve monthly statements for our account will be in error? Now use the BINOMDIST with True for cumulative to find the probability that *at least* two of the next twelve statements contain errors. Use this result with subtraction to find the probability that *more than* two of the next twelve statements contain errors. You can activate a cell and use the formula bar to do the required subtraction.

4. Some tables for the binomial distribution give values only up to 0.5 for the probability of success p. There is a symmetry between values of p greater than 0.5 and values of p less than 0.5.

   (a) Consider the binomial distribution with $n = 10$ and $p = .75$. Since there are anywhere from 0 to 10 successes possible, put the numbers 0 through 10 in Cells A2 through A12. Use Cell A1 for the label **r.** Use BINOMDIST with cumulative False option to generate the probabilities for $r = 0$ through 10. Store the results in Cells B2 through B12. Use Cell B1 for the label **p = 0.75.**

   (b) Now consider the binomial distribution with $n = 10$ and $p = .25$. Use BINOMDIST with cumulative False option to generate the probabilities for $r = 0$ through 10. Store the results in Cells C2 through C12. Use Cell C1 for the label **p = 0.25.**

   (c) Now compare the entries in Columns B and C. How does $P(r = 4$ successes with $p = .75)$ compare to $P(r = 6$ successes with $p = .25)$?

5. **(a)** Consider a binomial distribution with fifteen trials and probability of success on a single trial $p = 0.25$. Create a worksheet showing values of r and corresponding binomial probabilities. Generate a bar graph of the distribution.

   (b) Consider a binomial distribution with fifteen trials and probability of success on a single trial $p = 0.75$. Create a worksheet showing values of r and the corresponding binomial probabilities. Generate a bar graph.

   (c) Compare the graphs of parts (a) and (b). How are they skewed? Is one symmetric with the other?

CHAPTER 6 NORMAL DISTRIBUTIONS

GRAPHS OF NORMAL PROBABILITY DISTRIBUTIONS (SECTION 6.1 OF *UNDERSTANDABLE STATISTICS*)

A normal distribution is a continuous probability distribution governed by the parameters μ (the mean) and σ (the standard deviation), as discussed in Section 6.1 of *Understandable Statistics.* The Excel command that generates values for a normal distribution is

NORMDIST(x,mean,standard deviation,cumulative)

When we set the value of cumulative to FALSE, the command gives the values of the normal probability density function for the corresponding x value. You can type the command directly into the formula bar, or find it by using the Paste Function button on the standard toolbar, selecting Statistical in the left column and scrolling to NORMDIST in the right column to call up the dialog box below. We filled in the entries that we will use in the next example.

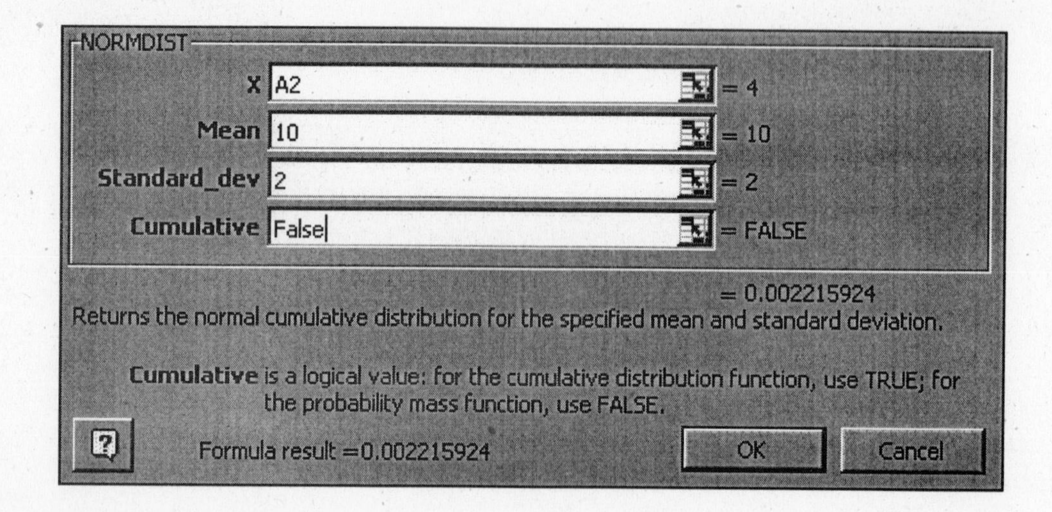

Example

Graph the normal distribution with mean $\mu = 10$ and standard deviation $\sigma = 2$.

Since most of the normal curve occurs over the values $\mu - 3\sigma$ to $\mu + 3\sigma$, we will start the graph at $10 - 3(2) = 4$ and end it at $10 + 3(2) = 16$. We will let Excel set the scale on the vertical axis automatically.

Generate the column of *x* values

To graph a normal distribution, we must have a column of x values and a column of corresponding y values. We begin by generating a column of x values ranging 4 to 16, with an increment of 0.25. To do this, select Cell A2 and enter the number 4. Select Cell A2 again and use the **➤Edit➤Fill➤Series** to open the dialogue box shown next. Set the options in the dialogue box as shown and then press Enter.

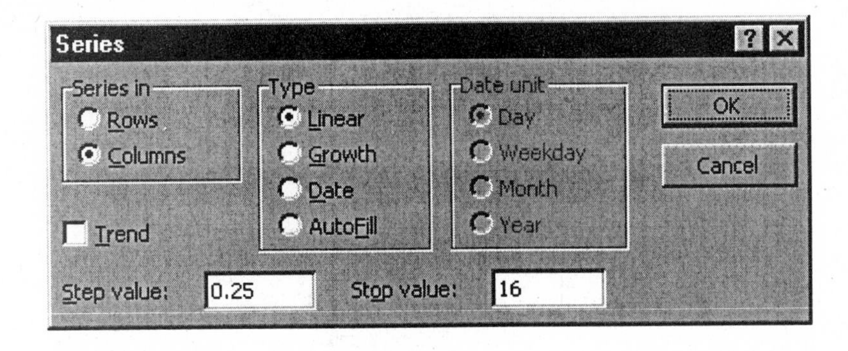

You will see that Column A now contains the numbers 4, 4.25, 4.50, … all the way up to 16.

Generate the column of *y* values

Select Cell B2, and enter

=NORMDIST(A2,10,2,False)

Press Enter. Select Cell B2 again and move the cursor to the lower right corner of the cell. When the cursor changes to a small black +, hold down the left mouse button and drag down the column until each Column-A entry has a corresponding Column-B entry. Release the left mouse button. All the *y* values should now appear.

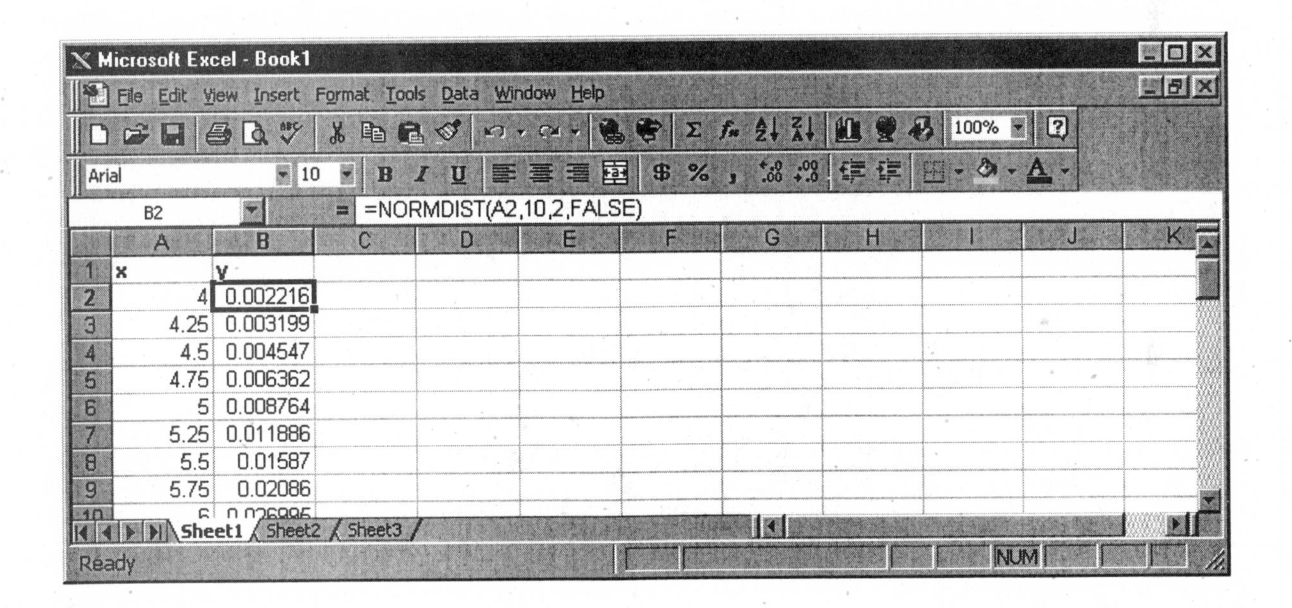

Create the graph of a normal distribution

We will use the Chart Wizard to create the graph of a normal distribution. On the standard toolbar, press the Chart Wizard button. Select Line Graph and choose the first chart sub-type. Click Next.

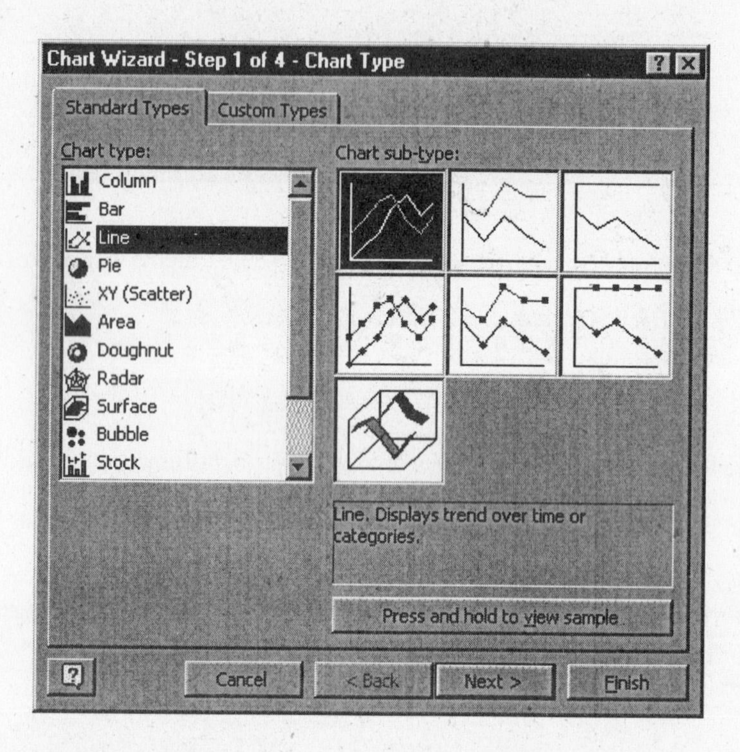

Enter all of Column B as the Data range.

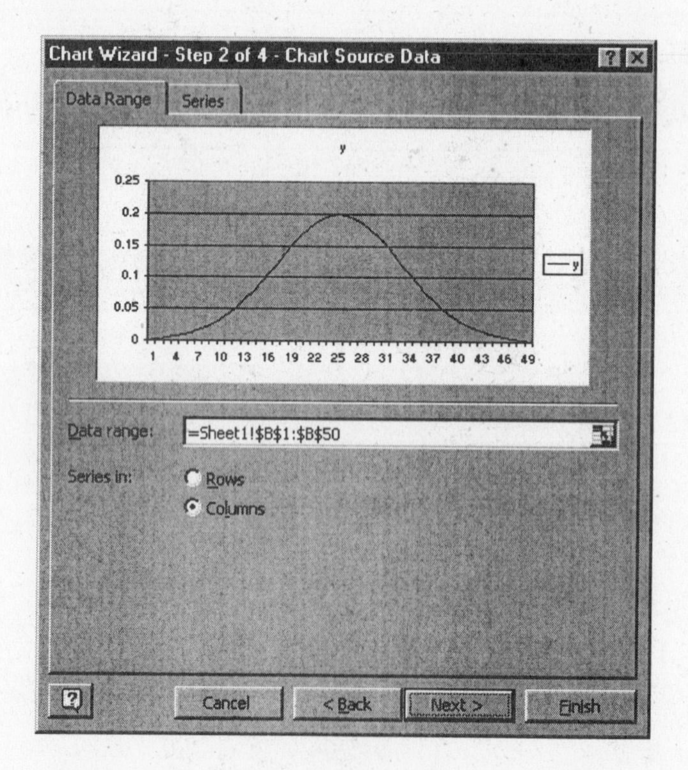

Click on the series tab. Click to place the cursor at Category (x) axis labels, and then, in the worksheet, select the cells in Column A, starting with Cell A2. Click Next.

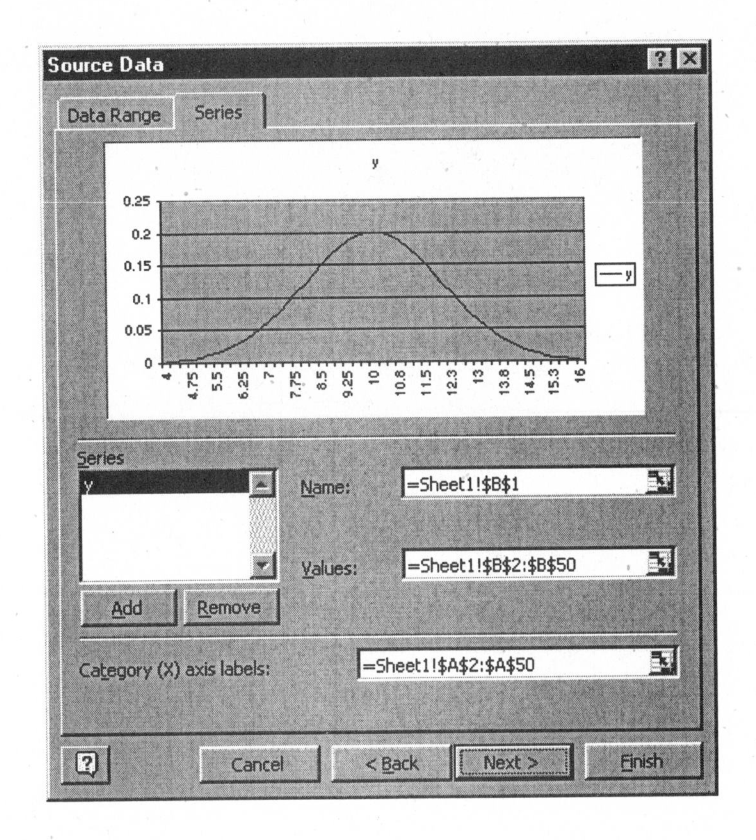

Next we will add a title and variable label to the x-axis. In the Chart Title, type

Normal Distribution, Mean = 10, St Dev = 2

For Category (X) axis, type x. Click Finish.

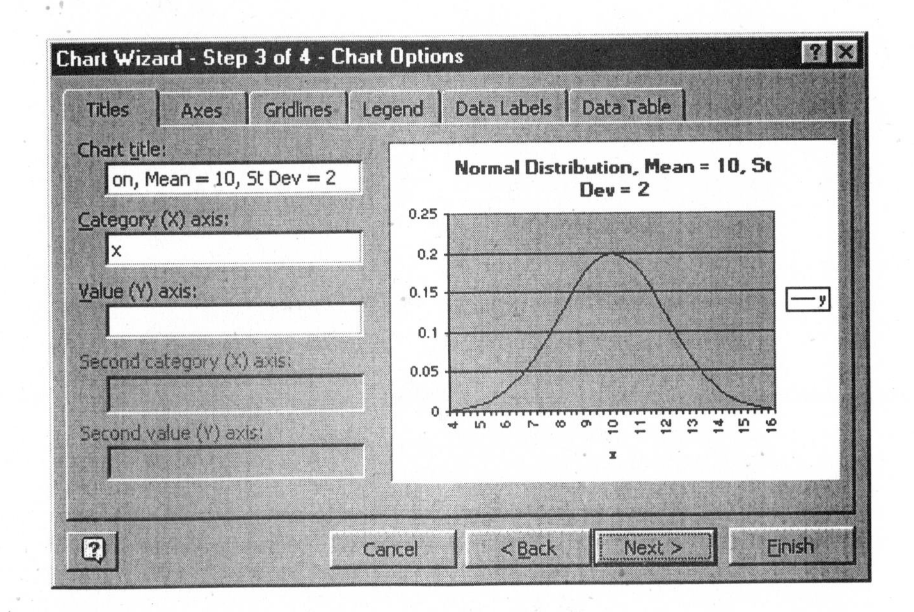

Now your worksheet will contain the graph of the described normal distribution. Move the graph and size it to your liking. Notice that as you make the graph wider or taller, the labels shown on the *x*-axis might change.

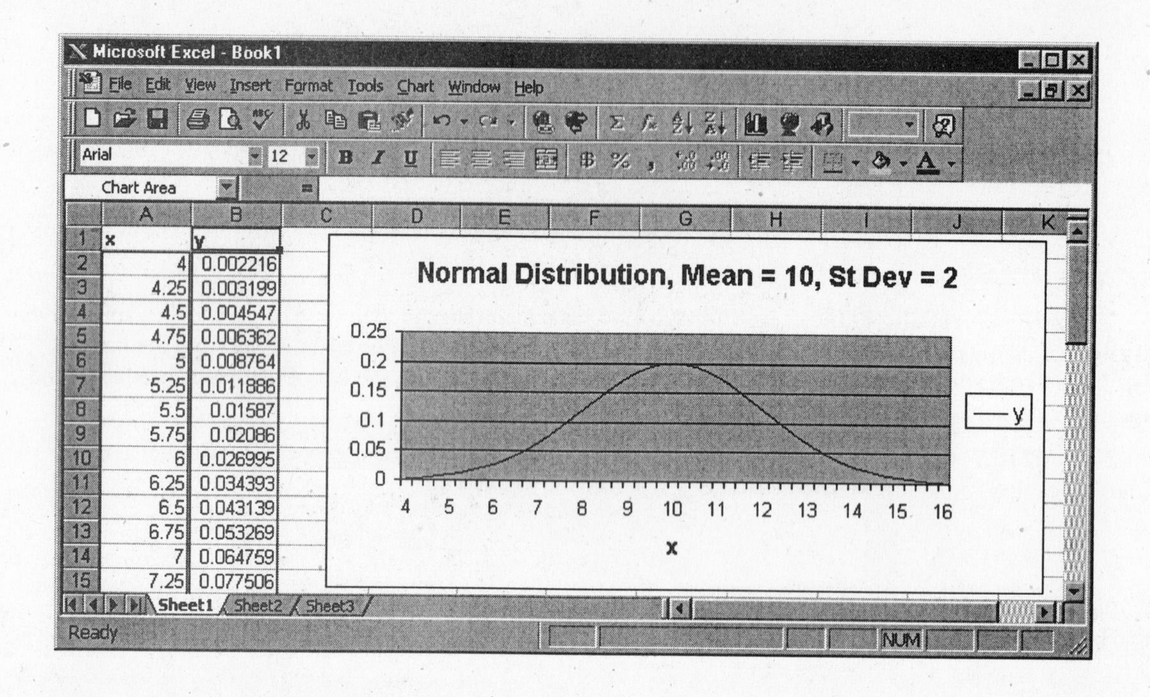

x	y
4	0.002216
4.25	0.003199
4.5	0.004547
4.75	0.006362
5	0.008764
5.25	0.011886
5.5	0.01587
5.75	0.02086
6	0.026995
6.25	0.034393
6.5	0.043139
6.75	0.053269
7	0.064759
7.25	0.077506

We can also graph two (or more) normal distributions on the same graph. In the next display we generated *y* values for a normal distribution with mean 10 and standard deviation 1 in Column C. Then, in the Data Range box of the Chart Wizard, we selected both Column B and C.

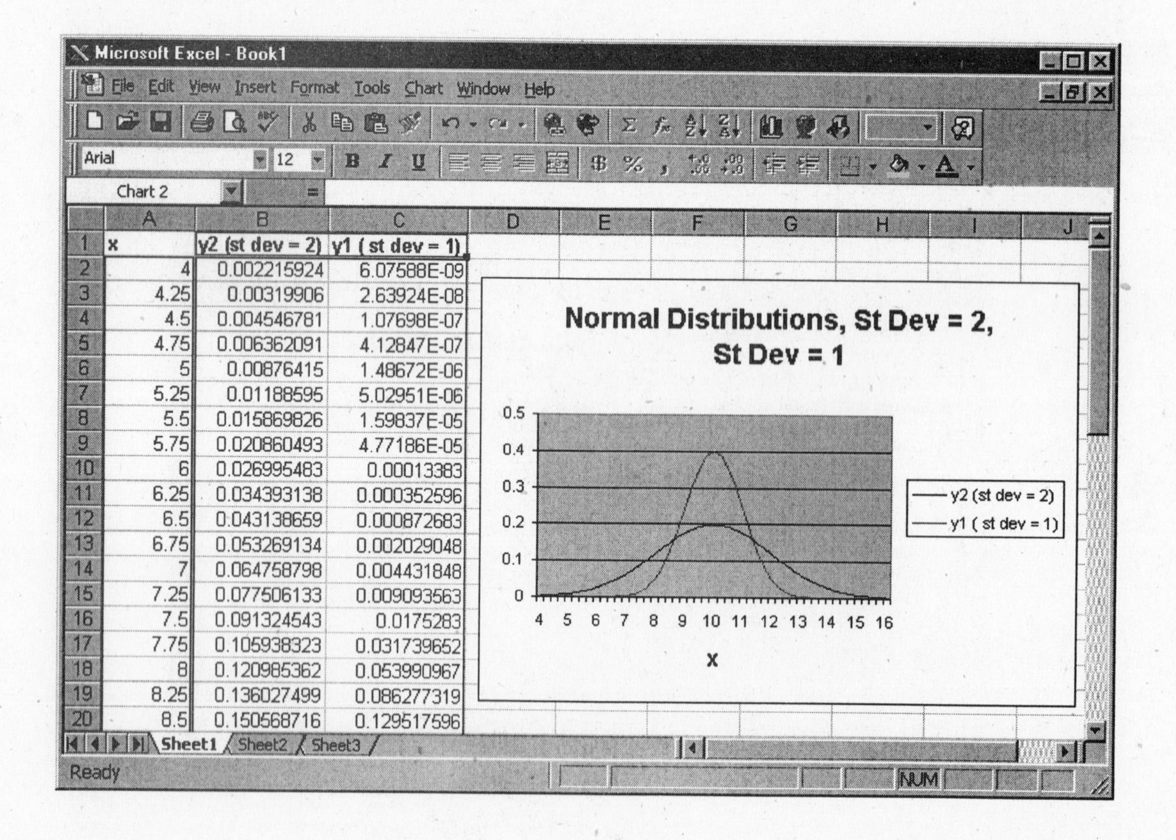

x	y2 (st dev = 2)	y1 (st dev = 1)
4	0.002215924	6.07588E-09
4.25	0.00319906	2.63924E-08
4.5	0.004546781	1.07698E-07
4.75	0.006362091	4.12847E-07
5	0.00876415	1.48672E-06
5.25	0.01188595	5.02951E-06
5.5	0.015869826	1.59837E-05
5.75	0.020860493	4.77186E-05
6	0.026995483	0.00013383
6.25	0.034393138	0.000352596
6.5	0.043138659	0.000872683
6.75	0.053269134	0.002029048
7	0.064758798	0.004431848
7.25	0.077506133	0.009093563
7.5	0.091324543	0.0175283
7.75	0.105938323	0.031739652
8	0.120985362	0.053990967
8.25	0.136027499	0.086277319
8.5	0.150568716	0.129517596

STANDARD SCORES AND NORMAL PROBABILITIES

Excel has several built-in functions relating to normal distributions.

STANDARDIZE(x,mean,standard deviation) which returns the z score for the given x value from a distribution with the specified mean and standard deviation.

NORMDIST(x_1,mean,standard deviation,cumulative) which when cumulative is TRUE, returns probability that a random value x selected from this distribution is $\leq x_1$, i.e. it returns $P(x \leq x_1)$. This is the same as the area to the left of the specified x_1 value under the described normal distribution. When cumulative is FALSE, it returns the height of the normal probability density function evaluated at x_1. We used this function to graph a normal distribution.

NORMINV(probability,mean,standard deviation) which returns the inverse of the normal cumulative distribution. In other words, when a probability is entered, the command returns the value from the normal distribution with specified mean and standard deviation so that the area to the left of that value is equal to the designated probability.

NORMSDIST(z_1) which returns the probability that a randomly selected z score is less or equal the specified value of z_1, i.e., it returns $P(z \leq z_1)$. This is the same as the area to the left of the specified z_1 value under the standard normal distribution. This command is equivalent to NORMDIST(x_1,0,1,true).

NORMSINV(probability) which returns the value such that the area to its left under the standard normal distribution is equal to the specified probability. This command is equivalent to NORMINV(probability,0,1).

Each of these commands can be typed directly into the formula bar for an active cell or accessed by using the Paste Function button.

Examples

(a) Consider a normal distribution with mean 100 and standard deviation 15. Find the z score corresponding to $x = 90$ and find the area to the left of 90 under the distribution.

First we place some headers and labels on the worksheet. Then,

in Cell B3, enter =STANDARDIZE(90,100,15), and

in Cell C3, enter =NORMDIST(90,100,15,true).

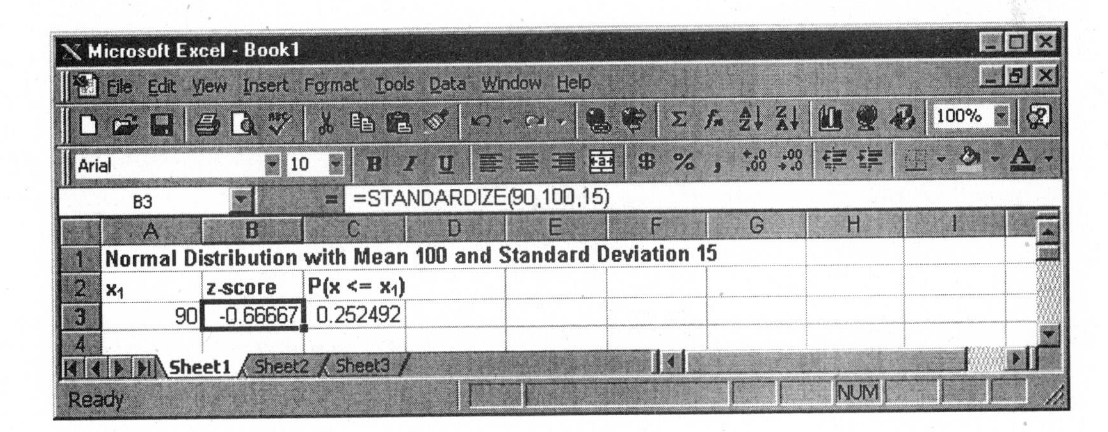

(b) Find the *z* score so that 10% of the area under the standard normal distribution is to the left of *z*.

Again, we put some labels on the worksheet. Then, since we are working with a standard normal distribution, we use NORMSINV(0.1).

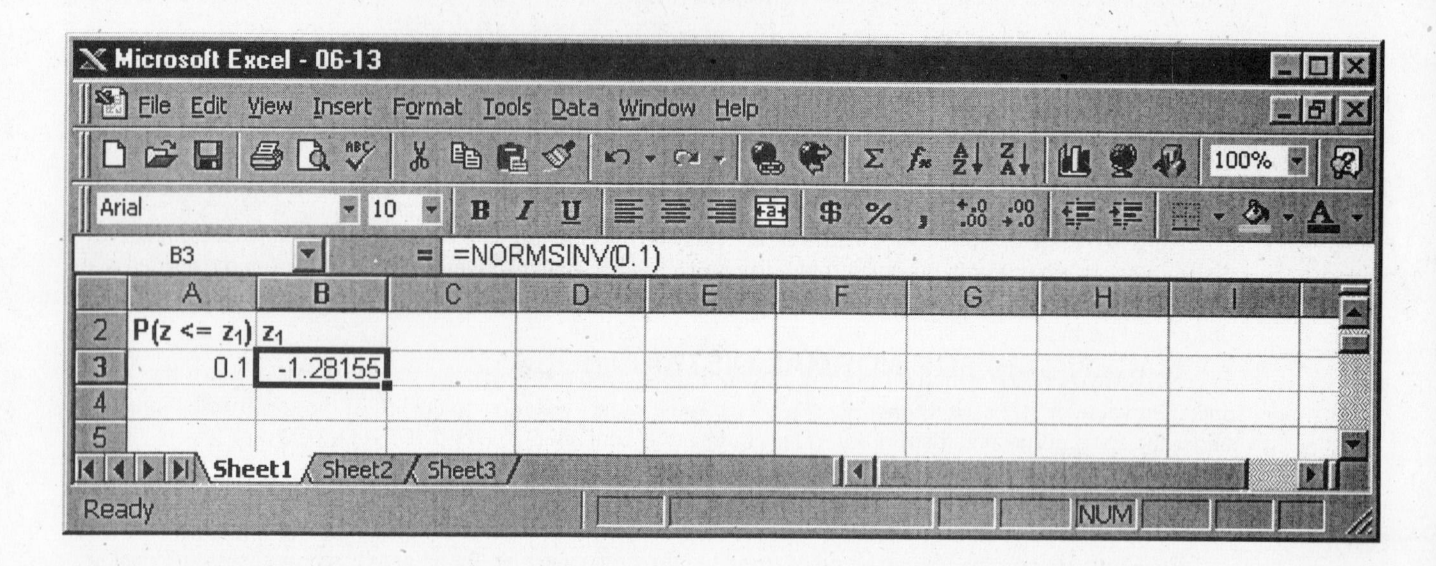

To find areas under normal curves between two values, we do simple arithmetic with the cumulative areas provided by Excel. For instance, to find the area under a standard normal distribution between –2 and 3, we would use NORMDIST(3) to find the cumulative area to the left of 3 and then subtract the cumulative area to the left of –2, found using NORMDIST(-2).

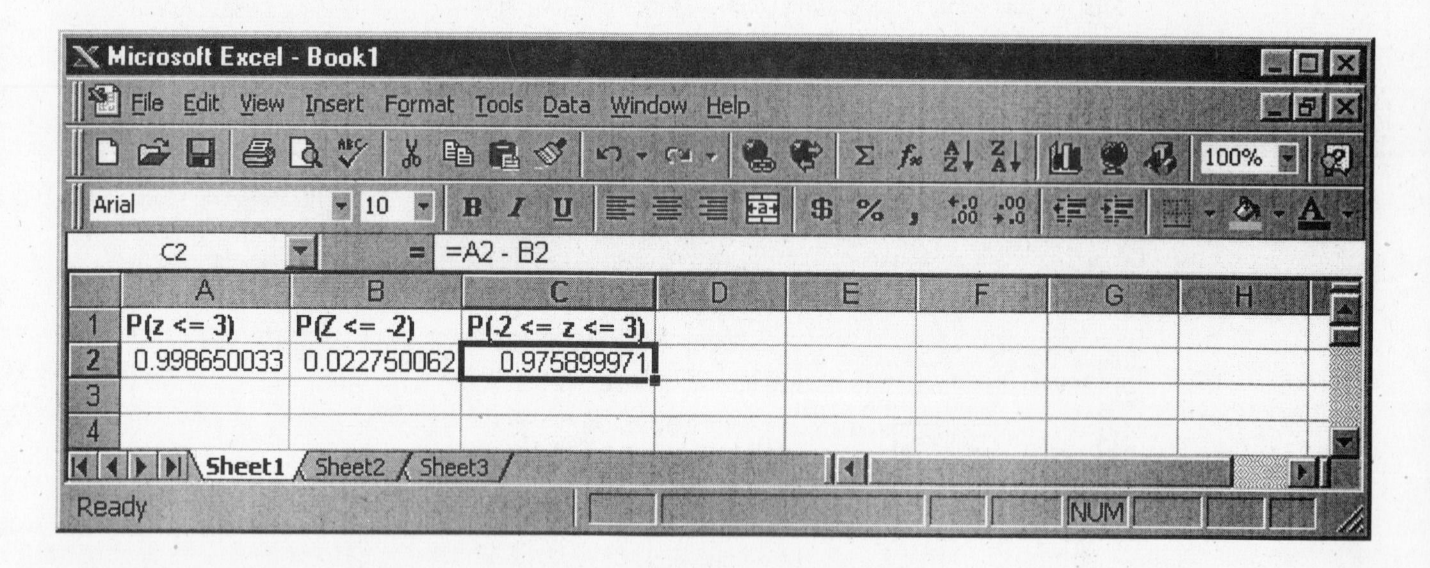

To find areas under normal curves to the right of a specified value, we subtract the cumulative area to the left of the value from 1. For instance, consider the normal distribution with mean 50 and standard deviation 5. At the top of the next page is a worksheet in which the area to the right of 60 is found.

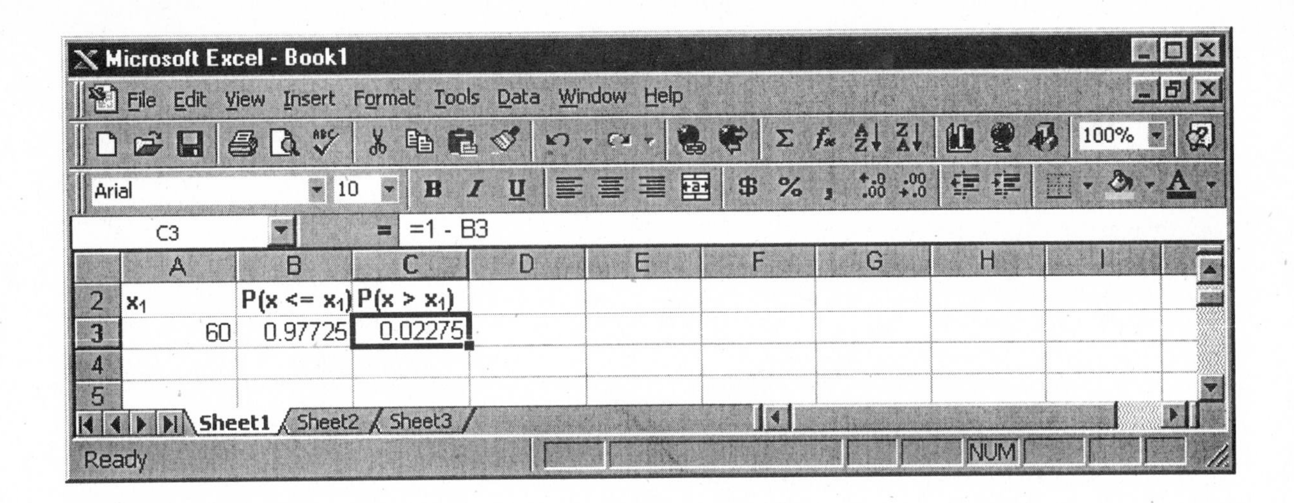

LAB ACTIVITIES FOR NORMAL DISTRIBUTIONS

1. **(a)** Use the Chart Wizard to sketch a graph of the standard normal distribution with a mean of 0 and a standard deviation of 1. Generate x values in column A ranging from –3 to 3 in increments of 0.5. Use NORMDIST to generate the y values in column B.

(b) Use the Chart Wizard to sketch a graph of a normal distribution with a mean of 10 and a standard deviation of 1. Generate x values in Column A ranging from 7 to 13 in increments of 0.5. Use NORMDIST to generate the y values in column B. Compare the graphs of parts (a) and (b). Do the height and spread of the graphs appear to be the same? What is different? Why would you expect this difference.

(c) Sketch a graph of a normal distribution with a mean of 0 and a standard deviation of 2. Generate x values in Column A ranging from –6 to 6 in increments of 0.5. Use NORMDIST to generate the y values in Column B. Compare that graph to that of part (a). Do the height and spread of the graphs appear to be the same? What is different? Why would you expect this difference? Note, to really compare the graphs, it is best to graph them using the same scales. Redo the graph of part (a) using x from –6 to 6. Then redo the graph in this part using the same x values as in part (a) and y values ranging from 0 to the high value in part (a).

2. Use NORMDIST or NORMSDIST plus arithmetic to find the specified area.

(a) Find the area to the left of 2 on a standard normal distribution.

(b) Find the area to the left of –1 on a standard normal distribution.

(c) Find the area between –1 and 2 on a standard normal distribution.

(d) Find the area to the right of 2 on a standard normal distribution.

(e) Find the area to the left of 40 on a normal distribution with $\mu = 50$ and $\sigma = 8$.

(f) Find the area to the left of 55 on a normal distribution with $\mu = 50$ and $\sigma = 8$.

(g) Find the area between 40 and 55 on a normal distribution with $\mu = 50$ and $\sigma = 8$.

(h) Find the area to the right of 55 on a normal distribution with $\mu = 50$ and $\sigma = 8$.

3. Use NORMINV or NORMSINV to find the specified x or z value.

(a) Find the z value so that 5% of the area under the standard normal curve falls to the left of z.

(b) Find the z value so that 15% of the area under the standard normal curve falls to the left of z.

(c) Consider a normal distribution with mean 10 and standard deviation 2. Find the x value so that 5% of the area under the normal curve falls to the left of x.

(d) Consider a normal distribution with mean 10 and standard deviation 2. Find the x value so that 15% of the area under the normal curve falls to the left of x.

CHAPTER 7
INTRODUCTION TO SAMPLING DISTRIBUTIONS

Excel has no commands that directly support the demonstration of sampling distributions. To do the class project in the "Using Technology" section of Chapter 7 in *Understandable Statistics,* use Random Number Generation (under ➤**Tools**➤**Data Analysis**) and the AVERAGE and STDEV functions.

CHAPTER 8 ESTIMATION

CONFIDENCE INTERVALS FOR THE MEAN – LARGE SAMPLES (SECTION 8.1 OF *UNDERSTANDABLE STATISTICS*)

Excel's function for computing confidence intervals for a population mean assumes a normal distribution, regardless of sample size. The command syntax is

CONFIDENCE(alpha,standard deviation,sample size)

where alpha equals 1 minus the confidence level. In other words, an alpha of 0.05 indicates a 95% confidence interval. To generate a 99% confidence interval, use alpha = 0.01. The standard deviation can be either population or sample standard deviation. To access a dialogue box for the command, use the Paste Function.

Recall from the discussion in *Understandable Statistics* that a confidence interval for the population mean has the form

$$\bar{x} - E \leq \mu \leq \bar{x} + E$$

Excel uses the formula

$$E = z_c \frac{\sigma \text{ or } s}{\sqrt{n}}$$

where z_c is the critical value for the chosen confidence level. For $c = 95\%$, $z_c = 1.96$ (see the table of Confidence Interval Critical Values in the Appendix of *Understandable Statistics*).

CONFIDENCE returns the value of E. To find the lower boundary of the confidence interval, you must subtract E from the sample mean $\bar{x}$ of your data; to find the upper boundary, you add E to the sample mean.

Example

Lucy decided to try to estimate the average number of miles she drives each day. For a three-month period, she selected a random sample of 35 days and kept a record of the distance driven on each of those sample days. The sample mean was 28.3 miles, and the sample standard deviation was $s = 5$ miles. Find a 95% confidence interval for the population mean of miles Lucy drove per day in the three-month period.

For a 95% confidence level, alpha is 0.05. In our Excel worksheet, after putting in some information and labels, we enter =CONFIDENCE(0.05,5,35) in Cell B3 to represent E. In Cell D4, we type =28.3–B3 to compute the lower value of the confidence interval, and we place the upper value of the confidence interval in Cell F4 using =28.3+B3.

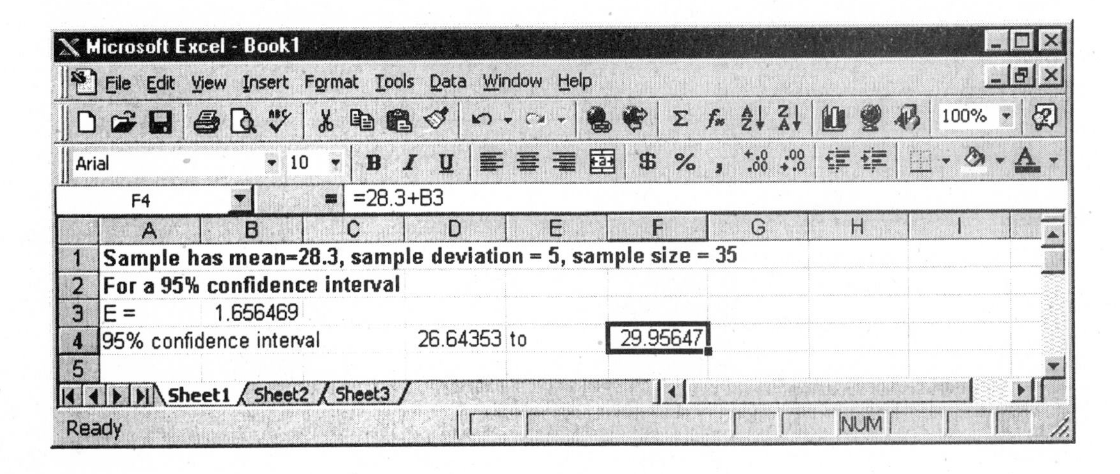

We can also find the E value for a confidence interval around a population mean in the Describe Statistics dialog box found by selecting **➤Tools➤Data Analysis➤Descriptive Statistics.** If you have data entered into a worksheet, you can use these menu selections to automatically compute the same mean $\bar{x}$ and the sample standard deviation s for the data. Note, however, that here Excel calculates E on the basis of Student's t distribution (see the following section, on small samples) no matter what the sample size is.

Example

Open the Excel workbook Svls02.xls. This workbook contains the weights in pounds of fifty randomly selected professional football linebackers.

Use the menu selection **➤Tools➤Data Analysis➤Descriptive Statistics** to access the following dialog box. Since the weights are in Column A, we select the cells containing the range and use these for the input range. We place the upper left corner of the output in Cell C1 and check that we want summary statistics and a 95% confidence interval.

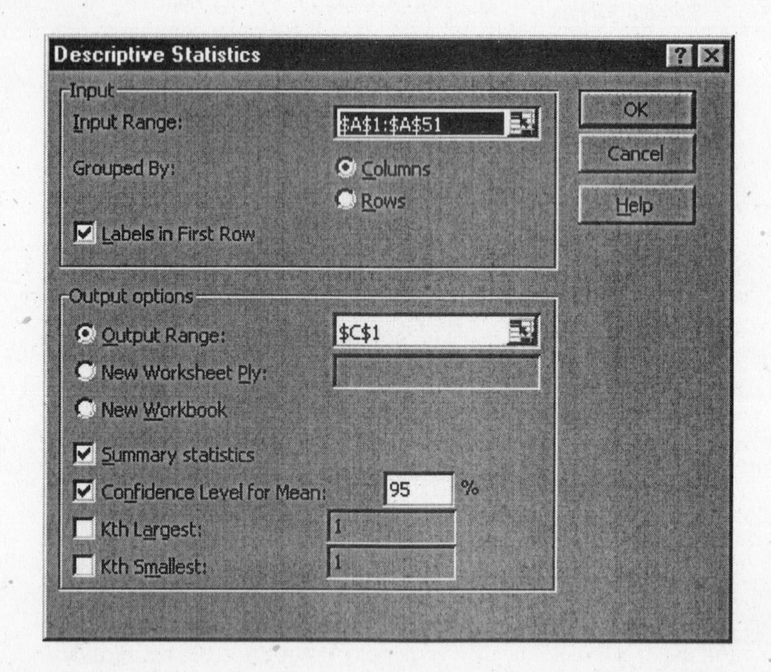

Next we widen cells in Column C and D to accommodate the output. Notice that the sample mean is in Cell D3 and the value of E for a 95% confidence interval (again, based on Student's t distribution, not the standard normal distribution) is in Cell D16. We put the confidence interval in Cells F2 to H2, by entering =D3–D16 in Cell F2 and =D3+D16 in Cell H2. The display should be similar to the one shown at the top of the next page.

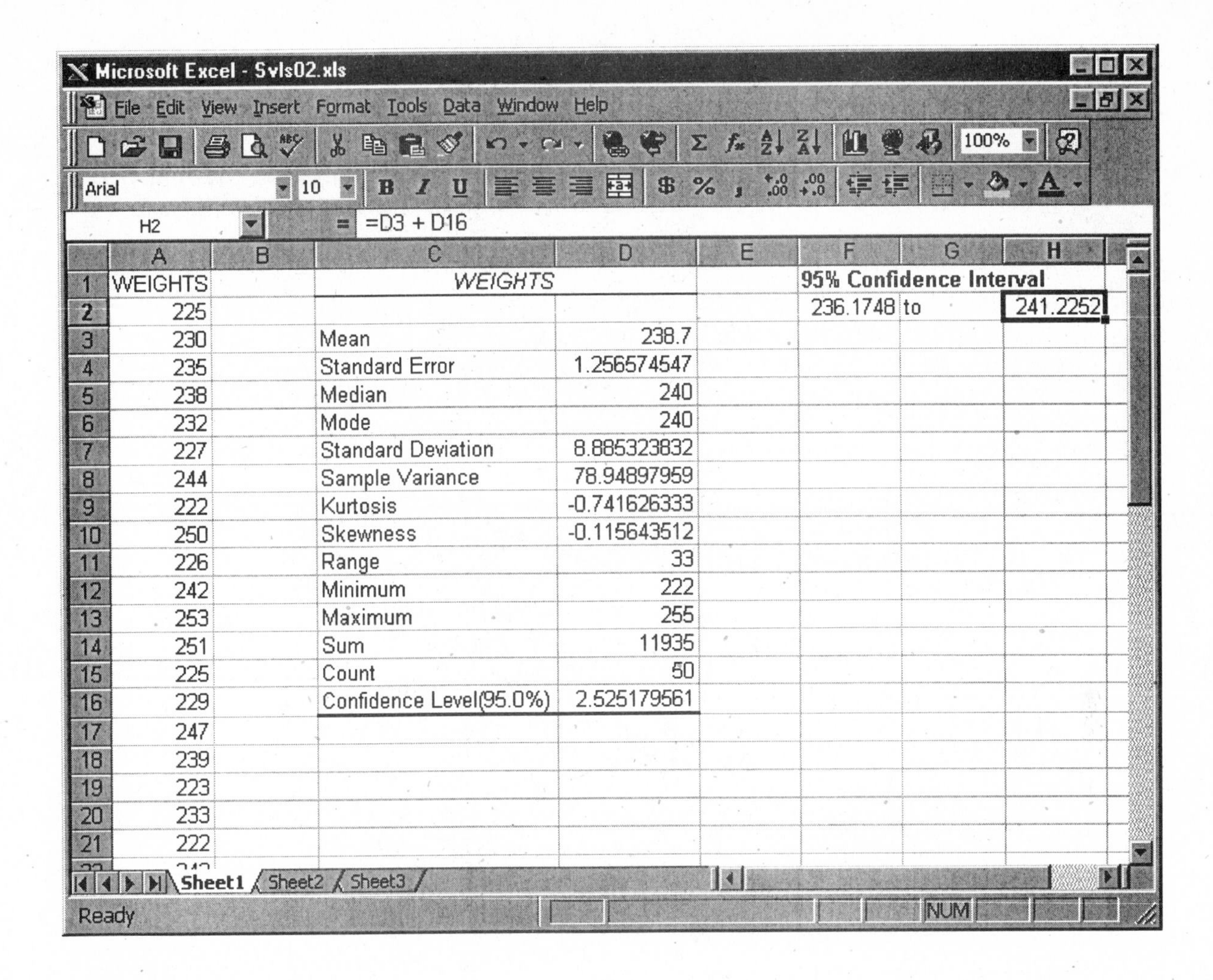

	A	B	C	D	E	F	G	H
1	WEIGHTS		*WEIGHTS*			95% Confidence Interval		
2	225					236.1748	to	241.2252
3	230		Mean	238.7				
4	235		Standard Error	1.256574547				
5	238		Median	240				
6	232		Mode	240				
7	227		Standard Deviation	8.885323832				
8	244		Sample Variance	78.94897959				
9	222		Kurtosis	-0.741626333				
10	250		Skewness	-0.115643512				
11	226		Range	33				
12	242		Minimum	222				
13	253		Maximum	255				
14	251		Sum	11935				
15	225		Count	50				
16	229		Confidence Level(95.0%)	2.525179561				
17	247							
18	239							
19	223							
20	233							
21	222							

LAB ACTIVITIES FOR CONFIDENCE INTERVALS FOR THE MEAN

1. Retrieve the worksheet Svls03.xls. This contains the heights (in feet) of 65 randomly selected pro basketball players. Use the Descriptive Statistics dialog box to get summary statistics for the data and to create a 90% confidence interval.

2. Retrieve the worksheet Svls01.xls from the Excel data disk. This worksheet contains the number of shares of Disney Stock (in hundreds of shares) sold for a random sample of sixty trading days in 1993 and 1994. Use the Descriptive Statistics dialog box to get summary statistics for the data and to create the following confidence intervals.
   (a) Find a 99% confidence interval for the population mean volume.
   (b) Find a 95% confidence interval for the population mean volume.
   (c) Find a 90% confidence interval for the population mean volume.
   (d) Find an 85% confidence interval for the population mean volume.
   (e) What do you notice about the lengths of the intervals as the confidence level decreases?

3. There are many types of errors that will cause a computer program to terminate or give incorrect results. One type of error is punctuation. For instance, if a comma is inserted in the wrong place, the program might not run. A study of programs written by students in a beginning programming course showed that 75 out of 300 errors selected at random were punctuation errors. Find a 99% confidence interval for the proportion of errors made by beginning programming students that are punctuation errors. Next find a 90% confidence interval. Use the CONFIDENCE command to find the interval. Is this interval longer or shorter?

Confidence Intervals for the Mean – Small Samples (Section 8.2 of *Understandable Statistics*)

Excel does not have a function comparable to CONFIDENCE that directly calculates confidence intervals for the mean using small samples. However, recall from the text that for small-sample confidence intervals we use Student's t distribution.

The confidence interval is computed as

$$\bar{x} - t\left(s/\sqrt{n}\right) \text{ to } \bar{x} + t\left(s/\sqrt{n}\right)$$

Excel has two commands for Student's t distribution under the statistical options of Paste Function.

TDIST(x,degrees of freedom,tails)

returns the area in the tail of Student's t distribution beyond the specified value of x, for the specified number of degrees of freedom and number of tails (1 or 2).

TINV(probability,degrees of freedom)

returns the t value such that the area in the two tails beyond the t value equals the specified probability for the specified degrees of freedom.

We can use the TINV command to find the t value to use in the confidence interval. For instance, if we have a sample of size 10 with mean $\bar{x} = 6$ and $s = 1.2$, then the t value we use in the computation of a 95% confidence interval is 2.262. Notice that for a 95% confidence interval, 5% of the area is in the two tails. The number of degrees of freedom is $10 - 1 = 9$.

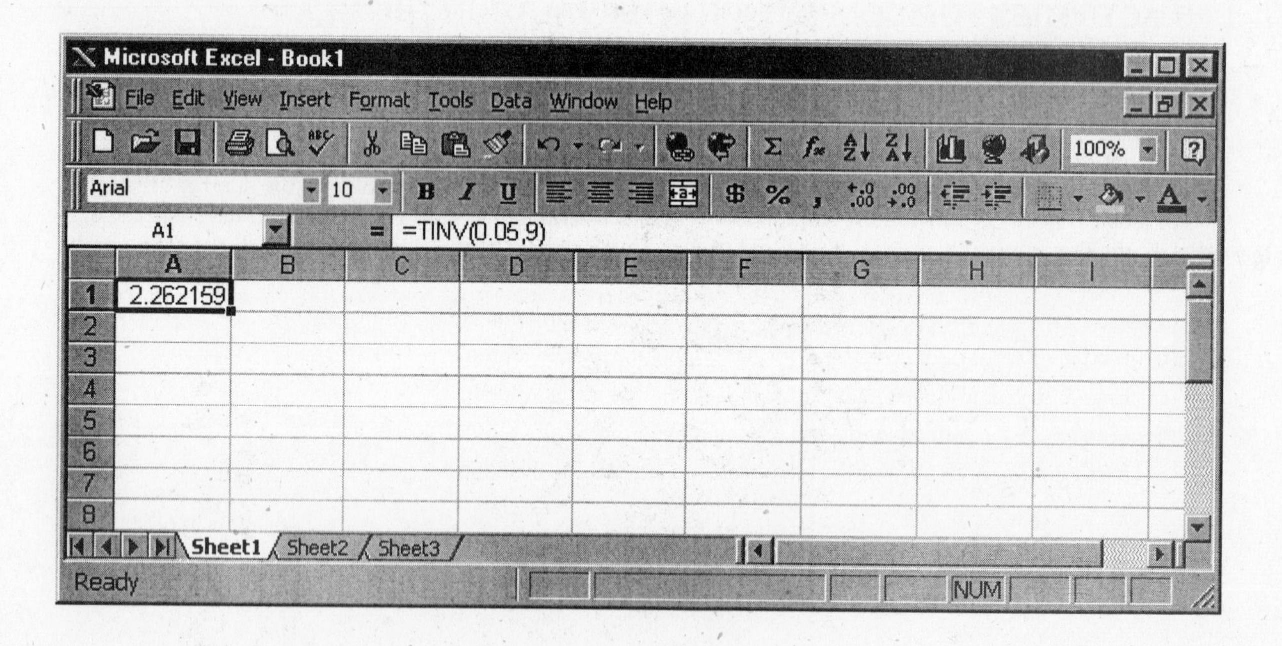

CHAPTER 9 HYPOTHESIS TESTING

TESTING A SINGLE POPULATION MEAN – LARGE SAMPLES (SECTIONS 9.2 AND 9.3 OF *UNDERSTANDABLE STATISTICS*)

Chapter 9 of *Understandable Statistics* introduces tests of hypotheses. Testing involving a single mean with a large sample are found in Sections 9.2 and 9.3. Hypothesis tests in these sections test the value of the population mean, μ, against some specified value, denoted by k.

One-sample z-tests are appropriate for testing the null hypothesis H_0: $\mu = k$ against one of the three alternative hypotheses H_1: $\mu > k$, H_1: $\mu < k$, or H_1: $\mu \neq k$ when (1) the data in the sample are known to be from a normal distribution (in which case any sample size will do) or when (2) the data distribution is unknown or the data are believed to be from a non-normal distribution, but the sample size, n, is large ($n \geq 30$). The z-test makes reference to the population standard deviation, σ, but if the sample size n is large, the sample standard deviation, s, is assumed to be close to σ and can be used instead.

In Excel, the **ZTEST** function finds the P value for an upper- or right-tailed test, used to decide between the hypotheses H_0: $\mu = k$ and H_1: $\mu > k$. The null hypothesis says that value of the population mean μ is k. A right-tailed test is used when the sample mean $\bar{x}$ is greater than k, suggesting that μ may in fact be greater than k, as the alternative hypothesis states. **Note, the Excel documentation for ZTEST should be ignored. It mistakenly says that ZTEST gives the result of a two-tailed test.**

The syntax is

ZTEST(array,x,sigma)

The array is the list of sample values; what Excel calls x is k, and sigma is the known value of σ, the population standard deviation. If the syntax used is ZTEST(array,x), i.e., if there is no sigma value given, then Excel calculates the sample standard deviation, s, from the sample data in array and uses that in place of σ.

The P value returned by ZTEST is the probability, given that the null hypothesis is true, of getting results at least as extreme as those observed in the sample. More precisely, ZTEST gives the probability of obtaining a sample mean greater than or equal to the observed sample mean, $\bar{x}$. When this probability is small, it means that the data in the observed sample would be surprising if H_0 were true. This is a reason to reject H_0.

ZTEST can also be used to apply a left-tailed test (H_0: $\mu = k$ versus H_1: $\mu < k$) or a two-tailed test (H_0: $\mu = k$ versus H_1: $\mu \neq k$). To apply a left-tailed test, for the case where the sample mean x is less than k, simply apply a right-tailed test and then subtract the result from 1. (When $\bar{x} < k$, the area found by ZTEST in the upper "tail" will be greater than 0.5, and 1 minus that area will be the area in the lower tail.) To apply a two-tailed test, either double the P value from a right-tailed test (when $\bar{x} > k$) or double the P value from a left-tailed test (when $\bar{x} < k$).

To call up the ZTEST dialog box, click the Paste Function button on the standard tool bar, select Statistical in the left column, and scroll to ZTEST in the right column. The dialog box should be similar to the one shown on the top of the next page.

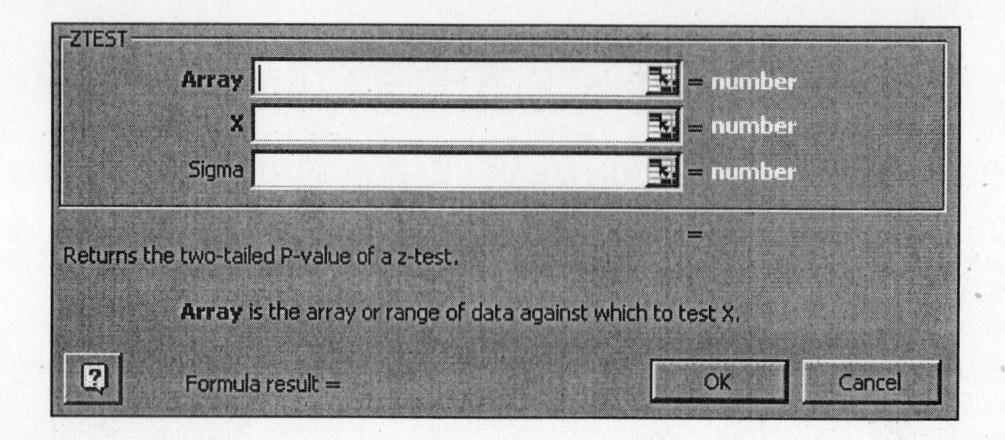

Enter the cell range containing the sample values in the Array blank, and in the blank for X, enter the mean given by the null hypothesis. In the Sigma blank, enter the value of the population standard deviation σ if it is known. Again: sigma is optional; if this box is left blank, Excel will compute the sample standard deviation for the data in the specified Array and use s instead of σ in the computation for z. Recall that if we are dealing with large samples, s and σ are fairly close, so this approximation produces reliable results. Finally, when you click on OK, the P value of the right-tailed test of x is computed.

You can also type the command directly into the formula bar using

ZTEST(data range,X,sigma)

where again, the sigma is optional.

Once the P value is computed, the user can then compare it with α, the level of significance of the test. If

P value $\leq \alpha$ we reject the null hypothesis.

P value $> \alpha$ we do not reject the null hypothesis

Example

Since ZTEST requires the use of large samples (size 30 or greater), let's use some data from the data CD. The Excel workbook Svls03.xls contains heights in feet of 65 randomly selected professional basketball players.

Assume that twenty years ago the average height of professional basketball players was 6.3 feet (that translates to 6 ft 3.6 inches). Let's use the sample data in Svls03.xls to consider whether the current population mean height of professional basketball players is greater than it was twenty years ago. The null hypothesis will be that their average height is the same. Given our alternative hypothesis ("greater than"), we will apply a right-tailed test.

Open the workbook Svls03.xls found on the data CD. The data will appear in Column A. Cell A1 contains the label Heights. The data are in cells A2:A66.

After typing in some labeling information, we want to display the P value provided by ZTEST in Cell F3. Activate Cell F3 and, in the Paste Function dialog box, select Statistical in the left column and ZTEST in the right column. The dialog box should be similar to the one shown at the top of the next page. **Ignore the dialog box statement that this is a two-tailed test. It is right-tailed.**

We will use the cell range A2:A66 for the Array and 6.3 as the value of X3, letting Excel compute s from the sample data. Notice that with the space for Sigma left blank, the dialog box tells us that the P value is 2.12826E-05. We interpret this as the probability that 65 data values could come out with a mean greater than or equal to that of the sample, given that they were taken from a normal distribution with a mean of 6.3.

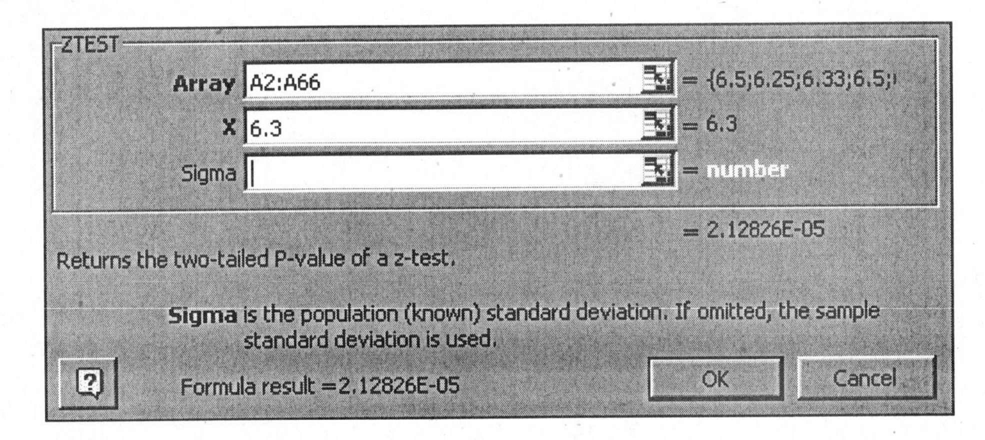

So the P value is about 0.00002. Since this is less than even the very restrictive $\alpha = 0.01$, we reject the null hypothesis and conclude that the population mean height of pro basketball players now is greater than it was twenty years ago.

For completeness, we also used the **➤Tools➤Data Analysis➤Descriptive statistics** menu choice and dialog box to generate the descriptive statistics for our data. We selected output range beginning in cell C5, and then widened the columns to fit the display.

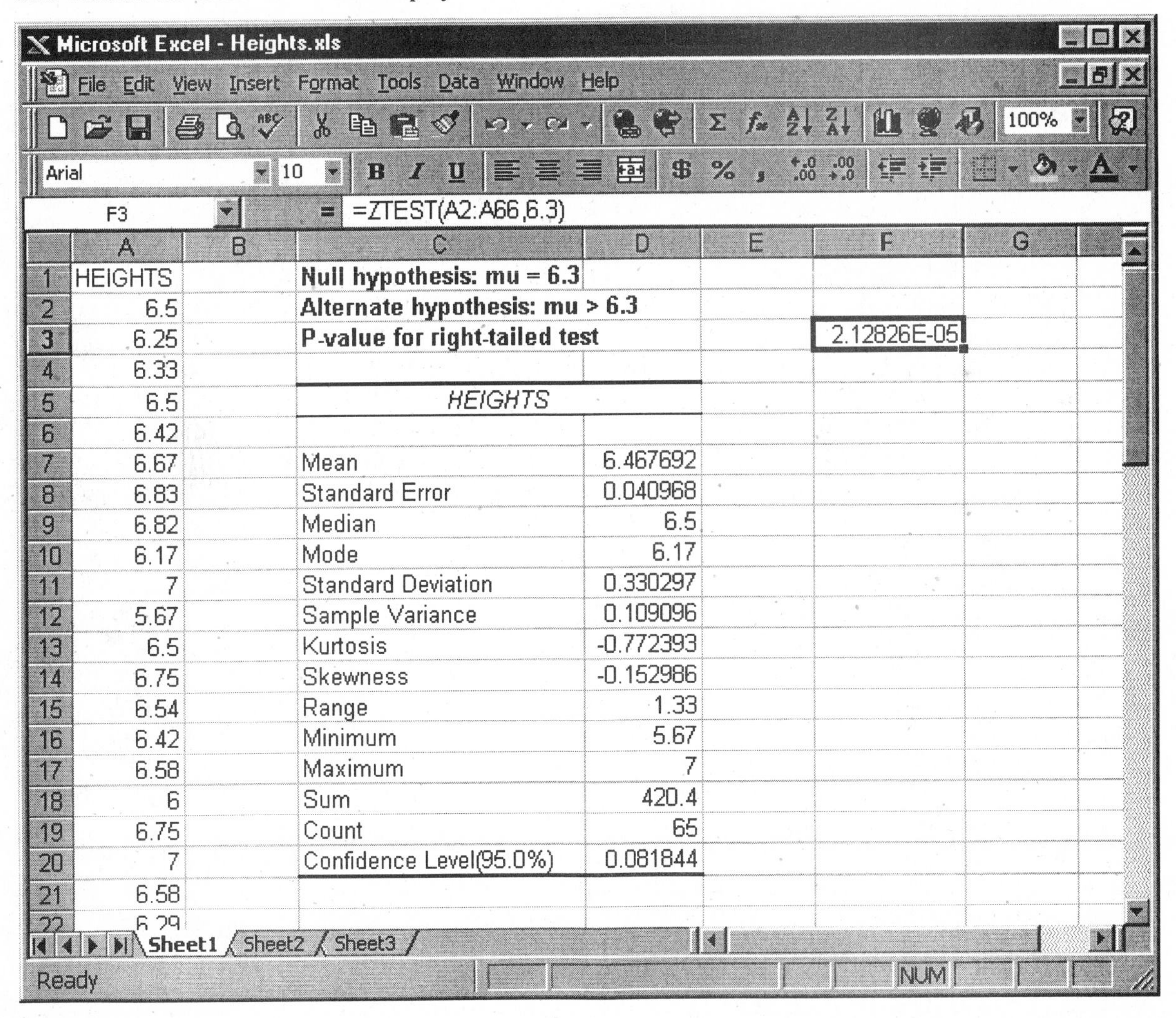

	A	B	C	D	E	F	G
1	HEIGHTS		Null hypothesis: mu = 6.3				
2	6.5		Alternate hypothesis: mu > 6.3				
3	6.25		P-value for right-tailed test			2.12826E-05	
4	6.33						
5	6.5		HEIGHTS				
6	6.42						
7	6.67		Mean	6.467692			
8	6.83		Standard Error	0.040968			
9	6.82		Median	6.5			
10	6.17		Mode	6.17			
11	7		Standard Deviation	0.330297			
12	5.67		Sample Variance	0.109096			
13	6.5		Kurtosis	-0.772393			
14	6.75		Skewness	-0.152986			
15	6.54		Range	1.33			
16	6.42		Minimum	5.67			
17	6.58		Maximum	7			
18	6		Sum	420.4			
19	6.75		Count	65			
20	7		Confidence Level(95.0%)	0.081844			
21	6.58						
22	6.29						

LAB ACTIVITIES FOR TESTING A SINGLE POPULATION MEAN

1. Open or retrieve the worksheet Svls04.xls from the data CD. The data in Column A of this worksheet represent the miles per gallon gasoline consumption (highway) for a random sample of 55 makes and models of passenger cars (source: Environmental Protection Agency).

30	27	22	25	24	25	24	15
35	35	33	52	49	10	27	18
20	23	24	25	30	24	24	24
18	20	25	27	24	32	29	27
24	27	26	25	24	28	33	30
13	13	21	28	37	35	32	33
29	31	28	28	25	29	31	

Test the hypothesis that the population mean mile per gallon gasoline consumption for such cars is greater than 25 mpg.

(a) Do we know σ for the mpg consumption? Can we estimate σ by s, the sample standard deviation? Can we use the normal distribution for the hypothesis test?

(b) State the null and alternate hypothesis, and type them on your worksheet.

(c) Use ZTEST with Sigma omitted.

(d) Look at the P value in the output. Compare it to α. Do we reject the null hypothesis or not? Does it depend on the level of significance?

(e) Use the Descriptive Statistics dialog box to generate the summary statistics for the data, and place the results on the worksheet.

TESTS INVOLVING PAIRED DIFFERENCES – DEPENDENT SAMPLES (SECTION 9.6 OF *UNDERSTANDABLE STATISTICS*)

The test for difference of means, dependent samples is presented in Section 9.6 of *Understandable Statistics.* Dependent samples arise from before-and after-studies, some studies of data taken from the same subjects, and some studies on identical twins.

In Excel there are two functions that produce the P value for a one- or two-tailed test of paired differences. The first command is **TTEST,** found using Paste Function with Statistical in the left column and TTEST in the right column. You can also activate a cell and type the command in the formula bar. This command returns only the P value for the test. The syntax is

TTEST(data range of sample 1,data range of sample 2, tails, type)

If tails = 1, then TTEST returns the P value for a one-tailed test, and if tails = 2, then TTEST returns the two-tailed value. For the parameter called type, there are three choices:

type	Test performed using Student's t distribution
1	Paired difference test
2	Difference of means test for two samples with equal variances
3	Difference of means test for two samples with unequal variances

The other Excel command, ➤**Tools**➤**Data Analysis**➤**t-Test: Paired Two Sample for Means,** gives much more information than TTEST. We will use this command in the next example.

Example

Promoters of a state lottery decided to advertise the lottery heavily on television for one week during the middle of one of the lottery games. To see if the advertising improved ticket sales, they surveyed a random sample of 8 ticket outlets and recorded weekly sales for one week before the television campaign and for one week after the campaign. The results follow (in ticket sales) where row A gives sales prior to the campaign and row B gives sales afterward.

A	3201	4529	1425	1272	1784	1733	2563	3129
B	3762	4851	1202	1131	2172	1802	2492	3151

Test the claim that the television campaign increased lottery ticket sales at the 0.05 level of significance.

We enter the data in Columns A and B, with appropriate headers. Next, open the dialog box below, using ➤**Tools**➤**Data Analysis**➤**t-Test: Paired Two Sample for Means**.

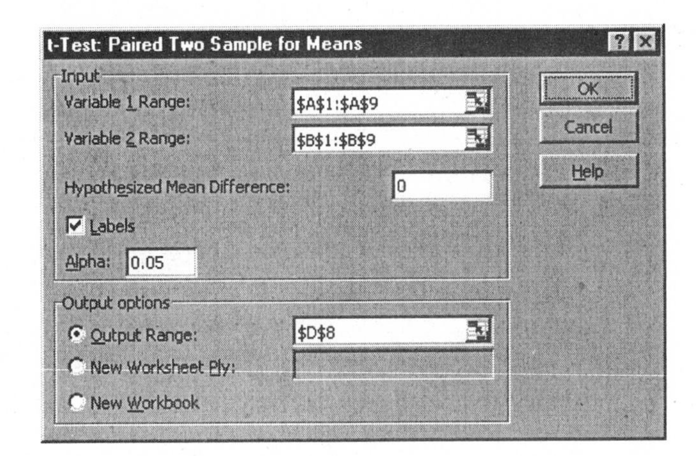

Notice that we use Column A cells for Variable 1 Range, Column B cells for Variable 2 range, and we check the Labels box. The null hypothesis is H_0: $\mu = 0$, so we enter 0 as the value for the Hypothesized Mean difference. We select Cell D8 as the upper left cell for the Output Range, and we widen the output columns to fit the display.

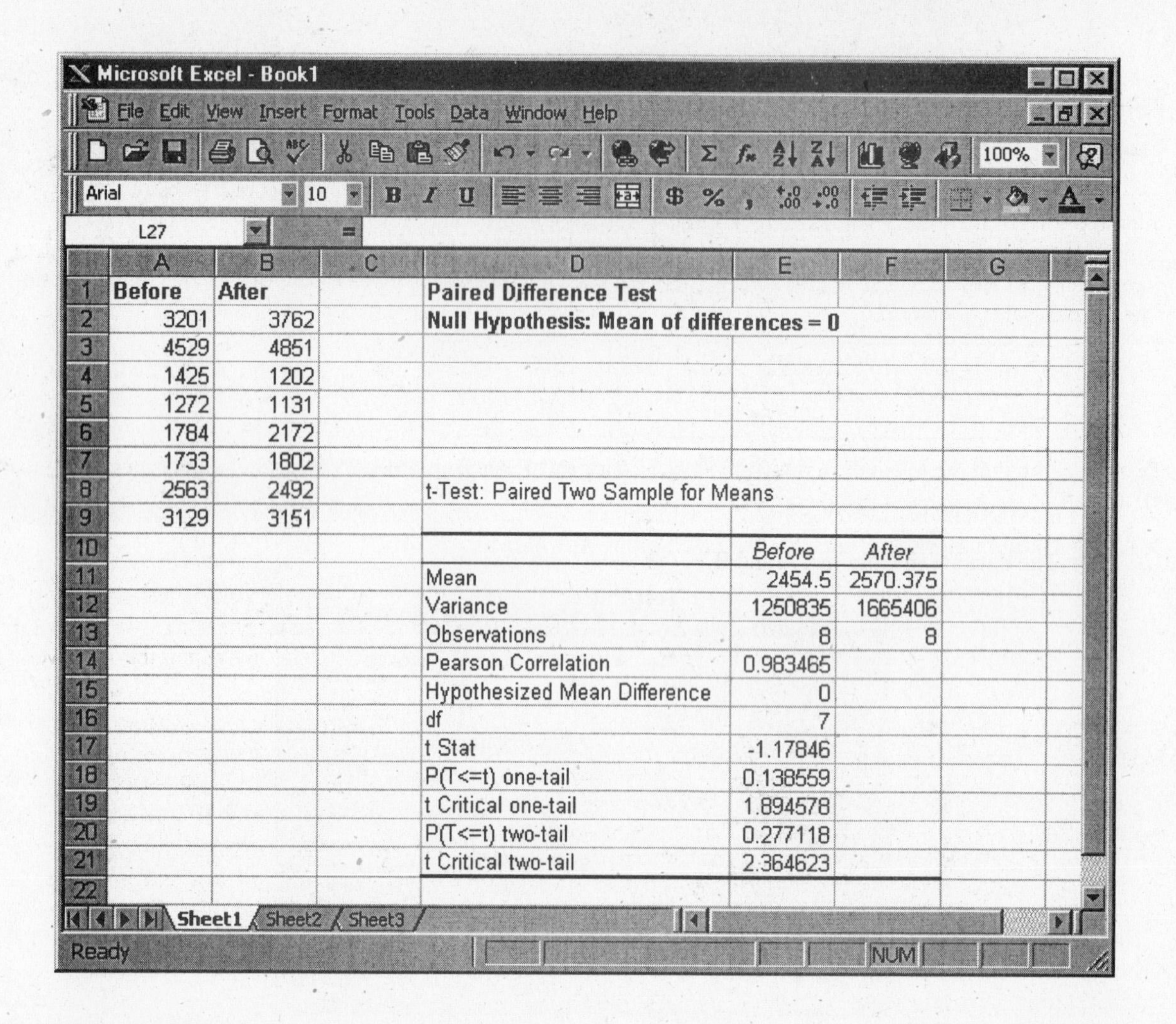

	A	B	C	D	E	F
1	**Before**	**After**		**Paired Difference Test**		
2	3201	3762		**Null Hypothesis: Mean of differences = 0**		
3	4529	4851				
4	1425	1202				
5	1272	1131				
6	1784	2172				
7	1733	1802				
8	2563	2492		t-Test: Paired Two Sample for Means		
9	3129	3151				
10					*Before*	*After*
11				Mean	2454.5	2570.375
12				Variance	1250835	1665406
13				Observations	8	8
14				Pearson Correlation	0.983465	
15				Hypothesized Mean Difference	0	
16				df	7	
17				t Stat	-1.17846	
18				P(T<=t) one-tail	0.138559	
19				t Critical one-tail	1.894578	
20				P(T<=t) two-tail	0.277118	
21				t Critical two-tail	2.364623	

Notice that we get $P = 0.1386$ for a one-tailed test. Since this value is larger than the level of significance, we do not reject the null hypothesis. The same output gives the P value for a two-tailed test as well. In addition, we see the sample t value of -1.17846, together with the critical values for a one- or two-tailed test using $\alpha = 0.05$.

LAB ACTIVITIES FOR TESTS INVOLVING PAIRED DIFFERENCES

1. Open or retrieve the worksheet Tvds01.xls from the data CD-ROM. The data are pairs of values where the entries in Column A represents average salary ($1000/yr) for male faculty members at an institution and those in Column B represent the average salary for female faculty members ($1000/yr) at the same institution. A random sample of 22 U.S. colleges and universities was used (source: Academe, Bulletin of the American Association of University Professors).

(34.5, 33.9) (30.5, 31.2) (35.1, 35.0) (35.7, 34.2) (31.5, 32.4)
(34.4, 34.1) (32.1, 32.7) (30.7, 29.9) (33.7, 31.2) (35.3, 35.5)
(30.7, 30.2) (34.2, 34.8) (39.6, 38.7) (30.5, 30.0) (33.8, 33.8)
(31.7, 32.4) (32.8, 31.7) (38.5, 38.9) (40.5, 41.5) (25.3, 25.5)
(28.6, 28.0) (35.8, 35.1)

(a) The data are in Columns A and B.

(b) Use the **➤Tools➤Data Analysis➤t-Test Paired Two Sample for Means** dialog box to test the hypothesis that there is a difference in salary. What is the *P* value of the sample test statistic? Do we reject or fail to reject the null hypothesis at the 5% level of significance? What about at the 1% level of significance?

(c) Use the **➤Tools➤Data Analysis➤t-Test Paired Two Sample for Means** dialog box to test the hypothesis that female faculty members have a lower average salary than male faculty members. What is the test conclusion at the 5% level of significance? At the 1% level of significance?

2. An audiologist is conducting a study on noise and stress. Twelve subjects selected at random were given a stress test in a room that was quiet. Then the same subjects were given another stress test, this time in a room with high-pitched background noise. The results of the stress tests were scores 1 through 20 with 20 indicating the greatest stress. The results follow, where A represents the score of the test administered in the quiet room and B represents the scores of the test administered in the room with the high-pitched background noise.

Subject	1	2	4	5	6	7	8	9	10	11	12
A	13	12	16	19	7	13	9	15	17	6	14
B	18	15	14	18	10	12	11	14	17	8	16

Test the hypothesis that the stress level was greater during exposure to high-pitched background noise. Look at the *P* value. Should you reject the null hypothesis at the 1% level of significance? At the 5% level?

TESTING OF DIFFERENCES OF MEANS (SECTION 9.7 OF *UNDERSTANDABLE STATISTICS*)

Tests of difference of means for independent samples are presented in Section 9.7 of *Understandable Statistics*. We consider the $\bar{x}_1 - \bar{x}_2$ distribution. The null hypothesis is that there is no difference between means, so $H_0 : \mu_1 = \mu_2$ or $H_0 : \mu_1 - \mu_2 = 0$.

Large Samples

When we are testing the difference of means using large samples, the text uses the normal distribution even if the population variance of each population is unknown. Because we have large samples, the population variances may be approximated by the sample variances. If you don't know the population variances, create some labels on your worksheet, then use Paste Function, and select Statistical in the left column, VAR in the right column. We did this to get the variances shown in the next worksheet.

The menu selection **➤Tools➤Data Analysis➤z-Test Two Sample for Means** provides the sample z statistic, P values for a one- or two-tailed test, and critical z values for a one- or two-tailed test at the specified level of significance.

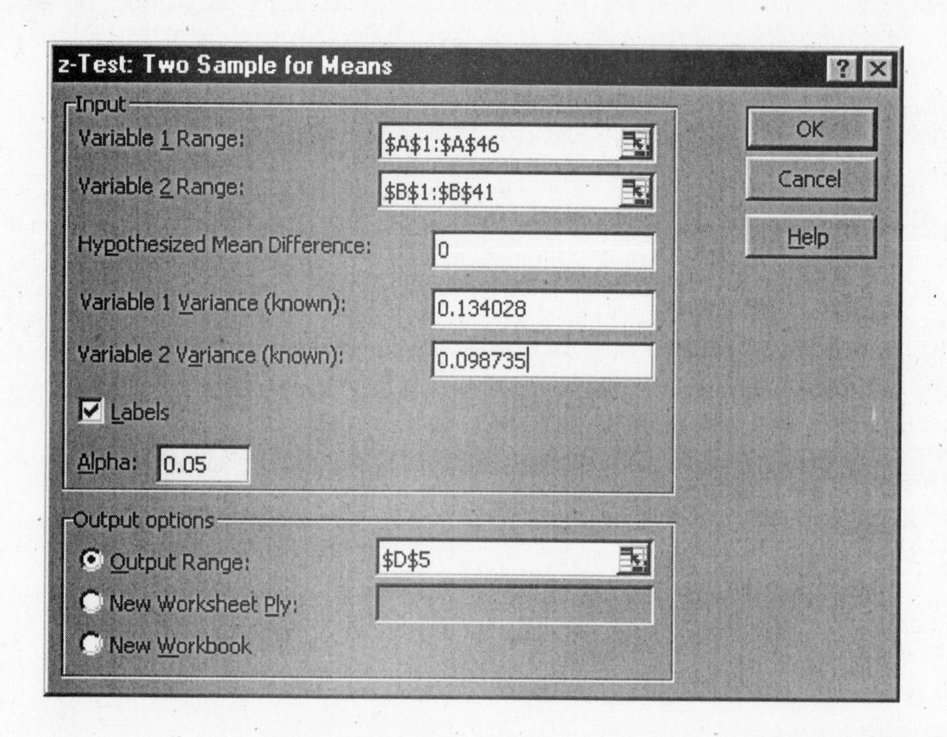

We used the Excel worksheet Tvis01.xls to generate the worksheet that follows. This data gives the heights of a random sample of football players (Column A) and the heights of a random sample of basketball players (Column B).

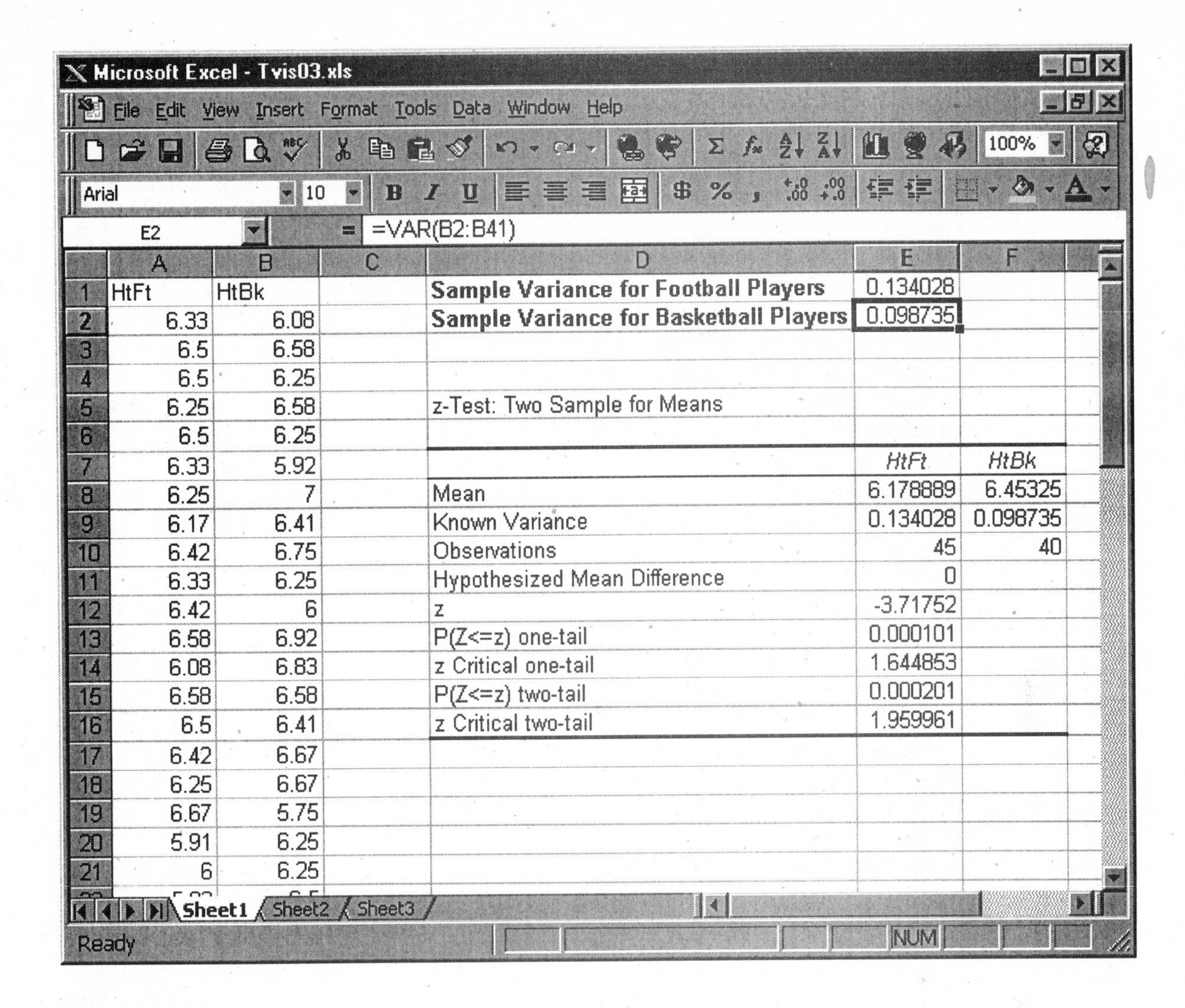

Microsoft Excel - Tvis03.xls

E2 =VAR(B2:B41)

	A	B	C	D	E	F
1	HtFt	HtBk		**Sample Variance for Football Players**	0.134028	
2	6.33	6.08		**Sample Variance for Basketball Players**	0.098735	
3	6.5	6.58				
4	6.5	6.25				
5	6.25	6.58		z-Test: Two Sample for Means		
6	6.5	6.25				
7	6.33	5.92			*HtFt*	*HtBk*
8	6.25	7		Mean	6.178889	6.45325
9	6.17	6.41		Known Variance	0.134028	0.098735
10	6.42	6.75		Observations	45	40
11	6.33	6.25		Hypothesized Mean Difference	0	
12	6.42	6		z	-3.71752	
13	6.58	6.92		P(Z<=z) one-tail	0.000101	
14	6.08	6.83		z Critical one-tail	1.644853	
15	6.58	6.58		P(Z<=z) two-tail	0.000201	
16	6.5	6.41		z Critical two-tail	1.959961	
17	6.42	6.67				
18	6.25	6.67				
19	6.67	5.75				
20	5.91	6.25				
21	6	6.25				

Small Samples

To do a test of difference of sample means with small samples, with the assumption that the samples come from populations with the same standard deviation, use **➤Tools➤Data Analysis➤t-Test: Two-Sample Assuming Equal Variances.**

Example

Sellers of microwave French fry cookers claim that their process saves cooking time. The McDougle Fast Food Chain is considering the purchase of these new cookers, but wants to test the claim.

Six batches of French fries were cooked in the traditional way. The cooking times (in minutes) were

15 17 14 15 16 13

Six batches of French fries of the same weight were cooked using the new microwave cooker. These cooking times (in minutes) were

11 14 12 10 11 15

Test the claim that the microwave process takes less time. Use $\alpha = 0.05$.

We will enter the traditional data in Column A and the new data in Column B. Then we use **➤Tools➤Data Analysis➤t-Test: Two-Sample Assuming Equal Variances.** The hypothesized mean difference is zero.

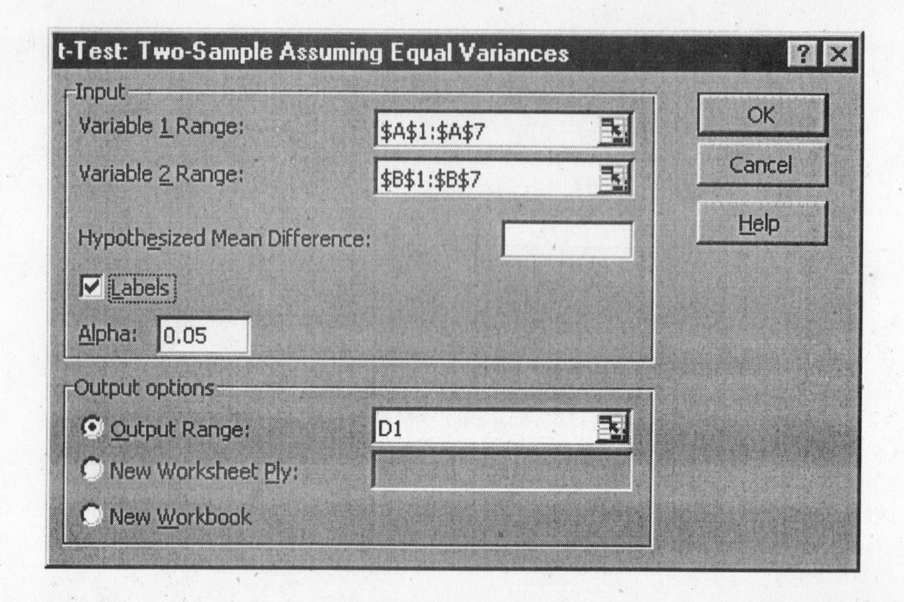

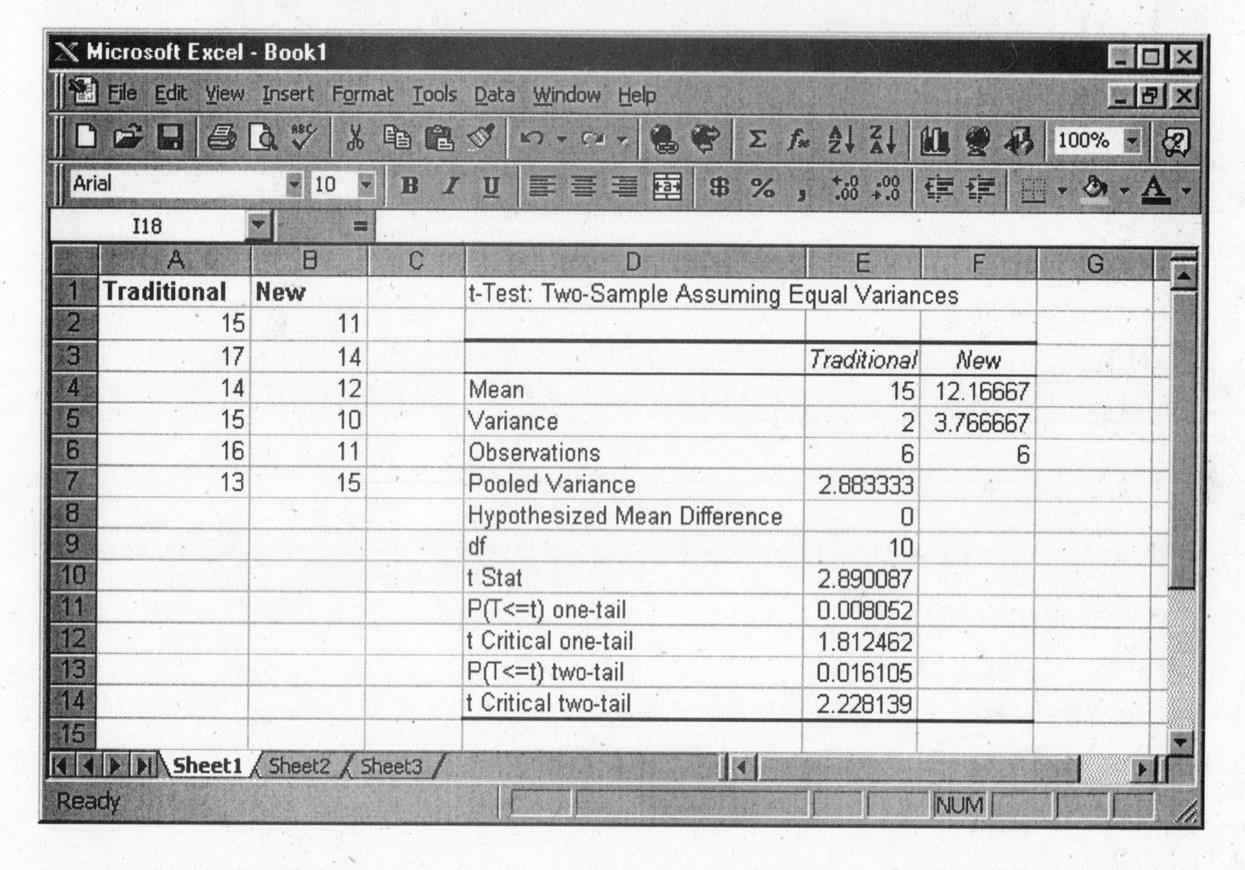

	A	B	C	D	E	F
1	Traditional	New		t-Test: Two-Sample Assuming Equal Variances		
2	15	11				
3	17	14			*Traditional*	*New*
4	14	12		Mean	15	12.16667
5	15	10		Variance	2	3.766667
6	16	11		Observations	6	6
7	13	15		Pooled Variance	2.883333	
8				Hypothesized Mean Difference	0	
9				df	10	
10				t Stat	2.890087	
11				P(T<=t) one-tail	0.008052	
12				t Critical one-tail	1.812462	
13				P(T<=t) two-tail	0.016105	
14				t Critical two-tail	2.228139	
15						

We see that the P value for a one-tail test is 0.00805. Since this value is less than 0.05, we reject the null hypothesis and conclude that the new method takes less time on average.

LAB ACTIVITIES FOR TESTING DIFFERENCES OF MEANS

1. Calm Cough Medicine is testing a new ingredient to see if its addition will lengthen the effective cough relief time of a single dose. A random sample of fifteen doses of the standard medicine was tested, and the effective relief times (in minutes) were

   42 35 40 32 30 26 51 39 33 28
   37 22 36 33 41

   Then a random sample of twenty doses with the new ingredient was tested. The effective relief times (in minutes) were

   43 51 35 49 32 29 42 38 45 74
   31 31 46 36 33 45 30 32 41 25

   Assume that the standard deviations of the relief times are equal for the two populations. Test the claim that the effective relief time is longer when the new ingredient is added. Use $\alpha = 0.01$.

2. Retrieve the worksheet Tvis06.xls from the data CD-ROM. The data represent numbers of cases of red fox rabies for a random sample of sixteen areas in each of two different regions of southern Germany.

   Number of Cases in Region 1

   10 2 2 5 3 4 3 3 4 0 2 6 4 8 7 4

   Number of Cases in Region 2

   1 1 2 1 3 9 2 2 4 5 4 2 2 0 0 2

   Test the hypothesis that the average number of cases in Region 1 is greater than the average number of cases in Region 2. Use a 1% level of significance.

3. Retrieve the Excel worksheet Tvis02.xls from the data CD-ROM. The data represent the petal length (in centimeters) for a random sample of 35 Iris *Virginica* plants and for a random sample of 38 *Iris Setosa* plants (source: Anderson, E., Bull. Amer. Iris Soc).

   Petal Length of Iris Virginica

   5.1 5.8 6.3 6.1 5.1 5.5 5.3 5.5 6.9 5.0 4.9 6.0 4.8 6.1 5.6 5.1
   5.6 4.8 5.4 5.1 5.1 5.9 5.2 5.7 5.4 4.5 6.1 5.3 5.5 6.7 5.7 4.9
   4.8 5.8 5.1

   Petal Length of Iris Setosa

   1.5 1.7 1.4 1.5 1.5 1.6 1.4 1.1 1.2 1.4 1.7 1.0 1.7 1.9 1.6 1.4
   1.5 1.4 1.2 1.3 1.5 1.3 1.6 1.9 1.4 1.6 1.5 1.4 1.6 1.2 1.9 1.5
   1.6 1.4 1.3 1.7 1.5 1.7

   Test the hypothesis that the average petal length for *Iris Setosa* is shorter than the average petal length for *Iris Virginica*.

CHAPTER 10 REGRESSION AND CORRELATION

LINEAR REGRESSION – TWO VARIABLES (SECTIONS 10.1–10.4 OF *UNDERSTANDABLE STATISTICS*)

Chapter 10 of *Understandable Statistics* introduces linear regression. Formulas to find the equation of the least squares line,

$$y = a + bx$$

are given in Section 10.2. This section also contains the equation for the standard error of estimate as well as the procedure to find a confidence interval for the predicted value of y. The formula for the correlation coefficient r and coefficient of determination r^2 are given in Section 10.3.

Excel supports several functions related to linear regression. To use these, first enter the paired data values in two columns. Put the explanatory variable in a column labeled with x, or an appropriate descriptive name, and put the response variable in a column labeled with y, or an appropriate descriptive name.

The functions and corresponding syntax are

LINEST(y range,x range) which returns the slope b and y-intercept a of the least-squares line, in that order. Although this command can be found under the Paste Function button menu, it is best to type it in because it is an array formula. (The full LINEST function involves two more, optional parameters, but we will ignore these.) To use LINEST,

1. Activate two cells, the first to hold the slope b, the second for the intercept a.
2. In the formula bar, type =LINEST(y range,x range) with the appropriate cell ranges in place of x range and y range.
3. Instead of pressing Enter, press **Ctrl+Shift+Enter.** This key combination activates the array formula features so that you get the outputs for both b and a. Otherwise, you will get only the slope b of the least-squares line.

The other functions are employed in the usual way, by activating a cell and then either typing the command directly in the formula bar, followed by Enter, or by using the Paste Function dialog box.

SLOPE(y range,x range) which returns the slope b of the least-squares line.

INTERCEPT(y range,x range) which returns the intercept a of the least-squares line.

CORREL(y range,x range) which returns the correlation coefficient r.

FORECAST(x value,y range,x range) which returns the predicted y value for the specified x value, using extrapolation from the given pairs of x and y values. Note that you need to use a new FORECAST command for each different x value.

STEYX(y range,x range) which returns the standard error of estimate, S_e.

We will now use the Chart Wizard to generate a scatter diagram and then add the results of the least-squares regression.

Example

In retailing, merchandise loss due to shoplifting, damage, and other causes is called shrinkage. The managers at H.R. Merchandise think that there is a relationship between shrinkage and the number of clerks on duty. To explore this relationship, a random sample of seven weeks was selected. During each week, the staffing level of sales clerks was held constant and the dollar value (in hundreds of dollars) of the shrinkage was recorded.

X	10	12	11	15	9	13	8	Staffing level
Y	19	15	20	9	25	12	31	(in hundreds)

Open a worksheet. Place the X values in Column A with a corresponding label and the Y values in Column B.

Create a Scatter Diagram

Click on the Chart Wizard and select XY (Scatter). Choose the first subtype, which shows only points. Click Next.

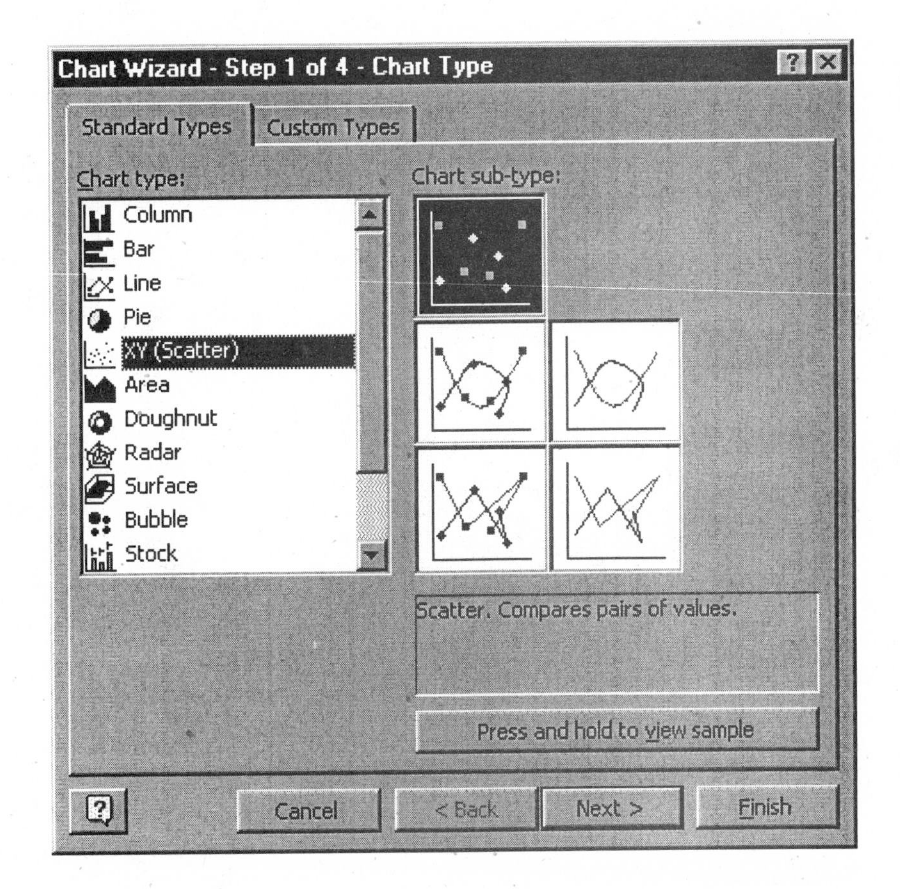

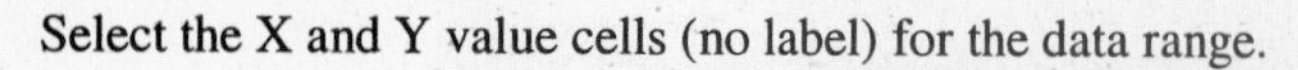

Select the X and Y value cells (no label) for the data range.

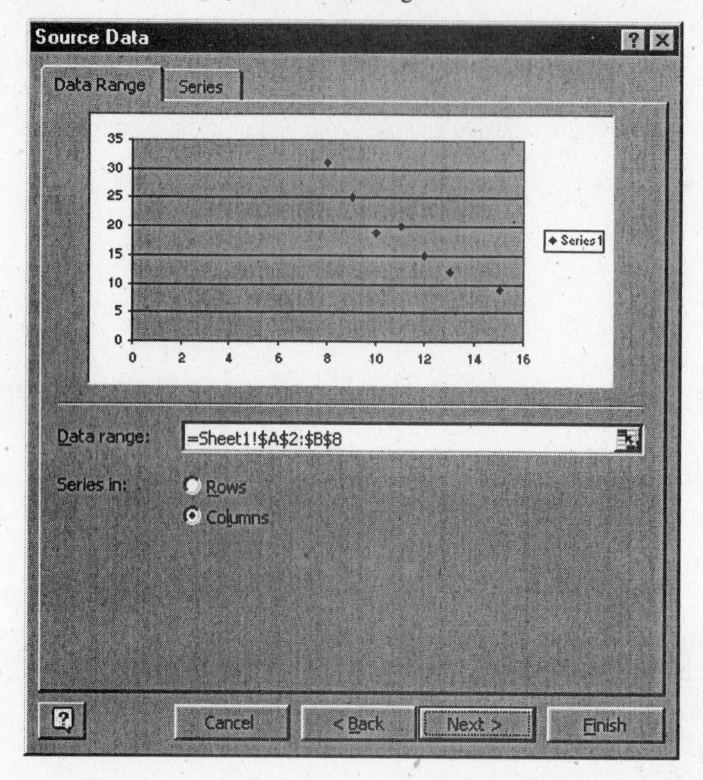

Click the Series tab to verify that the X values are being taken from Column A and the Y values from Column B.

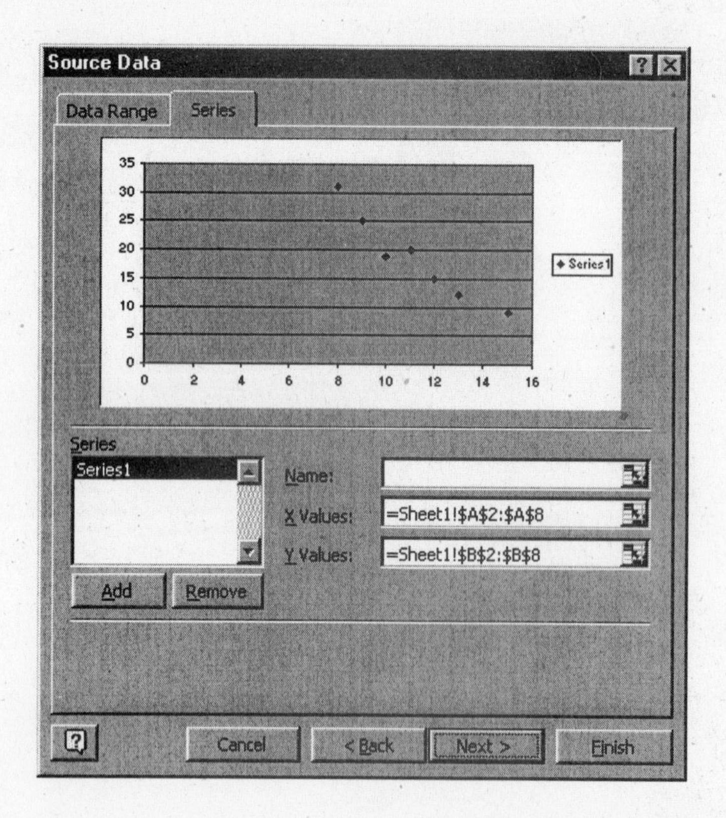

Give the chart a title and give the axes labels. Then click on the Legend tab and turn off Legend.

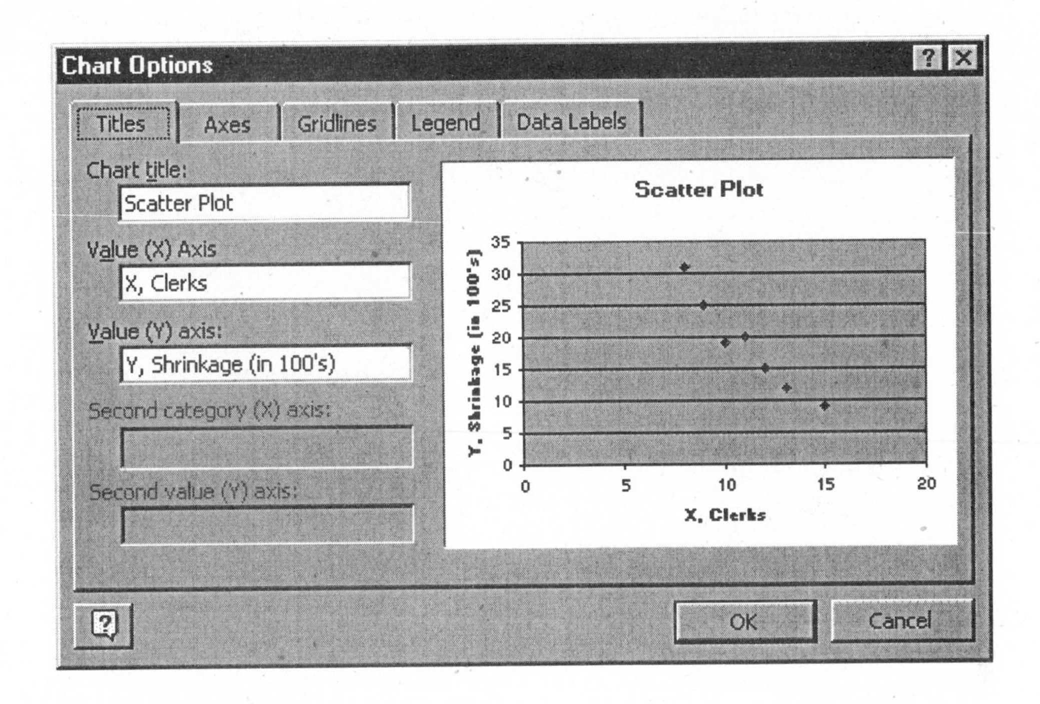

Click Finish to see the scatter plot on your worksheet.

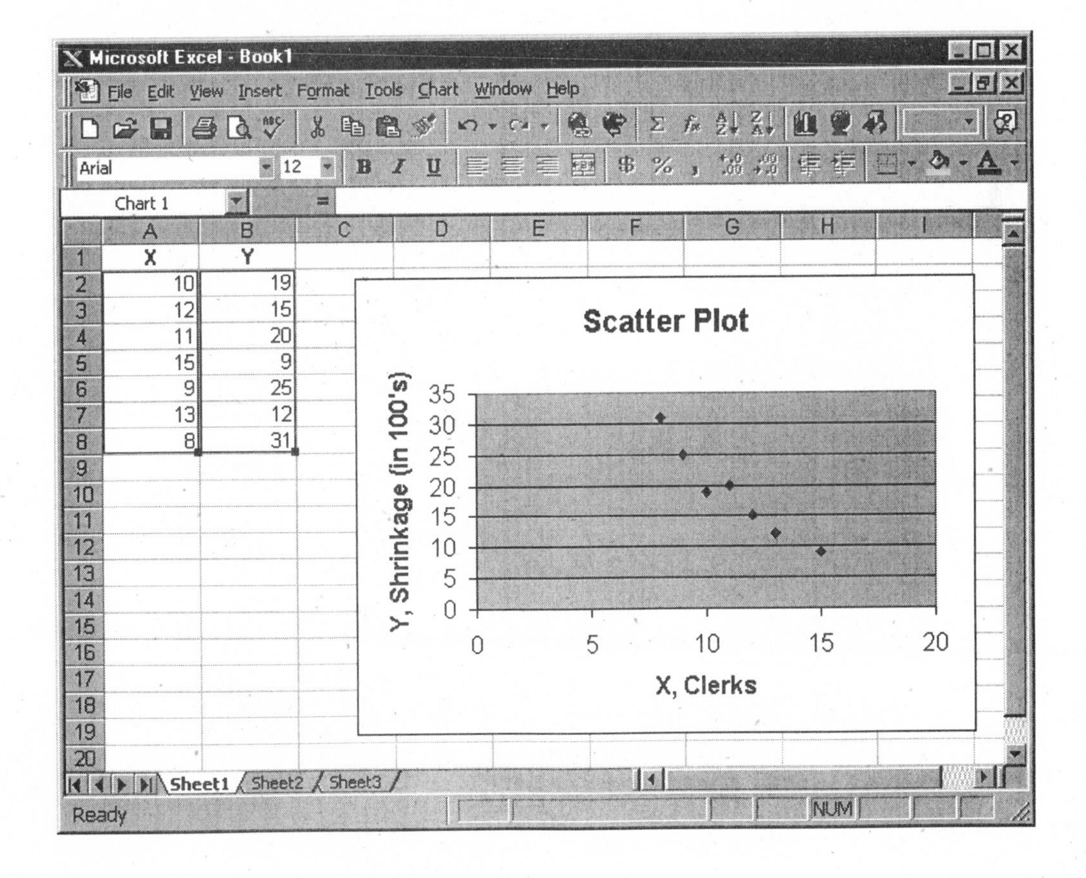

Add least-squares results to the plot

The least-squares line can be added to the plot, along with its equation and the value of r^2. Right-click on one of the data points shown in the scatter diagram. A drop-down menu will appear. Select Add Trendline to call up a dialog box.

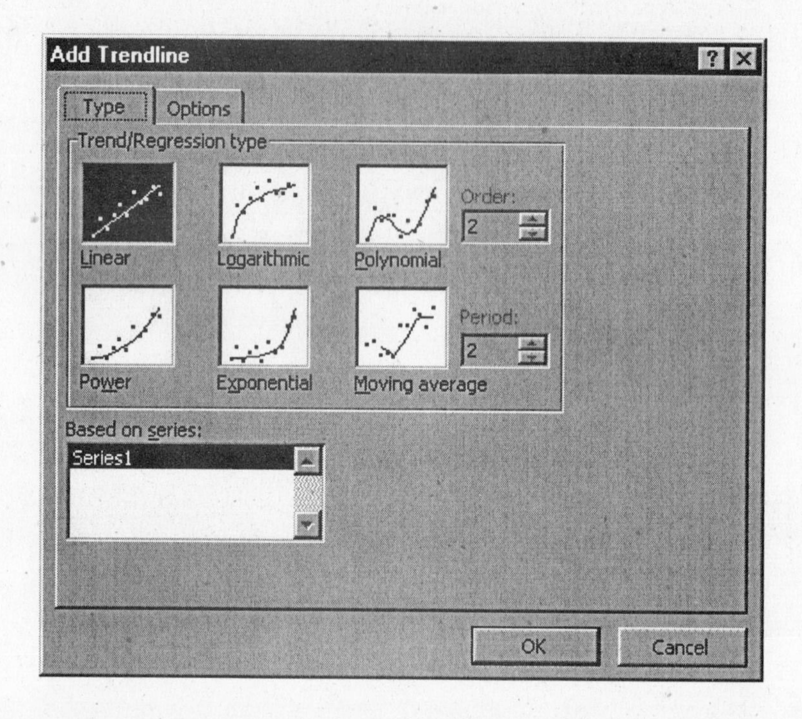

Be sure Linear is selected as the Type. Click on the Options tab.

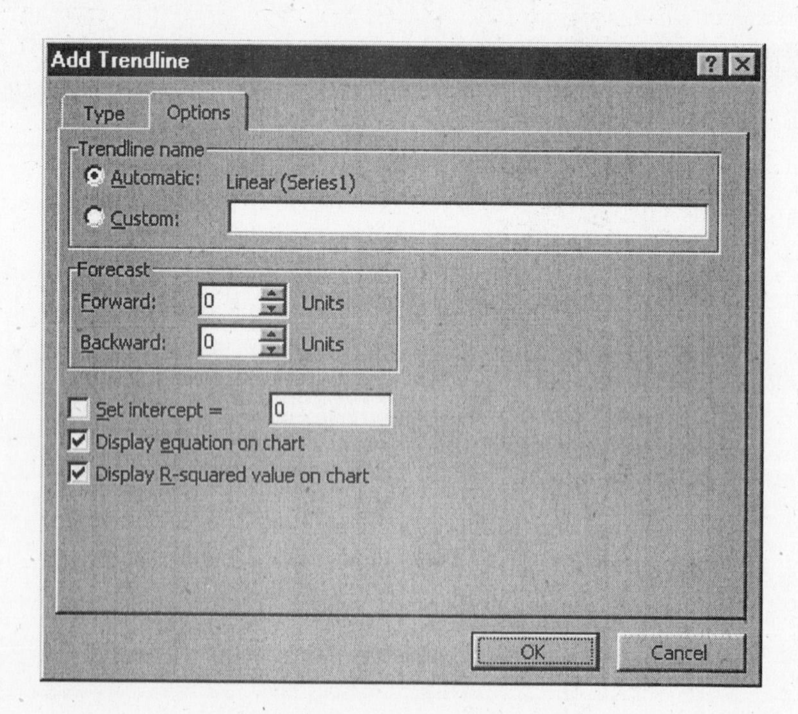

Check Display equation on chart and Display R-squared on chart, then click OK. Now our scatter diagram shows the graph of the least squares-line and the equation. You can move the equation out of the way of the graph by clicking on it and dragging the resulting box to a convenient location.

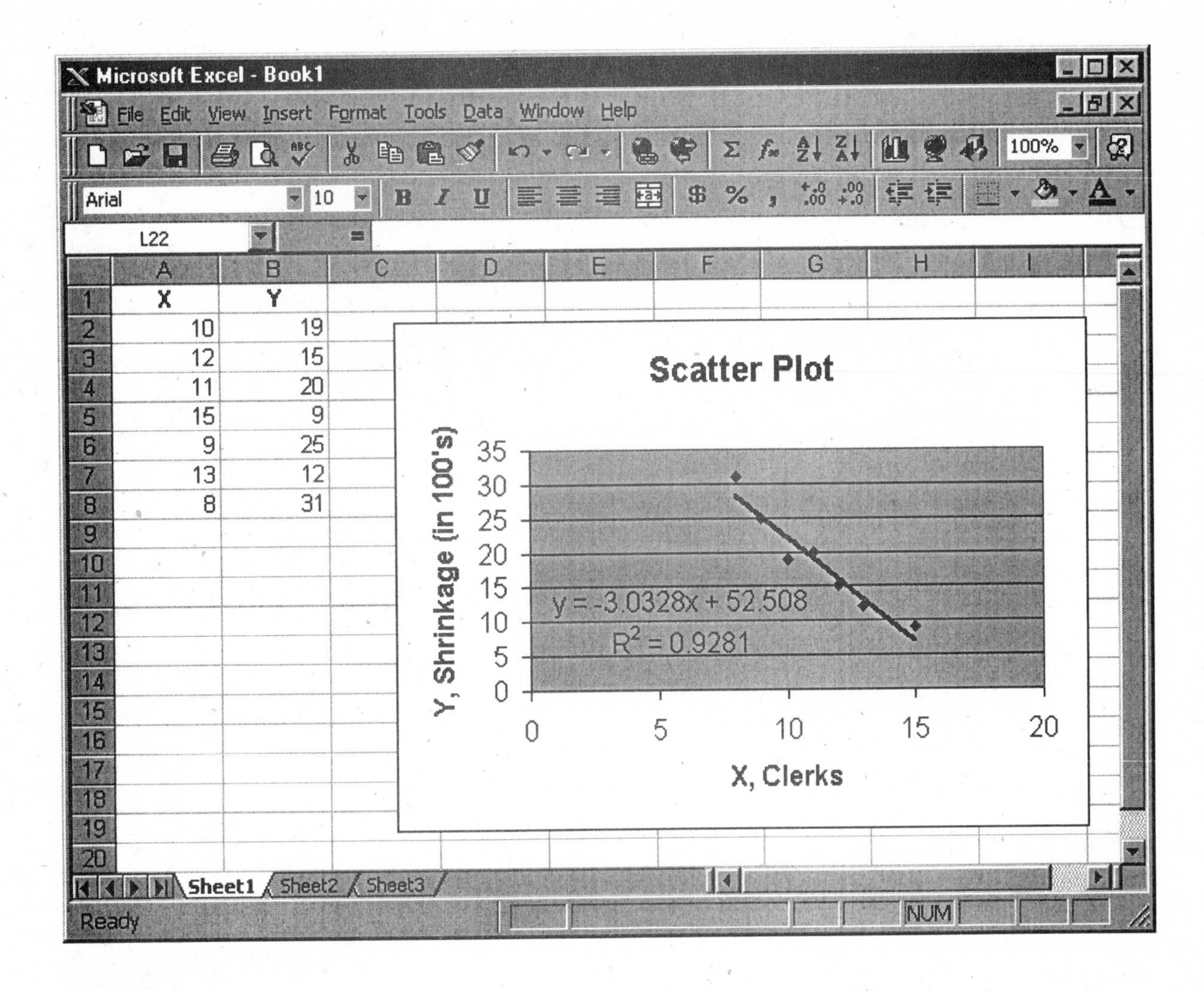

Scale the axes

Sometimes all the points of a scatter diagram are in a corner, and we want to rescale the axes to reflect the data range. To do so,

1. Right-click on the *X*-axis, select Format Axes.
2. Click on the Scale tab. Change the minimum and maximum values for X. You may retain 0 as the value for Value (Y) axis Crosses at.

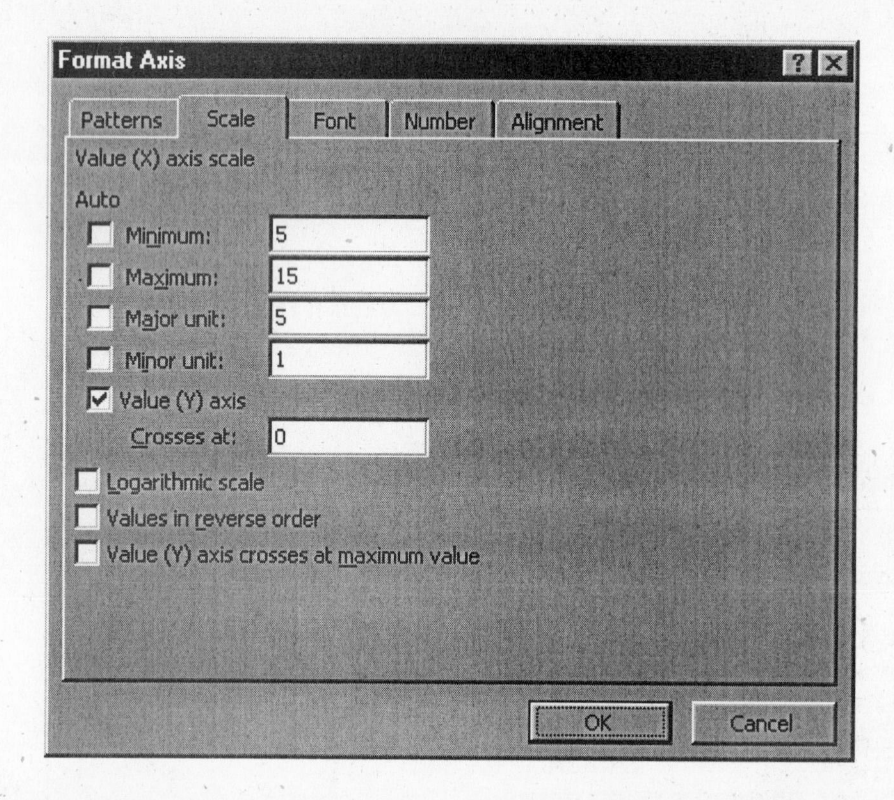

Go through a similar procedure to rescale the *Y*-axis. The result of our changes appear as shown at the top of the next page.

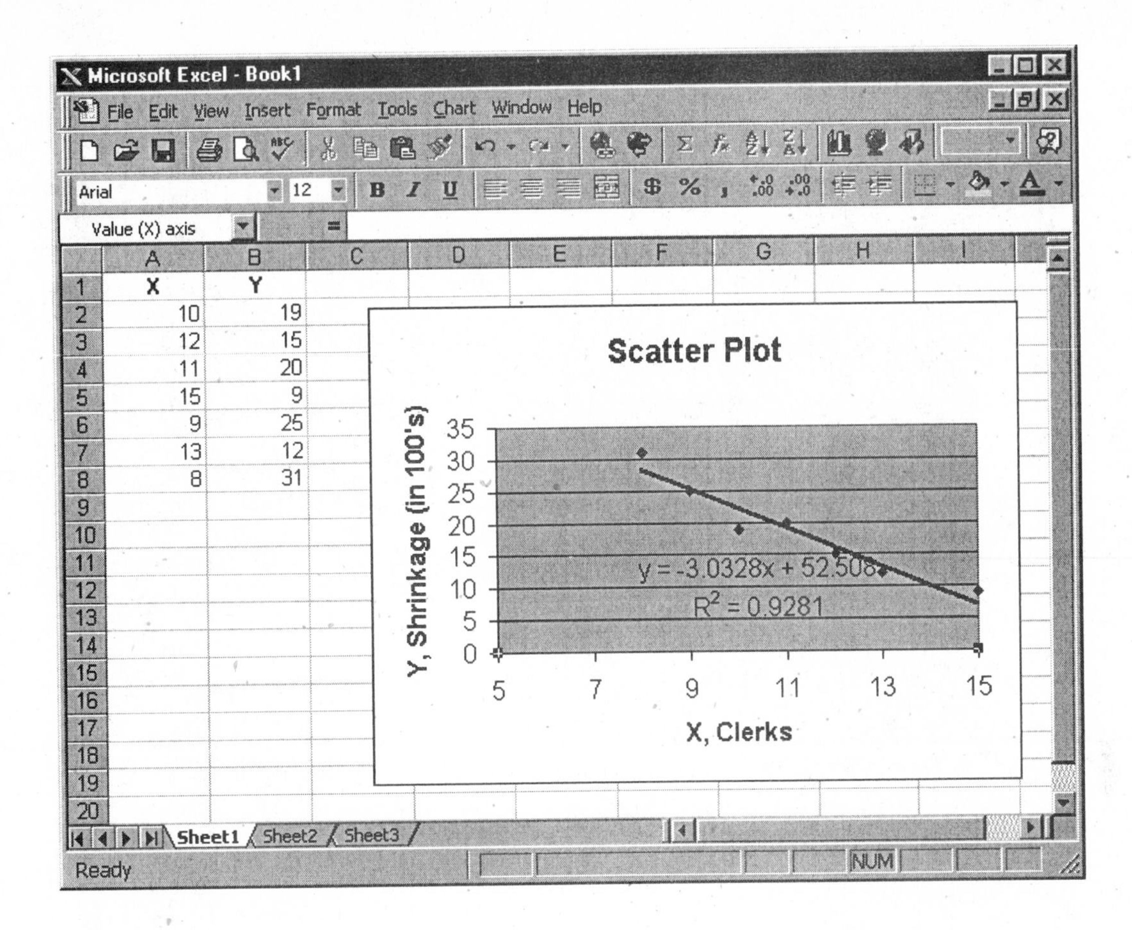

Forecast a value

Let's predict the shrinkage when fourteen clerks are available, using FORECAST. Click Paste Function on the standard tool bar, then select Statistical in the left column and Forecast in the right column. Fill in the dialog box as shown.

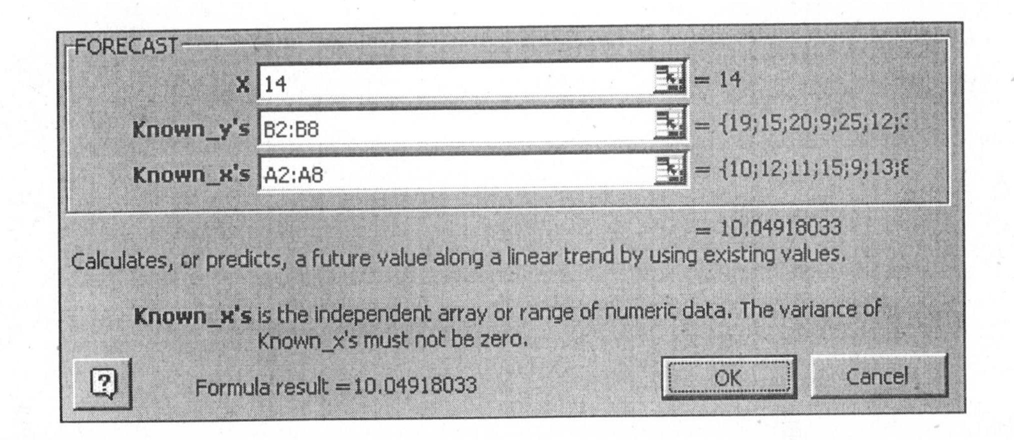

The predicted *Y* value is about 10.05. Since the unit for *Y* is hundreds of dollars, this represents a predicted shrinkage of $1005 when fourteen clerks are on duty.

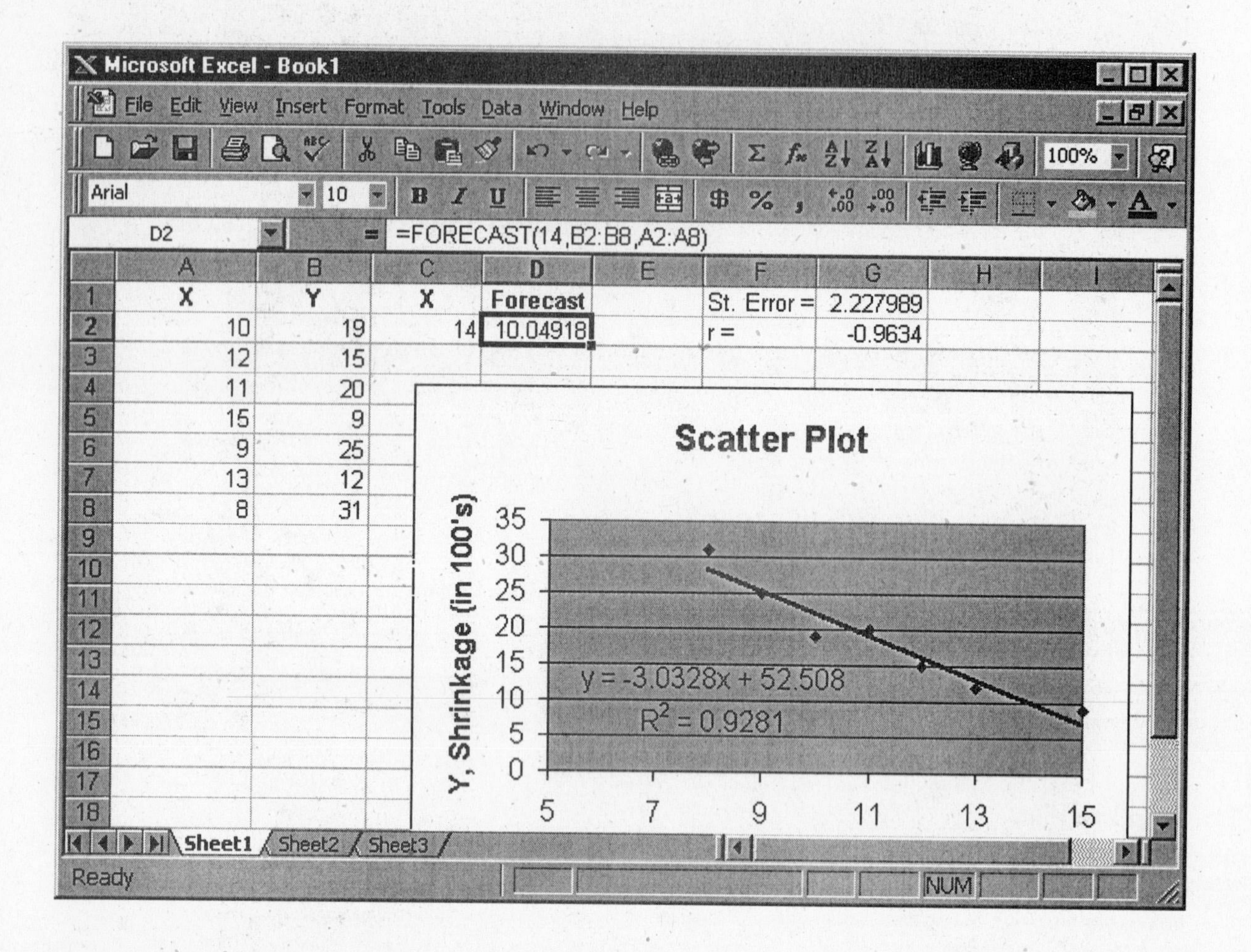

Find the standard error of estimate and the value of *r*

We use Paste Function, Statistical and select STEYX and CORREL to find the standard error and the correlation coefficient.

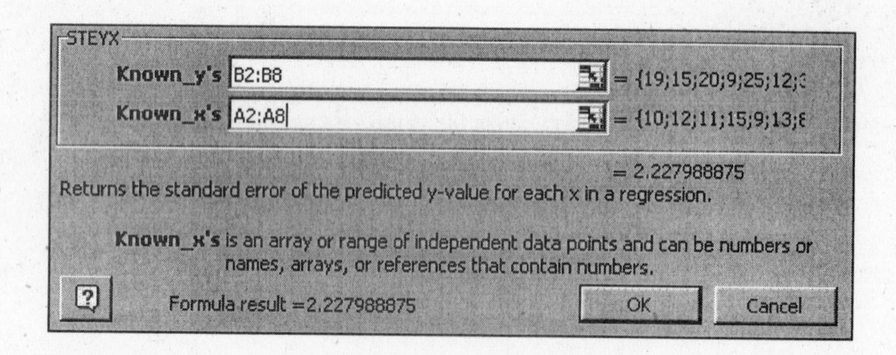

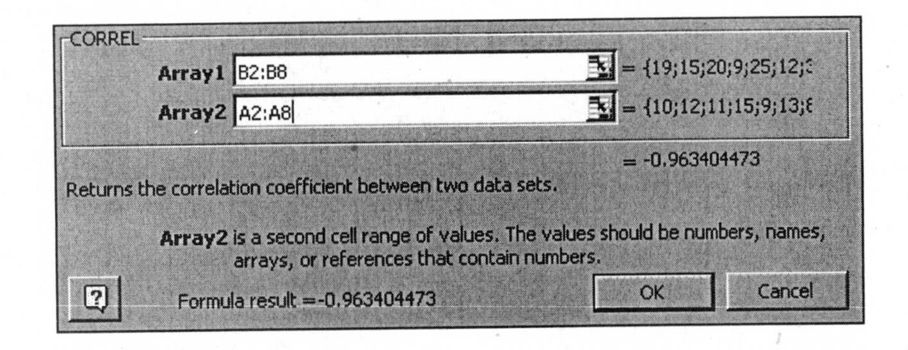

The worksheet shows the results.

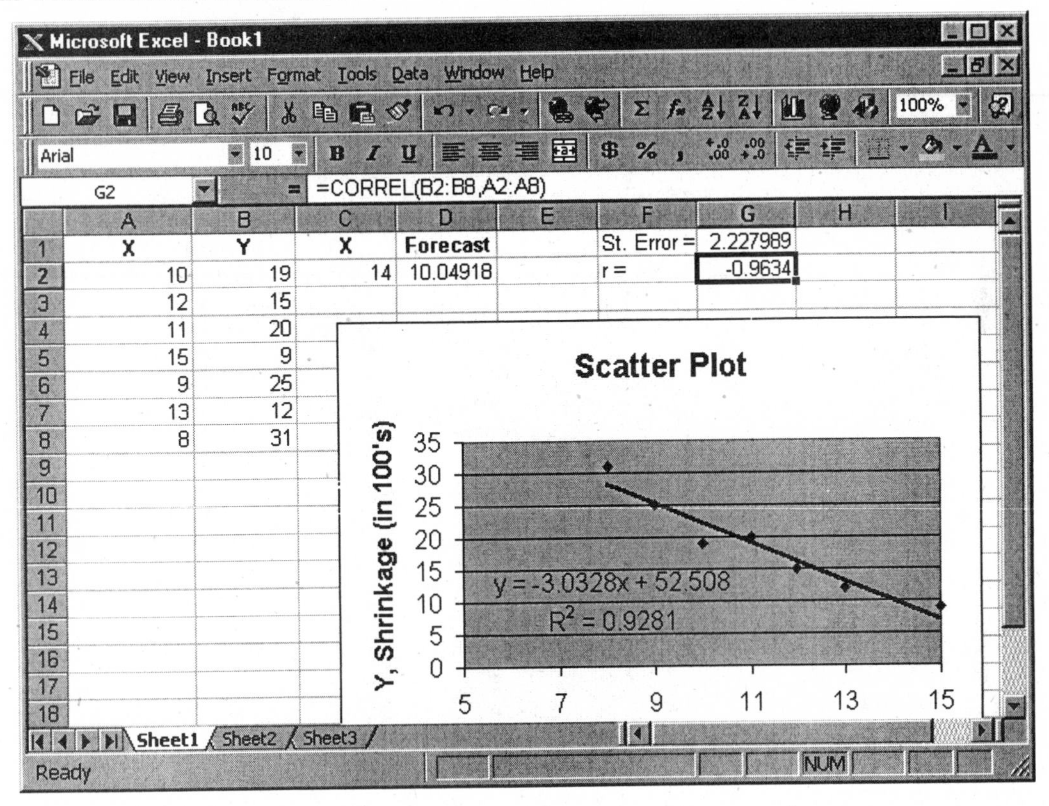

	A	B	C	D	E	F	G
1	X	Y	X	Forecast		St. Error =	2.227989
2	10	19	14	10.04918		r =	-0.9634
3	12	15					
4	11	20					
5	15	9					
6	9	25					
7	13	12					
8	8	31					

If we want to obtain the values of b and a in the least-squares line without using the Chart Wizard, we can use LINEST(y range, x range). Activate *two* cells on the worksheet. Type =LINEST(B2:B8,A2:A8) in the formula bar, and press **Ctrl+Shift+Enter** to generate the values of both b and a.

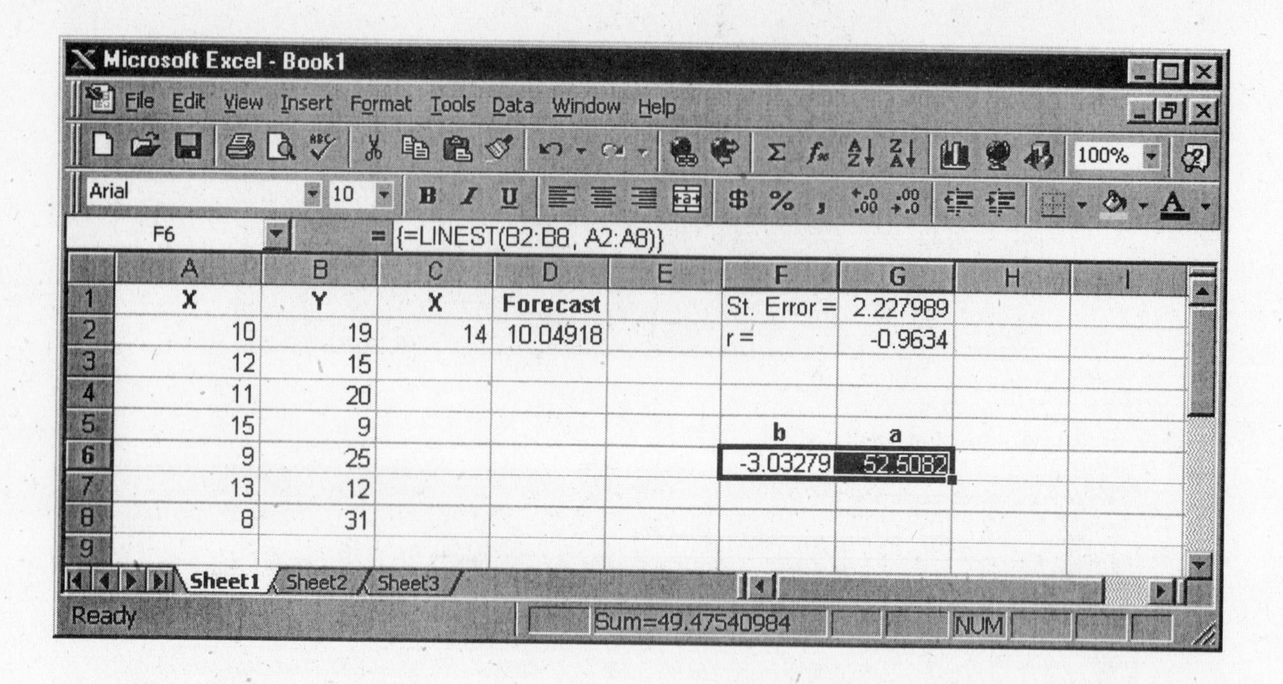

Another way to get a great deal of information at once is with **➤Tools➤Data Analysis➤Regression.**

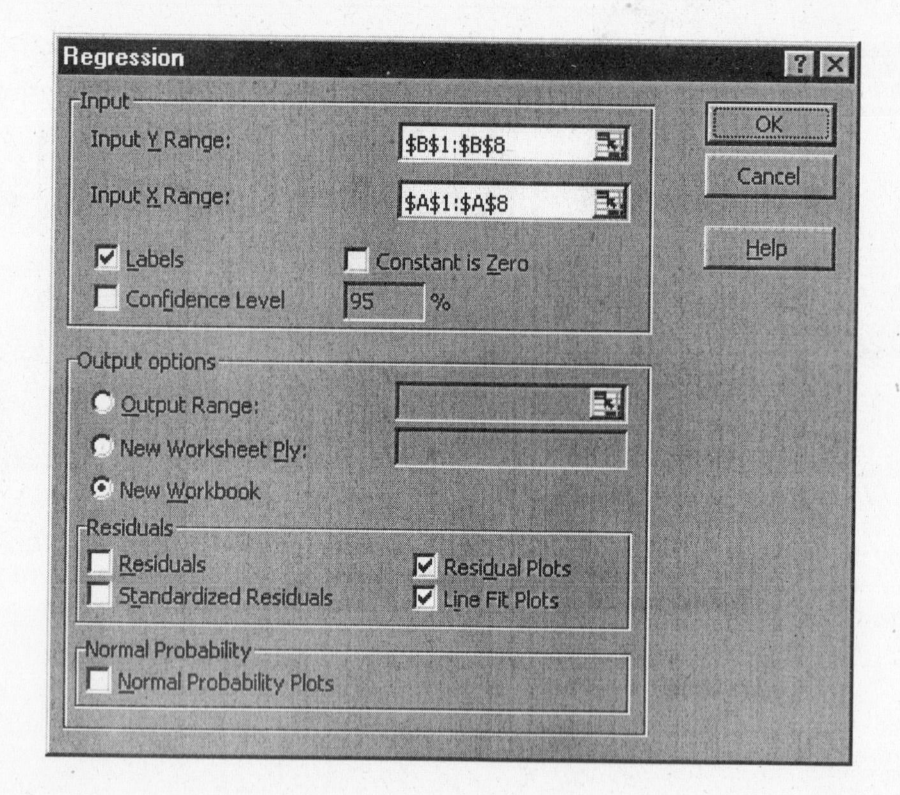

We checked Residuals Plot and Line Fit Plot. Notice that the output goes to a new worksheet. We used **➤Format➤Column➤AutoFit Selection** to adjust the column widths of the output.

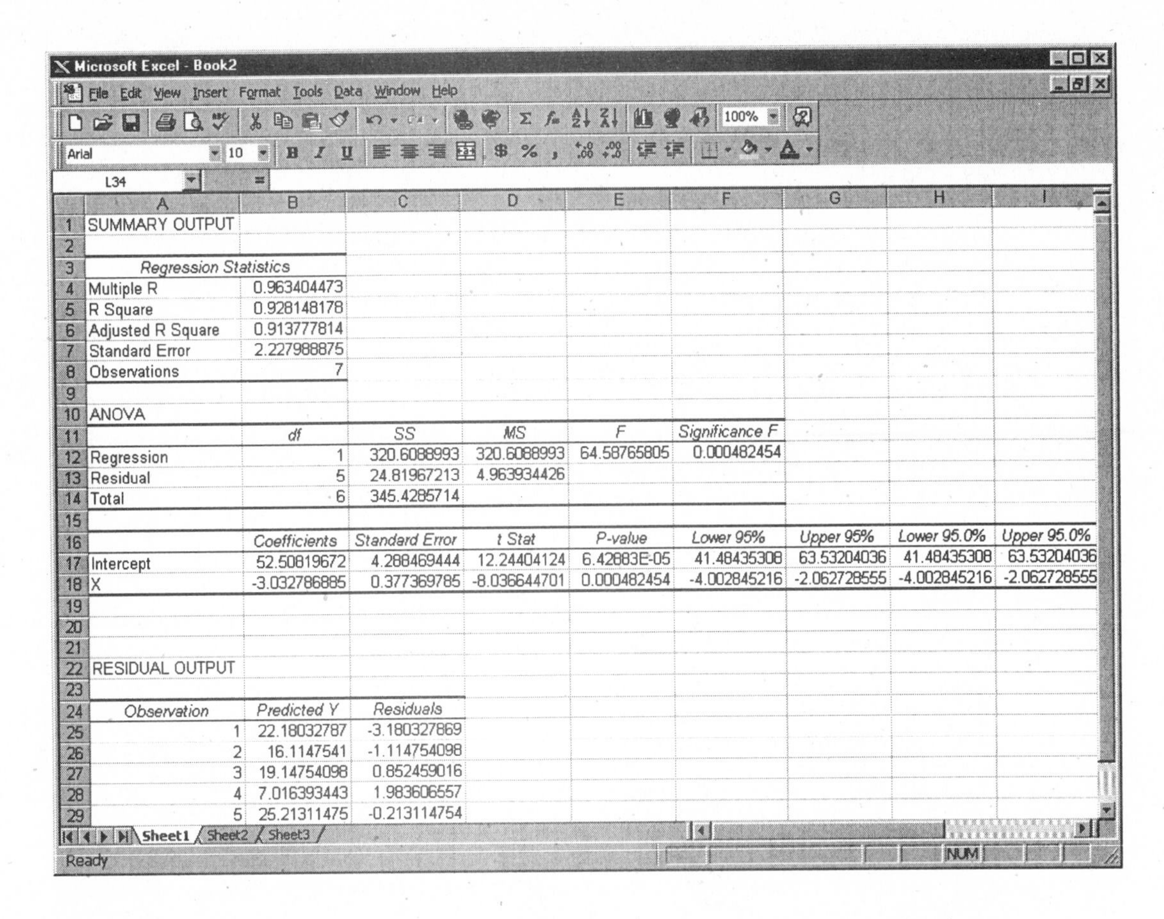

	A	B	C	D	E	F	G	H	I
1	SUMMARY OUTPUT								
2									
3	*Regression Statistics*								
4	Multiple R	0.963404473							
5	R Square	0.928148178							
6	Adjusted R Square	0.913777814							
7	Standard Error	2.227988875							
8	Observations	7							
9									
10	ANOVA								
11		*df*	*SS*	*MS*	*F*	*Significance F*			
12	Regression	1	320.6088993	320.6088993	64.58765805	0.000482454			
13	Residual	5	24.81967213	4.963934426					
14	Total	6	345.4285714						
15									
16		*Coefficients*	*Standard Error*	*t Stat*	*P-value*	*Lower 95%*	*Upper 95%*	*Lower 95.0%*	*Upper 95.0%*
17	Intercept	52.50819672	4.288469444	12.24404124	6.42883E-05	41.48435308	63.53204036	41.48435308	63.53204036
18	X	-3.032786885	0.377369785	-8.036644701	0.000482454	-4.002845216	-2.062728555	-4.002845216	-2.062728555
19									
20									
21									
22	RESIDUAL OUTPUT								
23									
24	*Observation*	*Predicted Y*	*Residuals*						
25	1	22.18032787	-3.180327869						
26	2	16.1147541	-1.114754098						
27	3	19.14754098	0.852459016						
28	4	7.016393443	1.983606557						
29	5	25.21311475	-0.213114754						

Scrolling down would show the rest of the residual output. Scrolling right shows the charts.

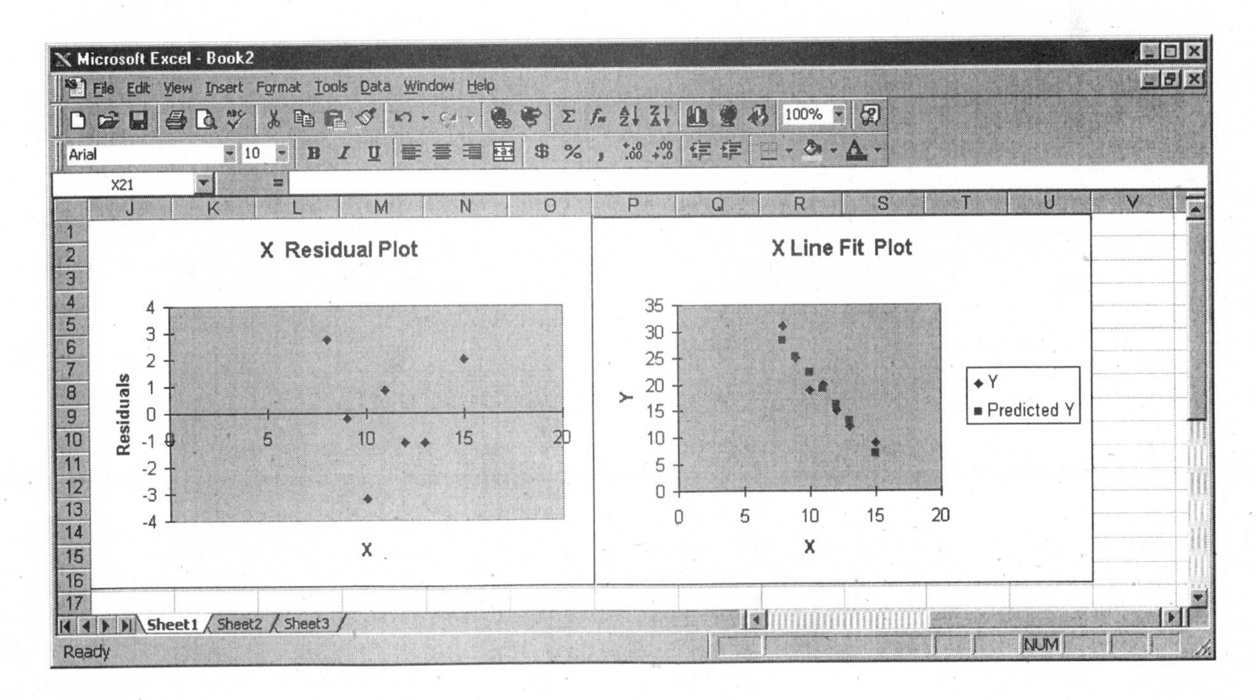

LAB ACTIVITIES FOR TWO-VARIABLE LINEAR REGRESSION

1. Open or retrieve the worksheet Slr01.xls from the data CD-ROM. This worksheet contains the following data, with the list price in Column C1 and the best price in Column C2. The best price is the best price negotiated by a team from the magazine.

LIST PRICE VERSUS BEST PRICE FOR A NEW GMC PICKUP TRUCK

In the following data pairs (*X*, *Y*),

X = List Price (in $1000) for a GMC Pickup Truck

Y = Best Price (in $1000) for a GMC Pickup Truck

Source: Consumers Digest, February 1994

(12.400), 11.200)	(14.300, 12.500)	(14.500, 12.700)
(14.900, 13.100)	(16.100, 14.100)	(16.900, 14.800)
(16.500, 14.400)	(15.400, 13.400)	(17.000, 14.900)
(17.900, 15.600)	(18.800, 16.400)	(20.300, 17.700)
(22.400, 19.600)	(19.400, 16.900)	(15.500, 14.000)
(16.700, (14.600)	(17.300, 15.100)	(18.400, 16.100)
(19.200, 16.800)	(17.400, 15.200)	(19.500, 17.000)
(19.700, 17.200)	(21.200, 18.600)	

(a) Use the Chart Wizard to create a scatter plot for the data

(b) Right-click on a data point and use the Add Trendline option to show the least-squares line on the scatter diagram, along with its equation and the value of r^2.

(c) What is the value of the standard error of estimate? (Use STEYX.)

(d) What is the value of the correlation coefficient *r*? (Use CORREL.)

(e) Use the least-squares model to predict the best price for a truck with a list price of $20,000. Note: Enter this value as 20, since *X* is assumed to be in thousands of dollars. (Use FORECAST.)

2. Other Excel worksheets appropriate to use for simple linear regression are

Cricket Chirps Versus Temperature: Slr02.xls

Source: *The Song of Insects* by Dr. G.W. Pierce, Harvard Press

The chirps per second for the striped grouped cricket are stored in C1; the corresponding temperature in degrees Fahrenheit is stored in C2.

Diameter of Sand Granules Versus Slope on a Natural Occurring Ocean Beach: Slr03.xls

Source *Physical Geography* by A.M. King, Oxford press

The median diameter (MM) of granules of sand is stored in C1; the corresponding gradient of beach slope in degrees is stored in C2.

National Unemployment Rate Male Versus Female: Slr04.xls

Source: *Statistical Abstract of the United States*

The national unemployment rate for adult males is stored in C1; the corresponding unemployment rate for adult females for the same period of time is stored in C2.

Select these worksheets and repeat Parts (a)–(d) of Problem 1, using Column A as the explanatory variable and Column B as the response variable.

3. A psychologist studying the correlation between interruptions and job stress rated a group of jobs for interruption level. She selected a random sample of twelve people holding jobs from among those rated, and analyzed the people's stress level. The results follow, with X being interruption level of the job on a scale of 1 (fewest interruptions) to 20 and Y the stress level on a scale of 1 (lowest stress) to 50.

Person	1	2	3	4	5	6	7	8	9	10	11	12
X	9	15	12	18	20	9	5	3	17	12	17	6
Y	20	37	45	42	35	40	20	10	15	39	32	25

(a) Enter the X values into Column A and the Y values into Column B.

(b) Follow parts (a) through (d) of Problem 1 using the X values as the explanatory data values and the Y values as response data values.

(c) Redo Part (b). This time change the X values to the response data values and the Y values to the explanatory data values (i.e. exchange headers for the X and Y columns) How does the scatter diagram compare? How does the least-squares equation compare? How does the correlation coefficient compare? How does the standard error of estimate compare? Does it seem to make a difference which variable is the response variable and which is the explanatory?

4. The researcher of Problem 3 was able to add to her data. Another random sample of eleven people had their jobs rated for interruption level and were then evaluated for stress level.

Person	13	14	15	16	17	18	19	20	21	22	23
X	4	15	19	13	10	9	3	11	12	15	4
Y	20	35	42	37	40	23	15	32	28	38	12

Add this data to the data in problem 3, and repeat Parts (a) and (b). Be sure the label column A as the X values and column B as the Y values. Compare the new standard error of estimate with the old one. Does more data tend to reduce the value of standard error of estimate? What about the value of r?

MULTIPLE REGRESSION

An introduction to multiple regression is presented in Section 10.5 of *Understandable Statistics*. **➤Tools➤Data Analysis➤Regression** calls up a dialog box that supports multiple regression (and simple regression as well). The data must be entered in adjacent columns, so that one data range includes the data for all the explanatory variables. Data for the response variable can be entered in any other column or row.

Example

Bowman Brothers, a large sporting goods store in Denver, has a giant ski sale every October. The chief executive officer at Bowman Brothers is studying the following variables regarding the ski sale

x_1 = Total dollar receipts from October ski sale

x_2 = Total dollar amount spend advertising ski sale on local TV

x_3 = Total dollar amount spend advertising ski sale on local radio

x_4 = Total dollar amount spend advertising ski sale in Denver newspapers

Data for the past eight years is shown below (in thousands of dollars).

Year	1	2	3	4	5	6	7	8
x_1	751	768	801	832	775	718	739	780
x_2	19	23	27	32	25	18	20	24
x_3	14	17	20	24	19	9	10	19
x_4	11	15	16	18	12	5	7	14

Enter the data

Since we will be using x_1 as the response variable, let's enter the x_1 data in Column A and the other data in Columns B through D.

Look at descriptive statistics for each column of data

Use **➤Tools➤Data Analysis➤Descriptive Statistics** to open the Descriptive Statistics dialog box. Specify the Input Range as shown and check the box labeled Summary Statistics.

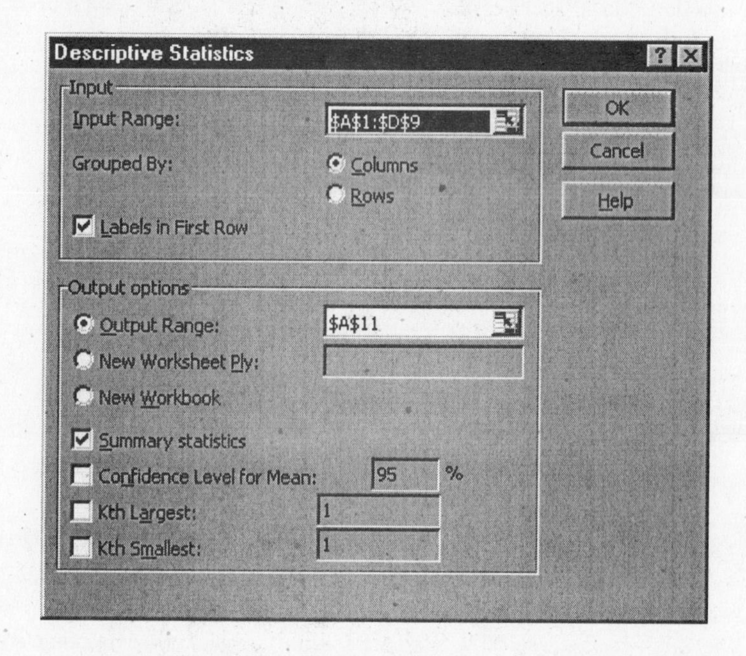

The following worksheet shows the data and the descriptive statistics. The column width was adjusted to show all the measurements on one page.

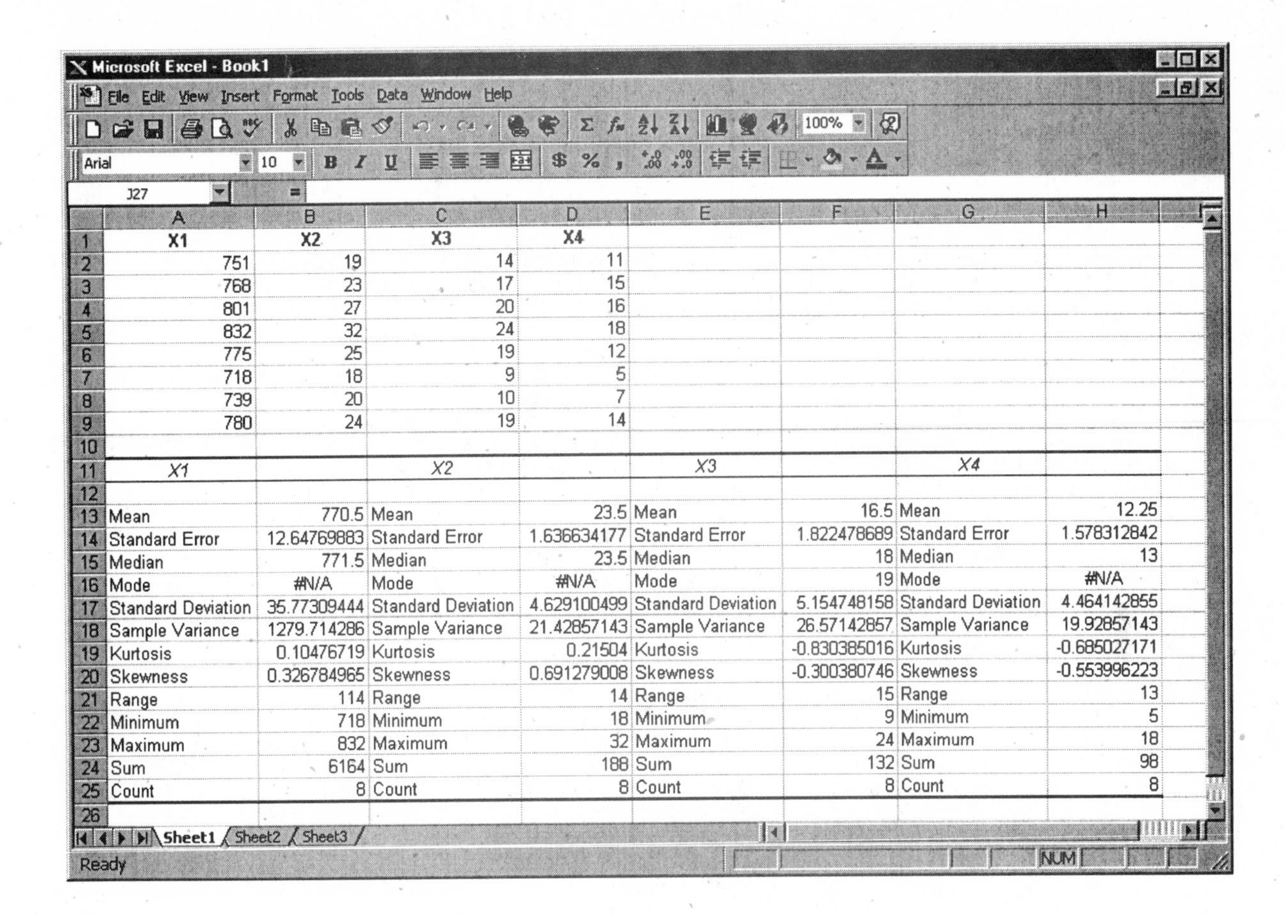

X1	X2	X3	X4
751	19	14	11
768	23	17	15
801	27	20	16
832	32	24	18
775	25	19	12
718	18	9	5
739	20	10	7
780	24	19	14

X1		X2		X3		X4	
Mean	770.5	Mean	23.5	Mean	16.5	Mean	12.25
Standard Error	12.64769883	Standard Error	1.636634177	Standard Error	1.822478689	Standard Error	1.578312842
Median	771.5	Median	23.5	Median	18	Median	13
Mode	#N/A	Mode	#N/A	Mode	19	Mode	#N/A
Standard Deviation	35.77309444	Standard Deviation	4.629100499	Standard Deviation	5.154748158	Standard Deviation	4.464142855
Sample Variance	1279.714286	Sample Variance	21.42857143	Sample Variance	26.57142857	Sample Variance	19.92857143
Kurtosis	0.10476719	Kurtosis	0.21504	Kurtosis	-0.830385016	Kurtosis	-0.685027171
Skewness	0.326784965	Skewness	0.691279008	Skewness	-0.300380746	Skewness	-0.553996223
Range	114	Range	14	Range	15	Range	13
Minimum	718	Minimum	18	Minimum	9	Minimum	5
Maximum	832	Maximum	32	Maximum	24	Maximum	18
Sum	6164	Sum	188	Sum	132	Sum	98
Count	8	Count	8	Count	8	Count	8

Examine the correlation between each pair of columns of data

To make a table of correlation coefficients between columns of data, use **➤Tools➤Data Analysis➤ Correlation.**

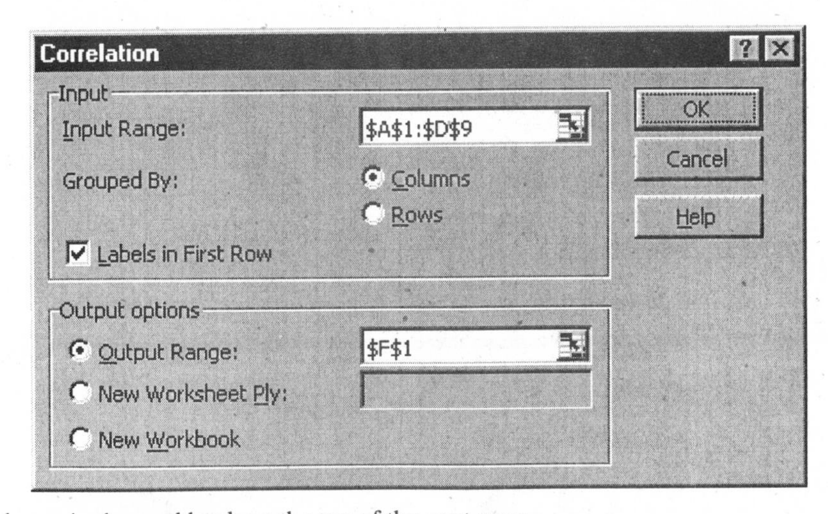

The results are shown in the workbook on the top of the next page.

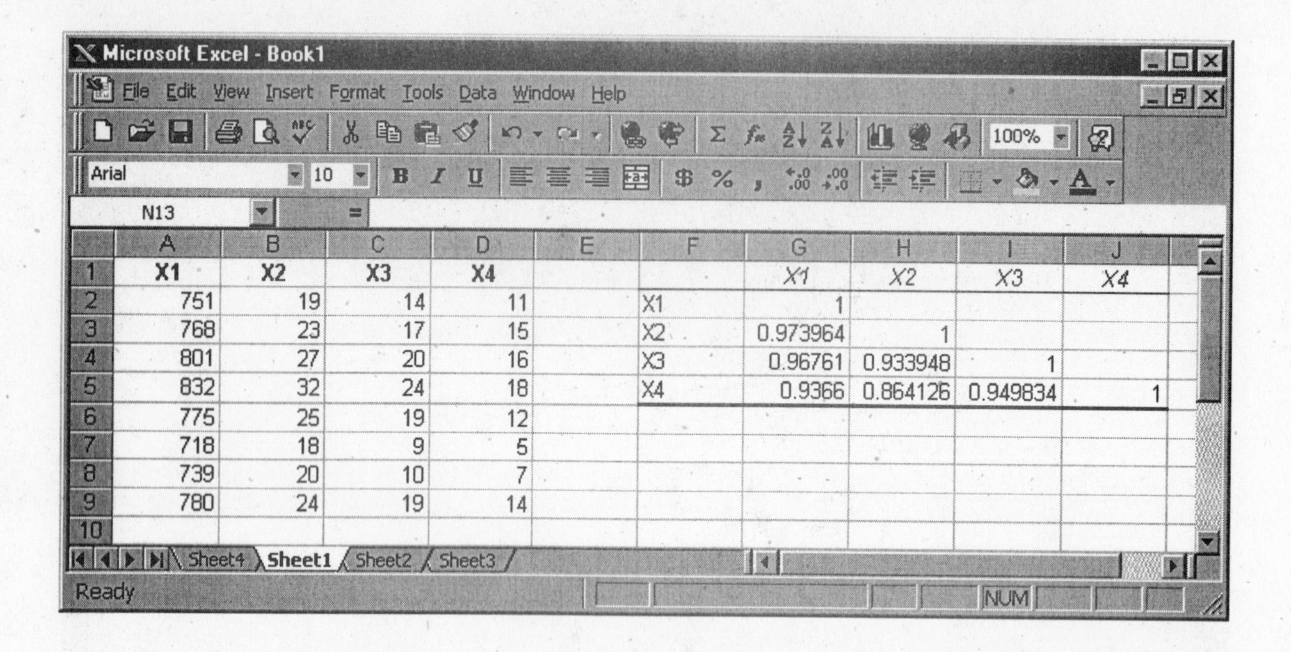

	A	B	C	D	E	F	G	H	I	J
1	X1	X2	X3	X4			X1	X2	X3	X4
2	751	19	14	11		X1	1			
3	768	23	17	15		X2	0.973964	1		
4	801	27	20	16		X3	0.96761	0.933948	1	
5	832	32	24	18		X4	0.9366	0.864126	0.949834	1
6	775	25	19	12						
7	718	18	9	5						
8	739	20	10	7						
9	780	24	19	14						
10										

Find the linear regression formula with x_1 as the response variable and x_2, x_3, x_4 as the explanatory variables.

We use **➤Tools➤Data Analysis➤Regression** to find the coefficients of the linear regression formula as well as some other useful statistics relative to the model.

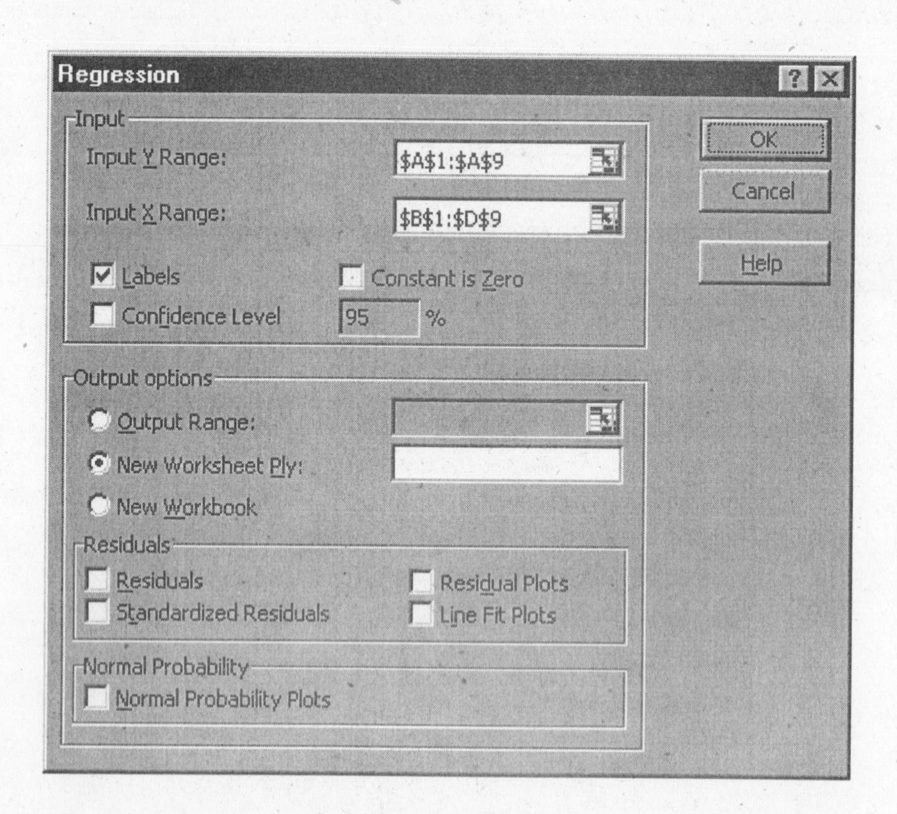

We use ➤**Format**➤**Column**➤**Auto Fit Selection** to adjust the column width.

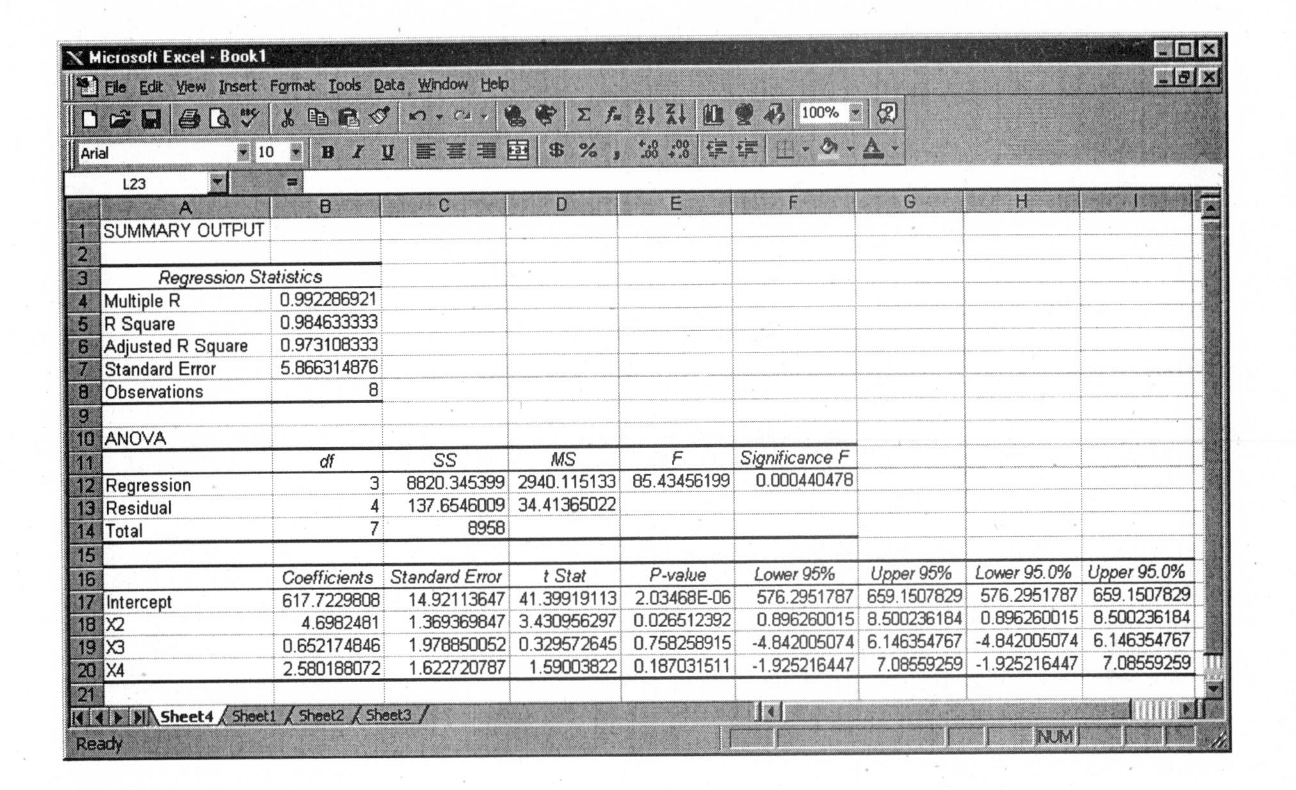

SUMMARY OUTPUT

Regression Statistics	
Multiple R	0.992286921
R Square	0.984633333
Adjusted R Square	0.973108333
Standard Error	5.866314876
Observations	8

ANOVA

	df	SS	MS	F	Significance F
Regression	3	8820.345399	2940.115133	85.43456199	0.000440478
Residual	4	137.6546009	34.41365022		
Total	7	8958			

	Coefficients	Standard Error	t Stat	P-value	Lower 95%	Upper 95%	Lower 95.0%	Upper 95.0%
Intercept	617.7229808	14.92113647	41.39919113	2.03468E-06	576.2951787	659.1507829	576.2951787	659.1507829
X2	4.6982481	1.369369847	3.430956297	0.026512392	0.896260015	8.500236184	0.896260015	8.500236184
X3	0.652174846	1.978850052	0.329572645	0.758258915	-4.842005074	6.146354767	-4.842005074	6.146354767
X4	2.580188072	1.622720787	1.59003822	0.187031511	-1.925216447	7.08559259	-1.925216447	7.08559259

The coefficients of the regression equation are given in the last box. The equation is

$$x_1 = 617.72 + 4.70x_2 + 0.65x_3 + 2.58x_4.$$

Notice that the value of coefficient of multiple determination R square is 0.9846, and the standard error of estimate is 5.866. The *P* value for each coefficient is given. Remember, we are testing the null hypothesis H_0: $\beta = 0$ against the alternate hypothesis H_1: $\beta \neq 0$. Finally, a 95% confidence interval is given for each coefficient.

Note that we do not use the results of the Analysis of Variance.

Forecast a value

Supply some labels on the worksheet, and then for the forecast value, type in the linear regression equation using the specified values for x_2, x_3, x_4. For instance, to forecast the total receipts for October (x_1) given that $21,000 dollars is spent on local TV ads, $11,000 is spent on local radio ads, and $8000 is spent on newspaper ads, we use the corresponding values in the regression equation.

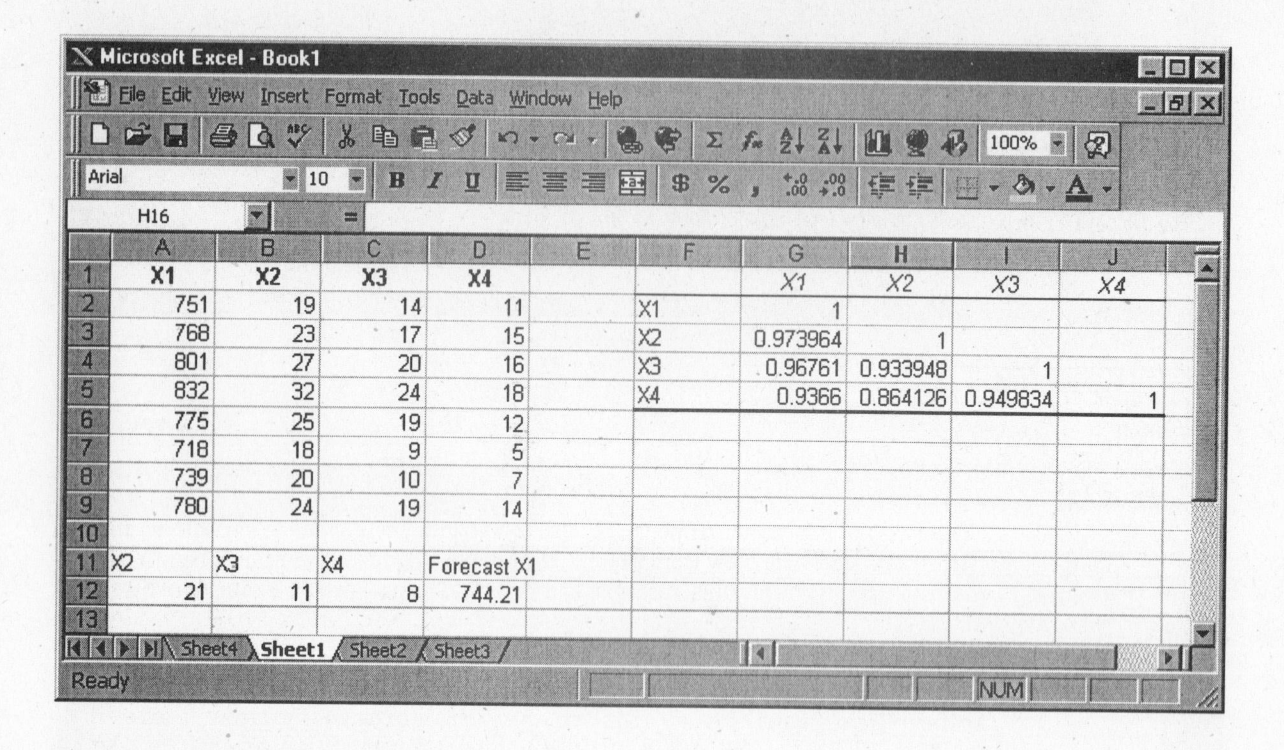

	A	B	C	D	E	F	G	H	I	J
1	X1	X2	X3	X4			X1	X2	X3	X4
2	751	19	14	11		X1	1			
3	768	23	17	15		X2	0.973964	1		
4	801	27	20	16		X3	0.96761	0.933948	1	
5	832	32	24	18		X4	0.9366	0.864126	0.949834	1
6	775	25	19	12						
7	718	18	9	5						
8	739	20	10	7						
9	780	24	19	14						
10										
11	X2	X3	X4	Forecast X1						
12	21	11	8	744.21						
13										

Change the response variable

To change the response variable to x_2, and use x_1, x_3, x_4 as explanatory variables, we first need to move the x_2 column to the far left and put the x_1 column next to the other explanatory variables. Use **➤Edit➤Cut** and **➤Edit➤Paste** to move the data columns.

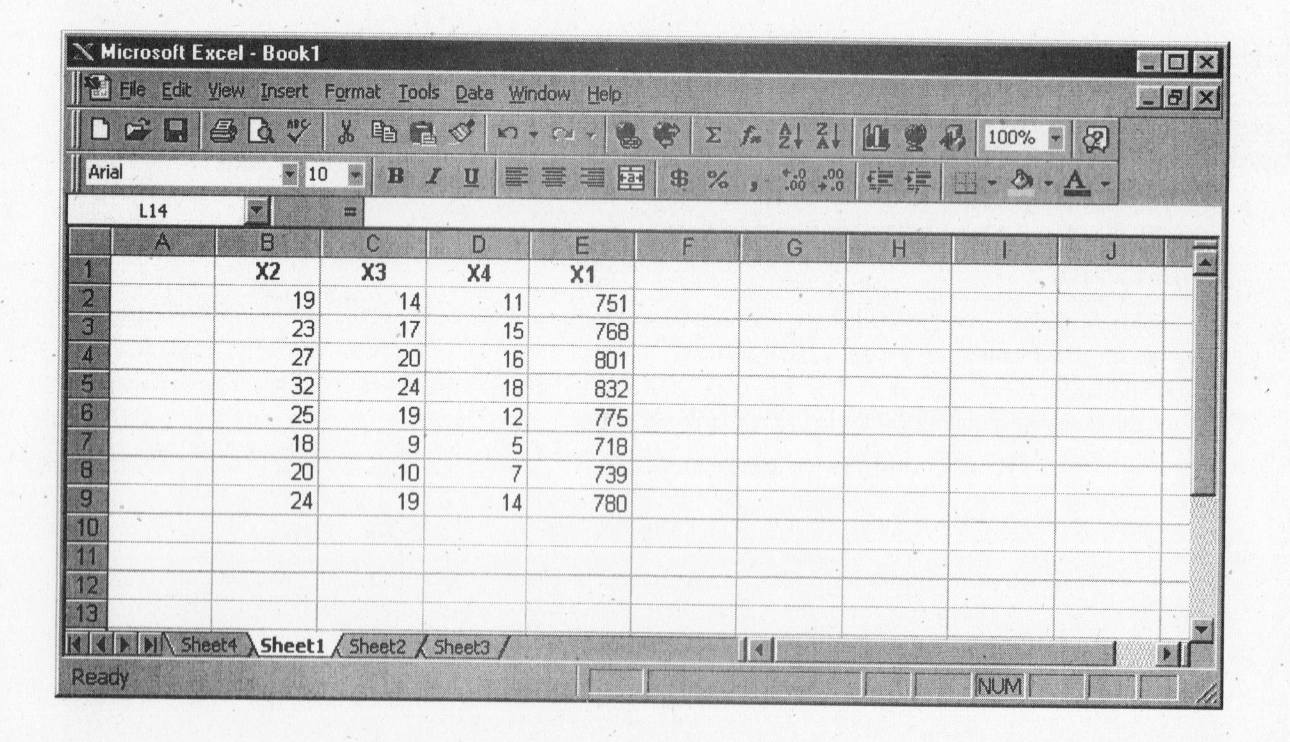

	A	B	C	D	E	F	G	H	I	J
1		X2	X3	X4	X1					
2		19	14	11	751					
3		23	17	15	768					
4		27	20	16	801					
5		32	24	18	832					
6		25	19	12	775					
7		18	9	5	718					
8		20	10	7	739					
9		24	19	14	780					

LAB ACTIVITIES FOR MULTIPLE REGRESSION

For 1–6, use the data provided on Excel worksheets stored on the data CD-ROM to explore the relationships among the variables. Activities 1–4 come from Section 10.5 Problems 3–6 respectfully. Activities 5 and 6 are two additional case studies on the data CD-ROM.

1. Systolic Blood Pressure Data
   Excel CD-ROM worksheet Mlr02.xls
2. Test Scores for General Psychology
   Excel CD-ROM worksheet Mlr03.xls
3. Hollywood Movies
   Excel CD-ROM worksheet Mlr04.xls
4. All Greens Franchise
   Excel CD-ROM worksheet Mlr05.xls
5. Crime
   This data is a case study of education, crime, and police funding for small cities in ten Eastern and Southeastern states. The states are New Hampshire, Connecticut, Rhode Island, Maine, New York, Virginia, North Carolina, South Carolina, Georgia, and Florida. The data are for a sample of 50 small cities in these states.

   x_1 = Total overall reported crime rate per 1 million residents

   x_2 = Reported violent crime rate per 100,000 residents

   x_3 = Annual police funding in dollars per resident

   x_4 = Percent of people 25 years and older that have had four years of high school

   x_5 = Percent of 16- to 19-year-olds not in high school and not high school graduates

   x_6 = Percent of 18- to 24-year-olds enrolled in college

   x_7 = Percent of people 25 years and older with at least four years of college

   Excel data CD-ROM worksheet Mlr06.xls
6. Health
   This data is a case study of public health, income, and population density for small cities in eight Midwestern states: Ohio, Indiana, Illinois, Iowa, Missouri, Nebraska, Kansas, and Oklahoma. The data are for a sample of 53 small cities in these states.

   x_1 = Death rate per 1000 residents

   x_2 = Doctor availability per 100,000 residents

   x_3 = Hospital availability per 1000,000 residents

   x_4 = Annual per capita income in thousands of dollars

   x_5 = Population density people per square mile

   Excel data CD-ROM worksheet Mlr07.xls

CHAPTER 11 CHI-SQUARE AND *F* DISTRIBUTIONS

CHI-SQUARE TEST OF INDEPENDENCE (SECTION 11.1 OF *UNDERSTANDABLE STATISTICS*)

Use of the chi-square distribution to test independence is discussed in Section 11.1 of *Understandable Statistics.* In such tests we use hypotheses

H_0: The variables are independent

H_1: The variables are not independent

In Excel, the applicable command (accessed using the Paste Function button) is

CHITEST(set of observed values,set of expected values)

which returns the *P* value of the sample X^2 value, where the sample X^2 value is computed as

$$X^2 = \sum \frac{(O-E)^2}{E}$$

Here, *E* stands for the expected count in a cell, and *O* stands for the observed count in that same cell. The sum is taken over all cells.

In our Excel worksheet, we first enter in the contingency table of observed values. If the table does not contain column sums or row sums, use the Sum button on the tool bar to generate the sums. We need to create the table of expected values, where the expected value *E* for a cell is

$$E = (\text{column total})\left(\frac{\text{row total}}{\text{grand total}}\right)$$

By careful use of absolute and relative cell addresses, we can type the formula once and then copy it to different positions in the contingency table of expected values. Recall that an absolute cell address has $ symbols preceding the column and row designators.

Example

A computer programming aptitude test has been developed for high school seniors. The test designers claim that scores on the test are independent of the type of school the student attends: rural, suburban, urban. A study involving a random sample of students from these types of institutions yielded the following contingency table. Use the CHITEST command to compute the *P* value of the sample chi-square value. Then determine if type of school and test score are independent at the $\alpha = 0.05$ level of significance.

	School Type		
Score	Rural	Suburban	Urban
200-299	33	65	83
300-399	45	79	95
400-500	21	47	63

First we enter the table into a worksheet and use the sum button Σ on the standard toolbar to generate the column, row, and grand total sums.

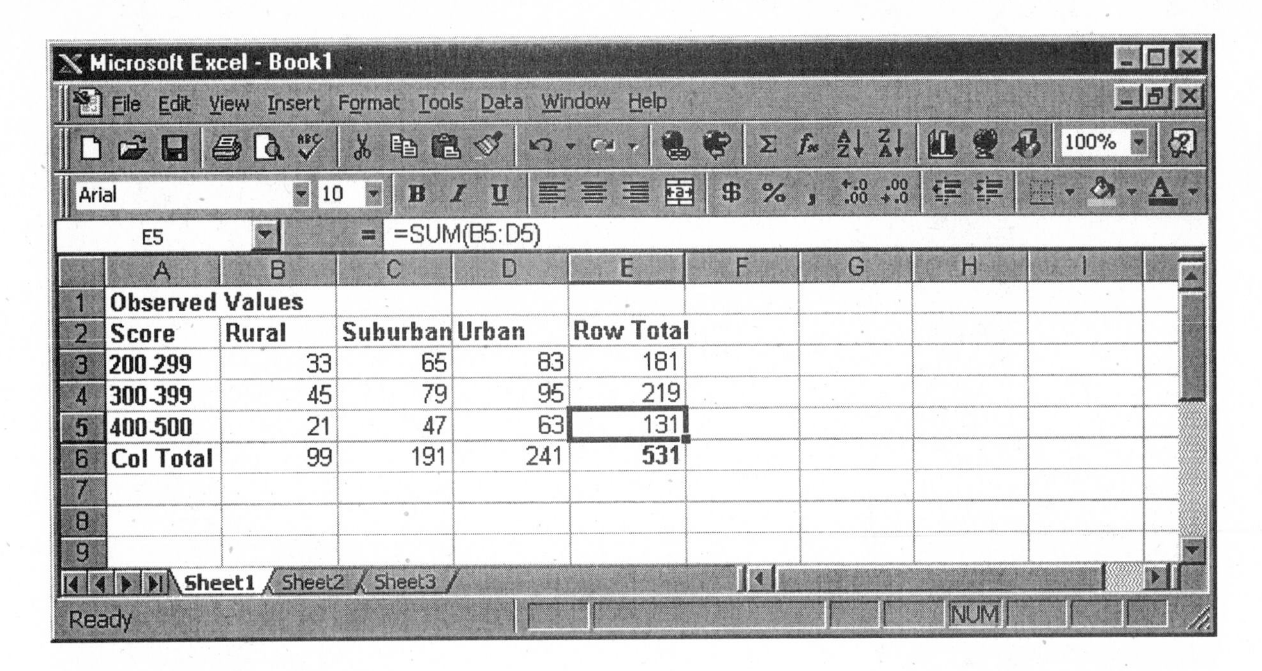

Microsoft Excel - Book1

E5 =SUM(B5:D5)

	A	B	C	D	E
1	Observed Values				
2	Score	Rural	Suburban	Urban	Row Total
3	200-299	33	65	83	181
4	300-399	45	79	95	219
5	400-500	21	47	63	131
6	Col Total	99	191	241	531

Next we create the contingency table of expected values, where the expected value for Cell B3 will go in Cell H3. Notice that in the formula

$$E = (\text{row total})\left(\frac{\text{row total}}{\text{grand total}}\right)$$

the grand total stays the same for each expected value. The grand total is in Cell E6. Since we want this to be an absolute address used in each computation, we use the cell label $E$6. (Alternatively, we could just type in the grand total of 531 in the formula bar.) The column totals are all in Row 6, so when we refer to a column total, we will fix the row address by using $6 and let the column names vary. The row totals are all in Column E, so we will fix the column address as $E and let the row address vary when we use row totals. So the formula as entered in Cell H3 should be

= B$6*($E3/$E$6)

Now move the cursor to the lower right corner of Cell H3. When the small + appears, drag it to the lower right corner of cell J5. The calculations for all the cells will automatically be done.

We now have both the observed values and the expected values.

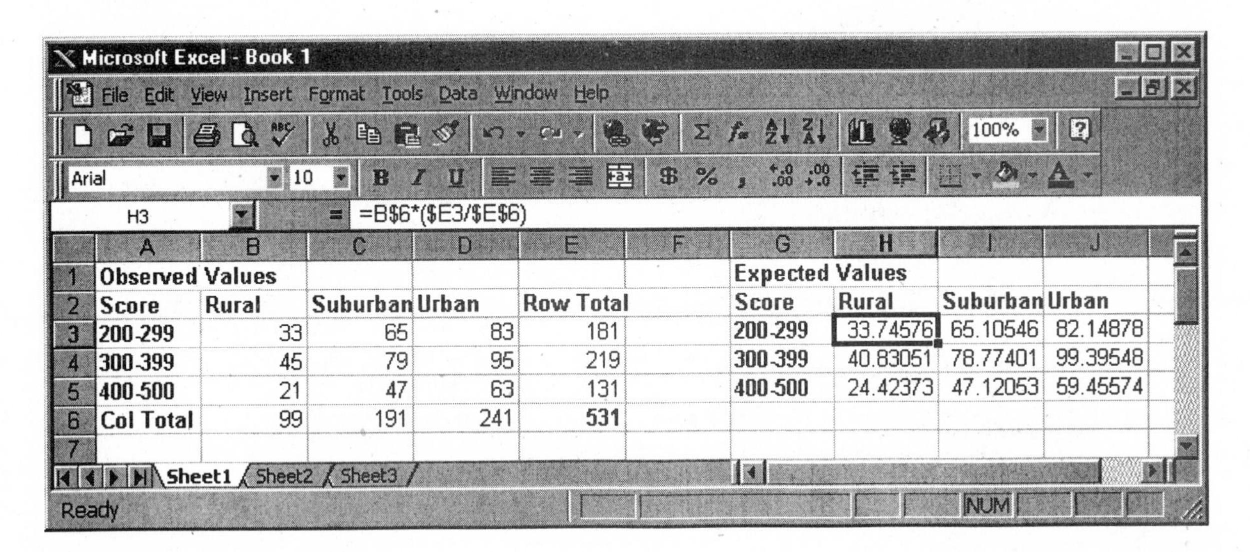

Microsoft Excel - Book 1

H3 =B$6*($E3/$E$6)

	A	B	C	D	E	F	G	H	I	J
1	Observed Values						Expected Values			
2	Score	Rural	Suburban	Urban	Row Total		Score	Rural	Suburban	Urban
3	200-299	33	65	83	181		200-299	33.74576	65.10546	82.14878
4	300-399	45	79	95	219		300-399	40.83051	78.77401	99.39548
5	400-500	21	47	63	131		400-500	24.42373	47.12053	59.45574
6	Col Total	99	191	241	531					

Now use the CHITEST command. After clicking the Paste Function button on the tool bar, select the CHITEST function and, in the dialog box that appears, enter the required ranges of values as shown.

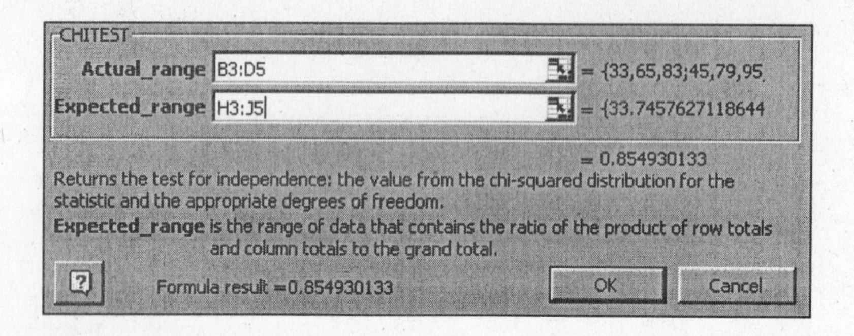

The resulting *P* value is 0.8549. Place appropriate labels on the worksheet

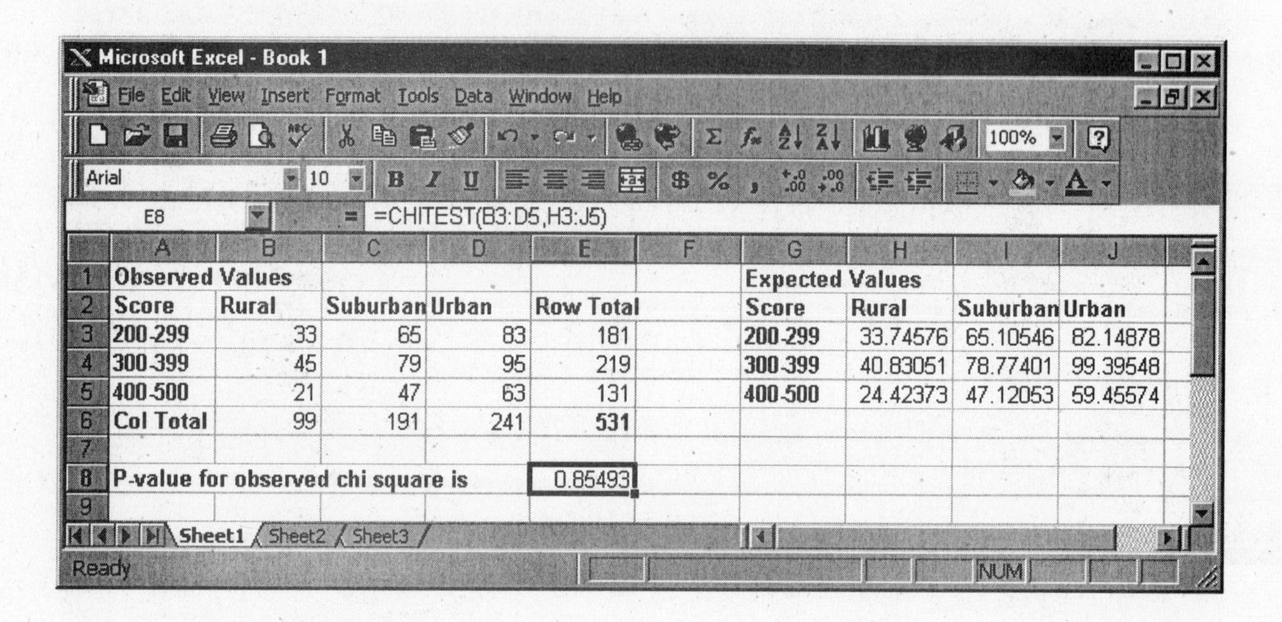

	A	B	C	D	E	F	G	H	I	J
1	Observed Values						Expected Values			
2	Score	Rural	Suburban	Urban	Row Total		Score	Rural	Suburban	Urban
3	200-299	33	65	83	181		200-299	33.74576	65.10546	82.14878
4	300-399	45	79	95	219		300-399	40.83051	78.77401	99.39548
5	400-500	21	47	63	131		400-500	24.42373	47.12053	59.45574
6	Col Total	99	191	241	531					
7										
8	P-value for observed chi square is				0.85493					
9										

Since the *P* value is greater than $\alpha = 0.05$, we do not reject the null hypothesis. There is insufficient evidence to conclude that school type and test scores are not independent. Intuitively, we can confirm this by observing that the values we would expect, assuming independence (the values in the right table) are not very different from the values observed (the values in the left table).

LAB ACTIVITIES FOR CHI-SQUARE TEST OF INDEPENDENCE

In each activity, enter the contingency tables into a worksheet, then use the Sum button to generate the required row and column sums. Create a table of expected values. Finally, use CHITEST to find the *P* value of the sample statistic and draw the appropriate conclusion.

1. We Care Auto Insurance had its staff of actuaries conduct a study to see if vehicle type and loss claim are independent. A random sample of auto claims over the first six months gives the information in this contingency table.

	Total Loss Claims per Year per Vehicle			
Type of Vehicle	$0–999	$1000–2999	$3000–5999	$6000+
Sports Car	20	10	16	8
Truck	16	25	33	9
Family Sedan	40	68	17	7
Compact	52	73	48	12

Test the claim that car type and loss claim are independent. Use $\alpha = 0.05$.

2. An educational specialist is interested in comparing three methods of instruction:

SL – standard lecture with discussion

TV – video taped lectures with no discussion

IM – individualized method with reading assignments and tutoring, but no lectures.

The specialist conducted a study of these three methods to see if they were independent. A course was taught using each of the three methods, and a standard final exam given at the end. Students were put into the different method sections at random. The course type and test results are shown in the contingency table below.

	Final Exam Score				
Course Type	<60	60–69	70–79	80–89	90–100
SL	10	4	70	31	25
TV	8	3	62	27	23
IM	7	2	58	25	22

Test the claim that the instruction method and final exam test scores are independent, using $\alpha = 0.01$.

Note: If you have raw data entered in columns, you can use the Pivot Wizard to construct a contingency table. See the Excel help menu or other manuals for details.

TESTING TWO VARIANCES (SECTION 11.4 OF *UNDERSTANDABLE STATISTICS*)

In Excel there are two commands that give the *P* value for testing two variances.

FTEST(data range of first variable,data range of second variable) which returns the *P* value for a test with the alternate hypothesis $H_1: \sigma_1^2 \neq \sigma_2^2$. To find this command, use the Paste Function button.

F-Test: Two Sample for Variances which returns the *P* value for a one-tailed test as well as some summary statistics. The dialog box for this command is found using **➤Tools➤Data Analysis➤F-Test.**

Example

Two processes for manufacturing paint are under study. The useful life (in years) of the paint for a random sample produced by method A is

5.2 5.9 6.2 4.8 5.3 5.2

With method B, the useful life of a random sample of test patches is

5.1 4.9 4.6 5.8 6.7 5.2

Use a 5% level of significance to test if the variances are equal. First enter the data and use the **FTEST** command from Paste Function. The results are

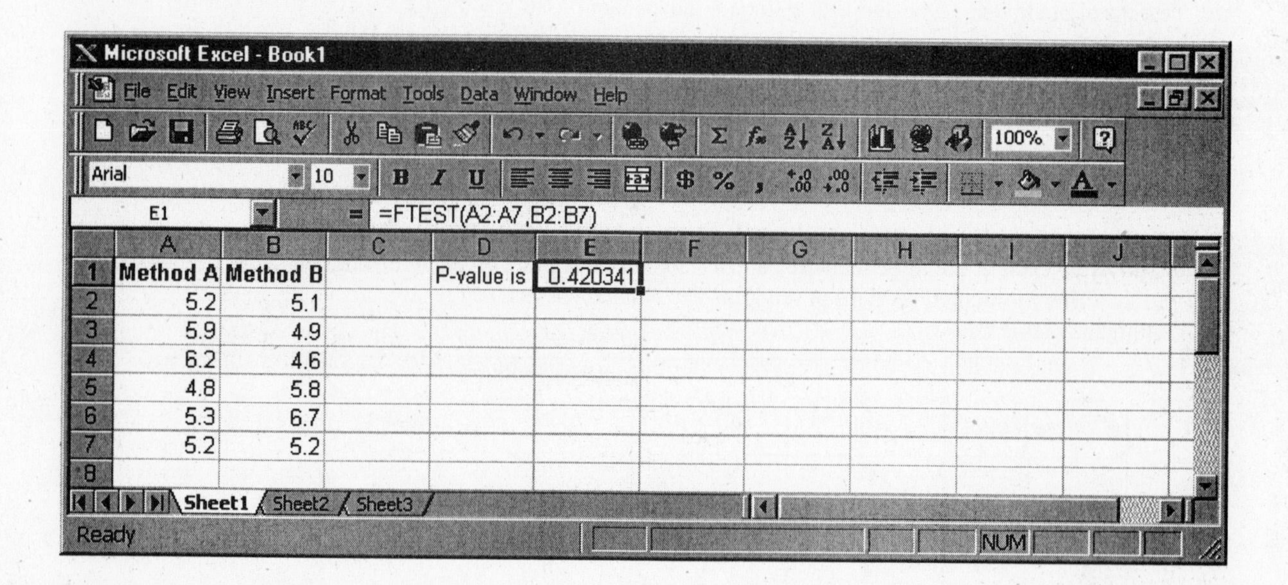

Since the *P* value is greater than 0.05, we do not reject H_0, and we conclude that there is not enough evidence to judge the variances unequal.

Next use the F-Test dialog box found under **➤Tools➤Data Analysis➤F-Test.**

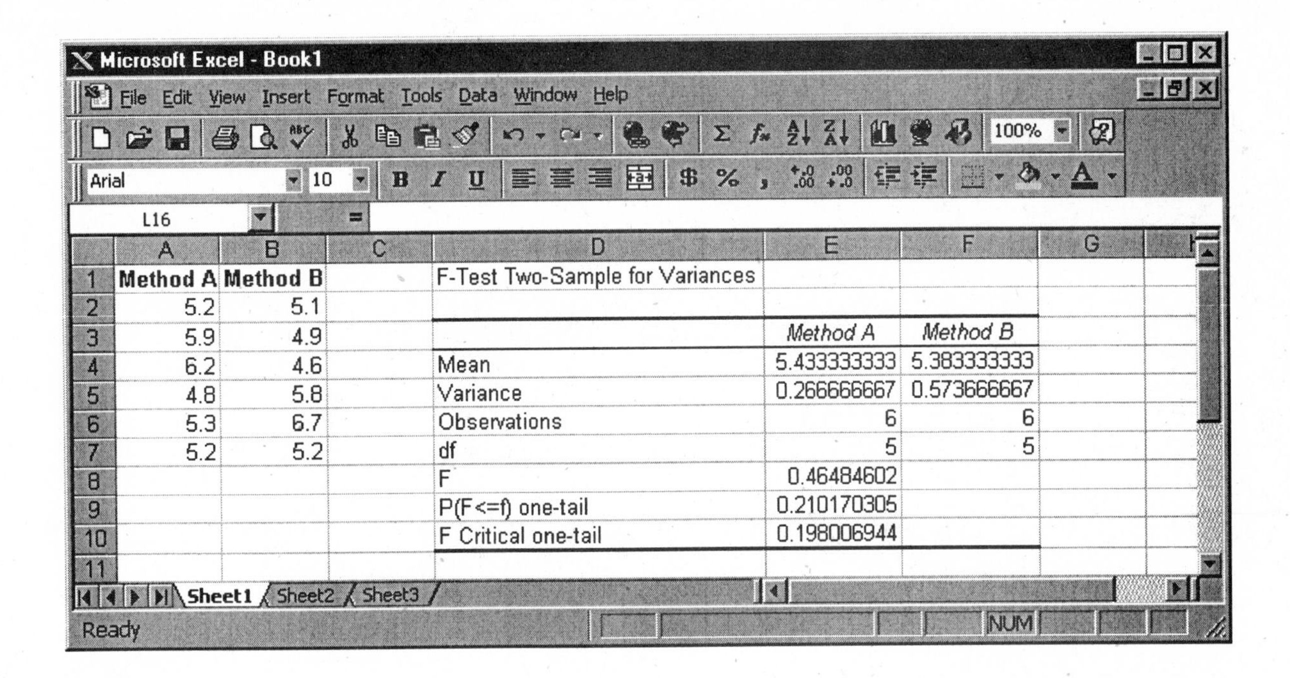

Method A	Method B		F-Test Two-Sample for Variances		
5.2	5.1				
5.9	4.9			*Method A*	*Method B*
6.2	4.6		Mean	5.433333333	5.383333333
4.8	5.8		Variance	0.266666667	0.573666667
5.3	6.7		Observations	6	6
5.2	5.2		df	5	5
			F	0.46484602	
			P(F<=f) one-tail	0.210170305	
			F Critical one-tail	0.198006944	

Notice that this output gives the *P* value for a one-tailed test. Double the value to get the results for a two-tailed test. Again, the *P* value is too large to reject the null hypothesis.

LAB ACTIVITIES FOR TESTING TWO VARIANCES

Select several exercises from 11.4 of the text *Understandable Statistics.*

ANALYSIS OF VARIANCE – ONE-WAY (SECTION 11.5 OF *UNDERSTANDABLE STATISTICS*)

Section 11.5 of *Understandable Statistics* introduces single-factor analysis of variance (also called one-way ANOVA). We consider several populations that are assumed to follow a normal distribution. The standard deviations of the populations are assumed to be approximately equal. ANOVA provides a method to compare several different populations to see if the means are the same. Let population 1 have mean μ_1, population 2 have mean μ_2, and so on. The hypotheses of ANOVA are

$$H_0: \mu_1 = \mu_2 = \ldots = \mu_n$$
H_1: not all the means are equal

In Excel we use **➤Tools➤Data Analysis➤Anova: Single Factor.** The output provides summary statistics of the groups, and a summary table giving the degrees of freedom, sum of squares, mean squares, the value of *F*, and the *P* value of *F*.

Example

A psychologist has developed a series of tests to measure a person's level of depression. The composite scores range from 50 to 100, with 100 representing the most severe depression level. A random sample of twelve patients with approximately the same depression level (as measured by the tests) was divided into three different treatment groups. Then, one month after treatment was competed, the depression of level of each patient was again evaluated. The after-treatment depression levels are as given.

Treatment 1	70	65	82	83	71
Treatment 2	75	62	81		
Treatment 3	77	60	80	75	

Enter the data in Columns A, B, and C. Then access the ANOVA Single Factor dialog box by using the menu selections **➤Tools➤Data Analysis➤Anova: Single Factor.**

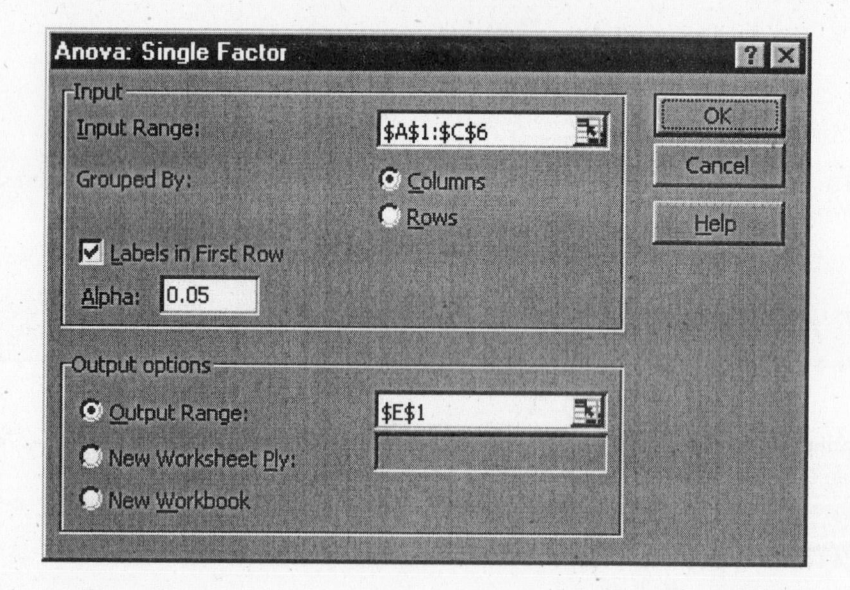

The output is

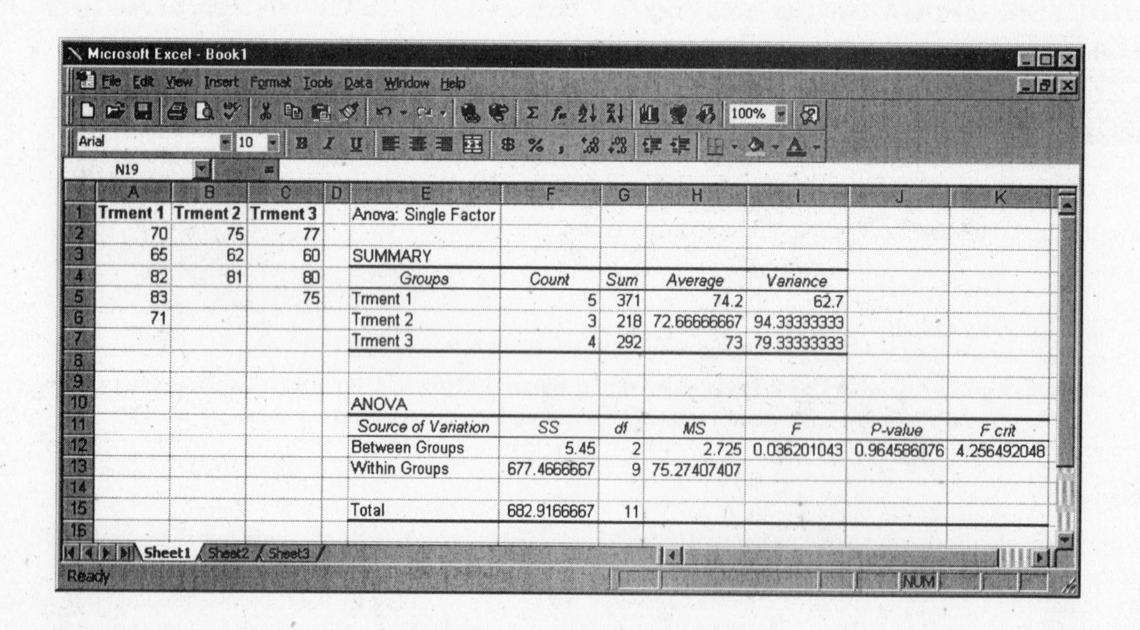

Trment 1	Trment 2	Trment 3
70	75	77
65	62	60
82	81	80
83		75
71		

Anova: Single Factor

SUMMARY

Groups	Count	Sum	Average	Variance
Trment 1	5	371	74.2	62.7
Trment 2	3	218	72.66666667	94.33333333
Trment 3	4	292	73	79.33333333

ANOVA

Source of Variation	SS	df	MS	F	P-value	F crit
Between Groups	5.45	2	2.725	0.036201043	0.964586076	4.256492048
Within Groups	677.4666667	9	75.27407407			
Total	682.9166667	11				

LAB ACTIVITIES FOR ANALYSIS OF VARIANCE – ONE-WAY

1. A random sample of twenty overweight adults was randomly divided into four equal groups. Each group was given a different diet plan, and the weight loss for each individual (in pounds) was measured after three months:

Plan 1	18	10	20	25	17
Plan 2	28	12	22	17	16
Plan 3	16	20	24	8	17
Plan 4	14	17	18	5	16

Test the claim that the population mean weight loss is the same for the four diet plans, at the 5% level of significance.

2. A psychologist is studying the time it takes rats to respond to stimuli after being given doses of different tranquilizing drugs. A random sample of eighteen rats were divided into three groups. Each group was given a different drug. The time of response to stimuli was measured (in seconds).

Drug A	3.1	2.5	2.2	1.5	0.7	2.4
Drug B	4.2	2.5	1.7	3.5	1.2	3.1
Drug C	3.3	2.6	1.7	3.9	2.8	3.5

Test the claim that the population mean response times for the three drugs is the same at the 5% level of significance.

3. A research group is testing various chemical combinations designed to neutralize and buffer the effects of acid rain on lakes. A random sample of eighteen lakes of similar size in the same region have all been affected in the same way by acid rain. The lakes are divided into four groups, and each group of lakes is sprayed with a different combination of chemicals. An acidity index is then taken after treatment. The index ranges from 60 to 100, with 100 indicating the greatest acid rain pollution. The results follow.

Combination I	63	55	72	81	75
Combination II	78	56	75	73	82
Combination III	59	72	77	60	
Combination IV	72	81	66	71	

Test the claim that the population mean acidity index after each of the four treatments is the same, at the 0.01 level of significance.

ANALYSIS OF VARIANCE – TWO-WAY (SECTION 11.6 OF *UNDERSTANDABLE STATISTICS*)

Excel has two commands for two-way ANOVA under the **➤Tools➤Data Analysis** menu choices.

Anova: Two-Factor With Replication is used when two or more sample measurements are available for each factor combination. Each factor combination must contain the same number of data values.

Anova: Two-Factor Without Replication is used when there is exactly one sample measurement for each factor combination.

Example (with replication)

This data set is from Example 7 of Section 11.6 of the text. The example gives customer satisfaction data with regard to time of day and type of customer contact. The data are listed on the spreadsheet.

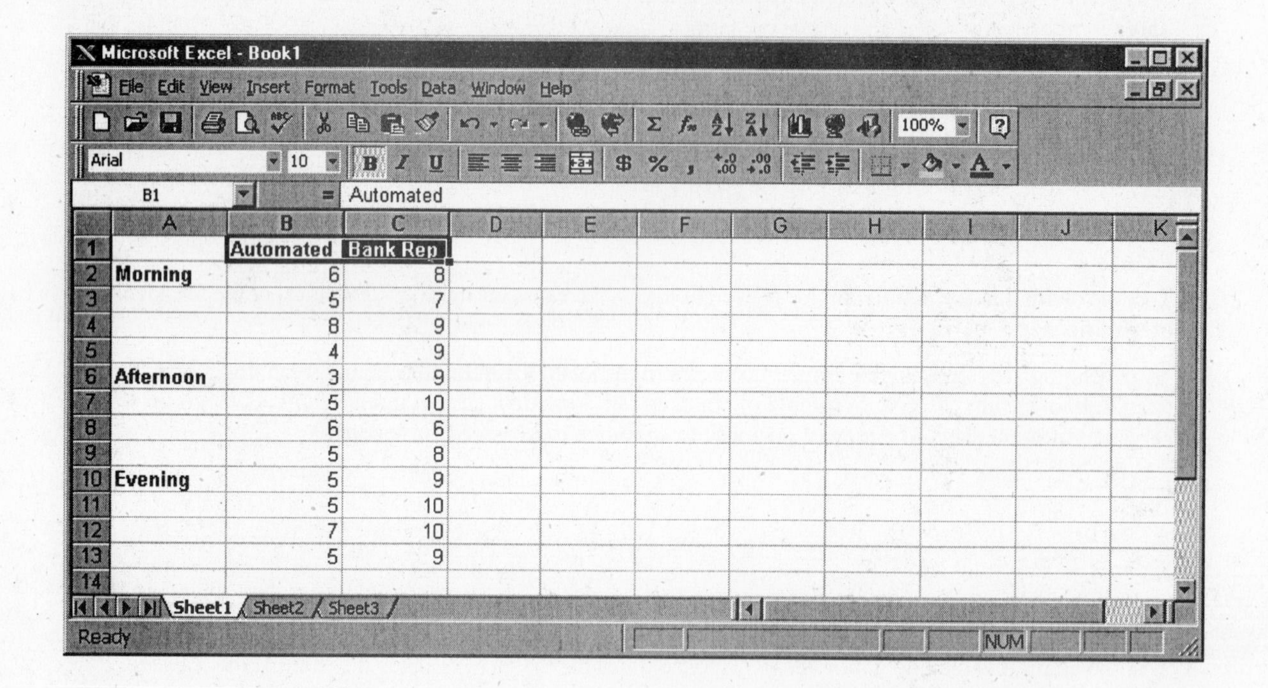

Open the **Anova: Two-Factor With Replication** dialog box and fill in the designated boxes.

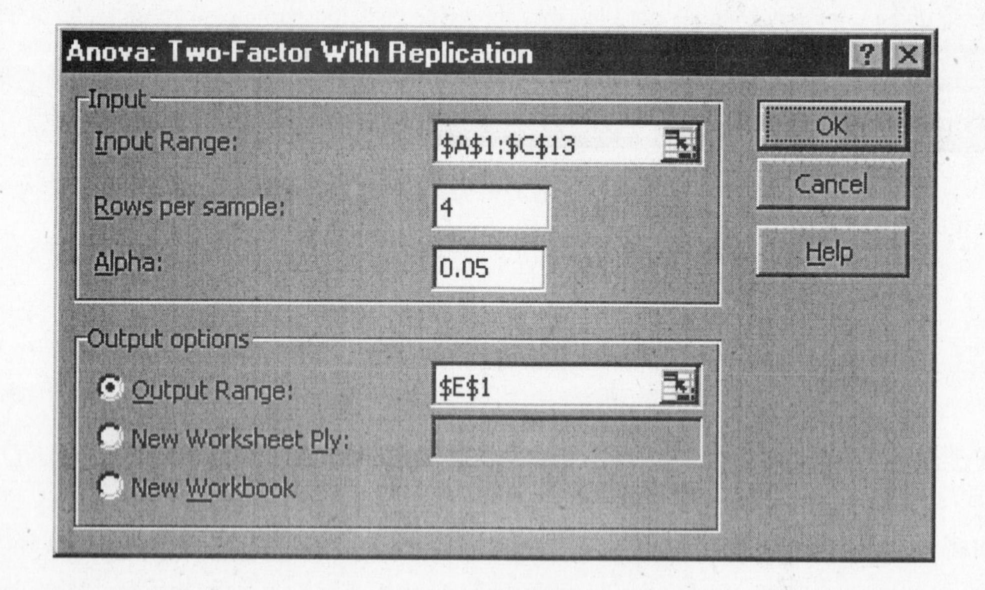

The output covers two pages:

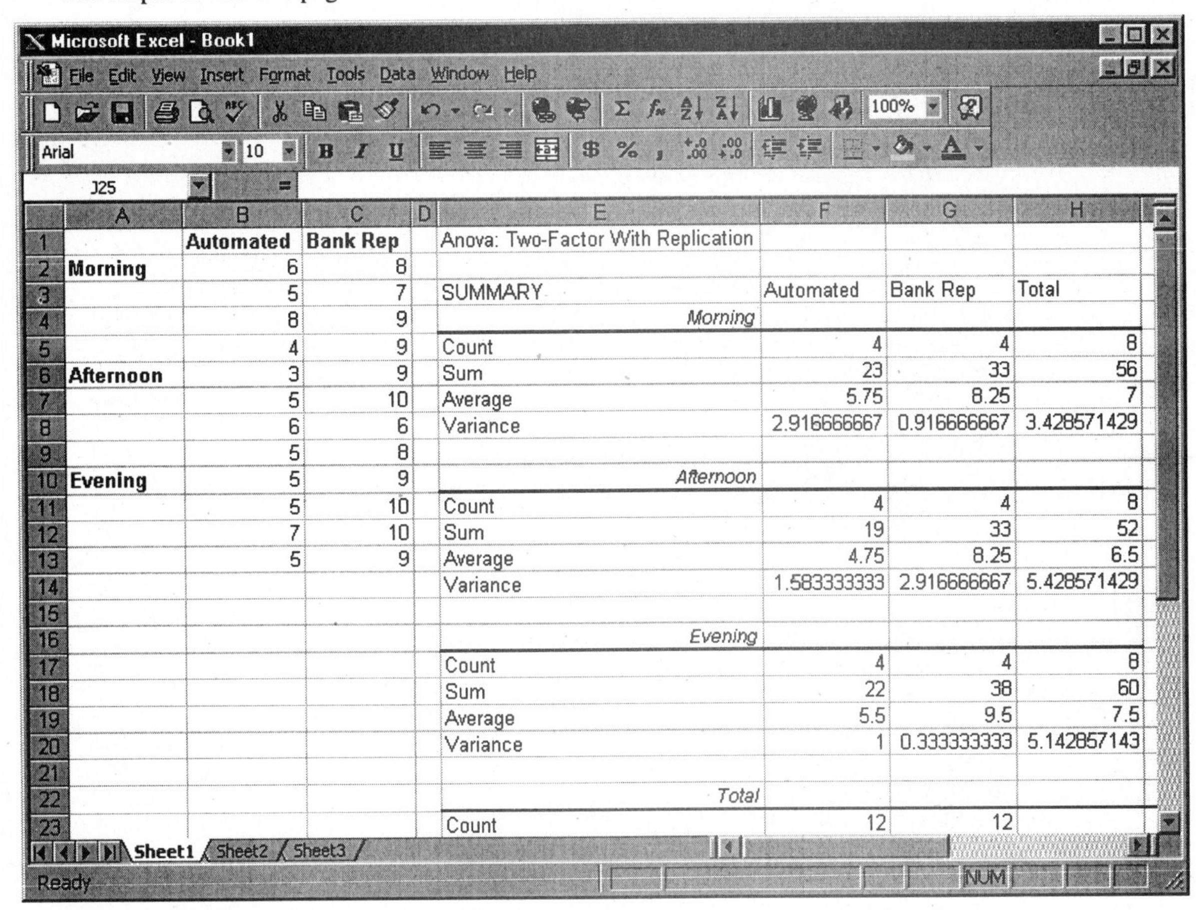

Microsoft Excel - Book1

	A	B	C	D	E	F	G	H
1		**Automated**	**Bank Rep**		Anova: Two-Factor With Replication			
2	**Morning**	6	8					
3		5	7		SUMMARY	Automated	Bank Rep	Total
4		8	9		*Morning*			
5		4	9		Count	4	4	8
6	**Afternoon**	3	9		Sum	23	33	56
7		5	10		Average	5.75	8.25	7
8		6	6		Variance	2.916666667	0.916666667	3.428571429
9		5	8					
10	**Evening**	5	9		*Afternoon*			
11		5	10		Count	4	4	8
12		7	10		Sum	19	33	52
13		5	9		Average	4.75	8.25	6.5
14					Variance	1.583333333	2.916666667	5.428571429
15								
16					*Evening*			
17					Count	4	4	8
18					Sum	22	38	60
19					Average	5.5	9.5	7.5
20					Variance	1	0.333333333	5.142857143
21								
22					*Total*			
23					Count	12	12	

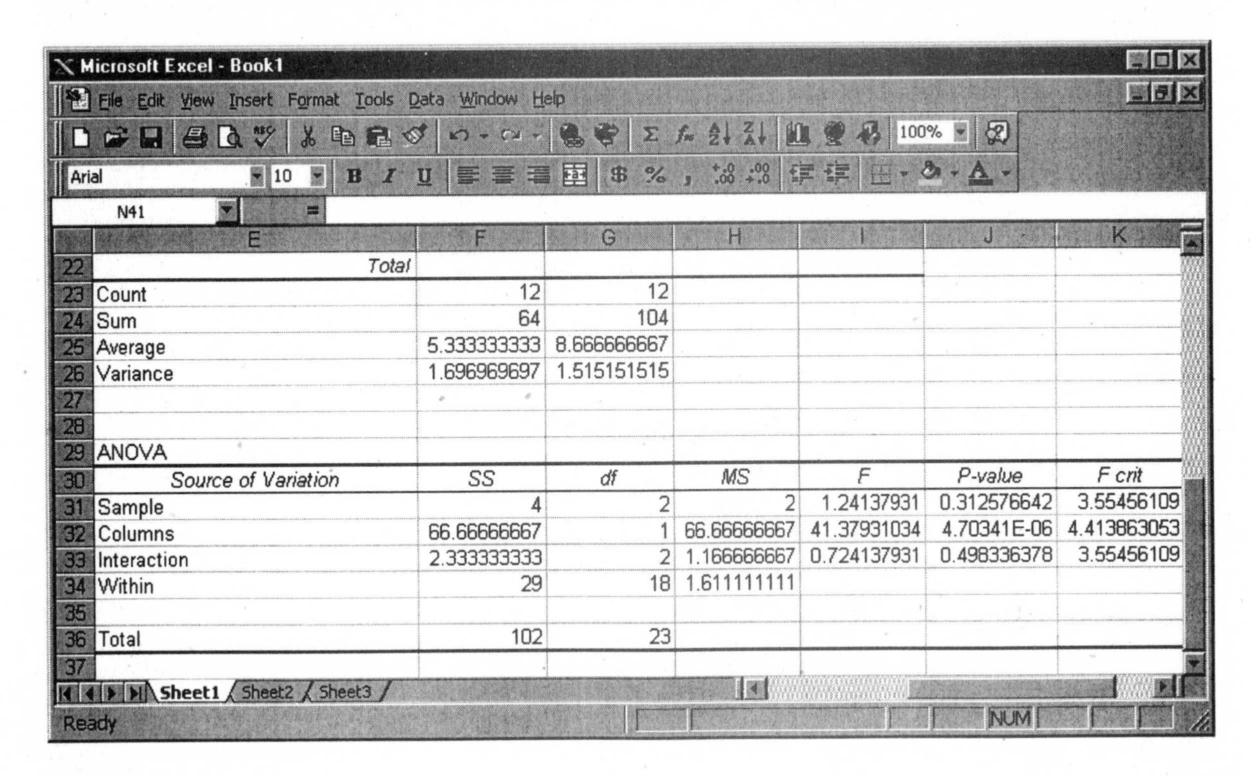

Microsoft Excel - Book1

	E	F	G	H	I	J	K
22	*Total*						
23	Count	12	12				
24	Sum	64	104				
25	Average	5.333333333	8.666666667				
26	Variance	1.696969697	1.515151515				
27							
28							
29	ANOVA						
30	*Source of Variation*	*SS*	*df*	*MS*	*F*	*P-value*	*F crit*
31	Sample	4	2	2	1.24137931	0.312576642	3.55456109
32	Columns	66.66666667	1	66.66666667	41.37931034	4.70341E-06	4.413863053
33	Interaction	2.333333333	2	1.166666667	0.724137931	0.498336378	3.55456109
34	Within	29	18	1.611111111			
35							
36	Total	102	23				
37							

The "Columns" data is for type of contact, and the "Sample" data is for time of contact. We see the sample F values for each factor and for the interaction and the corresponding P value. The F critical values are critical values for $\alpha = 0.05$ (as specified in the dialog box).

Example (without replication)

For this example, let's look at the example in Guided Exercises 12 of Section 11.6 of *Understandable Statistics*. In this example we have the average grams of fat in 3-oz servings of potato chips, as measured by three labs from three brands of chips.

The data are entered in the worksheet. Since there is only one measurement for each factor combination, we use **➤Tools➤Data Analysis➤Anova: Two-Factor without Replication.**

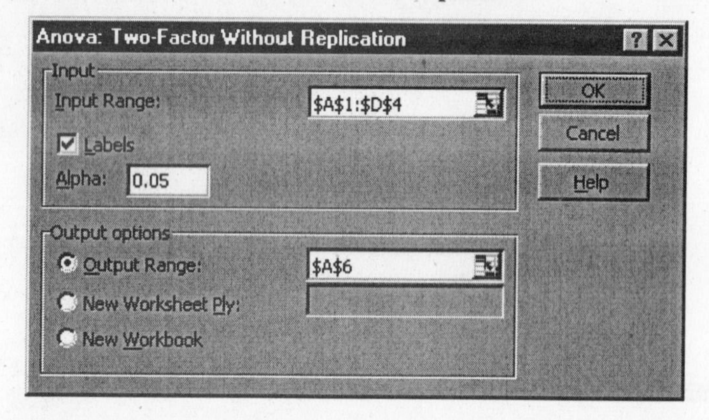

The output is

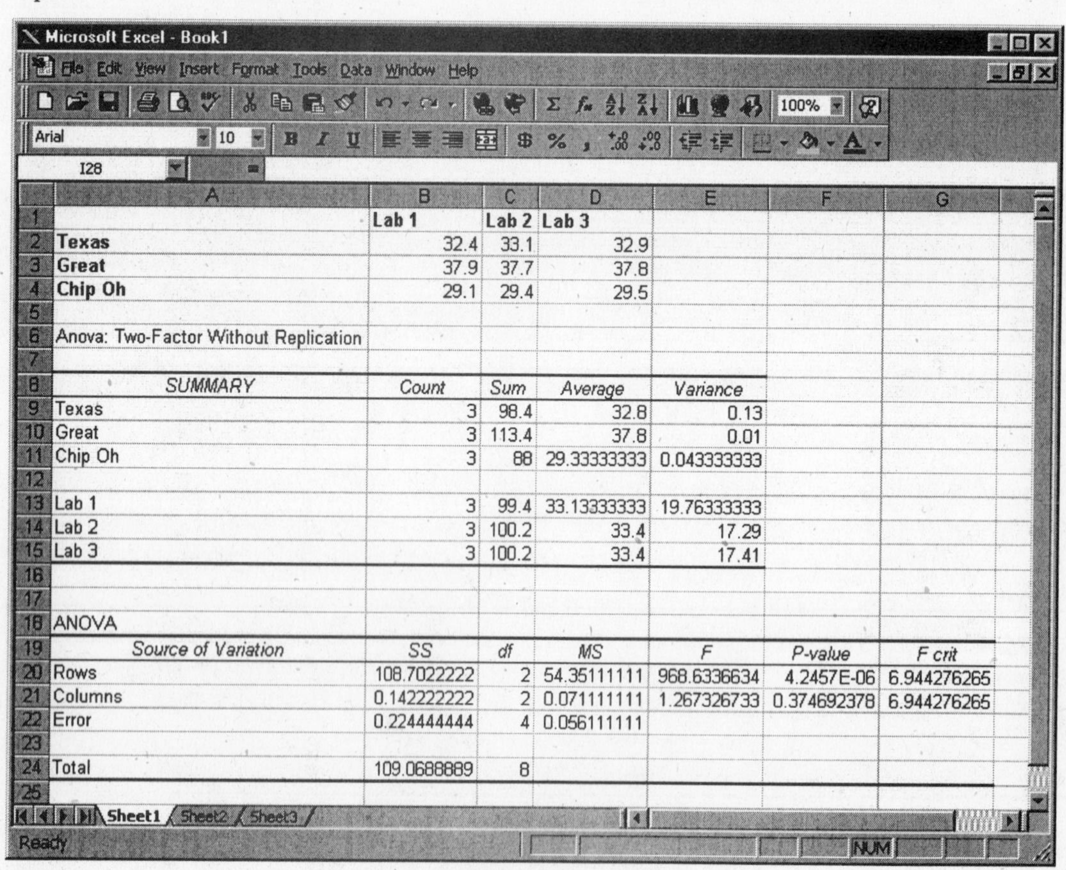

	Lab 1	Lab 2	Lab 3
Texas	32.4	33.1	32.9
Great	37.9	37.7	37.8
Chip Oh	29.1	29.4	29.5

Anova: Two-Factor Without Replication

SUMMARY	Count	Sum	Average	Variance
Texas	3	98.4	32.8	0.13
Great	3	113.4	37.8	0.01
Chip Oh	3	88	29.33333333	0.043333333
Lab 1	3	99.4	33.13333333	19.76333333
Lab 2	3	100.2	33.4	17.29
Lab 3	3	100.2	33.4	17.41

ANOVA

Source of Variation	SS	df	MS	F	P-value	F crit
Rows	108.7022222	2	54.35111111	968.6336634	4.2457E-06	6.944276265
Columns	0.142222222	2	0.071111111	1.267326733	0.374692378	6.944276265
Error	0.224444444	4	0.056111111			
Total	109.0688889	8				

The "Columns" data involve the laboratory factor, and the "Rows" data involve the chip brand factor. We see the sample *F* for each factor and the corresponding *P* value. The *F* critical values are for the designated level of significance, $\alpha = 0.05$.

LAB ACTIVITIES FOR ANALYSIS OF VARIANCE – TWO-WAY

See *Understandable Statistics* Section 11.6 Problems. Enter the data for the problems into an Excel worksheet and use the appropriate two-factor command to generate the computer output. Use the computer-generated output to draw conclusions.

TABLE OF EXCEL FUNCTIONS

DESCRIPTIVE STATISTICS

Can be entered by using the Paste Function button on the standard toolbar, or by directly typing the function in the formula bar.

=AVERAGE(cells containing data) returns the arithmetic mean of data

=COUNT(cells containing data) returns the number of data items

=COUNTIF(cells containing data,criteria) returns the number of data items satisfying the criteria

=MAX(cells containing data) returns the maximum value in the data

=MEDIAN(cells containing data) returns the median value of the data

=MIN(cells containing data) returns the minimum value in the data

=MODE(cells containing data) returns the mode of the data

=QUARTILE(cells containing data,quartile) returns the indicated quartile of the data

=STDEV(cells containing data) returns the sample standard deviation of the data

=STDEVP(cells containing data) returns the population standard deviation of the data

=TRIMMEAN(cells containing data,percent) returns the mean of the data trimmed by the total indicated percent, half from the bottom and half from the top.

=VAR(cells containing data) returns the sample variance of the data

=VARP(cells containing data) returns the population variance of the data

Dialog boxes found using the menu selections **➤Tools➤Data Analysis➤Descriptive Statistics** dialog box with Summary Statistics checked returns the mean standard error of mean, median, mode, standard deviation, variance, kurtosis, skewness, range, minimum, maximum, sum, count of the data. Checking the confidence level box returns the error E for a confidence interval $\overline{x}-E$ to $\overline{x}+E$ at the designated confidence level.

GRAPHICS

Use the Chart Wizard on the standard tool bar to create graphs for column charts (bar graphs), pie charts (circle graphs), line graphs (for time series), or scatter diagrams. Right-click a data point and click Add trend line to show a regression line and formula. Use **➤Tools➤Data Analysis➤Histogram** to open the histogram dialog box.

RANDOM SAMPLES

Use the Paste Function button on the standard tool bar or type directly

=RAND( ) returns a random number between 0 and 1.

=RANDBETWEEN(bottom,top) returns a random number between the designated values.

Use the menu selection **➤Tools➤Data Analysis** to access the dialog box.

Sampling returns a random sample from a designated cell range.

Random Number Generator returns a random sample from a designated distribution (uniform, normal, binomial, poisson, patterned, discrete).

PROBABILITY

Use the Paste Function button on the standard tool bar or type directly.

=BINOMDIST(# of success,# of trails,probability of success,cumulative)

returns the probability of exactly r success if the value of cumulative is false the probability of at most *r* successes if the value of cumulative is true.

=CHIDIST(x degrees of freedom)

returns the area to the right of *x* under a chi-square distribution with the designated degrees of freedom. The area is the probability that a value is greater than or equal to *x*.

=CHIINV(probability,degrees of freedom)

returns the chi-square value x such that the probability a value falls to the right of *x* is the designated probability.

=FDIST(x,degrees of freedom numerator,degrees of freedom denominator)

returns area in the right tail of the distribution beyond *x*.

=FINV(probability,degrees of freedom numerator,degrees of freedom denominator)

returns the value *x* such that the probability of a value falling to the right of *x* is the designated probability.

=HYPGEOMDIST(# of success in sample,size of sample,number of successes in population,population size)

returns the probability that the designated number of successes in the sample occur.

=NORMDIST(x,mean,standard deviation,cumulative)

returns the probability that a value is less than or equal x for true as the value of cumulative.

returns the density function value of *x* for false as the value of cumulative.

=NORMINV(probability,mean,standard deviation)

returns the *x* value such that the area under the normal distribution to the left of *x* equals the designated probability.

=NORMSDIST(z)

returns the area to the left of *z* under the standard normal.

=NORMSINV(probability)

returns the *z* value such that the area to the left of *z* is equal to the specified probability.

=POISSON(x,mean,cumulative)

returns the probability that the number of random events occurring will be between zero and *x* inclusive when the value of cumulative is true.

the density function value that the number of events occurring will be exactly *x* when the value of cumulative is false.

=TDIST(x,degrees of freedom,tails)

returns the area in the tail to the right of x when the value of tails is 1. When the value of tails is 2, returns the total area in the tail to the right of *x* and the tail to the left of $-x$.

=TINV(probability,degree of freedom)

returns the *x* value that the total area to the right of *x* and that to the left of $-x$ equals the designated probability.

CONFIDENCE INTERVAL

Use Paste Function or type directly

=CONFIDENCE(alpha,standard deviation,size)

returns the value of E in the confidence interval for a mean $\overline{x}-E$ to $\overline{x}+E$. The confidence level equals $100(1-\alpha)\%$. The value of E is computed using a normal distribution.

Confidence intervals for other parameters are included in some of the outputs for certain dialog boxes contained in the **➤Tools➤Data Analysis** choices.

HYPOTHESIS TESTING

Use the Paste Function on the standard tool bar or type directly

=CHITEST(observed value data cells,expected value data cells)

returns the P value of the sample chi-square statistics for a test of independence.

=FTEST(cells containing the data of first sample,cells containing data of second sample)

returns P value for a two -tailed test of variances.

=TTEST(cells containing first sample,cells containing second sample,tails,type)

returns the P value of a one-tailed test if the value of tails is 1 and a two-tailed test if the value of tails is 2.

The type of test performed is as follows:

type = 1: a paired test is performed.
type = 2: a two-sample equal variance test is performed.
type = 3: a two-sample unequal variance test is performed.

=ZTEST(cells containing data,x,sigma)

returns the P value for a two tailed test where $H_0: \mu = x$ is the null hypothesis and $H_0: \mu \neq x$ is the alternate hypothesis. For sigma, use the population standard deviation, if it is known. Otherwise leave out sigma, and Excel will use the sample standard deviation computed from the data. The normal distribution is the sampling distribution used.

These dialog boxes are under the menu choice **➤Tools➤Data Analysis.**

F-Test: Two Sample for Variances

returns the P value for a one-tailed test as well as some summary statistics for the data.

t-Test: Paired Two Sample for Means

returns P values for a one-tailed test and P values for a two-tailed test, the t value of the sample test statistic, critical one-tail or two-tail values, and summary statistics for the data.

t-Test: Two-Sample Assuming Equal Variances

returns P values for a one-tailed test and P values for a two-tailed test, the t value of the sample test statistic, critical one-tailed or two-tailed values, and summary statistics for the data.

t-Test: Two-Sample Assuming Unequal Variances

returns P values for a one-tailed test and P values for a two-tailed test, the t value of the sample test statistic, critical one-tailed or two-tailed values, and summary statistics for the data.

z-Test: Two-Sample for Means

returns *P* values for a one-tailed test and *P* values for a two-tailed test, the *z* value of the sample test statistic, critical one-tailed or two-tailed values, and summary statistics for the data.

ANALYSIS OF VARIANCE

These dialog boxes are under the menu choice **➤Tools➤Data Analysis.**

Anova: Single Factor

Anova: Two-Factor With Replication

(equal number greater than 1 of measurements per factor combination)

Anova: Two-Factor Without Replication

(one measurement per factor combination)

Each of these dialog boxes returns summary statistics for the factors and a summary table giving degrees of freedom, sum of squares, mean squares, *F* values, *P* values.

LINEAR REGRESSION

Use Paste Function on the standard tool bar or type the command directly into the formula bar.

=CORREL(y range,x range)

returns the correlation coefficient *r* between two data sets.

=FORECAST(x value,y range,x range)

returns the y value for the specified *x* as computed using the least-squares regression equation.

=INTERCEPT(y range,x range)

returns the *y*-intercept of the least -squares regression line.

=LINEST(y range,x range)

returns the slope and *y*-intercept of the least-squares line. (We are ignoring two optional parameters.) Since this is an array formula, two cells need to be activated to receive the output. The command needs to be typed into the formula bar and entered with the **Ctrl+Shift+Enter** combination.

=PEARSON(y range,x range)

returns the Pearson product moment correlation coefficient *r* for the two data sets.

=RSQ(y range,x range)

returns r^2 (the square of the Pearson product moment correlation coefficient).

=SLOPE(y range,x range)

returns the slope of the least-squares line.

=STEYX(y range,x range)

returns the standard error of estimate for the predicted *y* value.

These dialog boxes are under the menu choice **➤Tools➤Data Analysis.**

Correlation

returns the correlation between all variables in a multiple linear regression model.

Regression

returns the coefficients for a simple or multiple linear regression model. Other options provide for a table of residuals, a residual plot a line fit plot, a normal probability plot, and an ANOVA table. An output table including coefficients, standard error of *y* estimates, r^2 values, number of observations, and standard error of coefficients is provided.

MISCELLANEOUS

Under the Paste Function button on the standard menu bar

=STANDARDIZE(x,mean,standard deviation)

returns the z value for the specified *x* value.

On the tool bars

Σ button gives the sum of the selected cells.

Sort buttons AZ↓ or **ZA↑** sort data in increasing or decreasing order.

Chart Wizard button opens the chart-making tools.

$ button formats numbers in selected cells in dollar and cent format.

% button formats numbers in selected cells to percents.

, button formats numbers in selected cells to comma format.

←.0 button formats numbers in selected cells with one more digit after the decimal each time the button is pushed.

→.00 button formats numbers in selected cells with one less digit after the decimal each.

Descriptions of Data Sets on the HM StatPass CD-ROM

I. General

There are over 100 data sets saved in Excel, Minitab Portable, and TI-83 Plus/ASCII formats to accompany *Understandable Statistics,* 7th edition. These files can be found on the HM StatPass CD-ROM packaged with the student textbook. You may also visit the Brase/Brase statistics site at http://math.college.hmco.com/students to view these data sets online. The data sets are organized by category.

A. The following are provided for each data set:
   1. The category
   2. A brief description of the data and variables with a reference when appropriate
   3. File names for Excel, Minitab, and TI-83Plus/ASCII formats

B. The categories are
   1. **Single variable large sample** ($n \geq 30$)
      File name prefix **Svls** followed by the data set number
      There are 30 data sets.. page 109
   2. **Single variable small sample** ($n < 30$)
      File name prefix **Svss** followed by the data set number
      There are 11 data sets.. page 120
   3. **Time series data** for control chart about the mean or for P-Charts
      File name prefix **Tscc** followed by the data set number
      There are 10 data sets.. page 123
   4. **Two variable independent samples** (large and small sample)
      File name prefix **Tvis** followed by the data set number
      There are 10 data sets.. page 127
   5. **Two variable dependent samples** appropriate for t-tests
      File name prefix **Tvds** followed by the data set number
      There are 10 data sets.. page 132
   6. **Simple linear regression**
      File name prefix **Slr** followed by the data set number
      There are 12 data sets.. page 137
   7. **Multiple linear regression**
      File name prefix **Mlr** followed by the data set number
      There are 10 data sets.. page 144
   8. **One-way ANOVA**
      File name prefix **Owan** followed by the data set number
      There are 5 data sets.. page 158
   9. **Two-way ANOVA**
      File name prefix **Twan** followed by the data set number
      There are 5 data sets.. page 163

C. The formats are
   1. Excel files in subdirectory Excel_7e. These files have suffix .xls
   2. Minitab portable files in subdirectory Minitab_7e. These files have suffix .mtp
   3. TI-83Plus/ASCII files in subdirectory TI83_7e. These files have suffix .txt
   4. Some of the data sets are also built-in to ComputerStat, which is included on the HM StatPass CD-ROM.

II. Suggestions for using the data sets

1. Single variable large sample (file name prefix Svls)
   These data sets are appropriate for
   Graphs: Histograms, box plots
   Descriptive statistics: Mean, median, mode, variance, standard deviation, coefficient of variation, 5 number summary
   Inferential statistics: Confidence intervals for the population mean, hypothesis tests of a single mean

2. Single variable small sample (file name prefix Svss)
   Graphs: Histograms, box plots,
   Descriptive statistics: Mean, median, mode, variance, standard deviation, coefficient of variation, 5 number summary
   Inferential statistics: Confidence intervals for the population mean, hypothesis tests of a single mean

3. Time series data (file name prefix Tsccc)
   Graphs: Time plots, control charts about the mean utilizing individual data for the data sets so designated, *P* charts for the data sets so designated

4. Two independent data sets (file name prefix Tvis)
   Graphs: Histograms, box plots for each data set
   Descriptive statistics: Mean, median, mode, variance, standard deviation, coefficient of variation, 5-number summary for each data set
   Inferential statistics: Confidence intervals for the difference of means, hypothesis tests for the difference of means

5. Paired data, dependent samples (file name prefix Tvds)
   Descriptive statistics: Mean, median, mode, variance, standard deviation, coefficient of variation, 5 number summary for the difference of the paired data values.
   Inferential statistics: Hypothesis tests for the difference of means (paired data)

6. Data pairs for simple linear regression (file name prefix Slr)
   Graphs: Scatter plots, for individual variables histograms and box plots
   Descriptive statistics:
   (a) Mean, median, mode, variance, standard deviation, coefficient of variation, 5 number summary for individual variables.
   (b) Least squares line, sample correlation coefficient, sample coefficient of determination
   Inferential statistics: Testing ρ, confidence intervals for β, testing β

7. Data for multiple linear regression (file name prefix Mlr)
   Graphs:
   Descriptive statistics: Histograms, box plots for individual variables
   (a) Mean, median, mode, variance, standard deviation, coefficient of variation, 5 number summary for individual variables.
   (b) Least squares line, sample coefficient of determination
   Inferential statistics: confidence intervals for coefficients, testing coefficients

8. Data for one-way ANOVA (file name prefix Owan)
    Graphs: Histograms, box plots for individual samples
    Descriptive statistics: Mean, median, mode, variance, standard deviation, coefficient of variation, 5 number summary for individual samples.
    Inferential statistics: One-way ANOVA

9. Data for two-way ANOVA (file name prefix Twan)
    Graphs: Histograms, box plots for individual samples
    Descriptive statistics: Mean, median, mode, variance, standard deviation, coefficient of variation, 5 number summary for data in individual cells.
    Inferential statistics: Two-way ANOVA

Single Variable Large Sample ($n \geq 30$)
File name prefix: Svls followed by the number of the data file

01. Disney Stock Volume (Single Variable Large Sample $n \geq 30$)

The following data represents the number of shares of Disney stock (in hundreds of shares) sold for a random sample of 60 trading days

Reference: *The Denver Post*, Business section

12584	9441	18960	21480	10766	13059	8589	4965
4803	7240	10906	8561	6389	14372	18149	6309
13051	12754	10860	9574	19110	29585	21122	14522
17330	18119	10902	29158	16065	10376	10999	17950
15418	12618	16561	8022	9567	9045	8172	13708
11259	10518	9301	5197	11259	10518	9301	5197
6758	7304	7628	14265	13054	15336	14682	27804
16022	24009	32613	19111				

File names — Excel: Svls01.xls
Minitab: Svls01.mtp
TI-83Plus/ASCII: Svls01.txt

02. Weights of Pro Football Players (Single Variable Large Sample $n \geq 30$)

The following data represents weights in pounds of 50 randomly selected pro football linebackers.

Reference: The Sports Encyclopedia Pro Football

225	230	235	238	232	227	244	222
250	226	242	253	251	225	229	247
239	223	233	222	243	237	230	240
255	230	245	240	235	252	245	231
235	234	248	242	238	240	240	240
235	244	247	250	236	246	243	255
241	245						

File names — Excel: Svls02.xls
Minitab: Svls02.mtp
TI-83Plus/ASCII: Svls02.txt

03. Heights of Pro Basketball Players (Single Variable Large Sample $n \geq 30$)
The following data represents heights in feet of 65 randomly selected pro basketball players.
Reference: All-Time Player Directory, The Official NBA Encyclopedia

6.50	6.25	6.33	6.50	6.42	6.67	6.83	6.82
6.17	7.00	5.67	6.50	6.75	6.54	6.42	6.58
6.00	6.75	7.00	6.58	6.29	7.00	6.92	6.42
5.92	6.08	7.00	6.17	6.92	7.00	5.92	6.42
6.00	6.25	6.75	6.17	6.75	6.58	6.58	6.46
5.92	6.58	6.13	6.50	6.58	6.63	6.75	6.25
6.67	6.17	6.17	6.25	6.00	6.75	6.17	6.83
6.00	6.42	6.92	6.50	6.33	6.92	6.67	6.33
6.08							

File names
Excel: Svls03.xls
Minitab: Svls03.mtp
TI-83Plus/ASCII: Svls03.txt

04. Miles per Gallon Gasoline Consumption (Single Variable Large Sample $n \geq 30$)
The following data represents miles per gallon gasoline consumption (highway) for a random sample of 55 makes and models of passenger cars.
Reference: Environmental Protection Agency

30	27	22	25	24	25	24	15
35	35	33	52	49	10	27	18
20	23	24	25	30	24	24	24
18	20	25	27	24	32	29	27
24	27	26	25	24	28	33	30
13	13	21	28	37	35	32	33
29	31	28	28	25	29	31	

File names
Excel: Svls04.xls
Minitab: Svls04.mtp
TI-83Plus/ASCII: Svls04.txt

05. Fasting Glucose Blood Tests (Single Variable Large Sample $n \geq 30$)
The following data represents glucose blood level (mg/100ml) after a 12-hour fast for a random sample of 70 women.
Reference: American J. Clin. Nutr. Vol. 19, 345-351

45	66	83	71	76	64	59	59
76	82	80	81	85	77	82	90
87	72	79	69	83	71	87	69
81	76	96	83	67	94	101	94
89	94	73	99	93	85	83	80
78	80	85	83	84	74	81	70
65	89	70	80	84	77	65	46
80	70	75	45	101	71	109	73
73	80	72	81	63	74		

File names
Excel: Svls05.xls
Minitab: Svls05.mtp
TI-83Plus/ASCII: Svls05.txt

06. Number of Children in Rural Canadian Families (Single Variable Large Sample $n \geq 30$)
The following data represents the number of children in a random sample of 50 rural Canadian families.
Reference: American Journal Of Sociology Vol. 53, 470-480

11	13	4	14	10	2	5	0
0	3	9	2	5	2	3	3
3	4	7	1	9	4	3	3
2	6	0	2	6	5	9	5
4	3	2	5	2	2	3	5
14	7	6	6	2	5	3	4
6	1						

File names Excel: Svls06.xls
Minitab: Svls06.mtp
TI-83Plus/ASCII: Svls06.txt

07. Children as a % of Population (Single Variable Large Sample $n \geq 30$)
The following data represent percentage of children in the population for a random sample of 72 Denver neighborhoods.
Reference: The Piton Foundation, Denver, Colorado

30.2	18.6	13.6	36.9	32.8	19.4	12.3	39.7	22.2	31.2
36.4	37.7	38.8	28.1	18.3	22.4	26.5	20.4	37.6	23.8
22.1	53.2	6.8	20.7	31.7	10.4	21.3	19.6	41.5	29.8
14.7	12.3	17.0	16.7	20.7	34.8	7.5	19.0	27.2	16.3
24.3	39.8	31.1	34.3	15.9	24.2	20.3	31.2	30.0	33.1
29.1	39.0	36.0	31.8	32.9	26.5	4.9	19.5	21.0	24.2
12.1	38.3	39.3	20.2	24.0	28.6	27.1	30.0	60.8	39.2
21.6	20.3								

File names Excel: Svls07.xls
Minitab: Svls07.mtp
TI-83Plus/ASCII: Svls07.txt

08. Percentage Change in Household Income (Single Variable Large Sample $n \geq 30$)
The following data represent the percentage change in household income over a five-year period for a random sample of $n = 78$ Denver neighborhoods.
Reference: The Piton Foundation, Denver, Colorado

27.2	25.2	25.7	80.9	26.9	20.2	25.4	26.9	26.4	26.3
27.5	38.2	20.9	31.3	23.5	26.0	35.8	30.9	15.5	24.8
29.4	11.7	32.6	32.2	27.6	27.5	28.7	28.0	15.6	20.0
21.8	18.4	27.3	13.4	14.7	21.6	26.8	20.9	32.7	29.3
21.4	29.0	7.2	25.7	25.5	39.8	26.6	24.2	33.5	16.0
29.4	26.8	32.0	24.7	24.2	29.8	25.8	18.2	26.0	26.2
21.7	27.0	23.7	28.0	11.2	26.2	21.6	23.7	28.3	34.1
40.8	16.0	50.5	54.1	3.3	23.5	10.1	14.8		

File names Excel: Svls08.xls
Minitab: Svls08.mtp
TI-83Plus/ASCII: Svls08.txt

09. Crime Rate per 1,000 Population (Single Variable Large Sample $n \geq 30$)
The following data represent the crime rate per 1,000 population for a random sample of 70 Denver neighborhoods.
Reference: The Piton Foundation, Denver, Colorado

84.9	45.1	132.1	104.7	258.0	36.3	26.2	207.7
58.5	65.3	42.5	53.2	172.6	69.2	179.9	65.1
32.0	38.3	185.9	42.4	63.0	86.4	160.4	26.9
154.2	111.0	139.9	68.2	127.0	54.0	42.1	105.2
77.1	278.0	73.0	32.1	92.7	704.1	781.8	52.2
65.0	38.6	22.5	157.3	63.1	289.1	52.7	108.7
66.3	69.9	108.7	96.9	27.1	105.1	56.2	80.1
59.6	77.5	68.9	35.2	65.4	123.2	130.8	70.7
25.1	62.6	68.6	334.5	44.6	87.1		

File names
Excel: Svls09.xls
Minitab: Svls09.mtp
TI-83Plus/ASCII: Svls09.txt

10. Percentage Change in Population (Single Variable Large Sample $n \geq 30$)
The following data represent the percentage change in population over a nine-year period for a random sample of 64 Denver neighborhoods.
Reference: The Piton Foundation, Denver, Colorado

6.2	5.4	8.5	1.2	5.6	28.9	6.3	10.5	-1.5	17.3
21.6	-2.0	-1.0	3.3	2.8	3.3	28.5	-0.7	8.1	32.6
68.6	56.0	19.8	7.0	38.3	41.2	4.9	7.8	7.8	97.8
5.5	21.6	32.5	-0.5	2.8	4.9	8.7	-1.3	4.0	32.2
2.0	6.4	7.1	8.8	3.0	5.1	-1.9	-2.6	1.6	7.4
10.8	4.8	1.4	19.2	2.7	71.4	2.5	6.2	2.3	10.2
1.9	2.3	-3.3	2.6						

File names
Excel: Svls10.xls
Minitab: Svls10.mtp
TI-83Plus/ASCII: Svls10.txt

11. Thickness of the Ozone Column (Single Variable Large Sample $n \geq 30$)
The following data represent the January mean thickness of the ozone column above Arosa, Switzerland (Dobson units: one milli-centimeter ozone at standard temperature and pressure). The data is from a random sample of years from 1926 on.
Reference: Laboratorium fuer Atmosphaerensphysik, Switzerland

324	332	362	383	335	349	354	319	360	329
400	341	315	368	361	336	349	347	338	332
341	352	342	361	318	337	300	352	340	371
327	357	320	377	338	361	301	331	334	387
336	378	369	332	344					

File names
Excel: Svls11.xls
Minitab: Svls11.mtp
TI-83Plus/ASCII: Svls11.txt

12. Sun Spots (Single Variable Large Sample $n \geq 30$)

The following data represent the January mean number of sunspots. The data is taken from a random sample of Januarys from 1749 to 1983.

Reference: Waldmeir, M, *Sun Spot Activity*, International Astronomical Union Bulletin

12.5	14.1	37.6	48.3	67.3	70.0	43.8	56.5	59.7	24.0
12.0	27.4	53.5	73.9	104.0	54.6	4.4	177.3	70.1	54.0
28.0	13.0	6.5	134.7	114.0	72.7	81.2	24.1	20.4	13.3
9.4	25.7	47.8	50.0	45.3	61.0	39.0	12.0	7.2	11.3
22.2	26.3	34.9	21.5	12.8	17.7	34.6	43.0	52.2	47.5
30.9	11.3	4.9	88.6	188.0	35.6	50.5	12.4	3.7	18.5
115.5	108.5	119.1	101.6	59.9	40.7	26.5	23.1	73.6	165.0
202.5	217.4	57.9	38.7	15.3	8.1	16.4	84.3	51.9	58.0
74.7	96.0	48.1	51.1	31.5	11.8	4.5	78.1	81.6	68.9

File names

Excel: Svls12.xls
Minitab: Svls12.mtp
TI-83Plus/ASCII: Svls12.txt

13. Motion of Stars (Single Variable Large Sample $n \geq 30$)

The following data represent the angular motions of stars across the sky due to the stars own velocity. A random sample of stars from the M92 global cluster was used. Units are arc seconds per century.

Reference: Cudworth, K.M., Astronomical Journal, Vol. 81, p 975-982

0.042	0.048	0.019	0.025	0.028	0.041	0.030	0.051	0.026
0.040	0.018	0.022	0.048	0.045	0.019	0.028	0.029	0.018
0.033	0.035	0.019	0.046	0.021	0.026	0.026	0.033	0.046
0.023	0.036	0.024	0.014	0.012	0.037	0.034	0.032	0.035
0.015	0.027	0.017	0.035	0.021	0.016	0.036	0.029	0.031
0.016	0.024	0.015	0.019	0.037	0.016	0.024	0.029	0.025
0.022	0.028	0.023	0.021	0.020	0.020	0.016	0.016	0.016
0.040	0.029	0.025	0.025	0.042	0.022	0.037	0.024	0.046
0.016	0.024	0.028	0.027	0.060	0.045	0.037	0.027	0.028
0.022	0.048	0.053						

File names

Excel: Svls13.xls
Minitab: Svls13.mtp
TI-83Plus/ASCII: Svls13.txt

14. Arsenic and Ground Water (Single Variable Large Sample $n \geq 30$)

The following data represent (naturally occurring) concentration of arsenic in ground water for a random sample of 102 Northwest Texas wells. Units are parts per billion.
Reference: Nichols, C.E. and Kane, V.E., Union Carbide Technical Report K/UR-1

7.6	10.4	13.5	4.0	19.9	16.0	12.0	12.2	11.4	12.7
3.0	10.3	21.4	19.4	9.0	6.5	10.1	8.7	9.7	6.4
9.7	63.0	15.5	10.7	18.2	7.5	6.1	6.7	6.9	0.8
73.5	12.0	28.0	12.6	9.4	6.2	15.3	7.3	10.7	15.9
5.8	1.0	8.6	1.3	13.7	2.8	2.4	1.4	2.9	13.1
15.3	9.2	11.7	4.5	1.0	1.2	0.8	1.0	2.4	4.4
2.2	2.9	3.6	2.5	1.8	5.9	2.8	1.7	4.6	5.4
3.0	3.1	1.3	2.6	1.4	2.3	1.0	5.4	1.8	2.6
3.4	1.4	10.7	18.2	7.7	6.5	12.2	10.1	6.4	10.7
6.1	0.8	12.0	28.1	9.4	6.2	7.3	9.7	62.1	15.5
6.4	9.5								

File names
Excel: Svls14.xls
Minitab: Svls14.mtp
TI-83Plus/ASCII: Svls14.txt

15. Uranium In Ground Water (Single Variable Large Sample $n \geq 30$)

The following data represent (naturally occurring) concentrations of uranium in ground water for a random sample of 100 Northwest Texas wells. Units are parts per billion.
Reference: Nichols, C.E. and Kane, V.E., Union Carbide Technical Report K/UR-1

8.0	13.7	4.9	3.1	78.0	9.7	6.9	21.7	26.8
56.2	25.3	4.4	29.8	22.3	9.5	13.5	47.8	29.8
13.4	21.0	26.7	52.5	6.5	15.8	21.2	13.2	12.3
5.7	11.1	16.1	11.4	18.0	15.5	35.3	9.5	2.1
10.4	5.3	11.2	0.9	7.8	6.7	21.9	20.3	16.7
2.9	124.2	58.3	83.4	8.9	18.1	11.9	6.7	9.8
15.1	70.4	21.3	58.2	25.0	5.5	14.0	6.0	11.9
15.3	7.0	13.6	16.4	35.9	19.4	19.8	6.3	2.3
1.9	6.0	1.5	4.1	34.0	17.6	18.6	8.0	7.9
56.9	53.7	8.3	33.5	38.2	2.8	4.2	18.7	12.7
3.8	8.8	2.3	7.2	9.8	7.7	27.4	7.9	11.1
24.7								

File names
Excel: Svls15.xls
Minitab: Svls15.mtp
TI-83Plus/ASCII: Svls15.txt

16. Ground Water pH (Single Variable Large Sample $n \geq 30$)

A pH less than 7 is acidic, and a pH above 7 is alkaline. The following data represent pH levels in ground water for a random sample of 102 Northwest Texas wells.
Reference: Nichols, C.E. and Kane, V.E., Union Carbide Technical Report K/UR-1

7.6	7.7	7.4	7.7	7.1	8.2	7.4	7.5	7.2	7.4
7.2	7.6	7.4	7.8	8.1	7.5	7.1	8.1	7.3	8.2
7.6	7.0	7.3	7.4	7.8	8.1	7.3	8.0	7.2	8.5
7.1	8.2	8.1	7.9	7.2	7.1	7.0	7.5	7.2	7.3
8.6	7.7	7.5	7.8	7.6	7.1	7.8	7.3	8.4	7.5
7.1	7.4	7.2	7.4	7.3	7.7	7.0	7.3	7.6	7.2
8.1	8.2	7.4	7.6	7.3	7.1	7.0	7.0	7.4	7.2
8.2	8.1	7.9	8.1	8.2	7.7	7.5	7.3	7.9	8.8
7.1	7.5	7.9	7.5	7.6	7.7	8.2	8.7	7.9	7.0
8.8	7.1	7.2	7.3	7.6	7.1	7.0	7.0	7.3	7.2
7.8	7.6								

File names
Excel: Svls16.xls
Minitab: Svls16.mtp
TI-83Plus/ASCII: Svls16.txt

17. Static Fatigue 90% Stress Level (Single Variable Large Sample $n \geq 30$)

Kevlar Epoxy is a material used on the NASA space shuttle. Strands of this epoxy were tested at 90% breaking strength. The following data represent time to failure in hours at the 90% stress level for a random sample of 50 epoxy strands.
Reference: R.E. Barlow University of California, Berkeley

0.54	1.80	1.52	2.05	1.03	1.18	0.80	1.33	1.29	1.11
3.34	1.54	0.08	0.12	0.60	0.72	0.92	1.05	1.43	3.03
1.81	2.17	0.63	0.56	0.03	0.09	0.18	0.34	1.51	1.45
1.52	0.19	1.55	0.02	0.07	0.65	0.40	0.24	1.51	1.45
1.60	1.80	4.69	0.08	7.89	1.58	1.64	0.03	0.23	0.72

File names
Excel: Svls17.xls
Minitab: Svls17.mtp
TI-83Plus/ASCII: Svls17.txt

18. Static Fatigue 80% Stress Level (Single Variable Large Sample $n \geq 30$)

Kevlar Epoxy is a material used on the NASA space shuttle. Strands of this epoxy were tested at 80% breaking strength. The following data represent time to failure in hours at the 80% stress level for a random sample of 54 epoxy strands.
Reference: R.E. Barlow University of California, Berkeley

152.2	166.9	183.8	8.5	1.8	118.0	125.4	132.8	10.6
29.6	50.1	202.6	177.7	160.0	87.1	112.6	122.3	124.4
131.6	140.9	7.5	41.9	59.7	80.5	83.5	149.2	137.0
301.1	329.8	461.5	739.7	304.3	894.7	220.2	251.0	269.2
130.4	77.8	64.4	381.3	329.8	451.3	346.2	663.0	49.1
31.7	116.8	140.2	334.1	285.9	59.7	44.1	351.2	93.2

File names
Excel: Svls18.xls
Minitab: Svls18.mtp
TI-83Plus/ASCII: Svls18.txt

19. Tumor Recurrence (Single Variable Large Sample $n \geq 30$)

Certain kinds of tumors tend to recur. The following data represents the length of time in months for a tumor to recur after chemotherapy (sample size, 42).
Reference: Byar, D.P, *Urology* Vol. 10, p 556-561

19	18	17	1	21	22	54	46	25	49
50	1	59	39	43	39	5	9	38	18
14	45	54	59	46	50	29	12	19	36
38	40	43	41	10	50	41	25	19	39
27	20								

File names
Excel: Svls19.xls
Minitab: Svls19.mtp
TI-83Plus/ASCII: Svls19.txt

20. Weight of Harvest (Single Variable Large Sample $n \geq 30$)

The following data represent the weights in kilograms of maize harvest from a random sample of 72 experimental plots on the island of St Vincent (Caribbean).
Reference: Springer, B.G.F. *Proceedings, Caribbean Food Corps. Soc.* Vol. 10 p 147-152

24.0	27.1	26.5	13.5	19.0	26.1	23.8	22.5	20.0
23.1	23.8	24.1	21.4	26.7	22.5	22.8	25.2	20.9
23.1	24.9	26.4	12.2	21.8	19.3	18.2	14.4	22.4
16.0	17.2	20.3	23.8	24.5	13.7	11.1	20.5	19.1
20.2	24.1	10.5	13.7	16.0	7.8	12.2	12.5	14.0
22.0	16.5	23.8	13.1	11.5	9.5	22.8	21.1	22.0
11.8	16.1	10.0	9.1	15.2	14.5	10.2	11.7	14.6
15.5	23.7	25.1	29.5	24.5	23.2	25.5	19.8	17.8

File names
Excel: Svls20.xls
Minitab: Svls20.mtp
TI-83Plus/ASCII: Svls20.txt

21. Apple Trees (Single Variable Large Sample $n \geq 30$)

The following data represent trunk girth (mm) of a random sample of 60 four-year-old apple trees at East Malling Research Station (England)
Reference: S.C. Pearce, University of Kent at Canterbury

108	99	106	102	115	120	120	117	122	142
106	111	119	109	125	108	116	105	117	123
103	114	101	99	112	120	108	91	115	109
114	105	99	122	106	113	114	75	96	124
91	102	108	110	83	90	69	117	84	142
122	113	105	112	117	122	129	100	138	117

File names
Excel: Svls21.xls
Minitab: Svls21.mtp
TI-83Plus/ASCII: Svls21.txt

22. Black Mesa Archaeology (Single Variable Large Sample $n \geq 30$)
The following data represent rim diameters (cm) of a random sample of 40 bowls found at Black Mesa archaeological site. The diameters are estimated from broken pot shards.
Reference: Michelle Hegmon, Crow Canyon Archaeological Center, Cortez, Colorado

17.2	15.1	13.8	18.3	17.5	11.1	7.3	23.1	21.5	19.7
17.6	15.9	16.3	25.7	27.2	33.0	10.9	23.8	24.7	18.6
16.9	18.8	19.2	14.6	8.2	9.7	11.8	13.3	14.7	15.8
17.4	17.1	21.3	15.2	16.8	17.0	17.9	18.3	14.9	17.7

File names
Excel: Svls22.xls
Minitab: Svls22.mtp
TI-83Plus/ASCII: Svls22.txt

23. Wind Mountain Archaeology (Single Variable Large Sample $n \geq 30$)
The following data represent depth (cm) for a random sample of 73 significant archaeological artifacts at the Wind Mountain excavation site.
Reference: Woosley, A. and McIntyre, A. *Mimbres Mogolion Archaology*, University New Mexico press.

85	45	75	60	90	90	115	30	55	58
78	120	80	65	65	140	65	50	30	125
75	137	80	120	15	45	70	65	50	45
95	70	70	28	40	125	105	75	80	70
90	68	73	75	55	70	95	65	200	75
15	90	46	33	100	65	60	55	85	50
10	68	99	145	45	75	45	95	85	65
65	52	82							

File names
Excel: Svls23.xls
Minitab: Svls23.mtp
TI-83Plus/ASCII: Svls23.txt

24. Arrow Heads (Single Variable Large Sample $n \geq 30$)
The following data represent length (cm) of a random sample of 61 projectile points found at the Wind Mountain Archaeological site.
Reference: Woosley, A. and McIntyre, A. *Mimbres Mogolion Archaology*, University New Mexico press.

3.1	4.1	1.8	2.1	2.2	1.3	1.7	3.0	3.7	2.3
2.6	2.2	2.8	3.0	3.2	3.3	2.4	2.8	2.8	2.9
2.9	2.2	2.4	2.1	3.4	3.1	1.6	3.1	3.5	2.3
3.1	2.7	2.1	2.0	4.8	1.9	3.9	2.0	5.2	2.2
2.6	1.9	4.0	3.0	3.4	4.2	2.4	3.5	3.1	3.7
3.7	2.9	2.6	3.6	3.9	3.5	1.9	4.0	4.0	4.6
1.9									

File names
Excel: Svls24.xls
Minitab: Svls24.mtp
TI-83Plus/ASCII: Svls24.txt

25. Anasazi Indian Bracelets (Single Variable Large Sample $n \geq 30$)
The following data represent the diameter (cm) of shell bracelets and rings found at the Wind Mountain archaeological site.
Reference: Woosley, A. and McIntyre, A. *Mimbres Mogolion Archaology*, University New Mexico press.

5.0	5.0	8.0	6.1	6.0	5.1	5.9	6.8	4.3	5.5
7.2	7.0	5.0	5.6	5.3	7.0	3.4	8.2	4.3	5.2
1.5	6.1	4.0	6.0	5.5	5.2	5.2	5.2	5.5	7.2
6.0	6.2	5.2	5.0	4.0	5.7	5.1	6.1	5.7	7.3
7.3	6.7	4.2	4.0	6.0	7.1	7.3	5.5	5.8	8.9
7.5	8.3	6.8	4.9	4.0	6.2	7.7	5.0	5.2	6.8
6.1	7.2	4.4	4.0	5.0	6.0	6.2	7.2	5.8	6.8
7.7	4.7	5.3							

File names Excel: Svls25.xls
Minitab: Svls25.mtp
TI-83Plus/ASCII: Svls25.txt

26. Pizza Franchise Fees (Single Variable Large Sample $n \geq 30$)
The following data represent annual franchise fees (in thousands of dollars) for a random sample of 36 pizza franchises.
Reference: *Business Opportunities Handbook*

25.0	15.5	7.5	19.9	18.5	25.5	15.0	5.5	15.2	15.0
14.9	18.5	14.5	29.0	22.5	10.0	25.0	35.5	22.1	89.0
17.5	33.3	17.5	12.0	15.5	25.5	12.5	17.5	12.5	35.0
30.0	21.0	35.5	10.5	5.5	20.0				

File names Excel: Svls26.xls
Minitab: Svls26.mtp
TI-83Plus/ASCII: Svls26.txt

27. Pizza Franchise Start-up Requirement (Single Variable Large Sample $n \geq 30$)
The following data represent annual start-up cost (in thousands of dollars) for a random sample of 36 pizza franchises.
Reference: *Business Opportunities Handbook*

40	25	50	129	250	128	110	142	25	90
75	100	500	214	275	50	128	250	50	75
30	40	185	50	175	125	200	150	150	120
95	30	400	149	235	100				

File names Excel: Svls27.xls
Minitab: Svls27.mtp
TI-83Plus/ASCII: Svls27.txt

28. College Degrees (Single Variable Large Sample $n \geq 30$)

The following data represent percentages of the adult population with college degrees. The sample is from a random sample of 68 Midwest counties.

Reference: *County and City Data Book* 12th edition, U.S. Department of Commerce

9.9	9.8	6.8	8.9	11.2	15.5	9.8	16.8	9.9	11.6
9.2	8.4	11.3	11.5	15.2	10.8	16.3	17.0	12.8	11.0
6.0	16.0	12.1	9.8	9.4	9.9	10.5	11.8	10.3	11.1
12.5	7.8	10.7	9.6	11.6	8.8	12.3	12.2	12.4	10.0
10.0	18.1	8.8	17.3	11.3	14.5	11.0	12.3	9.1	12.7
5.6	11.7	16.9	13.7	12.5	9.0	12.7	11.3	19.5	30.7
9.4	9.8	15.1	12.8	12.9	17.5	12.3	8.2		

File names
Excel: Svls28.xls
Minitab: Svls28.mtp
TI-83Plus/ASCII: Svls28.txt

29. Poverty Level (Single Variable Large Sample $n \geq 30$)

The following data represent percentages of all persons below the poverty level. The sample is from a random collection of 80 cities in the Western U.S.

Reference: *County and City Data Book* 12th edition, U.S. Department of Commerce

12.1	27.3	20.9	14.9	4.4	21.8	7.1	16.4	13.1
9.4	9.8	15.7	29.9	8.8	32.7	5.1	9.0	16.8
21.6	4.2	11.1	14.1	30.6	15.4	20.7	37.3	7.7
19.4	18.5	19.5	8.0	7.0	20.2	6.3	12.9	13.3
30.0	4.9	14.4	14.1	22.6	18.9	16.8	11.5	19.2
21.0	11.4	7.8	6.0	37.3	44.5	37.1	28.7	9.0
17.9	16.0	20.2	11.5	10.5	17.0	3.4	3.3	15.6
16.6	29.6	14.9	23.9	13.6	7.8	14.5	19.6	31.5
28.1	19.2	4.9	12.7	15.1	9.6	23.8	10.1	

File names
Excel: Svls29.xls
Minitab: Svls29.mtp
TI-83Plus/ASCII: Svls29.txt

30. Working at Home (Single Variable Large Sample $n \geq 30$)

The following data represent percentages of adults whose primary employment involves working at home. The data is from a random sample of 50 California cities.

Reference: *County and City Data Book* 12th edition, U.S. Department of Commerce

4.3	5.1	3.1	8.7	4.0	5.2	11.8	3.4	8.5	3.0
4.3	6.0	3.7	3.7	4.0	3.3	2.8	2.8	2.6	4.4
7.0	8.0	3.7	3.3	3.7	4.9	3.0	4.2	5.4	6.6
2.4	2.5	3.5	3.3	5.5	9.6	2.7	5.0	4.8	4.1
3.8	4.8	14.3	9.2	3.8	3.6	6.5	2.6	3.5	8.6

File names
Excel: Svls30.xls
Minitab: Svls30.mtp
TI-83Plus/ASCII: Svls30.txt

Single Variable Small Sample ($n < 30$)
File name prefix: SVSS followed by the number of the data file

01. Number of Pups in Wolf Den (Single Variable Small Sample $n < 30$)
The following data represent the number of wolf pups per den from a random sample of 16 wolf dens.
Reference: *The Wolf in the Southwest: The Making of an Endangered Species*, Brown, D.E., University of Arizona Press

5 8 7 5 3 4 3 9
5 8 5 6 5 6 4 7

File names Excel: Svss01.xls
Minitab: Svss01.mtp
TI-83plus/ASCII: Svss01.txt

02. Glucose Blood Level (Single Variable Small Sample $n < 30$)
The following data represent glucose blood level (mg/100ml) after a 12-hour fast for a random sample of 6 tests given to an individual adult female.
Reference: *American J. Clin. Nutr. Vol. 19*, p345-351

83 83 86 86 78 88

File names Excel: Svss02.xls
Minitab: Svss02.mtp
TI-83plus/ASCII: Svss02.txt

03. Length of Remission (Single Variable Small Sample $n < 30$)
The drug 6-mP (6-mercaptopurine) is used to treat leukemia. The following data represent the length of remission in weeks for a random sample of 21 patients using 6-mP.
Reference: E.A. Gehan, University of Texas Cancer Center

10 7 32 23 22 6 16 34 32 25
11 20 19 6 17 35 6 13 9 6
10

File names Excel: Svss03.xls
Minitab: Svss03.mtp
TI-83plus/ASCII: Svss03.txt

04. Entry Level Jobs (Single Variable Small Sample $n < 30$)
The following data represent percentage of entry-level jobs in a random sample of 16 Denver neighborhoods.
Reference: The Piton Foundation, Denver, Colorado

8.9 22.6 18.5 9.2 8.2 24.3 15.3 3.7
9.2 14.9 4.7 11.6 16.5 11.6 9.7 8.0

File names Excel: Svss04.xls
Minitab: Svss04.mtp
TI-83plus/ASCII: Svss04.txt

05. Licensed Child Care Slots (Single Variable Small Sample $n < 30$)

The following data represents the number of licensed childcare slots in a random sample of 15 Denver neighborhoods.
Reference: The Piton Foundation, Denver, Colorado

523	106	184	121	357	319	656	170
241	226	741	172	266	423	212	

File names
Excel: Svss05.xls
Minitab: Svss05.mtp
TI-83plus/ASCII: Svss05.txt

06. Subsidized Housing (Single Variable Small Sample $n < 30$)

The following data represent the percentage of subsidized housing in a random sample of 14 Denver neighborhoods.
Reference: The Piton Foundation, Denver, Colorado

10.2	11.8	9.7	22.3	6.8	10.4	11.0
5.4	6.6	13.7	13.6	6.5	16.0	24.8

File names
Excel: Svss06.xls
Minitab: Svss06.mtp
TI-83plus/ASCII: Svss06.txt

07. Sulfate in Ground Water (Single Variable Small Sample $n < 30$)

The following data represent naturally occurring amounts of sulfate $S0_4$ in well water. Units: parts per million. The data is from a random sample of 24 water wells in Northwest Texas.
Reference: Union Carbide Corporation Technical Report K/UR-1

1850	1150	1340	1325	2500	1060	1220	2325	460
2000	1500	1775	620	1950	780	840	2650	975
860	495	1900	1220	2125	990			

File names
Excel: Svss07.xls
Minitab: Svss07.mtp
TI-83plus/ASCII: Svss07.txt

08. Earth's Rotation Rate (Single Variable Small Sample $n < 30$)

The following data represent changes in the earth's rotation (i.e. day length). Units 0.00001 second. The data is for a random sample of 23 years.
Reference: *Acta Astron. Sinica* Vol. 15, p79-85

-12	110	78	126	-35	104	111	22	-31	92
51	36	231	-13	65	119	21	104	112	-15
137	139	101							

File names
Excel: Svss08.xls
Minitab: Svss08.mtp
TI-83plus/ASCII: Svss08.txt

09. Blood Glucose (Single Variable Small Sample $n < 30$)

The following data represent glucose levels (mg/100ml) in the blood for a random sample of 27 non-obese adult subjects.

Reference: *Diabetologia*, Vol. 16, p 17-24

80	85	75	90	70	97	91	85	90	85
105	86	78	92	93	90	80	102	90	90
99	93	91	86	98	86	92			

File names
Excel: Svss09.xls
Minitab: Svss09.mtp
TI-83plus/ASCII: Svss09.txt

10. Plant Species (Single Variable Small Sample $n < 30$)

The following data represent the observed number of native plant species from random samples of study plots on different islands in the Galapagos Island chain.

Reference: *Science*, Vol. 179, p 893-895

23	26	33	73	21	35	30	16	3	17
9	8	9	19	65	12	11	89	81	7
23	95	4	37	28					

File names
Excel: Svss10.xls
Minitab: Svss10.mtp
TI-83plus/ASCII: Svss10.txt

11. Apples (Single Variable Small Sample $n < 30$)

The following data represent mean fruit weight (grams) of apples per tree for a random sample of 28 trees in an agricultural experiment.

Reference: *Aust. J. Agric res.*, Vol. 25, p783-790

85.3	86.9	96.8	108.5	113.8	87.7	94.5	99.9	92.9
67.3	90.6	129.8	48.9	117.5	100.8	94.5	94.4	98.9
96.0	99.4	79.1	108.5	84.6	117.5	70.0	104.4	127.1
135.0								

File names
Excel: Svss11.xls
Minitab: Svss11.mtp
TI-83plus/ASCII: Svss11.txt

Time Series Data for Control Charts or P Charts
File name prefix: Tscc followed by the number of the data file

01. Yield of Wheat (Time Series for Control Chart)

The following data represent annual yield of wheat in tonnes (one ton = 1.016 tonne) for an experimental plot of land at Rothamsted experiment station U.K. over a period of thirty consecutive years.
Reference: Rothamsted Experiment Station U.K.

We will use the following target production values:
target mu = 2.6 tonnes
target sigma = 0.40 tonnes

1.73	1.66	1.36	1.19	2.66	2.14	2.25	2.25	2.36	2.82
2.61	2.51	2.61	2.75	3.49	3.22	2.37	2.52	3.43	3.47
3.20	2.72	3.02	3.03	2.36	2.83	2.76	2.07	1.63	3.02

File names   Excel: Tscc01.xls
Minitab: Tscc01.mtp
TI-83plus/ASCII: Tscc01.txt

02. Pepsico Stock Closing Prices (Time Series for Control Chart)

The following data represent a random sample of 25 weekly closing prices in dollars per share of Pepsico stock for 25 consecutive days.
Reference: *The Denver Post*
The long term estimates for weekly closings are
target mu = 37 dollars per share
target sigma = 1.75 dollars per share

37.000	36.500	36.250	35.250	35.625	36.500	37.000	36.125
35.125	37.250	37.125	36.750	38.000	38.875	38.750	39.500
39.875	41.500	40.750	39.250	39.000	40.500	39.500	40.500
37.875							

File names   Excel: Tscc02.xls
Minitab: Tscc02.mtp
TI-83plus/ASCII: Tscc02.txt

03. Pepsico Stock Volume Of Sales (Time Series for Control Chart)

The following data represent volume of sales (in hundreds of thousands of shares) of Pepsico stock for 25 consecutive days.
Reference: The Denver Post, business section
For the long term mu and sigma use
target mu = 15
target sigma = 4.5

19.00	29.63	21.60	14.87	16.62	12.86	12.25	20.87
23.09	21.71	11.14	5.52	9.48	21.10	15.64	10.79
13.37	11.64	7.69	9.82	8.24	12.11	7.47	12.67
12.33							

File names
Excel: Tscc03.xls
Minitab: Tscc03.mtp
TI-83plus/ASCII: Tscc03.txt

04. Futures Quotes For The Price Of Coffee Beans (Time Series for Control Chart)

The following data represent futures options quotes for the price of coffee beans (dollars per pound) for 20 consecutive business days.
Use the following estimated target values for pricing
target mu = $2.15
target sigma = $0.12

2.300	2.360	2.270	2.180	2.150	2.180	2.120	2.090	2.150	2.200
2.170	2.160	2.100	2.040	1.950	1.860	1.910	1.880	1.940	1.990

File names
Excel: Tscc04.xls
Minitab: Tscc04.mtp
TI-83plus/ASCII: Tscc04.txt

05. Incidence Of Melanoma Tumors (Time Series for Control Chart)

The following data represent number of cases of melanoma skin cancer (per 100,000 population) in Connecticut for each of the years 1953 to 1972.
Reference: *Inst. J. Cancer*, Vol. 25, p95-104
Use the following long term values (mu and sigma)
target mu = 3
target sigma = 0.9

2.4	2.2	2.9	2.5	2.6	3.2	3.8	4.2	3.9	3.7
3.3	3.7	3.9	4.1	3.8	4.7	4.4	4.8	4.8	4.8

File names
Excel: Tscc05.xls
Minitab: Tscc05.mtp
TI-83plus/ASCII: Tscc05.txt

06. Percent Change In Consumer Price Index (Time Series for Control Chart)

The following data represent annual percent change in consumer price index for a sequence of recent years.

Reference: *Statistical Abstract Of The United States*

Suppose an economist recommends the following long term target values for mu and sigma.

target mu = 4.0%
target sigma = 1.0%

1.3	1.3	1.6	2.9	3.1	4.2	5.5	5.7	4.4	3.2
6.2	11.0	9.1	5.8	6.5	7.6	11.3	13.5	10.3	6.2
3.2	4.3	3.6	1.9	3.6	4.1	4.8	5.4	4.2	3.0

File names Excel: Tscc06.xls
Minitab: Tscc06.mtp
TI-83plus/ASCII: Tscc06.txt

07. Broken Eggs (Time Series for *P* Chart)

The following data represent the number of broken eggs in a case of 10 dozen eggs (120 eggs). The data represent 21 days or 3 weeks of deliveries to a small grocery store.

14	23	18	9	17	14	12	11	10	17
12	25	18	15	19	22	14	22	15	10
13									

File names Excel: Tscc07.xls
Minitab: Tscc07.mtp
TI-83plus/ASCII: Tscc07.txt

08. Theater Seats (Time Series for *P* Chart)

The following data represent the number of empty seats at each show of a Community Theater production. The theater has 325 seats. The show ran 18 times.

28	19	41	38	32	47	53	17	29
32	31	27	25	33	26	62	15	12

File names Excel: Tscc08.xls
Minitab: Tscc08.mtp
TI-83plus/ASCII: Tscc08.txt

09. Rain (Time Series for *P* Chart)

The following data represents the number of rainy days at Waikiki beach, Hawaii during the prime tourist season of December and January (62 days). The data was taken over a 20-year period.

21	27	19	17	6	9	25	36	23	26
12	16	27	41	18	8	10	22	15	24

File names Excel: Tscc09.xls
Minitab: Tscc09.mtp
TI-83plus/ASCII: Tscc09.txt

10. Quality Control (Time Series for *P* Chart)

The following data represent the number of defective toys in a case of 500 toys coming off a production line. Every day for 35 consecutive days, a case was selected at random.

26	23	33	49	28	42	29	41	27	25
35	21	48	12	5	15	36	55	13	16
93	8	38	11	39	18	7	33	29	42
26	19	47	53	61					

File names

Excel: Tscc10.xls
Minitab: Tscc10.mtp
TI-83plus/ASCII: Tscc10.txt

Two Variable Independent Samples
File name prefix: Tvis followed by the number of the data file

01. Heights of Football Players Versus Heights of Basketball Players
(Two variable independent large samples)
The following data represent heights in feet of 45 randomly selected pro football players, and 40 randomly selected pro basketball players.
Reference: Sports Encyclopedia Pro Football, and Official NBA Basketball Encyclopedia

X1 = heights (ft.) of pro football players
6.33 6.50 6.50 6.25 6.50 6.33 6.25 6.17 6.42 6.33
6.42 6.58 6.08 6.58 6.50 6.42 6.25 6.67 5.91 6.00
5.83 6.00 5.83 5.08 6.75 5.83 6.17 5.75 6.00 5.75
6.50 5.83 5.91 5.67 6.00 6.08 6.17 6.58 6.50 6.25
6.33 5.25 6.67 6.50 5.83

X2 = heights (ft.) of pro basketball players
6.08 6.58 6.25 6.58 6.25 5.92 7.00 6.41 6.75 6.25
6.00 6.92 6.83 6.58 6.41 6.67 6.67 5.75 6.25 6.25
6.50 6.00 6.92 6.25 6.42 6.58 6.58 6.08 6.75 6.50
6.83 6.08 6.92 6.00 6.33 6.50 6.58 6.83 6.50 6.58

File names Excel: Tvis01.xls
Minitab: Tvis02.mtp
TI-83plus/ASCII: X1 data is stored in Tvis01L1.txt
X2 data is stored in Tvis01L2.txt

02. Petal Length for Iris Virginica Versus Petal Length for Iris Setosa
(Two variable independent large samples)
The following data represent petal length (cm.) for a random sample of 35 iris virginica and a random sample of 38 iris setosa
Reference: Anderson, E., *Bull. Amer. Iris Soc.*

X1 = petal length (c.m.) iris virginica
5.1 5.8 6.3 6.1 5.1 5.5 5.3 5.5 6.9 5.0 4.9 6.0 4.8 6.1 5.6 5.1
5.6 4.8 5.4 5.1 5.1 5.9 5.2 5.7 5.4 4.5 6.1 5.3 5.5 6.7 5.7 4.9
4.8 5.8 5.1

X2 = petal length (c.m.) iris setosa
1.5 1.7 1.4 1.5 1.5 1.6 1.4 1.1 1.2 1.4 1.7 1.0 1.7 1.9 1.6 1.4
1.5 1.4 1.2 1.3 1.5 1.3 1.6 1.9 1.4 1.6 1.5 1.4 1.6 1.2 1.9 1.5
1.6 1.4 1.3 1.7 1.5 1.7

File names Excel: Tvis02.xls
Minitab: Tvis02.mtp
TI-83plus/ASCII: X1 data is stored in Tvis02L1.txt
X2 data is stored in Tvis02L2.txt

03. Sepal Width Of Iris Versicolor Versus Iris Virginica (Two variable independent larage samples)

The following data represent sepal width (cm.) for a random sample of 40 iris versicolor and a random sample of 42 iris virginica

Reference: Anderson, E., *Bull. Amer. Iris Soc.*

X1 = sepal width (c.m.) iris versicolor

3.2 3.2 3.1 2.3 2.8 2.8 3.3 2.4 2.9 2.7 2.0 3.0 2.2 2.9 2.9 3.1
3.0 2.7 2.2 2.5 3.2 2.8 2.5 2.8 2.9 3.0 2.8 3.0 2.9 2.6 2.4 2.4
2.7 2.7 3.0 3.4 3.1 2.3 3.0 2.5

X2 = sepal width (c.m.) iris virginica

3.3 2.7 3.0 2.9 3.0 3.0 2.5 2.9 2.5 3.6 3.2 2.7 3.0 2.5 2.8 3.2
3.0 3.8 2.6 2.2 3.2 2.8 2.8 2.7 3.3 3.2 2.8 3.0 2.8 3.0 2.8 3.8
2.8 2.8 2.6 3.0 3.4 3.1 3.0 3.1 3.1 3.1

File names
Excel: Tvis03.xls
Minitab: Tvis03.mtp
TI-83plus/ASCII: X1 data is stored in Tvis03L1.txt
X2 data is stored in Tvis03L2.txt

04. Archaeology, Ceramics (Two variable independent large samples)

The following data represent independent random samples of shard counts of painted ceramics found at the Wind Mountain archaeological site.

Reference: Woosley and McIntyre, *Mimbres Mogollon Archaeology*, Univ. New Mexico Press

X1 = count Mogollon red on brown

52 10 8 71 7 31 24 20 17 5
16 75 25 17 14 33 13 17 12 19
67 13 35 14 3 7 9 19 16 22
7 10 9 49 6 13 24 45 14 20
3 6 30 41 26 32 14 33 1 48
44 14 16 15 13 8 61 11 12 16
20 39

X2 = count Mimbres black on white

61 21 78 9 14 12 34 54 10 15
43 9 7 67 18 18 24 54 8 10
16 6 17 14 25 22 25 13 23 12
36 10 56 35 79 69 41 36 18 25
27 27 11 13

File names
Excel: Tvis04.xls
Minitab: Tvis04.mtp
TI-83plus/ASCII: X1 data is stored in Tvis04L1.txt
X2 data is stored in Tvis04L2.txt

05. Agriculture, Water Content of Soil (Two variable independent large samples)

The following data represent soil water content (% water by volume) for independent random samples of soil from two experimental fields growing bell peppers.
Reference: *Journal of Agricultural, Biological, and Environmental Statistics*, Vol. 2, No. 2, p 149-155

X1 = soil water content from field I

15.1	11.2	10.3	10.8	16.6	8.3	9.1	12.3	9.1	14.3
10.7	16.1	10.2	15.2	8.9	9.5	9.6	11.3	14.0	11.3
15.6	11.2	13.8	9.0	8.4	8.2	12.0	13.9	11.6	16.0
9.6	11.4	8.4	8.0	14.1	10.9	13.2	13.8	14.6	10.2
11.5	13.1	14.7	12.5	10.2	11.8	11.0	12.7	10.3	10.8
11.0	12.6	10.8	9.6	11.5	10.6	11.7	10.1	9.7	9.7
11.2	9.8	10.3	11.9	9.7	11.3	10.4	12.0	11.0	10.7
8.8	11.1								

X2 = soil water content from field II

12.1	10.2	13.6	8.1	13.5	7.8	11.8	7.7	8.1	9.2
14.1	8.9	13.9	7.5	12.6	7.3	14.9	12.2	7.6	8.9
13.9	8.4	13.4	7.1	12.4	7.6	9.9	26.0	7.3	7.4
14.3	8.4	13.2	7.3	11.3	7.5	9.7	12.3	6.9	7.6
13.8	7.5	13.3	8.0	11.3	6.8	7.4	11.7	11.8	7.7
12.6	7.7	13.2	13.9	10.4	12.8	7.6	10.7	10.7	10.9
12.5	11.3	10.7	13.2	8.9	12.9	7.7	9.7	9.7	11.4
11.9	13.4	9.2	13.4	8.8	11.9	7.1	8.5	14.0	14.2

File names
Excel: Tvis05.xls
Minitab: Tvis05.mtp
TI-83plus/ASCII: X1 data is stored in Tvis05L1.txt
X2 data is stored in Tvis05L2.txt

06. Rabies (Two variable independent small samples)

The following data represent number of cases of red fox rabies for a random sample of 16 areas in each of two different regions of southern Germany.
Reference: Sayers, B., *Medical Informatics*, Vol. 2, 11-34

X1 = number cases in region 1
10 2 2 5 3 4 3 3 4 0 2 6 4 8 7 4

X2 = number cases in region 2
1 1 2 1 3 9 2 2 4 5 4 2 2 0 0 2

File names
Excel: Tvis06.xls
Minitab: Tvis06.mtp
TI-83plus/ASCII: X1 data is stored in Tvis06L1.txt
X2 data is stored in Tvis06L2.txt

07. Weight of Football Players Versus Weight of Basketball Players (Two variable independent small samples)

The following data represent weights in pounds of 21 randomly selected pro football players, and 19 randomly selected pro basketball players.

Reference: *Sports Encyclopedia of Pro Football*, and *Official **NBA** Basketball Encyclopedia*

X1 = weights (lb) of pro football players

245	262	255	251	244	276	240	265	257	252	282
256	250	264	270	275	245	275	253	265	270	

X2 = weights (lb) of pro basketball

205	200	220	210	191	215	221	216	228	207
225	208	195	191	207	196	181	193	201	

File names
Excel: Tvis07.xls
Minitab: Tvis07.mtp
TI-83plus/ASCII: X1 data is stored in Tvis07L1.txt
X2 data is stored in Tvis07L2.txt

08. Birth Rate (Two variable independent small samples)

The following data represent birth rate (per 1000 residential population) for independent random samples of counties in California and Maine.

Reference: *County and City Data Book* 12th edition, U.S. Dept. of Commerce

X1 = birth rate in California counties

14.1	18.7	20.4	20.7	16.0	12.5	12.9	9.6	17.6
18.1	14.1	16.6	15.1	18.5	23.6	19.9	19.6	14.9
17.7	17.8	19.1	22.1	15.6				

X2 = birth rate in Maine counties

15.1	14.0	13.3	13.8	13.5	14.2	14.7	11.8	13.5	13.8
16.5	13.8	13.2	12.5	14.8	14.1	13.6	13.9	15.8	

File names
Excel: Tvis08.xls
Minitab: Tvis08.mtp
TI-83plus/ASCII: X1 data is stored in Tvis08L1.txt
X2 data is stored in Tvis08L2.txt

09. Death Rate (Two variable independent small samples)
The following data represents death rate (per 1000 resident population) for independent random samples of counties in Alaska and Texas.
Reference: *County and City Data Book* 12th edition, U.S. Dept. of Commerce

X1 = death rate in Alaska counties
1.4 4.2 7.3 4.8 3.2 3.4 5.1 5.4
6.7 3.3 1.9 8.3 3.1 6.0 4.5 2.5

X2 = death rate in Texas counties
7.2 5.8 10.5 6.6 6.9 9.5 8.6 5.9 9.1
5.4 8.8 6.1 9.5 9.6 7.8 10.2 5.6 8.6

File names Excel: Tvis09.xls
Minitab: Tvis09.mtp
TI-83plus/ASCII: X1 data is stored in Tvis09L1.txt
X2 data is stored in Tvis09L2.txt

10. Pickup Trucks (Two variable independent small samples)
The following data represents retail price (in thousands of dollars) for independent random samples of models of pickup trucks.
Reference: *Consumer Guide* Vol.681

X1 = prices for different GMC Sierra 1500 models
17.4 23.3 29.2 19.2 17.6 19.2 23.6 19.5 22.2
24.0 26.4 23.7 29.4 23.7 26.7 24.0 24.9

X2 = prices for different Chevrolet Silverado 1500 models
17.5 23.7 20.8 22.5 24.3 26.7 24.5 17.8
29.4 29.7 20.1 21.1 22.1 24.2 27.4 28.1

File names Excel: Tvis10.xls
Minitab: Tvis10.mtp
TI-83plus/ASCII: X1 data is stored in Tvis10L1.txt
X2 data is stored in Tvis10L2.txt

Two Variable Dependent Samples
File name prefix: Tvds followed by the number of the data file

01. Average Faculty Salary, Males vs Female (Two variable dependent samples)

In following data pairs

A = average salaries for males ($1000/yr)

B = average salaries for females ($1000/yr)

for assistant professors at the same college or university. A random sample of 22 US. colleges and universities was used.

Reference: *Academe, Bulletin of the American Association of University Professors*

A:	34.5	30.5	35.1	35.7	31.5	34.4	32.1	30.7	33.7	35.3
B:	33.9	31.2	35.0	34.2	32.4	34.1	32.7	29.9	31.2	35.5

A:	30.7	34.2	39.6	30.5	33.8	31.7	32.8	38.5	40.5	25.3
B:	30.2	34.8	38.7	30.0	33.8	32.4	31.7	38.9	41.2	25.5

A:	28.6	35.8
B:	28.0	35.1

File names

Excel: Tvds01.xls

Minitab: Tvds01.mtp

TI-83plus/ASCII: A data is stored in Tvds01L1.txt

B data is stored in Tvds01L2.txt

02. Unemployment for College Graduates Versus High School Only (Two variable dependent samples)

In the following data pairs

A = Percent unemployment for college graduates

B = Percent unemployment for high school only graduates

The data are paired by year

Reference: *Statistical Abstract of the United States*

A:	2.8	2.2	2.2	1.7	2.3	2.3	2.4	2.7	3.5	3.0	1.9	2.5
B:	5.9	4.9	4.8	5.4	6.3	6.9	6.9	7.2	10.0	8.5	5.1	6.9

File names

Excel: Tvds02.xls

Minitab: Tvds02.mtp

TI-83plus/ASCII: A data is stored in Tvds02L1.txt

B data is stored in Tvds02L2.txt

03. Number of Navajo Hogans versus Modern Houses (Two variable dependent samples)

In the following data pairs
A = Number of traditional Navajo hogans in a given district
B = Number of modern houses in a given district
The data are paired by districts on the Navajo reservation. A random sample of 8 districts were used.
Reference: *Navajo Architecture, Forms, History, Distributions* by S.C. Jett and V.E. Spencer, Univ. of Arizona Press

A:	13	14	46	32	15	47	17	18
B:	18	16	68	9	11	28	50	50

File names
Excel: Tvds03.xls
Minitab: Tvds03.mtp
TI-83plus/ASCII: A data is stored in Tvds03L1.txt
B data is stored in Tvds03L2.txt

04. Temperatures in Miami versus Honolulu (Two variable dependent samples)

In the following data pairs
A = Average monthly temperature in Miami
B = Average monthly temperature in Honolulu
The data are paired by month.
Reference: U.S. Department of Commerce Environmental Data Service

A:	67.5	68.0	71.3	74.9	78.0	80.9	82.2	82.7	81.6	77.8	72.3	68.5
B:	74.4	72.6	73.3	74.7	76.2	78.0	79.1	79.8	79.5	78.4	76.1	73.7

File names
Excel: Tvds04.xls
Minitab: Tvds04.mtp
TI-83plus/ASCII: A data is stored in Tvds04L1.txt
B data is stored in Tvds04L2.txt

05. January/February Ozone Column (Two variable dependent samples)

In the following pairs the data represents the thickness of the ozone column in Dobson units: one milli-centimeter ozone at standard temperature and pressure.
A = monthly mean thickness in January
B = monthly mean thickness in February
The data are paired by year for a random sample of 15 years.
Reference: Laboratorium für Atmospharensphysic, Switzerland

A:	360	324	377	336	383	361	369	349
B:	365	325	359	352	397	351	367	397

A:	301	354	344	329	337	387	378
B:	335	338	349	393	370	400	411

File names
Excel: Tvds05.xls
Minitab: Tvds05.mtp
TI-83plus/ASCII: A data is stored in Tvds05L1.txt
B data is stored in Tvds05L2.txt

06. Birth Rate/Death Rate (Two variable dependent samples)

In the following data pairs,

A = birth rate (per 1000 resident population)
B = death rate (per 1000 resident population)

The data are paired by county in Iowa
Reference: *County and City Data Book* 12th edition, U.S. Dept. of Commerce

A:	12.7	13.4	12.8	12.1	11.6	11.1	14.2
B:	9.8	14.5	10.7	14.2	13.0	12.9	10.9

A:	12.5	12.3	13.1	15.8	10.3	12.7	11.1
B:	14.1	13.6	9.1	10.2	17.9	11.8	7.0

File names Excel: Tvds06.xls
Minitab: Tvds06.mtp
TI-83plus/ASCII: A data is stored in Tvds06L1.txt
B data is stored in Tvds06L2.txt

07. Democrat/Republican (Two variable dependent samples)

In the following data pairs

A = percentage of voters who voted Democrat
B = percentage of voters who voted Republican

in a recent national election. The data are paired by county in Indiana
Reference: *County and City Data Book* 12th edition, U.S. Dept. of Commerce

A:	42.2	34.5	44.0	34.1	41.8	40.7	36.4	43.3	39.5
B:	35.4	45.8	39.4	40.0	39.2	40.2	44.7	37.3	40.8

A:	35.4	44.1	41.0	42.8	40.8	36.4	40.6	37.4
B:	39.3	36.8	35.5	33.2	38.3	47.7	41.1	38.5

File names Excel: Tvds07.xls
Minitab: Tvds07.mtp
TI-83plus/ASCII: A data is stored in Tvds07L1.txt
B data is stored in Tvds07L2.txt

08. Santiago Pueblo Pottery (Two variable dependent samples)

In the following data

A = percentage of utility pottery
B = percentage of ceremonial pottery

found at the Santiago Pueblo archaeological site. The data are paired by location of discovery.
Reference: Laboratory of Anthropology, Notes 475, Santa Fe, New Mexico

A:	41.4	49.6	55.6	49.5	43.0	54.6	46.8	51.1	43.2	41.4
B:	58.6	50.4	44.4	59.5	57.0	45.4	53.2	48.9	56.8	58.6

File names Excel: Tvds08.xls
Minitab: Tvds08.mtp
TI-83plus/ASCII: A data is stored in Tvds08L1.txt
B data is stored in Tvds08L2.txt

09. Poverty Level (Two variable dependent samples)

In the following data pairs

A = percentage of population below poverty level in 1998

B = percentage of population below poverty level in 1990

The data are grouped by state and District of Columbia

Reference: *Statistical Abstract of the United States*, 120th edition

A:	14.5	9.4	16.6	14.8	15.4	9.2	9.5	10.3	22.3	13.1
B:	19.2	11.4	13.7	19.6	13.9	13.7	6.0	6.9	21.1	14.4

A:	13.6	10.9	13.0	10.1	9.4	9.1	9.6	13.5	19.1	10.4
B:	15.8	11.0	14.9	13.7	13.0	10.4	10.3	17.3	23.6	13.1

A:	7.2	8.7	11.0	10.4	17.6	9.8	16.6	12.3	10.6	9.8
B:	9.9	10.7	14.3	12.0	25.7	13.4	16.3	10.3	9.8	6.3

A:	8.6	20.4	16.7	14.0	15.1	11.2	14.1	15.0	11.2	11.6
B:	9.2	20.9	14.3	13.0	13.7	11.5	15.6	9.2	11.0	7.5

A:	13.7	10.8	13.4	15.1	9.0	9.9	8.8	8.9	17.8	8.8	10.6
B:	16.2	13.3	16.9	15.9	8.2	10.9	11.1	8.9	18.1	9.3	11.0

File names

Excel: Tvds09.xls
Minitab: Tvds09.mtp
TI-83plus/ASCII: A data is stored in Tvds09L1.txt
B data is stored in Tvds09L2.txt

10. Cost of Living Index (Two variable dependent samples)

The following data pairs represent cost of living index for

A = grocery items

B = health care

The data are grouped by metropolitan areas.

Reference: *Statistical Abstract of the United States*, 120th edition

Grocery

A: 96.6	97.5	113.9	88.9	108.3	99.0	97.3	87.5	96.8
B: 91.6	95.9	114.5	93.6	112.7	93.6	99.2	93.2	105.9

A: 102.1	114.5	100.9	100.0	100.7	99.4	117.1	111.3	102.2
B: 110.8	127.0	91.5	100.5	104.9	104.8	124.1	124.6	109.1

A: 95.3	91.1	95.7	87.5	91.8	97.9	97.4	102.1	94.0
B: 98.7	95.8	99.7	93.2	100.7	96.0	99.6	98.4	94.0

A: 115.7	118.3	101.9	88.9	100.7	99.8	101.3	104.8	100.9
B: 121.2	122.4	110.8	81.2	104.8	109.9	103.5	113.6	94.6

A: 102.7	98.1	105.3	97.2	105.2	108.1	110.5	99.3	99.7
B: 109.8	97.6	109.8	107.4	97.7	124.2	110.9	106.8	94.8

File names

Excel: Tvds10.xls

Minitab: Tvds10.mtp

TI-83plus/ASCII: A data is stored in Tvds10L1.txt

B data is stored in Tvds10L2.txt

Simple Linear Regression
File name prefix: Slr followed by the number of the data file

01. List Price versus Best Price for a New GMC Pickup Truck (Simple Linear Regression)

In the following data

X = List price (in $1000) for a GMC pickup truck

Y = Best price (in $1000) for a GMC pickup truck

Reference: *Consumer's Digest*

X:	12.4	14.3	14.5	14.9	16.1	16.9	16.5	15.4	17.0	17.9
Y:	11.2	12.5	12.7	13.1	14.1	14.8	14.4	13.4	14.9	15.6

X:	18.8	20.3	22.4	19.4	15.5	16.7	17.3	18.4	19.2	17.4
Y:	16.4	17.7	19.6	16.9	14.0	14.6	15.1	16.1	16.8	15.2

X:	19.5	19.7	21.2
Y:	17.0	17.2	18.6

File names

Excel: Slr01.xls

Minitab: Slr01.mtp

TI-83plus/ASCII: X data is stored in Slr01L1.txt

Y data is stored in Slr01L2.txt

02. Cricket Chirps versus Temperature (Simple Linear Regression)

In the following data

X = chirps/sec for the striped ground cricket

Y = temperature in degrees Fahrenheit

Reference: T*he Song of Insects* by Dr.G.W. Pierce, Harvard College Press

X:	20.0	16.0	19.8	18.4	17.1	15.5	14.7	17.1
Y:	88.6	71.6	93.3	84.3	80.6	75.2	69.7	82.0

X:	15.4	16.2	15.0	17.2	16.0	17.0	14.4
Y:	69.4	83.3	79.6	82.6	80.6	83.5	76.3

File names

Excel: Slr02.xls

Minitab: Slr02.mtp

TI-83plus/ASCII: X data is stored in Slr02L1.txt

Y data is stored in Slr02L2.txt

03. Diameter of Sand Granules versus Slope on Beach (Simple Linear Regression)

In the following data pairs

X = median diameter (mm) of granules of sand

Y = gradient of beach slope in degrees

The data is for naturally occurring ocean beaches

Reference: *Physical geography* by A.M King, Oxford Press, England

X:	0.170	0.190	0.220	0.235	0.235	0.300	0.350	0.420	0.850
Y:	0.630	0.700	0.820	0.880	1.150	1.500	4.400	7.300	11.300

File names

Excel: Slr03.xls
Minitab: Slr03.mtp
TI-83plus/ASCII: X data is stored in Slr03L1.txt
Y data is stored in Slr03L2.txt

04. National Unemployment Male versus Female (Simple Linear Regression)

In the following data pairs

X = national unemployment rate for adult males

Y = national unemployment rate for adult females

Reference: *Statistical Abstract of the United States*

X:	2.9	6.7	4.9	7.9	9.8	6.9	6.1	6.2	6.0	5.1	4.7	4.4	5.8
Y:	4.0	7.4	5.0	7.2	7.9	6.1	6.0	5.8	5.2	4.2	4.0	4.4	5.2

File names

Excel: Slr04.xls
Minitab: Slr04.mtp
TI-83plus/ASCII: X data is stored in Slr04L1.txt
Y data is stored in Slr04L2.txt

05. Fire and Theft in Chicago (Simple Linear Regression)

In the following data pairs

X = fires per 1000 housing units

Y = thefts per 1000 population

within the same Zip code in the Chicago metro area

Reference: U.S. Commission on Civil Rights

X:	6.2	9.5	10.5	7.7	8.6	34.1	11.0	6.9	7.3	15.1
Y:	29	44	36	37	53	68	75	18	31	25

X:	29.1	2.2	5.7	2.0	2.5	4.0	5.4	2.2	7.2	15.1
Y:	34	14	11	11	22	16	27	9	29	30

X:	16.5	18.4	36.2	39.7	18.5	23.3	12.2	5.6	21.8	21.6
Y:	40	32	41	147	22	29	46	23	4	31

X:	9.0	3.6	5.0	28.6	17.4	11.3	3.4	11.9	10.5	10.7
Y:	39	15	32	27	32	34	17	46	42	43

X:	10.8	4.8
Y:	34	19

File names

Excel: Slr05.xls
Minitab: Slr05.mtp
TI-83plus/ASCII: X data is stored in Slr05L1.txt
Y data is stored in Slr05L2.txt

06. Auto Insurance in Sweden (Simple Linear Regression)

In the following data

X = number of claims

Y = total payment for all the claims in thousands of Swedish Kronor

for geographical zones in Sweden

Reference: Swedish Committee on Analysis of Risk Premium in Motor Insurance

X: 108	19	13	124	40	57	23	14	45	10
Y: 392.5	46.2	15.7	422.2	119.4	170.9	56.9	77.5	214.0	65.3

X: 5	48	11	23	7	2	24	6	3	23
Y: 20.9	248.1	23.5	39.6	48.8	6.6	134.9	50.9	4.4	113.0

X: 6	9	9	3	29	7	4	20	7	4
Y: 14.8	48.7	52.1	13.2	103.9	77.5	11.8	98.1	27.9	38.1

X: 0	25	6	5	22	11	61	12	4	16
Y: 0.0	69.2	14.6	40.3	161.5	57.2	217.6	58.1	12.6	59.6

X: 13	60	41	37	55	41	11	27	8	3
Y: 89.9	202.4	181.3	152.8	162.8	73.4	21.3	92.6	76.1	39.9

X: 17	13	13	15	8	29	30	24	9	31
Y: 142.1	93.0	31.9	32.1	55.6	133.3	194.5	137.9	87.4	209.8

X: 14	53	26
Y: 95.5	244.6	187.5

File names Excel: Slr06.xls

Minitab: Slr06.mtp

TI-83plus/ASCII: X data is stored in Slr06L1.txt

Y data is stored in Slr06L2.txt

07. Gray Kangaroos (Simple Linear Regression)

In the following data pairs

X = nasal length (mm ×10)

Y = nasal width (mm × 10)

for a male gray kangaroo from a random sample of such animals.

Reference: *Australian Journal of Zoology*, Vol. 28, p607-613

X: 609	629	620	564	645	493	606	660	630	672
Y: 241	222	233	207	247	189	226	240	215	231

X: 778	616	727	810	778	823	755	710	701	803
Y: 263	220	271	284	279	272	268	278	238	255

X: 855	838	830	864	635	565	562	580	596	597
Y: 308	281	288	306	236	204	216	225	220	219

X: 636	559	615	740	677	675	629	692	710	730
Y: 201	213	228	234	237	217	211	238	221	281

X: 763	686	717	737	816
Y: 292	251	231	275	275

File names

Excel: Slr07.xls
Minitab: Slr07.mtp
TI-83plus/ASCII: X data is stored in Slr07L1.txt
Y data is stored in Slr07L2.txt

08. Pressure and Weight in Cryogenic Flow Meters (Simple Linear Regression)

In the following data pairs

X = pressure (lb/sq in) of liquid nitrogen

Y = weight in pounds of liquid nitrogen passing through flow meter each second

Reference: *Technometrics*, Vol. 19, p353-379

X: 75.1	74.3	88.7	114.6	98.5	112.0	114.8	62.2	107.0
Y: 577.8	577.0	570.9	578.6	572.4	411.2	531.7	563.9	406.7

X: 90.5	73.8	115.8	99.4	93.0	73.9	65.7	66.2	77.9
Y: 507.1	496.4	505.2	506.4	510.2	503.9	506.2	506.3	510.2

X: 109.8	105.4	88.6	89.6	73.8	101.3	120.0	75.9	76.2
Y: 508.6	510.9	505.4	512.8	502.8	493.0	510.8	512.8	513.4

X: 81.9	84.3	98.0
Y: 510.0	504.3	522.0

File names

Excel: Slr08.xls
Minitab: Slr08.mtp
TI-83plus/ASCII: X data is stored in Slr08L1.txt
Y data is stored in Slr07L2.txt

09. Ground Water Survey (Simple Linear Regression)

In the following data

X = pH of well water

Y = Bicarbonate (parts per million) of well water

The data is by water well from a random sample of wells in Northwest Texas.

Reference: Union Carbide Technical Report K/UR-1

X:	7.6	7.1	8.2	7.5	7.4	7.8	7.3	8.0	7.1	7.5
Y:	157	174	175	188	171	143	217	190	142	190

X:	8.1	7.0	7.3	7.8	7.3	8.0	8.5	7.1	8.2	7.9
Y:	215	199	262	105	121	81	82	210	202	155

X:	7.6	8.8	7.2	7.9	8.1	7.7	8.4	7.4	7.3	8.5
Y:	157	147	133	53	56	113	35	125	76	48

X:	7.8	6.7	7.1	7.3
Y:	147	117	182	87

File names Excel: Slr09.xls
Minitab: Slr09.mtp
TI-83plus/ASCII: X data is stored in Slr09L1.txt
Y data is stored in Slr09L2.txt

10. Iris Setosa (Simple Linear Regression)

In the following data

X = sepal width (cm)

Y = sepal length (cm)

The data is for a random sample of the wild flower iris setosa.

Reference: Fisher, R.A., *Ann. Eugenics,* Vol. 7 Part II, p 179-188

X:	3.5	3.0	3.2	3.1	3.6	3.9	3.4	3.4	2.9	3.1
Y:	5.1	4.9	4.7	4.6	5.0	5.4	4.6	5.0	4.4	4.9

X:	3.7	3.4	3.0	4.0	4.4	3.9	3.5	3.8	3.8	3.4
Y:	5.4	4.8	4.3	5.8	5.7	5.4	5.1	5.7	5.1	5.4

X:	3.7	3.6	3.3	3.4	3.0	3.4	3.5	3.4	3.2	3.1
Y:	5.1	4.6	5.1	4.8	5.0	5.0	5.2	5.2	4.7	4.8

X:	3.4	4.1	4.2	3.1	3.2	3.5	3.6	3.0	3.4	3.5
Y:	5.4	5.2	5.5	4.9	5.0	5.5	4.9	4.4	5.1	5.0

X:	2.3	3.2	3.5	3.8	3.0	3.8	3.7	3.3
Y:	4.5	4.4	5.0	5.1	4.8	4.6	5.3	5.0

File names Excel: Slr10.xls
Minitab: Slr10.mtp
TI-83plus/ASCII: X data is stored in Slr10L1.txt
Y data is stored in Slr10L2.txt

11. Pizza Franchise (Simple Linear Regression)

In the following data

X = annual franchise fee ($1000)
Y = start up cost ($1000)

for a pizza franchise

Reference: *Business Opportunity Handbook*

X:	25.0	8.5	35.0	15.0	10.0	30.0	10.0	50.0	17.5	16.0
Y:	125	80	330	58	110	338	30	175	120	135

X:	18.5	7.0	8.0	15.0	5.0	15.0	12.0	15.0	28.0	20.0
Y:	97	50	55	40	35	45	75	33	55	90

X:	20.0	15.0	20.0	25.0	20.0	3.5	35.0	25.0	8.5	10.0
Y:	85	125	150	120	95	30	400	148	135	45

X:	10.0	25.0
Y:	87	150

File names
Excel: Slr11.xls
Minitab: Slr11.mtp
TI-83plus/ASCII: X data is stored in Slr11L1.txt
Y data is stored in Slr11L2.txt

12. Prehistoric Pueblos (Simple Linear Regression)

In the following data

X = estimated year of initial occupation
Y = estimated year of end of occupation

The data are for each prehistoric pueblo in a random sample of such pueblos in Utah, Arizona, and Nevada.

Reference *Prehistoric Pueblo World* by A. Adler, Univ. of Arizona Press

X:	1000	1125	1087	1070	1100	1150	1250	1150	1100
Y:	1050	1150	1213	1275	1300	1300	1400	1400	1250

X:	1350	1275	1375	1175	1200	1175	1300	1260	1330
Y:	1830	1350	1450	1300	1300	1275	1375	1285	1400

X:	1325	1200	1225	1090	1075	1080	1080	1180	1225
Y:	1400	1285	1275	1135	1250	1275	1150	1250	1275

X:	1175	1250	1250	750	1125	700	900	900	850
Y:	1225	1280	1300	1250	1175	1300	1250	1300	1200

File names
Excel: Slr12.xls
Minitab: Slr12.mtp
TI-83plus/ASCII: X data is stored in Slr12L1.txt
Y data is stored in Slr12L2.txt

Multiple Linear Regression
File name prefix: Mlr followed by the number of the data file

01. Thunder Basin Antelope Study (Multiple Linear Regression)

The data (X1, X2, X3, X4) are for each year.
X1 = spring fawn count/100
X2 = size of adult antelope population/100
X3 = annual precipitation (inches)
X4 = winter severity index (1=mild , 5=severe)

X1	X2	X3	X4
2.90	9.20	13.20	2.00
2.40	8.70	11.50	3.00
2.00	7.20	10.80	4.00
2.30	8.50	12.30	2.00
3.20	9.60	12.60	3.00
1.90	6.80	10.60	5.00
3.40	9.70	14.10	1.00
2.10	7.90	11.20	3.00

File names
Excel: Mlr01.xls
Minitab: Mlr01.mtp
TI-83plus/ASCII: X1 data is stored in Mlr01L1.txt
X2 data is stored in Mlr01L2.txt
X3 data is stored in Mlr01L3.txt
X4 data is stored in Mlr01L4.txt

02. Section 10.5, problem #3 Systolic Blood Pressure Data (Multiple Linear Regression)

The data (X1, X2, X3) are for each patient.
X1 = systolic blood pressure
X2 = age in years
X3 = weight in pounds

X1	X2	X3
132.00	52.00	173.00
143.00	59.00	184.00
153.00	67.00	194.00
162.00	73.00	211.00
154.00	64.00	196.00
168.00	74.00	220.00
137.00	54.00	188.00
149.00	61.00	188.00
159.00	65.00	207.00
128.00	46.00	167.00
166.00	72.00	217.00

File names
Excel: Mlr02.xls
Minitab: Mlr02.mtp
TI-83plus/ASCII: X1 data is stored in Mlr02L1.txt
X2 data is stored in Mlr02L2.txt
X3 data is stored in Mlr02L3.txt

03. Section 10.5, Problem #4 Test Scores for General Psychology (Multiple Linear Regression)

The data (X1, X2, X3, X4) are for each student.
X1 = score on exam #1
X2 = score on exam #2
X3 = score on exam #3
X4 = score on final exam

X1	X2	X3	X4
73	80	75	152
93	88	93	185
89	91	90	180
96	98	100	196
73	66	70	142
53	46	55	101
69	74	77	149
47	56	60	115
87	79	90	175
79	70	88	164
69	70	73	141
70	65	74	141
93	95	91	184
79	80	73	152
70	73	78	148
93	89	96	192
78	75	68	147
81	90	93	183
88	92	86	177
78	83	77	159
82	86	90	177
86	82	89	175
78	83	85	175
76	83	71	149
96	93	95	192

File names Excel: Mlr03.xls
Minitab: Mlr03.mtp
TI-83plus/ASCII: X1 data is stored in Mlr03L1.txt
X2 data is stored in Mlr03L2.txt
X3 data is stored in Mlr03L3.txt
X4 data is stored in Mlr03L4.txt

04. Section 10.5, Problem #5 Hollywood Movies (Multiple Linear Regression)

The data (X1, X2, X3, X4) are for each movie
X1 = first year box office receipts/millions
X2 = total production costs/millions
X3 = total promotional costs/millions
X4 = total book sales/millions

X1	X2	X3	X4
85.10	8.50	5.10	4.70
106.30	12.90	5.80	8.80
50.20	5.20	2.10	15.10
130.60	10.70	8.40	12.20
54.80	3.10	2.90	10.60
30.30	3.50	1.20	3.50
79.40	9.20	3.70	9.70
91.00	9.00	7.60	5.90
135.40	15.10	7.70	20.80
89.30	10.20	4.50	7.90

File names
Excel: Mlr04.xls
Minitab: Mlr04.mtp
TI-83plus/ASCII: X1 data is stored in Mlr04L1.txt
X2 data is stored in Mlr04L2.txt
X3 data is stored in Mlr04L3.txt
X4 data is stored in Mlr04L4.txt

05. Section 10.5, Problem #6 All Greens Franchise (Multiple Linear Regression)

The data (X1, X2, X3, X4, X5, X6) are for each franchise store.

X1 = annual net sales/$1000
X2 = number sq. ft./1000
X3 = inventory/$1000
X4 = amount spent on advertizing/$1000
X5 = size of sales district/1000 families
X6 = number of competing stores in district

X1	X2	X3	X4	X5	X6
231.00	3.00	294.00	8.20	8.20	11.00
156.00	2.20	232.00	6.90	4.10	12.00
10.00	0.50	149.00	3.00	4.30	15.00
519.00	5.50	600.00	12.00	16.10	1.00
437.00	4.40	567.00	10.60	14.10	5.00
487.00	4.80	571.00	11.80	12.70	4.00
299.00	3.10	512.00	8.10	10.10	10.00
195.00	2.50	347.00	7.70	8.40	12.00
20.00	1.20	212.00	3.30	2.10	15.00
68.00	0.60	102.00	4.90	4.70	8.00
570.00	5.40	788.00	17.40	12.30	1.00
428.00	4.20	577.00	10.50	14.00	7.00
464.00	4.70	535.00	11.30	15.00	3.00
15.00	0.60	163.00	2.50	2.50	14.00
65.00	1.20	168.00	4.70	3.30	11.00
98.00	1.60	151.00	4.60	2.70	10.00
398.00	4.30	342.00	5.50	16.00	4.00
161.00	2.60	196.00	7.20	6.30	13.00
397.00	3.80	453.00	10.40	13.90	7.00
497.00	5.30	518.00	11.50	16.30	1.00
528.00	5.60	615.00	12.30	16.00	0.00
99.00	0.80	278.00	2.80	6.50	14.00
0.50	1.10	142.00	3.10	1.60	12.00
347.00	3.60	461.00	9.60	11.30	6.00
341.00	3.50	382.00	9.80	11.50	5.00
507.00	5.10	590.00	12.00	15.70	0.00
400.00	8.60	517.00	7.00	12.00	8.00

File names

Excel: Mlr05.xls
Minitab: Mlr05.mtp
TI-83plus/ASCII: X1 data is stored in Mlr05L1.txt
X2 data is stored in Mlr05L2.txt
X3 data is stored in Mlr05L3.txt
X4 data is stored in Mlr05L4.txt
X5 data is stored in Mlr05L5.txt
X6 data is stored in Mlr05L6.txt

06. Crime (Multiple Linear Regression)

This is a case study of education, crime, and police funding for small cities in ten eastern and south eastern states. The states are New Hampshire, Connecticut, Rhode Island, Maine, New York, Virginia, North Carolina, South Carolina, Georgia, and Florida.

The data (X1, X2, X3, X4, X5, X6, X7) are for each city.
X1 = total overall reported crime rate per 1million residents
X2 = reported violent crime rate per 100,000 residents
X3 = annual police funding in dollars per resident
X4 = percent of people 25 years and older that have had 4 years of high school
X5 = percent of 16 to 19 year-olds not in highschool and not highschool graduates.
X6 = percent of 18 to 24 year-olds enrolled in college
X7 = percent of people 25 years and older with at least 4 years of college

Reference: *Life In America's Small Cities,* By G.S. Thomas

X1	X2	X3	X4	X5	X6	X7
478	184	40	74	11	31	20
494	213	32	72	11	43	18
643	347	57	70	18	16	16
341	565	31	71	11	25	19
773	327	67	72	9	29	24
603	260	25	68	8	32	15
484	325	34	68	12	24	14
546	102	33	62	13	28	11
424	38	36	69	7	25	12
548	226	31	66	9	58	15
506	137	35	60	13	21	9
819	369	30	81	4	77	36
541	109	44	66	9	37	12
491	809	32	67	11	37	16
514	29	30	65	12	35	11
371	245	16	64	10	42	14
457	118	29	64	12	21	10
437	148	36	62	7	81	27
570	387	30	59	15	31	16
432	98	23	56	15	50	15
619	608	33	46	22	24	8
357	218	35	54	14	27	13
623	254	38	54	20	22	11
547	697	44	45	26	18	8
792	827	28	57	12	23	11
799	693	35	57	9	60	18
439	448	31	61	19	14	12
867	942	39	52	17	31	10
912	1017	27	44	21	24	9
462	216	36	43	18	23	8
859	673	38	48	19	22	10
805	989	46	57	14	25	12

Data continued

X1	X2	X3	X4	X5	X6	X7
652	630	29	47	19	25	9
776	404	32	50	19	21	9
919	692	39	48	16	32	11
732	1517	44	49	13	31	14
657	879	33	72	13	13	22
1419	631	43	59	14	21	13
989	1375	22	49	9	46	13
821	1139	30	54	13	27	12
1740	3545	86	62	22	18	15
815	706	30	47	17	39	11
760	451	32	45	34	15	10
936	433	43	48	26	23	12
863	601	20	69	23	7	12
783	1024	55	42	23	23	11
715	457	44	49	18	30	12
1504	1441	37	57	15	35	13
1324	1022	82	72	22	15	16
940	1244	66	67	26	18	16

File names

Excel: Mlr06.xls
Minitab: Mlr06.mtp
TI-83plus/ASCII: X1 data is stored in Mlr06L1.txt
X2 data is stored in Mlr06L2.txt
X3 data is stored in Mlr06L3.txt
X4 data is stored in Mlr06L4.txt
X5 data is stored in Mlr06L5.txt
X6 data is stored in Mlr06L6.txt
X7 data is stored in Mlr06L7.txt

07. Health (Multiple Linear Regression)

This is a case study of public health, income, and population density for small cities in eight Midwestern states: Ohio, Indiana, Illinois, Iowa, Missouri, Nebraska, Kansas, and Oklahoma.

The data (X1, X2, X3, X4, X5) are by city.
X1 = death rate per 1000 residents
X2 = doctor availability per 100,000 residents
X3 = hospital availability per 100,000 residents
X4 = annual per capita income in thousands of dollars
X5 = population density people per square mile

Reference: *Life In America's Small Cities*, by G.S. Thomas

X1	X2	X3	X4	X5
8.0	78	284	9.1	109
9.3	68	433	8.7	144
7.5	70	739	7.2	113
8.9	96	1792	8.9	97
10.2	74	477	8.3	206
8.3	111	362	10.9	124
8.8	77	671	10.0	152
8.8	168	636	9.1	162
10.7	82	329	8.7	150
11.7	89	634	7.6	134
8.5	149	631	10.8	292
8.3	60	257	9.5	108
8.2	96	284	8.8	111
7.9	83	603	9.5	182
10.3	130	686	8.7	129
7.4	145	345	11.2	158
9.6	112	1357	9.7	186
9.3	131	544	9.6	177
10.6	80	205	9.1	127
9.7	130	1264	9.2	179
11.6	140	688	8.3	80
8.1	154	354	8.4	103
9.8	118	1632	9.4	101
7.4	94	348	9.8	117
9.4	119	370	10.4	88
11.2	153	648	9.9	78
9.1	116	366	9.2	102
10.5	97	540	10.3	95
11.9	1 76	680	8.9	80
8.4	75	345	9.6	92
5.0	134	525	10.3	126
9.8	161	870	10.4	108
9.8	111	669	9.7	77
10.8	114	452	9.6	60
10.1	142	430	10.7	71
10.9	238	822	10.3	86

Data continued

X1	X2	X3	X4	X5
9.2	78	190	10.7	93
8.3	196	867	9.6	106
7.3	125	969	10.5	162
9.4	82	499	7.7	95
9.4	125	925	10.2	91
9.8	129	353	9.9	52
3.6	84	288	8.4	110
8.4	183	718	10.4	69
10.8	119	540	9.2	57
10.1	180	668	13.0	106
9.0	82	347	8.8	40
10.0	71	345	9.2	50
11.3	118	463	7.8	35
11.3	121	728	8.2	86
12.8	68	383	7.4	57
10.0	112	316	10.4	57
6.7	109	388	8.9	94

File names

Excel: Mlr07.xls
Minitab: Mlr07.mtp
TI-83plus/ASCII: X1 data is stored in Mlr07L1.txt
X2 data is stored in Mlr07L2.txt
X3 data is stored in Mlr07L3.txt
X4 data is stored in Mlr07L4.txt
X5 data is stored in Mlr07L5.txt

08. Baseball (Multiple Linear Regression)

A random sample of major league baseball players was obtained.

The following data (X1, X2, X3, X4, X5, X6) are by player.
X1 = batting average
X2 = runs scored/times at bat
X3 = doubles/times at bat
X4 = triples/times at bat
X5 = home runs/times at bat
X6 = strike outs/times at bat
Reference: *The Baseball Encyclopedia* 9th edition, Macmillan

X1	X2	X3	X4	X5	X6
0.283	0.144	0.049	0.012	0.013	0.086
0.276	0.125	0.039	0.013	0.002	0.062
0.281	0.141	0.045	0.021	0.013	0.074
0.328	0.189	0.043	0.001	0.030	0.032
0.290	0.161	0.044	0.011	0.070	0.076
0.296	0.186	0.047	0.018	0.050	0.007
0.248	0.106	0.036	0.008	0.012	0.095
0.228	0.117	0.030	0.006	0.003	0.145
0.305	0.174	0.050	0.008	0.061	0.112
0.254	0.094	0.041	0.005	0.014	0.124
0.269	0.147	0.047	0.012	0.009	0.111
0.300	0.141	0.058	0.010	0.011	0.070
0.307	0.135	0.041	0.009	0.005	0.065
0.214	0.100	0.037	0.003	0.004	0.138
0.329	0.189	0.058	0.014	0.011	0.032
0.310	0.149	0.050	0.012	0.050	0.060
0.252	0.119	0.040	0.008	0.049	0.233
0.308	0.158	0.038	0.013	0.003	0.068
0.342	0.259	0.060	0.016	0.085	0.158
0.358	0.193	0.066	0.021	0.037	0.083
0.340	0.155	0.051	0.020	0.012	0.040
0.304	0.197	0.052	0.008	0.054	0.095
0.248	0.133	0.037	0.003	0.043	0.135
0.367	0.196	0.063	0.026	0.010	0.031
0.325	0.206	0.054	0.027	0.010	0.048
0.244	0.110	0.025	0.006	0.000	0.061
0.245	0.096	0.044	0.003	0.022	0.151
0.318	0.193	0.063	0.020	0.037	0.081
0.207	0.154	0.045	0.008	0.000	0.252
0.320	0.204	0.053	0.017	0.013	0.070
0.243	0.141	0.041	0.007	0.051	0.264
0.317	0.209	0.057	0.030	0.017	0.058
0.199	0.100	0.029	0.007	0.011	0.188
0.294	0.158	0.034	0.019	0.005	0.014
0.221	0.087	0.038	0.006	0.015	0.142
0.301	0.163	0.068	0.016	0.022	0.092
0.298	0.207	0.042	0.009	0.066	0.211
0.304	0.197	0.052	0.008	0.054	0.095

Data continued

X1	X2	X3	X4	X5	X6
0.297	0.160	0.049	0.007	0.038	0.101
0.188	0.064	0.044	0.007	0.002	0.205
0.214	0.100	0.037	0.003	0.004	0.138
0.218	0.082	0.061	0.002	0.012	0.147
0.284	0.131	0.049	0.012	0.021	0.130
0.270	0.170	0.026	0.011	0.002	0.000
0.277	0.150	0.053	0.005	0.039	0.115

File names

Excel: Mlr08.xls
Minitab: Mlr08.mtp
TI-83plus/ASCII: X1 data is stored in Mlr08L1.txt
X2 data is stored in Mlr08L2.txt
X3 data is stored in Mlr08L3.txt
X4 data is stored in Mlr08L4.txt
X5 data is stored in Mlr08L5.txt
X6 data is stored in Mlr08L6.txt

09. Basketball (Multiple Linear Regression)

A random sample of professional basketball players was obtained.

The following data (X1, X2, X3, X4, X5) are for each player.
X1 = height in feet
X2 = weight in pounds
X3 = percent of successful field goals (out of 100 attempted)
X4 = percent of successful free throws (out of 100 attempted)
X5 = average points scored per game
Reference: *The official NBA basketball Encyclopedia*, Villard Books

X1	X2	X3	X4	X5
6.8	225	0.442	0.672	9.2
6.3	180	0.435	0.797	11.7
6.4	190	0.456	0.761	15.8
6.2	180	0.416	0.651	8.6
6.9	205	0.449	0.900	23.2
6.4	225	0.431	0.780	27.4
6.3	185	0.487	0.771	9.3
6.8	235	0.469	0.750	16.0
6.9	235	0.435	0.818	4.7
6.7	210	0.480	0.825	12.5
6.9	245	0.516	0.632	20.1
6.9	245	0.493	0.757	9.1
6.3	185	0.374	0.709	8.1
6.1	185	0.424	0.782	8.6
6.2	180	0.441	0.775	20.3
6.8	220	0.503	0.880	25.0
6.5	194	0.503	0.833	19.2
7.6	225	0.425	0.571	3.3
6.3	210	0.371	0.816	11.2
7.1	240	0.504	0.714	10.5
6.8	225	0.400	0.765	10.1
7.3	263	0.482	0.655	7.2
6.4	210	0.475	0.244	13.6
6.8	235	0.428	0.728	9.0
7.2	230	0.559	0.721	24.6
6.4	190	0.441	0.757	12.6
6.6	220	0.492	0.747	5.6
6.8	210	0.402	0.739	8.7
6.1	180	0.415	0.713	7.7
6.5	235	0.492	0.742	24.1
6.4	185	0.484	0.861	11.7
6.0	175	0.387	0.721	7.7
6.0	192	0.436	0.785	9.6
7.3	263	0.482	0.655	7.2
6.1	180	0.340	0.821	12.3
6.7	240	0.516	0.728	8.9
6.4	210	0.475	0.846	13.6
5.8	160	0.412	0.813	11.2
6.9	230	0.411	0.595	2.8

Data continued

X1	X2	X3	X4	X5
7.0	245	0.407	0.573	3.2
7.3	228	0.445	0.726	9.4
5.9	155	0.291	0.707	11.9
6.2	200	0.449	0.804	15.4
6.8	235	0.546	0.784	7.4
7.0	235	0.480	0.744	18.9
5.9	105	0.359	0.839	7.9
6.1	180	0.528	0.790	12.2
5.7	185	0.352	0.701	11.0
7.1	245	0.414	0.778	2.8
5.8	180	0.425	0.872	11.8
7.4	240	0.599	0.713	17.1
6.8	225	0.482	0.701	11.6
6.8	215	0.457	0.734	5.8
7.0	230	0.435	0.764	8.3

File names

Excel: Mlr09.xls
Minitab: Mlr09.mtp
TI-83plus/ASCII: X1 data is stored in Mlr09L1.txt
X2 data is stored in Mlr09L2.txt
X3 data is stored in Mlr09L3.txt
X4 data is stored in Mlr09L4.txt
X5 data is stored in Mlr09L5.txt

10. Denver Neighborhoods (Multiple Linear Regression)
A random sample of Denver neighborhoods was obtained.

The data (X1, X2, X3, X4, X5, X6, X7) are for each neighborhood
X1 = total population (in thousands)
X2 = percentage change in population over past several years
X3 = percentage of children (under 18) in population
X4 = percentage free school lunch participation
X5 = percentage change in household income over past several years
X6 = crime rate (per 1000 population)
X7 = percentage change in crime rate over past several years
Reference: The Piton Foundation, Denver, Colorado

X1	X2	X3	X4	X5	X6	X7
6.9	1.8	30.2	58.3	27.3	84.9	-14.2
8.4	28.5	38.8	87.5	39.8	172.6	-34.1
5.7	7.8	31.7	83.5	26.0	154.2	-15.8
7.4	2.3	24.2	14.2	29.4	35.2	-13.9
8.5	-0.7	28.1	46.7	26.6	69.2	-13.9
13.8	7.2	10.4	57.9	26.2	111.0	-22.6
1.7	32.2	7.5	73.8	50.5	704.1	-40.9
3.6	7.4	30.0	61.3	26.4	69.9	4.0
8.2	10.2	12.1	41.0	11.7	65.4	-32.5
5.0	10.5	13.6	17.4	14.7	132.1	-8.1
2.1	0.3	18.3	34.4	24.2	179.9	12.3
4.2	8.1	21.3	64.9	21.7	139.9	-35.0
3.9	2.0	33.1	82.0	26.3	108.7	-2.0
4.1	10.8	38.3	83.3	32.6	123.2	-2.2
4.2	1.9	36.9	61.8	21.6	104.7	-14.2
9.4	-1.5	22.4	22.2	33.5	61.5	-32.7
3.6	-0.3	19.6	8.6	27.0	68.2	-13.4
7.6	5.5	29.1	62.8	32.2	96.9	-8.7
8.5	4.8	32.8	86.2	16.0	258.0	0.5
7.5	2.3	26.5	18.7	23.7	32.0	-0.6
4.1	17.3	41.5	78.6	23.5	127.0	-12.5
4.6	68.6	39.0	14.6	38.2	27.1	45.4
7.2	3.0	20.2	41.4	27.6	70.7	-38.2
13.4	7.1	20.4	13.9	22.5	38.3	-33.6
10.3	1.4	29.8	43.7	29.4	54.0	-10.0
9.4	4.6	36.0	78.2	29.9	101.5	-14.6
2.5	-3.3	37.6	88.5	27.5	185.9	-7.6
10.3	-0.5	31.8	57.2	27.2	61.2	-17.6
7.5	22.3	28.6	5.7	31.3	38.6	27.2
18.7	6.2	39.7	55.8	28.7	52.6	-2.9
5.1	-2.0	23.8	29.0	29.3	62.6	-10.3
3.7	19.6	12.3	77.3	32.0	207.7	-45.6
10.3	3.0	31.1	51.7	26.2	42.4	-31.9
7.3	19.2	32.9	68.1	25.2	105.2	-35.7
4.2	7.0	22.1	41.2	21.4	68.6	-8.8
2.1	5.4	27.1	60.0	23.5	157.3	6.2
2.5	2.8	20.3	29.8	24.1	58.5	-27.5
8.1	8.5	30.0	66.4	26.0	63.1	-37.4

Data continued

X1	X2	X3	X4	X5	X6	X7
10.3	-1.9	15.9	39.9	38.5	86.4	-13.5
10.5	2.8	36.4	72.3	26.0	77.5	-21.6
5.8	2.0	24.2	19.5	28.3	63.5	2.2
6.9	2.9	20.7	6.6	25.8	68.9	-2.4
9.3	4.9	34.9	82.4	18.4	102.8	-12.0
11.4	2.6	38.7	78.2	18.4	86.6	-12.8

File names
Excel: Mlr10.xls
Minitab: Mlr10.mtp
TI-83plus/ASCII: X1 data is stored in Mlr10L1.txt
X2 data is stored in Mlr10L2.txt
X3 data is stored in Mlr10L3.txt
X4 data is stored in Mlr10L4.txt
X5 data is stored in Mlr10L5.txt
X6 data is stored in Mlr10L6.txt
X7 data is stored in Mlr10L7.txt

11. Chapter 10 Using Technology: U.S. Economy Case Study (Multiple Linear Regression)

U.S. economic data 1976 to 1987
X1 = dollars/barrel crude oil
X2 = % interest on ten yr. U.S. treasury notes
X3 = foreign investments/billions of dollars
X4 = Dow Jones industrial average
X5 = gross national product/billions of dollars
X6 = purchasing power u.s. dollar (1983 base)
X7 = consumer debt/billions of dollars
Reference: *Statistical Abstract of the United States* 103rd and 109th edition

X1	X2	X3	X4	X5	X6	X7
10.90	7.61	31.00	974.90	1718.00	1.76	234.40
12.00	7.42	35.00	894.60	1918.00	1.65	263.80
12.50	8.41	42.00	820.20	2164.00	1.53	308.30
17.70	9.44	54.00	844.40	2418.00	1.38	347.50
28.10	11.46	83.00	891.40	2732.00	1.22	349.40
35.60	13.91	109.00	932.90	3053.00	1.10	366.60
31.80	13.00	125.00	884.40	3166.00	1.03	381.10
29.00	11.11	137.00	1190.30	3406.00	1.00	430.40
28.60	12.44	165.00	1178.50	3772.00	0.96	511.80
26.80	10.62	185.00	1328.20	4015.00	0.93	592.40
14.60	7.68	209.00	1792.80	4240.00	0.91	646.10
17.90	8.38	244.00	2276.00	4527.00	0.88	685.50

File names
Excel: Mlr11.xls
Minitab: Mlr11.mtp
TI-83plus/ASCII: X1 data is stored in Mlr11L1.txt
X2 data is stored in Mlr11L2.txt
X3 data is stored in Mlr113.txt
X4 data is stored in Mlr114.txt
X5 data is stored in Mlr115.txt
X6 data is stored in Mlr116.txt
X7 data is stored in Mlr117.txt

One-Way ANOVA
File name prefix: Owan followed by the number of the data file

01. Excavation Depth and Archaeology (One-Way ANOVA)

Four different excavation sites at an archeological area in New Mexico gave the following depths (cm) for significant archaeological discoveries.

X1 = depths at Site I
X2 = depths at Site II
X3 = depths at Site III
X4 = depths at Site IV

Reference: *Mimbres Mogollon Archaeology* by Woosley and McIntyre, Univ. of New Mexico Press

X1	X2	X3	X4
93	85	100	96
120	45	75	58
65	80	65	95
105	28	40	90
115	75	73	65
82	70	65	80
99	65	50	85
87	55	30	95
100	50	45	82
90	40	50	
78	45		
95	55		
93			
88			
110			

File names

Excel: Owan01.xls
Minitab: Owan01.mtp
TI-83plus/ASCII: X1 data is stored in Owan01L1.txt
X2 data is stored in Owan01L2.txt
X3 data is stored in Owan01L3.txt
X4 data is stored in Owan01L4.txt

02. Apple Orchard Experiment (One-Way ANOVA)

Five types of root-stock were used in an apple orchard grafting experiment. The following data represent the extension growth (cm) after four years.

X1 = extension growth for type I
X2 = extension growth for type II
X3 = extension growth for type III
X4 = extension growth for type IV
X5 = extension growth for type V
Reference: S.C. Pearce, University of Kent at Canterbury, England

X1	X2	X3	X4	X5
2569	2074	2505	2838	1532
2928	2885	2315	2351	2552
2865	3378	2667	3001	3083
3844	3906	2390	2439	2330
3027	2782	3021	2199	2079
2336	3018	3085	3318	3366
3211	3383	3308	3601	2416
3037	3447	3231	3291	3100

File names
Excel: Owan02.xls
Minitab: Owan02.mtp
TI-83plus/ASCII: X1 data is stored in Owan02L1.txt
X2 data is stored in Owan02L2.txt
X3 data is stored in Owan02L3.txt
X4 data is stored in Owan02L4.txt
X5 data is stored in Owan02L5.txt

03. Red Dye Number 40 (One-Way ANOVA)

S.W. Laagakos and F. Mosteller of Harvard University fed mice different doses of red dye number 40 and recorded the time of death in weeks. Results for female mice, dosage and time of death are shown in the data

X1 = time of death for control group
X2 = time of death for group with low dosage
X3 = time of death for group with medium dosage
X4 = time of death for group with high dosage
Reference: *Journal Natl. Cancer Inst.*, Vol. 66, p 197-212

X1	X2	X3	X4
70	49	30	34
77	60	37	36
83	63	56	48
87	67	65	48
92	70	76	65
93	74	83	91
100	77	87	98
102	80	90	102
102	89	94	
103		97	
96			

File names Excel: Owan03.xls
Minitab: Owan03.mtp
TI-83plus/ASCII: X1 data is stored in Owan03L1.txt
X2 data is stored in Owan03L2.txt
X3 data is stored in Owan03L3.txt
X4 data is stored in Owan03L4.txt

04. Business Startup Costs (One-Way ANOVA)

The following data represent business startup costs (thousands of dollars) for shops.
X1 = startup costs for pizza
X2 = startup costs for baker/donuts
X3 = startup costs for shoe stores
X4 = startup costs for gift shops
X5 = startup costs for pet stores
Reference: *Business Opportunities Handbook*

X1	X2	X3	X4	X5
80	150	48	100	25
125	40	35	96	80
35	120	95	35	30
58	75	45	99	35
110	160	75	75	30
140	60	115	150	28
97	45	42	45	20
50	100	78	100	75
65	86	65	120	48
79	87	125	50	20
35	90			50
85				75
120				55
				60
				85
				110

File names

Excel: Owan04.xls
Minitab: Owan04.mtp
TI-83plus/ASCII: X1 data is stored in Owan04L1.txt
X2 data is stored in Owan04L2.txt
X3 data is stored in Owan04L3.txt
X4 data is stored in Owan04L4.txt
X5 data is stored in Owan04L5.txt

05. Weights of Football Players (One-Way ANOVA)

The following data represent weights (pounds) of a random sample of professional football players on the following teams.
X1 = weights of players for the Dallas Cowboys
X2 = weights of players for the Green Bay Packers
X3 = weights of players for the Denver Broncos
X4 = weights of players for the Miami Dolphins
X5 = weights of players for the San Francisco Forty Niners
Reference: *The Sports Encyclopedia Pro Football*

X1	X2	X3	X4	X5
250	260	270	260	247
255	271	250	255	249
255	258	281	265	255
264	263	273	257	247
250	267	257	268	244
265	254	264	263	245
245	255	233	247	249
252	250	254	253	260
266	248	268	251	217
246	240	252	252	208
251	254	256	266	228
263	275	265	264	253
248	270	252	210	249
228	225	256	236	223
221	222	235	225	221
223	230	216	230	228
220	225	241	232	271

File names Excel: Owan05.xls
Minitab: Owan05.mtp
TI-83plus/ASCII: X1 data is stored in Owan05L1.txt
X2 data is stored in Owan05L2.txt
X3 data is stored in Owan05L3.txt
X4 data is stored in Owan05L4.txt
X5 data is stored in Owan05L5.txt

Two-Way ANOVA
File name prefix: Twan followed by the number of the data file

01. Political Affiliation (Two-Way ANOVA)
Response: Percent of voters for a recent National Election
Factor 1: counties in Montana
Factor 2: political affiliation
Reference: *County and City Data Book* U.S. Dept. of Commerce

County	Democrat	Republican
Jefferson	33.5	36.5
Lewis/Clark	42.5	35.7
Powder River	22.3	47.3
Stillwataer	32.4	38.2
Sweet Grass	21.9	48.8
Yellowstone	35.7	40.4

File names Excel: Twan01.xls
Minitab: Twan01.mtp
ASCII: Twan01.txt

02. Density of Artifacts (Two-Way ANOVA)
Response: Average density of artifacts, number of artifacts per cubic meter
Factor 1: archeological excavation site
Factor 2: depth (cm) at which artifacts are found
Reference: Museum of New Mexico, Laboratory of Antrhopology

Site	50-100	101-150	151-200
I	3.8	4.9	3.4
II	4.1	4.1	2.7
III	2.9	3.8	4.4
IV	3.5	3.3	3
V	5.2	5.1	5.3
VI	3.6	4.6	4.5
VII	4.5	3.7	2.8

File names Excel: Twan02.xls
Minitab: Twan02.mtp
ASCII: Twan02.txt

03. Spruce Moth Traps (Two-Way ANOVA)

Response: number of spruce moths found in trap after 48 hours
Factor 1: Location of trap in tree (top branches, middle branches, lower branches, ground)
Factor 2: Type of lure in trap (scent, sugar, chemical)

Location	Scent	Sugar	Chemical
Top	28	35	32
	19	22	29
	32	33	16
	15	21	18
	13	17	20
Middle	39	36	37
	12	38	40
	42	44	18
	25	27	28
	21	22	36
Lower	44	42	35
	21	17	39
	38	31	41
	32	29	31
	29	37	34
Ground	17	18	22
	12	27	25
	23	15	14
	19	29	16
	14	16	19

File names Excel: Twan03.xls
Minitab: Twan03.mtp
ASCII: Twan03.txt

04. Advertising in Local Newspapers (Two-Way ANOVA)

Response: Number of inquiries resulting from advertisement
Factor 1: day of week (Monday through Friday)
Factor 2: section of newspaper (news, business, sports)

Day	News	Business	Sports
Monday	11	10	4
	8	12	3
	6	13	5
	8	11	6
Tuesday	9	7	5
	10	8	8
	10	11	6
	12	9	7
Wednesday	8	7	5
	9	8	9
	9	10	7
	11	9	6
Thrusday	4	9	7
	5	6	6
	3	8	6
	5	8	5
Friday	13	10	12
	12	9	10
	11	9	11
	14	8	12

File names

Excel: Twan04.xls
Minitab: Twan04.mtp
ASCII: Twan04.txt

05. Prehistoric Ceramic Sherds (Two-Way ANOVA)

Response: number of sherds
Factor 1: region of archaeological excavation
Factor 2: type of ceramic sherd (three circle red on white, Mogollon red on brown, Mimbres corrugated, bold face black on white)
Reference: *Mimbres Mogollon Archaeology* by Woosley and McIntyre, University of New Mexico Press

Region	Red on White	Mogollon	Mimbres	Bold Face
I	68	49	78	95
	33	61	53	122
	45	52	35	133
II	59	71	54	78
	43	41	51	98
	37	63	69	89
III	54	67	44	41
	91	46	76	29
	81	51	55	63
IV	55	45	78	56
	53	58	49	81
	42	72	46	35
V	27	47	41	46
	31	39	36	22
	38	53	25	26

File names Excel: Twan05.xls
Minitab: Twan05.mtp
ASCII: Twan05.txt